The Latest Clinical Advances in Thrombocytopenia

The Latest Clinical Advances in Thrombocytopenia

Editors

Hugo ten Cate
Bernhard Lämmle

MDPI • Basel • Beijing • Wuhan • Barcelona • Belgrade • Manchester • Tokyo • Cluj • Tianjin

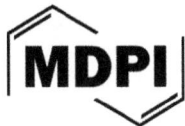

Editors
Hugo ten Cate
Maastricht University Medical Center
The Netherlands

Bernhard Lämmle
University of Bern
Switzerland
Johannes Gutenberg University
Germany
University College London
UK

Editorial Office
MDPI
St. Alban-Anlage 66
4052 Basel, Switzerland

This is a reprint of articles from the Special Issue published online in the open access journal *Journal of Clinical Medicine* (ISSN 2077-0383) (available at: https://www.mdpi.com/journal/jcm/special_issues/thrombocytopenia).

For citation purposes, cite each article independently as indicated on the article page online and as indicated below:

LastName, A.A.; LastName, B.B.; LastName, C.C. Article Title. *Journal Name* **Year**, *Volume Number*, Page Range.

ISBN 978-3-0365-2804-5 (Hbk)
ISBN 978-3-0365-2805-2 (PDF)

© 2021 by the authors. Articles in this book are Open Access and distributed under the Creative Commons Attribution (CC BY) license, which allows users to download, copy and build upon published articles, as long as the author and publisher are properly credited, which ensures maximum dissemination and a wider impact of our publications.

The book as a whole is distributed by MDPI under the terms and conditions of the Creative Commons license CC BY-NC-ND.

Contents

About the Editors . . . . **vii**

Hugo ten Cate and Bernhard Lämmle
Special Issue: "The Latest Clinical Advances in Thrombocytopenia"
Reprinted from: *J. Clin. Med.* **2021**, *10*, 3463, doi:10.3390/jcm10163463 . . . . **1**

Tanja Falter, Sibylle Böschen, Markus Schepers, Manfred Beutel, Karl Lackner, Inge Scharrer and Bernhard Lämmle
Influence of Personality, Resilience and Life Conditions on Depression and Anxiety in 104 Patients Having Survived Acute Autoimmune Thrombotic Thrombocytopenic Purpura
Reprinted from: *J. Clin. Med.* **2021**, *10*, 365, doi:10.3390/jcm10020365 . . . . **7**

Loredana Bury, Emanuela Falcinelli and Paolo Gresele
Learning the Ropes of Platelet Count Regulation: Inherited Thrombocytopenias
Reprinted from: *J. Clin. Med.* **2021**, *10*, 533, doi:10.3390/jcm10030533 . . . . **21**

Senthil Sukumar, Bernhard Lämmle and Spero R. Cataland
Thrombotic Thrombocytopenic Purpura: Pathophysiology, Diagnosis, and Management
Reprinted from: *J. Clin. Med.* **2021**, *10*, 536, doi:10.3390/jcm10030536 . . . . **45**

Benjamin Lardinois, Julien Favresse, Bernard Chatelain, Giuseppe Lippi and François Mullier
Pseudothrombocytopenia—A Review on Causes, Occurrence and Clinical Implications
Reprinted from: *J. Clin. Med.* **2021**, *10*, 594, doi:10.3390/jcm10040594 . . . . **69**

Enrico Squiccimarro, Federica Jiritano, Giuseppe Filiberto Serraino, Hugo ten Cate, Domenico Paparella and Roberto Lorusso
Quantitative and Qualitative Platelet Derangements in Cardiac Surgery and Extracorporeal Life Support
Reprinted from: *J. Clin. Med.* **2021**, *10*, 615, doi:10.3390/jcm10040615 . . . . **89**

Matteo Marchetti, Maxime G. Zermatten, Debora Bertaggia Calderara, Alessandro Aliotta and Lorenzo Alberio
Heparin-Induced Thrombocytopenia: A Review of New Concepts in Pathogenesis, Diagnosis, and Management
Reprinted from: *J. Clin. Med.* **2021**, *10*, 683, doi:10.3390/jcm10040683 . . . . **103**

Anurag Singh, Günalp Uzun and Tamam Bakchoul
Primary Immune Thrombocytopenia: Novel Insights into Pathophysiology and Disease Management
Reprinted from: *J. Clin. Med.* **2021**, *10*, 789, doi:10.3390/jcm10040789 . . . . **119**

Matthijs Raadsen, Justin Du Toit, Thomas Langerak, Bas van Bussel, Eric van Gorp and Marco Goeijenbier
Thrombocytopenia in Virus Infections
Reprinted from: *J. Clin. Med.* **2021**, *10*, 877, doi:10.3390/jcm10040877 . . . . **141**

Alessandro Aliotta, Debora Bertaggia Calderara, Maxime G. Zermatten, Matteo Marchetti and Lorenzo Alberio
Thrombocytopathies: Not Just Aggregation Defects—The Clinical Relevance of Procoagulant Platelets
Reprinted from: *J. Clin. Med.* **2021**, *10*, 894, doi:10.3390/jcm10050894 . . . . **175**

Nicolas Bonadies, Alicia Rovó, Naomi Porret and Ulrike Bacher
When Should We Think of Myelodysplasia or Bone Marrow Failure in a Thrombocytopenic Patient? A Practical Approach to Diagnosis
Reprinted from: *J. Clin. Med.* **2021**, *10*, 1026, doi:10.3390/jcm10051026 203

Kerstin Jurk and Yavar Shiravand
Platelet Phenotyping and Function Testing in Thrombocytopenia
Reprinted from: *J. Clin. Med.* **2021**, *10*, 1114, doi:10.3390/jcm10051114 223

Avi Leader, Liron Hofstetter and Galia Spectre
Challenges and Advances in Managing Thrombocytopenic Cancer Patients
Reprinted from: *J. Clin. Med.* **2021**, *10*, 1169, doi:10.3390/jcm10061169 245

Rüdiger E. Scharf
Thrombocytopenia and Hemostatic Changes in Acute and Chronic Liver Disease: Pathophysiology, Clinical and Laboratory Features, and Management
Reprinted from: *J. Clin. Med.* **2021**, *10*, 1530, doi:10.3390/jcm10071530 267

Annina Capraru, Katarzyna Aleksandra Jalowiec, Cesare Medri, Michael Daskalakis, Sacha Sergio Zeerleder and Behrouz Mansouri Taleghani
Platelet Transfusion—Insights from Current Practice to Future Development
Reprinted from: *J. Clin. Med.* **2021**, *10*, 1990, doi:10.3390/jcm10091990 285

About the Editors

Hugo ten Cate, M.D., PhD, Professor in Clinical Thrombosis and Hemostasis, Department of Internal Medicine and Thrombosis Expert Center, Maastricht University Medical Center; Adjunct Professor, Center of Thrombosis and Hemostasis, University Medical Center Mainz, Germany.

Bernhard Lämmle, M.D., Emeritus Professor and Director, Department of Hematology and Central Hematology Laboratory, Inselspital, University Hospital of Bern, Bern, Switzerland, retired in 2013, Senior Professor Center of Thrombosis and Hemostasis, University Medical Center Mainz, Germany, Visiting Professor Haemostasis Research Unit, University College London, London, UK, Senior Consultant Hämatologie Praxis Bern, Switzerland.

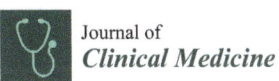

Editorial

Special Issue: "The Latest Clinical Advances in Thrombocytopenia"

Hugo ten Cate [1,2,3,*] and Bernhard Lämmle [3,4,5,6]

1. Thrombosis Expertise Center, Cardiovascular Research Institute Maastricht (CARIM), Maastricht University Medical Center, NL-P.O. Box 616, 6200 MD Maastricht, The Netherlands
2. Departments of Internal medicine and Biochemistry, Maastricht University Medical Center, NL-P.O. Box 616, 6200 MD Maastricht, The Netherlands
3. Center for Thrombosis and Hemostasis, University Medical Center Mainz, Johannes Gutenberg University, 55131 Mainz, Germany; bernhard.laemmle@uni-mainz.de
4. Central Hematology Laboratory, Department of Hematology, Inselspital, Bern University Hospital, University of Bern, CH 3010 Bern, Switzerland
5. Haemostasis Research Unit, University College London, London WC1E 6BT, UK
6. Schützenweg 3, CH 3065 Bolligen, Switzerland
* Correspondence: h.tencate@maastrichtuniversity.nl

Citation: ten Cate, H.; Lämmle, B. Special Issue: "The Latest Clinical Advances in Thrombocytopenia". *J. Clin. Med.* **2021**, *10*, 3463. https://doi.org/10.3390/jcm10163463

Received: 29 July 2021
Accepted: 2 August 2021
Published: 5 August 2021

Publisher's Note: MDPI stays neutral with regard to jurisdictional claims in published maps and institutional affiliations.

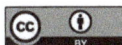

Copyright: © 2021 by the authors. Licensee MDPI, Basel, Switzerland. This article is an open access article distributed under the terms and conditions of the Creative Commons Attribution (CC BY) license (https://creativecommons.org/licenses/by/4.0/).

Platelets are critical elements in the blood stream, supporting hemostasis as well as performing even more complex tasks within networks of biological (immunity) and pathophysiological processes, such as cancer and ischemia/reperfusion injury. Changes in the number (and function) of platelets may have a substantial impact on any of these processes. The "simple" finding of a reduced platelet count (thrombocytopenia) has a history (origin) and a consequence (e.g., bleeding). The origin of thrombocytopenia can be unclear (idiopathic), can depend on associated illness (e.g., disseminated intravascular coagulation, heparin-induced thrombocytopenia, thrombotic thrombocytopenic purpura) with a different etiology depending on the illness (related to production, clustering, immune depletion, intravascular consumption, etc.), and can also be acquired (e.g., during extracorporeal circuits, such as "ECMO") or constitutional. In the current COVID-19 pandemic, thrombocytopenia is also a feature, although it is less severe than in other diseases, and the overall patient phenotype seems thrombotic rather than hemorrhagic. Thus, there are many possible causes for thrombocytopenia, and these are, quite often, poorly characterized. Since the clinical question is always whether or not the platelet deficit has consequences for the patient, it is important, and also timely (e.g., COVID-19), to discuss this topic in a Special Issue.

We, the editors, are extremely pleased that a large number of outstanding clinician-scientists were willing to contribute to this Special Issue! In times of substantial stress due to the COVID-19-related burden on society and work, the request to contribute a state-of-the-art paper for any journal is a major demand for any author, junior or experienced. To comply with strict timelines is a further challenge.

We consider ourselves very lucky that the authors we approached were, without exception, willing to do their best and to make it before the deadline. We are proud of the high quality of the papers we received. Now that this series is complete, at least according to our expectations, we hope that the readership will enjoy it. We observe that a number of these papers are already viewed at a high rate and even cited, supporting the value of this article series. For this issue, we acquired one original research article [1] and 13 reviews [2–14] that are shortly introduced below.

Falter, Böschen, Schepers, Beutel, Lackner, Scharrer, and Lämmle report their final analysis on a questionnaire study from 2015 and 2016 into neurocognitive and mental sequelae on 104 adult patients having survived at least one acute episode of autoimmune thrombotic thrombocytopenic purpura (iTTP) at the University Medical Center in Mainz or having consulted with this center [1]. Data on depressive symptoms and cognitive deficits in this cohort obtained in 2013 and 2014 had already been published before. Based on self-reporting using a series of validated questionnaires, iTTP survivors had a high prevalence of depression and anxiety, a more negative attitude to life, and low resilience as compared to controls. Quality of life and cognitive performance in patients were significantly reduced (see also the review article on thrombotic thrombocytopenic purpura by Sukumar et al. [3], introduced below).

Bury, Falcinelli, and Gresele comprehensively review the current knowledge of the inherited thrombocytopenias (ITs) [2]. As of today, more than 40 different disorders caused by defects of various genes involved in megakaryopoiesis and platelet production are known, and the field is rapidly evolving, not least by the diagnostic advances supported by modern next-generation sequencing techniques. Some ITs show isolated thrombocytopenia, others are associated with various clinical features (so-called syndromic ITs) and, importantly, some forms are associated with a tendency to develop a hematologic neoplasm during ensuing years. Bleeding diathesis is highly variable and generally more severe in ITs with associated functional platelet defects. Even though the general internist and hematologist may not have full knowledge on all individual ITs, it is mandatory to think of the possibility of a hereditary thrombocytopenia by obtaining a complete personal and family history and (in unclear cases) to proceed to genetic screening early in the diagnostic work-up in order to avoid misdiagnosis of immune thrombocytopenia (ITP) and unnecessary, potentially harmful immunosuppressive treatment. The ethical concerns of uncovering a potential premalignant condition are stressed by the authors.

Sukumar, Lämmle, and Cataland present an update on thrombotic thrombocytopenic purpura (TTP), a rare but potentially fatal disease caused by a severe autoantibody-mediated (iTTP) or congenital deficiency (cTTP) of the metalloprotease ADAMTS13 [3]. ADAMTS13 deficiency is associated with a defective proteolytic processing of the Von Willebrand factor (VWF), leading to the presence of unusually large, extremely adhesive VWF multimers in plasma and spontaneous widespread platelet clumping in the microcirculation. Severe thrombocytopenia and microangiopathic hemolytic anemia caused by erythrocyte fragmentation in the partially occluded microcirculation as well as ischemic organ dysfunction can rapidly lead to death if untreated. Besides, the established therapy with large-volume plasma exchange, fresh frozen plasma replacement and corticosteroids, new adjunctive therapeutic modalities with caplacizumab, inhibiting VWF–platelet interaction, and with the anti-CD20 antibody rituximab, inhibiting autoantibody production in iTTP, are described. Recombinant ADAMTS13 as a replacement for patients with cTTP is under investigation. Regular follow-up of iTTP and cTTP patients is imperative to minimize long-term sequelae (see also the article by Falter et al. [1] mentioned above).

Lardinois, Favresse, Chatelain, Lippi, and Mullier—starting from an observed case—review the not uncommon condition known as pseudothrombocytopenia (PTCP) [4]. It is of utmost relevance to recognize this laboratory phenomenon of an apparently decreased platelet count due to in vitro platelet clumping in order to avoid unnecessary and potentially harmful diagnostic and therapeutic measures. Best known is EDTA-induced PTCP, but multi-anticoagulant PTCP does exist, and they are best recognized by visual inspection of a peripheral blood smear. Of note, no specific disease is associated with or heralded by PTCP, even in patients followed for many years. Lardinois et al. provide a detailed discussion on the pathomechanism, the laboratory diagnostic approach including the use, if available, of various platelet counting techniques, different in vitro anticoagulants, and other analytical considerations. This overview is especially useful for the hematologic laboratory specialists confronted with this sometimes-challenging condition.

Squiccimarro, Jiritano, Serraino, ten Cate, Paparella, and Lorusso contribute a review on the quantitative and qualitative platelet derangements in cardiac surgery and extracorporeal life support [5]. Thrombocytopenia and simultaneous functional abnormalities of platelets are common in cardiac surgery using cardiopulmonary bypass (CPB) and extracorporeal membrane oxygenation (ECMO). The pathophysiologic mechanisms and complex interactions of platelets, other blood cells, activation of coagulation and complement systems, and release of cytokines and chemokines associated with heart surgery while blood is flowing over artificial surfaces are outlined. The need of heparinization may pose a high risk of heparin-induced thrombocytopenia for cardiac surgery patients (see also the review by Marchetti et al. [6] mentioned below).

Marchetti, Zermatten, Bertaggia Calderara, Aliotta, and Alberio review the still common and highly dangerous prothrombotic heparin-induced thrombocytopenia (HIT) [6]. They provide an update on the pathophysiology of this immunologic syndrome, which may be a "side effect" of a host immune mechanism intended to fight against Gram-negative bacterial infections. HIT pathophysiology involves monocytes, endothelial cells, and neutrophils, as well as platelets. The necessity of a Bayesian combined clinical and laboratory approach to diagnosis is stressed. Assessing clinical pretest probability and a combination of fast (semiquantitative) immunoassays may massively shorten diagnostic work-up and obviate the need for emergency testing of functional HIT antibodies. Finally, besides the current established treatment, emerging therapeutic concepts are discussed, including the difficult situation of cardiovascular surgery in patients with HIT or a history of HIT. The Lausanne HIT team exemplarily shows that each large medical center should have an established algorithm for the awareness and management of this condition.

Singh, Uzun, and Bakchoul provide an interesting review on the pathophysiology, diagnosis, and management of immune thrombocytopenia (ITP) [7]. They stress the multifactorial pathogenesis of this common condition, including the increased platelet sequestration and destruction as well as impaired platelet production. Autoantibodies against platelet glycoproteins lead to opsonization of platelets which are removed via Fc receptors on macrophages predominantly in the spleen. Autoantibodies may also promote de-sialylation of platelet glycoproteins, rendering these platelets susceptible to removal via the Ashwell-Morell receptors in the liver and, importantly, platelet production is compromised by autoantibodies. The authors suggest measuring anti-platelet glycoprotein autoantibodies with appropriate tests during initial diagnostic work-up even though current guidelines provide no firm recommendation. Treatment modalities are extensively discussed and some new drugs currently under investigation are presented as well.

Raadsen, Du Toit, Langerak, Van Bussel, Van Gorp, and Goeijenbier present a broad overview of the literature from the past 10 years on the relation/interaction of "platelets" with "viral infections" [8]. They complemented their extensive literature analysis by a second search performed in December 2020, focusing on the publications of the preceding year on SARS-CoV-2 and platelets. The role of platelets far exceeds the well-known hemostatic function, and they seem to have direct and indirect antiviral activity and are involved in the accompanying immunologic reactions. A large list of specific viral infections is discussed with highly varying degrees of thrombocytopenia. The most severe viral hemorrhagic fevers, e.g., Ebola, Marburg, and Lassavirus infections, are under-investigated because of the scarcity of laboratories with biosafety level 4 worldwide. Based on the current COVID-19 pandemic, the authors stress that any immunomodulating therapy potentially affecting platelets must be carefully evaluated because the immunothrombosis mechanisms may serve an important antiviral role which should not be compromised.

Aliotta, Bertaggia Calderara, Zermatten, Marchetti, and Alberio offer an in-depth review on thrombocytopathies [9]. They first outline the platelet activation endpoints, namely adhesion, secretion, and aggregation, discuss their classic defects such as Bernard-Soulier syndrome, platelet-type von Willebrand disease, alpha- and delta-storage pool deficiencies, and Glanzmann thrombasthenia respectively, and then highlight the major role of platelet procoagulant activity. The latter is primarily provided by the exposure of phosphatidylserine on the outer membrane of the phospholipid bilayer and the release of platelet microparticles. The technically demanding and difficult to standardize methodologies of assaying platelet procoagulant functions are explained. It is demonstrated that a low or high potential to generate procoagulant platelets in vitro may be associated with bleeding or thrombotic tendencies, respectively. A short summary of the thrombocytopathy associated with COVID-19 is added (for a discussion of platelet function testing, specifically in thrombocytopenic patients, see also the review by Jurk and Shiravand [11] introduced below).

Bonadies, Rovo, Porret, and Bacher expertly discuss thrombocytopenia in the context of hematologic diseases, i.e., myelodysplastic syndromes (MDS) and bone marrow failure syndromes (BMF) [10]. They describe the variable clinical presentations of patients with MDS and BMF, the latter consisting of acquired aplastic anemia and inherited forms of BMF, such as Fanconi anemia and several telomeropathies. The authors provide a detailed overview on the often-stepwise diagnostic approach, including cytologic investigation of peripheral blood and bone marrow aspirate, histopathology of bone marrow, flow cytometric immunophenotyping, and cytogenetic and next-generation sequencing analyses, obviously requiring specialized multidisciplinary teams. The authors remind us that an isolated thrombocytopenia, especially in the elderly, may herald either an evolving MDS or an aplastic anemia, and they stress the importance, especially in children, to consider an inherited BMF syndrome (see also the review by Bury et al. [2] in this issue for inherited thrombocytopenias predisposing to MDS and/or leukemia).

Jurk and Shiravand share their expertise on platelet phenotyping and function testing in thrombocytopenic patients [11]. Patients with inherited or acquired thrombocytopenia may additionally display functional platelet defects, contributing to the bleeding risk. The indications for such platelet function testing in thrombocytopenia are presented. The evaluation should start with a standardized assessment of the bleeding history and of the basic hematologic parameters, including inspection of a peripheral blood smear. The frequently used point-of-care tests (Multiplate® analyzer, Platelet function analyzer PFA-100® or PFA-200®, Impact R™, thromboelastography (TEG®), and rotational thromboelastometry (ROTEM®)) assess the global primary (and the latter two also the secondary) hemostasis and are not suitable to diagnose platelet dysfunction in thrombocytopenia. Light transmission aggregometry, lumi-aggregometry, flow cytometric platelet phenotyping and functional testing in vitro, and assay of platelet-dependent thrombin generation by calibrated automated thrombinography (CAT) allow the detailed characterization of platelet function defects. All these latter assays require expertise and are reserved for specialized laboratories. The same applies to microfluidic flow chamber assays of thrombus formation used for research purposes (see also the review by Aliotta et al. [9] introduced above).

Leader, Hofstetter, and Spectre provide an overview on the difficult topic of managing thrombocytopenic cancer patients by non-transfusion-based means [12]. Thrombocytopenia in patients with malignant neoplasms may be chemotherapy-induced or related to the malignant disease, e.g., in myelodysplastic syndromes (MDS) or acute leukemia (AML). First, the prophylactic and therapeutic roles of antifibrinolytic treatment with tranexamic acid and epsilon-amino caproic acid in various tumors are presented. Second, the efficacy and safety of thrombopoietin receptor agonists are outlined and results of performed and ongoing trials in MDS/AML and in chemotherapy-induced thrombocytopenia in solid tumors are summarized. Finally, the major dilemma of managing antithrombotic therapy with anticoagulants and/or antiplatelet agents in thrombocytopenic cancer patients who are often at high risk of both thromboembolic and bleeding complications is discussed. The authors also refer to the need for platelet transfusions in specific situations (see also the review by Capraru et al. [14], mentioned below).

Scharf provides an overview on thrombocytopenia, platelet dysfunction, and overall hemostatic changes in acute and chronic liver disease [13]. Thrombocytopenia is common and has a multifactorial pathophysiology in hepatopathies, involving splenomegaly with splenic sequestration of platelets, reduced hepatic thrombopoietin production, and increased platelet destruction. Plasmatic coagulation is impaired as well but is "rebalanced" by a concordant reduction of pro- and anti-hemostatic factors. The resulting low-level hemostatic balance predisposes not only to bleeding but also to thrombotic complications. Management of thrombocytopenia in liver disease may profit from newly available thrombopoietin receptor agonists, which allow to avoid platelet transfusions in many instances.

Limitations, risks, benefits, and general concepts for optimal hemotherapy of patients with liver disease are outlined.

Capraru, Jalowiec, Medri, Daskalakis, Zeerleder, and Taleghani review the current state of platelet transfusion and provide an outlook on ongoing and future developments from the perspective of transfusion medicine [14]. The authors explain the differences between apheresis platelet concentrates from single donors and pooled platelet concentrates from buffy coat or platelet-rich plasma. Next, storage media (platelet additive solutions) intended to increase the shelf life of platelet concentrates and reduce allergic reactions to contaminating plasma are discussed. Then, pathogen inactivation technologies aiming at decreasing the transmission of bacterial and viral infections by platelet transfusion are outlined. Cold storage (at 4 °C), cryopreservation (at −80 °C), and even lyophilization of thrombocyte preparations for transfusion are being studied. Finally, the authors discuss a series of alternatives to platelet transfusion that are under exploration, such as "thromboerythrocytes", "plateletsomes", in vitro production of platelets from pluripotent stem cells, and others, highlighting a very active research area in this field of transfusion medicine.

We hope that this compilation of articles and reviews on various pathophysiologic, diagnostic, and therapeutic aspects of thrombocytopenia is useful for clinicians and researchers from different specialities.

Author Contributions: Conceptualization, writing, review and editing: H.t.C. and B.L. Both authors have read and agreed to the published version of the manuscript.

Funding: This research received no external funding.

Conflicts of Interest: The authors declare no relevant conflict of interest.

References

1. Falter, T.; Böschen, S.; Schepers, M.; Beutel, M.; Lackner, K.; Scharrer, I.; Lämmle, B. Influence of Personality, Resilience and Life Conditions on Depression and Anxiety in 104 Patients Having Survived Acute Autoimmune Thrombotic Thrombocytopenic Purpura. *J. Clin. Med.* **2021**, *10*, 365. [CrossRef] [PubMed]
2. Bury, L.; Falcinelli, E.; Gresele, P. Learning the Ropes of Platelet Count Regulation: Inherited Thrombocytopenias. *J. Clin. Med.* **2021**, *10*, 533. [CrossRef] [PubMed]
3. Sukumar, S.; Lämmle, B.; Cataland, S.R. Thrombotic Thrombocytopenic Purpura: Pathophysiology, Diagnosis, and Management. *J. Clin. Med.* **2021**, *10*, 536. [CrossRef] [PubMed]
4. Lardinois, B.; Favresse, J.; Chatelain, B.; Lippi, G.; Mullier, F. Pseudothrombocytopenia-A Review on Causes, Occurrence and Clinical Implications. *J. Clin. Med.* **2021**, *10*, 594. [CrossRef] [PubMed]
5. Squiccimarro, E.; Jiritano, F.; Serraino, G.F.; Cate, H.T.; Paparella, D.; Lorusso, R. Quantitative and Qualitative Platelet Derangements in Cardiac Surgery and Extracorporeal Life Support. *J. Clin. Med.* **2021**, *10*, 615. [CrossRef] [PubMed]
6. Marchetti, M.; Zermatten, M.; Bertaggia, G.; Calderara, D.; Aliotta, A.; Alberio, L. Heparin-Induced Thrombocytopenia: A Review of New Concepts in Pathogenesis, Diagnosis, and Management. *J. Clin. Med.* **2021**, *10*, 683. [CrossRef] [PubMed]
7. Singh, A.; Uzun, G.; Bakchoul, T. Primary Immune Thrombocytopenia: Novel Insights into Pathophysiology and Disease Management. *J. Clin. Med.* **2021**, *10*, 789. [CrossRef] [PubMed]
8. Raadsen, M.; Toit, J.D.; Langerak, T.; Bussel, B.v.; Gorp, E.v.; Goeijenbier, M. Thrombocytopenia in Virus Infections. *J. Clin. Med.* **2021**, *10*, 877. [CrossRef] [PubMed]
9. Aliotta, A.; Calderara, D.B.; Zermatten, M.G.; Marchetti, M.; Alberio, L. Thrombocytopathies: Not Just Aggregation Defects-The Clinical Relevance of Procoagulant Platelets. *J. Clin. Med.* **2021**, *10*, 894. [CrossRef] [PubMed]
10. Bonadies, N.; Rovó, A.; Porret, N.; Bacher, U. When Should We Think of Myelodysplasia or Bone Marrow Failure in a Thrombocytopenic Patient? A Practical Approach to Diagnosis. *J. Clin. Med.* **2021**, *10*, 1026. [CrossRef] [PubMed]
11. Jurk, K.; Shiravand, Y. Platelet Phenotyping and Function Testing in Thrombocytopenia. *J. Clin. Med.* **2021**, *10*, 1114. [CrossRef] [PubMed]
12. Leader, A.; Hofstetter, L.; Spectre, G. Challenges and Advances in Managing Thrombocytopenic Cancer Patients. *J. Clin. Med.* **2021**, *10*, 1169. [CrossRef] [PubMed]
13. Scharf, R.E. Thrombocytopenia and Hemostatic Changes in Acute and Chronic Liver Disease: Pathophysiology, Clinical and Laboratory Features, and Management. *J. Clin. Med.* **2021**, *10*, 1530. [CrossRef] [PubMed]
14. Capraru, A.; Jalowiec, K.A.; Medri, C.; Daskalakis, M.; Zeerleder, S.S.; Taleghani, M.B. Platelet Transfusion-Insights from Current Practice to Future Development. *J. Clin. Med.* **2021**, *10*, 1990. [CrossRef] [PubMed]

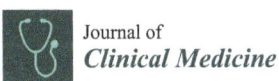

Article

Influence of Personality, Resilience and Life Conditions on Depression and Anxiety in 104 Patients Having Survived Acute Autoimmune Thrombotic Thrombocytopenic Purpura

Tanja Falter [1,*], Sibylle Böschen [1], Markus Schepers [2], Manfred Beutel [3], Karl Lackner [1], Inge Scharrer [4] and Bernhard Lämmle [4,5,6]

1. Institute of Clinical Chemistry and Laboratory Medicine, University Medical Center of the Johannes Gutenberg University, 55131 Mainz, Germany; Sibylle.boeschen@web.de (S.B.); Karl.Lackner@unimedizin-mainz.de (K.L.)
2. Institute of Medical Biostatistics, Epidemiology and Informatics (IMBEI), University Medical Center of the Johannes Gutenberg University, 55131 Mainz, Germany; Markus.Schepers@uni-mainz.de
3. Department of Psychosomatic Medicine and Psychotherapy, University Medical Center of the Johannes Gutenberg University, 55131 Mainz, Germany; Manfred.Beutel@unimedizin-mainz.de
4. Center for Thrombosis and Hemostasis (CTH), University Medical Center of the Johannes Gutenberg University, 55131 Mainz, Germany; Inge.scharrer@unimedizin-mainz.de (I.S.); Bernhard.laemmle@uni-mainz.de (B.L.)
5. Department of Hematology and Central Hematology Laboratory, Inselspital, Bern University Hospital, University of Bern, CH 3010 Bern, Switzerland
6. Haemostasis Research Unit, University College London, London WC1E 6BT, UK
* Correspondence: tanja.falter@unimedizin-mainz.de; Tel.: +49-6131-17-3263

Abstract: Autoimmune thrombotic thrombocytopenic purpura (iTTP) is a life-threatening, relapsing disease in which an acquired deficiency of the enzyme ADAMTS13 leads to generalised microvascular thrombosis. Survivors have a high prevalence of depression and impaired cognitive function. The aim of this study was to determine whether life circumstances and personality have an influence on the development and severity of depression and anxiety in iTTP patients and how they impact the quality of life. With validated questionnaires, we examined the prevalence of depression and anxiety symptoms in 104 iTTP patients, as well as parameters of subjective cognitive deficits, quality of life, attitude to life and resilience. iTTP patients had significantly more depressive symptoms ($p < 0.001$), a tendency to have anxiety disorders ($p = 0.035$) and a significantly worse cognitive performance ($p = 0.008$) compared to the controls. Sex, age, physical activity and partnership status had no significant influence on depression, whereas the number of comorbidities did. Lower scores of resilience, attitude to life and quality of life were reported by patients compared to controls. iTTP patients had a high prevalence of depression and anxiety, as well as a more negative attitude to life and low resilience. Resilience correlated negatively with the severity of the depression. Furthermore, quality of life and cognitive performance were significantly reduced.

Keywords: thrombotic thrombocytopenic purpura; depression; resilience; quality of life

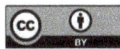

1. Introduction

Autoimmune thrombotic thrombocytopenic purpura (iTTP) is a potentially life-threatening, relapsing disease in which an acquired deficiency of the von Willebrand factor (VWF)-cleaving protease, ADAMTS13, leads to generalised microvascular thrombosis in various organs [1]. The characteristic features are thrombocytopenia due to the consumption of platelets and microangiopathic haemolytic anaemia with destruction of erythrocytes [2]. As soon as the laboratory parameters return to normal after treatment of an acute bout, the patient is often regarded as cured but lives with the risk of suffering an acute relapse at any time [3]. In recent years, some studies have shown that iTTP is much more than just an acute disease; not only potential relapses but also long-term consequences of the past acute episode should be in focus. Besides neurological impairments [4–7], depression is a prevalent sequela [6–10]. The occurrence of depression and anxiety disorders has been documented in numerous other acute and chronic diseases, e.g., stroke, multiple sclerosis and cancer [11–15]. Depression itself is considered a risk factor for cardiovascular disease [16] and leads to increased morbidity and mortality, regardless of its severity [15,17]. Furthermore, depression causes a reduced quality of life for patients and lower resilience. In turn, individuals with low resilience are more prone to develop psychiatric disorders [18]. However, resilience is also significantly influenced by other factors, such as alexithymia [19].

We [10], as well as others [6,9,20], have shown that the prevalence of depression is significantly increased in patients that have survived acute iTTP. In addition, our results revealed that the severity of the acute iTTP episode is not the determining factor for the development and severity of depression [10].

The aim of the present study was to determine whether life circumstances (e.g., partnership, employment and physical activity), personality and resilience are associated with the development and severity of depression and anxiety in iTTP patients and how they influence their quality of life.

2. Materials and Methods

The results are part of a five-year prospective cohort study that was approved by German law (Landeskrankenhausgesetz §36 and §37) in accordance with the Declaration of Helsinki and by the local Ethics Committee of "Landesärztekammer Rheinland-Pfalz" (837.265.14 (9504-F)), where all participants gave written consent to participate.

The study was divided into two main themes. The first part referred to evaluations in 2013 and 2014 that have already been published [10]. In brief, the iTTP patients displayed a high prevalence of depression and cognitive deficits via self-reporting questionnaires. However, we did not detect a significant correlation between the severity of depression or cognitive deficits and the number or severity of acute TTP episodes. Nevertheless, we could demonstrate a highly significant correlation between the severity of depression and the degree to which cognitive performance was reduced [10].

The second part had a focus on the long-term psychological consequences, where the personality structure and the influence on the quality of life were examined in more detail here (Figure S1).

In 2015 and 2016, using validated questionnaires, we examined the prevalence of depressive (PHQ-9) and anxiety symptoms (GAD-7) in 104 iTTP patients, as well as parameters of subjective cognitive deficits (FLei), resilience (RS-11), attitude to life (LOT-R) and quality of life (QLQ-C30) at two observation points one year apart. At the second observation time, an age- and sex-matched healthy control group was simultaneously interviewed.

2.1. Patients and Controls

The patient cohort for this study was recruited from the iTTP patients that were treated directly at the University Hospital Mainz, as well as from external patients for whom the University Hospital Mainz was asked for medical advice by external clinics. The external patients that presented themselves personally at the University Hospital Mainz at least once were asked to participate in the study. Since October 2012, all patients over 18 years of age with a confirmed iTTP diagnosis (defined as microangiopathic haemolytic anaemia, thrombocytopenia (<150,000/µL), severe acquired ADAMTS13 deficiency (activity < 10%) and an ADAMTS13 inhibitor (>0.5 Bethesda units/mL)) in the acute TTP episode have been included.

The healthy controls were 300 randomly selected people that were age- and gender-matched to the iTTP collective, whose contact details were received from the residents' registration office. We received 134 evaluable questionnaires.

2.2. Psychometric Assessment

TTP patients were invited to participate in the study twice with an interval of 10 to 12 months. At both time points, psychometric questionnaires were either sent by regular mail to the patients' home or directly given to patients when they presented at the outpatients ward.

One patient was excluded from this study (in 2015/2016) because of an inability to answer the questionnaires after having suffered from ischemic brain damage during an acute TTP episode.

2.2.1. Patient Health Questionnaire 9 Items (PHQ-9)

The Patient Health Questionnaire 9 (PHQ-9) was developed in 2001 by Spitzer et al. and is indicated for the self-assessment of depressive symptoms and their classification into degrees of severity [21]. It consists of nine questions, each of which is attributed 0, 1, 2 or 3 points. The final score is calculated from the sum of all answers. A high score indicates that patients often show depressive symptoms. If the patient receives 0 to 4 points, it can be assumed that there is no depression. Mild depressive symptoms are present at 5 to 9 points, moderate symptoms at 10 to 14 points and moderate-to-severe depression at 15 to 19 points. A score $\geq$ 20 points signals severe depressive symptomatology. The presence of major depression can be assumed at a cut-off of $\geq$10 points.

2.2.2. Generalized Anxiety Disorder 7 (GAD-7)

The "Generalized Anxiety Disorder 7", which is a self-assessment questionnaire with seven items, was developed to diagnose and classify generalised anxiety disorders [22]. The GAD-7 examines the symptoms of anxiety, such as nervousness or irritability in seven items. The patient must evaluate how often these symptoms have been experienced in the last 2 weeks. Depending on the answer, the patient receives between 0 and 3 points. The sum of all seven items corresponds to the total score. If the total score is between 0 and 4 points, no anxiety disorder can be assumed. A score of 5 points or more indicates a mild anxiety disorder, 10 points or more indicates a moderate anxiety disorder and 15 points or more indicates a severe anxiety disorder.

2.2.3. FLei

Cognitive deficits were assessed using the German questionnaire for complaints of cognitive disturbances (FLei), which is a self-report measure with 30 items covering the domains of deficient attention, memory and executive functions, with 10 items each. All items are rated on a five-point Likert-scale (0 = at no time; 4 = very frequent). Accordingly, the total score for all 30 items ranges between 0 and 120 points. The internal consistencies of the three subscores (Cronbach's alpha and split-half reliability) are all >0.87 [23]. Healthy controls reported in the literature showed a mean of 29.1 (SD 18.7), whereas controls with major depression (ICD.10) had a mean of 56.5 (SD 23.1) [23].

2.2.4. Resilience Scale 11 (RS-11)

The Resilience Scale 11 (RS-11) was developed as a tool to measure the mental resistance of patients [24]. The self-assessment questionnaire consists of 11 questions, each of which is rated with 1 to 7 points. From these scales, an overall score is formed, with values from 11 to 77. The higher the total score, the higher the presumed resilience of the respondent.

2.2.5. Life Orientation Test–Revised (LOT-R)

The Life Orientation Test–Revised (LOT-R) is a questionnaire with 10 items, each with five possible answers, which serves to assess the attitude to life. It evaluates general character features, such as the tendency toward optimism and pessimism, for both of which, a subscore is given. In addition, an overall score can be calculated [25].

2.2.6. Quality of Life Questionnaire C 30 (QLQ-C30)

The Quality of Life Questionnaire C 30 (QLQ-C30) was developed in 1993 by the European Organisation for Research and Treatment of Cancer to specifically evaluate the quality of life of cancer patients [26,27]. Fifteen subscales are formed from the 30 items. The subscales consist of five function scales (physical, role, cognitive, emotional and social function), three symptom scales (fatigue, pain and nausea or vomiting) and a global health status/quality of life scale, as well as six individual items with specific symptoms (dyspnea, loss of appetite, insomnia, constipation and diarrhea, and a question on the financial impact of the disease). Each item has four response alternatives, except for the global health status/quality of life scale, which has response options ranging from 1 to 7.

2.3. Covariates

In addition to the questionnaires, personal information, such as age, gender and life circumstances such as partnership and number of children, were also collected. Furthermore, data on physical fitness and other chronic and acute illnesses were obtained. The participants were able to specify their physical fitness themselves with the help of five predefined answer options (from not at all or only a little bit (1–2 times per month) to extremely active (more than 5 times per week)). Fifteen comorbidities were specifically asked for and further comorbidities could be indicated.

2.4. Statistical Analyses

Statistical analyses were performed using SPSS version 22.0 (IBM GmbH, Ehningen, Germany). Missing data were imputed using median imputation. The descriptive statistics included frequency, mean, standard deviation, median, interquartile range (IQR), minimum and maximum. The differences between the two groups were tested using Student's *t*-test for normally distributed data and the non-parametric Mann–Whitney *U* test for non-normally distributed data. For comparing changes in the different scores of patients who completed both surveys (in 2015 and 2016), a dependent *t*-test was used, as well as the dependent Wilcoxon test. Spearman's rank correlation coefficient (r_s) was calculated to estimate the relationship between depressive symptoms and resilience, respectively. The correlations between age, gender, comorbidities, physical activity and depressive symptoms were determined using Pearson's correlation coefficient (*r*). Any *p*-values less than 0.05 were considered to be statistically significant.

3. Results

3.1. Study Population

From June 2015 until July 2016, 147 patients with an acquired TTP that was diagnosed prior to starting this study were asked to participate. Between the 2015 and 2016 surveys, five of the 147 participants were lost to follow-up. Accordingly, 142 TTP patients were sent the questionnaires in the 2016 survey, about one year after the first inquiry. We received 89 responses in the 2015 survey, with 89 of those being evaluable for RS-11, 88 for PHQ-9, 87 for GAD-7 and LOT-R and 85 for FLei (Figure 1). Eighty-four responses were obtained in the 2016 survey, with 83 of those being evaluable for Flei, 81 for PHQ-9, RS-11 and QLQ-C30 and 80 for GAD-7 and LOT-R (Figure 1).

Overall, we received responses from 104 individual iTTP patients, 69 answered both surveys, 20 participated only in 2015 and 15 only in 2016 (Figure 1). The depression, anxiety, impairment of cognitive performance, resilience, attitude of life and quality of life results of the iTTP patients were compared with those from 134 healthy controls.

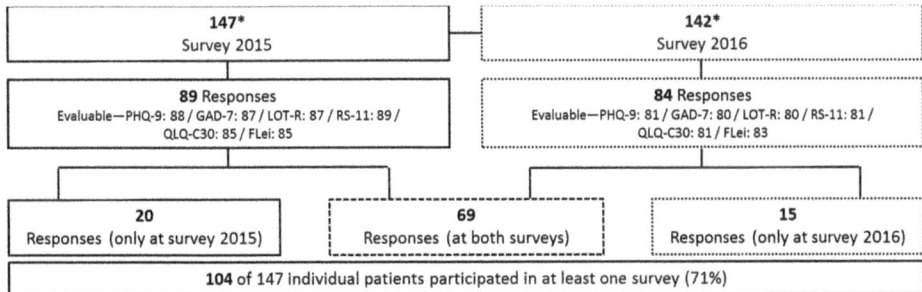

Figure 1. Patient recruitment and response rates in two surveys of the cohort of autoimmune thrombotic thrombocytopenic purpura (iTTP) patients from Mainz. A total of 147 eligible iTTP patients in remission were invited to fill in the various questionnaires used in two surveys each (2015 and 2016). * Between the first and second survey five patients were lost to follow-up. Questionnaires concerned: depression (PHQ-9), anxiety (GAD-7), attitude of life (LOT-R), resilience (RS-11), quality of life (QLQ-C30) and cognitive disturbance (FLei).

3.2. Patient Characteristics

A total of 147 (2015) and 142 (2016) iTTP patients could be reached for the surveys. The response rate was 60% in the 2015 survey and 59% in the 2016 survey (Figure 1). The characteristics of the patients and the healthy controls are shown in Table 1.

Table 1. Characteristics of the responding and evaluable autoimmune thrombotic thrombocytopenic purpura (iTTP) patients in both surveys and of the healthy controls.

Heading	iTTP Patients		Healthy Controls
Time of survey	2015	2016	2016
Number (n)	89	84	134
Gender and age			
Female	69 (76%)	69 (82%)	108 (81%)
Male	20 (24%)	15 (18%)	26 (19%)
Age (years) median (min, IQR, max)	48 (18, 37–59, 86)	51 (21, 38–59, 87)	48 (19, 30–60, 79)
Data for age missing	6	7	0
Current partnership			
Yes	62 (73%)	60 (75%)	96 (74%)
No	23 (27%)	20 (25%)	34 (26%)
Data missing	4	4	4
Occupation, BMI, smoking status			
Employed	45 (51%)	41 (50%)	72 (55%)
Studying	3 (3%)	1 (1%)	14 (11%)
Retired	26 (30%)	22 (27%)	27 (21%)
Unemployed	2 (2%)	4 (5%)	2 (1%)
Working at home	4 (5%)	7 (8.5%)	5 (4%)
Other	8 (9%)	7 (8.5%)	10 (8%)
Data missing	1	2	4
BMI median (min, IQR, max)	26 (18, 23–31, 48)	28 (18, 24–32, 47)	24 (18, 21–26, 42)
Obesity (BMI ≥ 30)	24 (27%)	29 (35%)	12 (9%)
Data missing	0	2	4
Smoking	22 (25%)	21 (25%)	18 (14%)
Data missing	0	1	2
Physical activity			
Hardly active (1–2×/month)	25 (29%)	32 (39%)	22 (17%)
Quite active (3–4×/month)	10 (12%)	13 (16%)	24 (18%)
Active (1–2×/week)	33 (39%)	24 (30%)	45 (34%)

Table 1. Cont.

Heading	iTTP Patients		Healthy Controls
Very active (3–4×/week)	14 (16%)	8 (10%)	32 (24%)
Extremely active (>5×/week)	3 (4%)	4 (5%)	9 (7%)
Data missing	4	3	2
Number of comorbidities [1]			
0	20 (22%)	10 (12%)	48 (36%)
1	25 (28%)	20 (24%)	43 (33%)
2	14 (16%)	23 (28%)	18 (14%)
≥3	30 (34%)	30 (36%)	23 (17%)
Data missing	0	1	2

[1] Includes cardiovascular diseases, hypertension, gastrointestinal diseases, rheumatoid arthritis, diabetes mellitus, skin diseases, metabolic disorders, allergies, multiple sclerosis, chronic pulmonary diseases, chronic pain, thyroid diseases, obesity, cancer and other.

About 80% of the patients were female and the median ages were 48 and 51 years in 2015 and 2016, respectively. Half of the participating patients were employed and one third were retired. The majority of patients lived in a partnership and 63% and 65% in 2015 and 2016, respectively, had children. One-third of patients each took part in low, intermediate or high physical activity. The median body mass index (BMI) was 26 and 28 kg/m^2, respectively, in the two surveys, with 27% and 35% being obese. Overall, the iTTP collective had several other diseases besides iTTP (78% had comorbidities in 2015 and 88% in 2016). On average, the iTTP patients had one additional disease in 2015 (min 0, IQR 1–3, max 9) and two additional comorbidities in 2016 (min 0, IQR 1–3, max 9). The control group had substantially fewer diseases (median 1, min 0, IQR 0–2, max 7). The comorbidities that were explicitly asked for were chronic heart diseases, hypertension, gastrointestinal diseases, rheumatoid arthritis, diabetes mellitus, skin diseases, metabolic disorders, allergies, multiple sclerosis, chronic pulmonary diseases, chronic pain, thyroid diseases, obesity and cancer. In addition, comorbidities not listed could be indicated. Both in iTTP patients and the control group, the most frequent health problems were hypertension and thyroid diseases, followed by allergies. Compared to the control collective, the iTTP patients were significantly more overweight, were more often smokers and had more comorbidities (Table 1).

3.3. Depression (PHQ-9)

In 2015, 54 (61.4%) of 88 iTTP patients were scored as having current depressive symptoms by the PHQ-9 (score ≥ 5) and the proportion of patients with major depression (score ≥ 10) was 21.6%. The median score was 5 (IQR 2–10), ranging from 0 to 23 (Figure 2a). Thirty-four (38.6%) patients had no depression, 31 (35.2%) had mild depression, 13 (14.8%) had moderate depression, nine (10.2%) had moderate-to-severe depression and 1 (1.1%) had severe depression.

In 2016, 51 (63.0%) of 81 iTTP patients were scored as having current depressive symptoms by the PHQ-9 (score ≥ 5) and the proportion of patients with major depression (score ≥ 10) was 34.5%. The median total score was 7 (IQR 2.5–12.5), ranging from 0 to 23 points (Figure 2a). Regarding the severity of depression, 30 (37.0%) patients had no depression, 23 (28.4%) had mild depression, 14 (17.3%) had moderate depression, 13 (16.0%) had moderate-to-severe depression and 1 (1.2%) had severe depression.

Forty-five of 133 (33.8%) healthy controls had depressive symptoms as scored by the PHQ-9 (score ≥ 5) (Figure 2a). Six (4.6%) of the 133 controls had clinically relevant depression (score ≥ 10). The median total score was 3 (IQR 1–6), ranging from 0 to 18 points (Figure 2a). The prevalence of depression in iTTP patients was significantly higher in both surveys (2015 $p < 0.001$; 2016 $p < 0.0001$) than in the controls (Figure 2a). No difference in the prevalence or severity of depression in the iTTP patients was found between the two surveys.

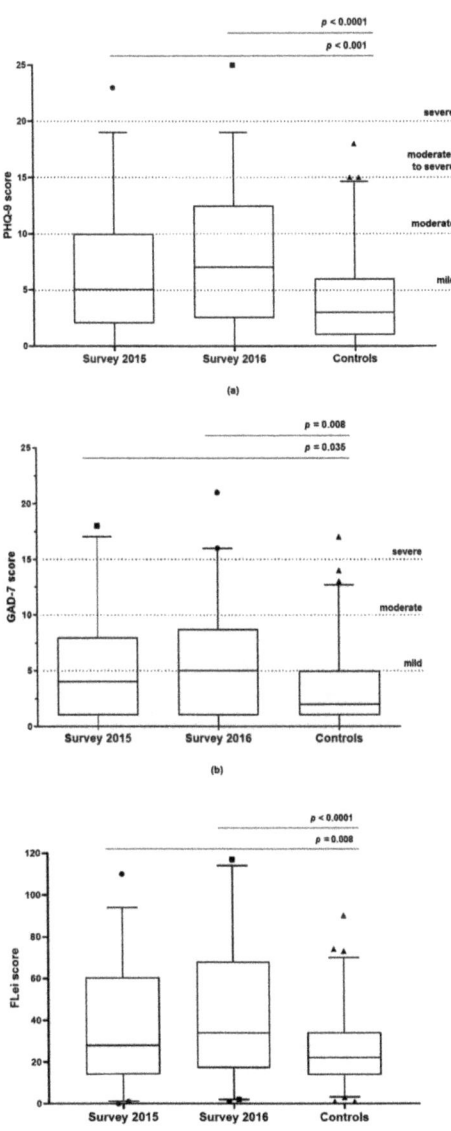

Figure 2. Results of the depression (PHQ-9), anxiety disorder (GAD-7) and cognitive performance (FLei score) questionnaires from the iTTP patients in two surveys (2015 and 2016) and the healthy controls (median, box 25th and 75th percentiles, whiskers 2.5th and 97.5th percentiles, •, ■, ▲ denote outliers above 97.5th percentiles or below 2.5th percentiles outliers). (**a**) PHQ-9: For the first survey ($n = 88$), the median evaluated score was 5 (IQR 2–10), for the second survey ($n = 81$), the median score was 7 (IQR 2.5–12.5), and for the healthy controls, the median score was 3 (IQR 1–6). (**b**) GAD-7: For the first survey ($n = 87$), the median evaluated score was 4 (IQR 1–8), for the second survey ($n = 80$), the median score was 5 (IQR 1–8.75), and for the healthy controls ($n = 131$), the median score was 2 (IQR 1–5). (**c**) FLei: For the first survey ($n = 85$), the median evaluated score was 28.0 (IQR 14–60.5), for the second survey ($n = 81$), the median score was 34.0 (IQR 17–68), and for the healthy controls ($n = 130$), the median score was 22.0 (IQR 13.75–34.25).

3.4. Anxiety Disorder (GAD-7)

In 2015, 49 (56.3%) of 87 iTTP patients had no symptoms of anxiety, whereas 21 (24.1%) had mild anxiety (score 5–9), 12 (13.8%) had moderate anxiety (score 10–14) and five (5.7%) had severe anxiety (score 15–21). The median evaluated score was 4 (IQR 1–8), ranging from 0 to 18 (Figure 2b).

In 2016, 37 (46.3%) of 80 iTTP patients had no symptoms of anxiety, whereas 29 (36.3%) patients had mild anxiety (score 5–9), 11 (13.8%) had moderate anxiety (score 10–14) and three (3.8%) had severe anxiety (score 15–21). The median evaluated score was 5 (IQR 1–9), ranging from 0 to 21 (Figure 2b). Ninety-five of the 132 controls (72.0%) did not show any symptoms of anxiety (Figure 2b). The prevalence of anxiety disorders in the overall iTTP cohort was higher in both surveys (2015 $p < 0.035$; 2016 $p < 0.008$) than in the control group (Figure 2b). In particular, the proportion of clinically relevant anxiety disorders (score ≥ 10) in the iTTP cohort was significantly higher in 2015 (19.5%) and in 2016 (17.6%) than in the control group (8.4%).

3.5. Cognitive Performance (FLei Score)

Eighty-five iTTP patients in 2015 and 81 in 2016 were evaluable for their cognitive performance using FLei (Figure 2c). The total scores in both surveys were normally distributed and showed a median of 28.0 (IQR 14–60.5) in the 2015 survey and a median of 34.0 (IQR 17–68) in the 2016 survey, ranging from 0 to 117 (Figure 2c). Cognitive performance was significantly worse for iTTP patients in both surveys ($p = 0.008$ for 2015, $p < 0.0001$ for 2016) in comparison to the healthy cohort (median 22.0, IQR 13.75–34.25) (Figure 2c).

3.6. Resilience (RS-11)

The 89 iTTP patients in the first survey in 2015 showed a median score of 60 (min 22, IQR 49.5–68.5, max 77) and the 81 iTTP patients in the second survey 2016 showed a median score of 55 (min 21, IQR 45–66, max 77) (Figure 3a). The control collective of 129 persons had a median score of 64 (min 33, IQR 56–69, max 77) (Figure 3a). Thus, the survivors of iTTP, both in the first ($p < 0.04$) and second ($p < 0.0001$) surveys, exhibited a lower resilience than the control collective (Figure 3a).

3.7. Attitude to Life (LOT-R)

The questionnaire on the attitude to life (LOT-R) was answered by 87 patients in 2015 and 80 patients in 2016. The results in the categories of optimism, pessimism and the total score could be compared with 134 control persons. In the first survey, no significant difference ($p = 0.088$) between the patients (median 15, IQR 12–19) and controls (median 17, IQR 14–19) was found in the total score, but in the second survey, a significant difference ($p = 0.009$) between the patients (median 17, IQR 11–18) and controls was found (Figure 3b). In the optimism score, the patients showed significantly worse results than the control group in both rounds (2015 survey $p = 0.011$, 2016 survey $p = 0.006$) (Figure 3b). Within the pessimism score, no large differences between the patients and controls could be detected (2015 survey $p = 0.49$, 2016 survey $p = 0.63$) (Figure 3b).

3.8. Quality of Life (QLQ-C30)

Eighty-five TTP patients in 2015 and 81 patients in 2016 were evaluable regarding their quality of life using the QLQ-C30 (Figure 3c). They could be compared with 134 healthy controls (Figure 3c). In all five functional scales (physical, cognitive, role and social function $p < 0.0001$ for both 2015 and 2016; emotional function $p = 0.001$ for 2015/$p = 0.007$ for 2016), as well as in the global quality of life scale ($p = 0.001$ for 2015/$p = 0.007$ for 2016), the iTTP patients showed significantly worse results in both rounds than the control group (Figure 3c, not all five functional scales are shown).

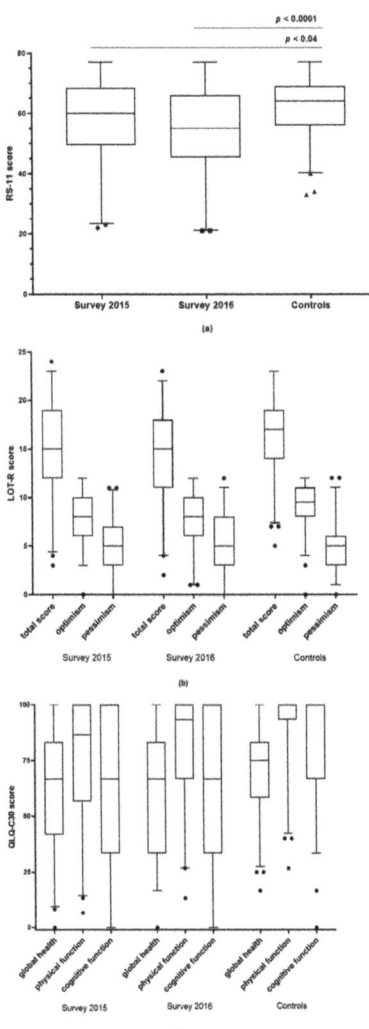

Figure 3. Results of the resilience (RS-11), attitude to life (LOT-R) and quality of life (QLQ-C30) questionnaires from the autoimmune thrombotic thrombocytopenic purpura (iTTP) patients in two surveys (2015 and 2016) and the healthy controls (median, box 25th and 75th percentiles, whiskers 2.5th and 97.5th percentiles, •, ■, ▲ outliers above the 97.5th percentiles or below the 2.5th percentiles). (**a**) RS-11: For the survey in 2015, the median evaluated score was 60 (IQR 49.5–68.5), for the survey in 2016, the score was 55 (IQR 45–66), and for healthy controls, the score was 64 (IQR 56–69). (**b**) LOT-R: In the optimism score, the patients showed significantly worse results than the control group in both rounds (2015 survey $p = 0.011$, 2016 survey $p = 0.006$). Within the pessimism score, no large differences between the patients and controls could be detected (2015 survey $p = 0.49$, 2016 survey $p = 0.63$). In the first round, no significant difference ($p = 0.088$) between the patients and controls was found in the total score, but in the second round, a significant difference ($p = 0.009$) between the patients and controls was found. (**c**) QLQ-C30: In the "global health", "physical function" and "cognitive function" scores, the patients had significantly worse results than the control group in both rounds (2015 and 2016 surveys $p < 0.0001$).

3.9. Correlation of Life Circumstances and Personality with Depression

Sex, age, physical activity and partnership status were not significantly correlated with depression. Using Pearson's correlation (age, physical activity, partnership status) and Mann–Whitney U analysis (sex), no significant correlation was established for any of these parameters in 2015 or 2016 with the degree of depression (PHQ-9 score) (Table S1). The comorbidities were associated with the PHQ-9 score. Only the number of co-morbidities was considered, not the specific diseases. If a patient had more co-morbidities, the PHQ-9 score showed a higher value, i.e., a more severe depressive state ($p = 0.015$ for 2015/$p = 0.006$ for 2016) (Table S1). Furthermore, the correlation between the QLQ-C30 score (quality of life) and the PHQ-9 score was significant ($p < 0.0001$ for both 2015 and 2016) (Table S1).

3.10. Correlation of Resilience with Depression

Our data revealed that the degree of depression (PHQ-9) was negatively associated with resilience (RS-11). Spearman's rank correlation coefficient (r_s) for 88 iTTP patients in the 2015 survey was -0.5346 ($p < 0.0001$), and for the 78 participants in the 2016 survey, $r_s = -0.6447$ ($p < 0.0001$). In Figure 4, the RS-11 and PHQ-9 data for 102 individual iTTP patients (only the first survey was considered for patients who participated in both surveys) revealed an r_s of -0.5878 ($p < 0.0001$) (Figure 4). Seventy iTTP patients without major depression (PHQ-9 score points < 10) had a median of 62 for the RS-11 score, which was comparable to the controls (median RS-11 score: 64, $p = 0.65$). The 32 iTTP patients with major depression (PHQ-9 score ≥ 10) had a median of 41.5 for the RS-11 score, which was significantly lower than that of the controls and the iTTP patients without major depression ($p < 0.0001$).

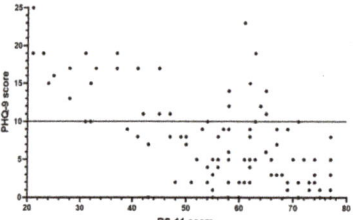

Figure 4. Correlation of the PHQ-9 score (depressive symptoms) with the resilience score. The correlation of the degree of depression (PHQ-9) with resilience (RS-11) was analysed for 102 iTTP patients ($r_s = -0.588$, $p < 0.0001$) (every iTTP patient was analysed only once, the first evaluation of those that participated in both surveys was considered). The horizontal line indicates the cut-off for major depression (PHQ-9 score ≥ 10).

4. Discussion

For a long time, the survival of acute iTTP bouts was the main concern, but in recent years, the long-term consequences in survivors of iTTP have become more important. The prevalence of major depression in our iTTP patients was 21.6% and 34.5% for 2015 and 2016, respectively, far above the prevalence in our population controls (4.6%) and the reported 12-month prevalence in the German population (9.3%) [28]. These results are consistent with our previous findings [10] and with other studies showing a significantly increased point prevalence of depression from 19% up to 65% in iTTP survivors [6,8,9,29,30]. A strong association between chronic physical illness and depression has been reported [15,31]. Independent from the disease, the rate of 21.1% mood disorders in patients is significantly higher than in healthy individuals with 9.4% [31]. In addition, anxiety disorders have been documented, for example, in patients after a heart attack or stroke and with cancer [15,31]. Anxiety disorders in those with serious illnesses are just as common (22.9%) as depression (21.1%) [31]. Within the general population, anxiety disorders are the most common mental disorder, affecting about 15% [28]. Our examination of 87 iTTP patients revealed clinically relevant anxiety disorders in 19.5% and 17.6% for 2015 and 2016, respectively, as compared to a prevalence of 8.4% in the controls. Riva et al. found that 20% had anxiety disorders in their 35 TTP patients [7]. Regarding iTTP, survivors depression seems to be more common than anxiety disorders [7,32]. Gender, age and partnership [33] did not seem to be related to depression in our patients, whereas comorbidities did. This is congruent with the data of Härter et al. [31]. This is important since more than two-thirds of iTTP patients suffer from at least one other disease. Long-term data from the Oklahoma TTP registry showed a significantly higher prevalence of obesity, systemic lupus erythematosus, diabetes mellitus, arterial hypertension and major depression in survivors of iTTP [8,20,30]. Depression and anxiety are associated with increased morbidity and mortality. Martin-Subero et al. demonstrated for 803 inpatients over a follow-up period of 18 years that major depression was associated with a 2.4-times higher risk of mortality [34], independent of their disease. According to Cuijpers and Smit, mortality is increased regardless of the severity of depression [17]. Given that depressive symptoms affected up to 60% of our iTTP patients, together with low quality of life scores, antidepressive therapy seems mandatory. Lewis et al. [35], Cataland et al. [5] and Riva et al. [7] also reported a significantly compromised quality of life in iTTP patients. The number and severity of survived acute episodes do not seem to have a significant influence on the development and severity of depression [10]. An abnormal cerebral MRI scan during an acute episode does not implicate an increased likelihood of the development of depression or an anxiety disorder [32]. The survey on the attitude to life and resilience of our iTTP patients suggests that the patients were less resilient and optimistic, but nevertheless, not more pessimistic than the control group. The resilience of our iTTP patients was negatively related to the severity of their depressive symptoms. This is congruent with the findings, for example, in dry eye disease or cardiovascular disease [36,37]. According to other studies, more resilient individuals develop less depression and anxiety overall, regardless of whether they have a severe underlying disease [38–41]. The resilience may be reduced by the experience of a life-threatening disease and cognitive deficits, which further increases the risk of depression in iTTP.

Limitations of the Study

Our study has limitations: First, we used self-report questionnaires. There was no examination by a clinician, such as in the studies by Han et al. [6]. However, we used questionnaires that have been widely validated in large cohorts of healthy subjects and patients. Second, only about 60% of our iTTP survivors participated in the self-evaluation study. Symptomatic patients may have been more motivated to answer the survey compared to asymptomatic patients. On the other hand, severely depressive patients may also have declined participation. The exact clinical data on the severity of the iTTP were not fully available for all patients, and comorbidities were not confirmed beyond the self-reporting. Finally, we do not have data on mental illness or resilience prior to the iTTP diagnosis.

5. Conclusions

The survivors of acute iTTP are significantly more likely to suffer from depressive and anxiety disorders as compared to the general population. The patients also reported a significantly compromised quality of life and perceived their cognitive performance as being significantly reduced. Overall, the iTTP patients were less optimistic and showed a significantly lower resilience, which in turn correlated strongly with the severity of the depression. It remains to be investigated whether psychological counseling in these long-term patients helps to improve neuropsychiatric disorders during long-term follow-ups. Furthermore, there is hope that new treatment strategies aiming at a fast resolution of the microvascular thrombotic process may improve long-term outcomes [42].

Supplementary Materials: The following are available online at https://www.mdpi.com/2077-0383/10/2/365/s1, Figure S1: Patient recruitment and response rates for the four surveys of the cohort of iTTP patients from Mainz, Table S1: Correlation of the PHQ-9 score (depressive symptoms) with sex, age, physical activity, partnership status and comorbidities in the 2015 and 2016 questionnaires.

Author Contributions: Conceptualization, T.F., M.B. and I.S.; methodology, M.B. and T.F.; formal analysis, M.S. and T.F.; investigation, S.B.; writing—original draft preparation, T.F.; writing—review and editing, B.L., M.B., K.L. and I.S. All authors have read and agreed to the published version of the manuscript.

Funding: This study (BMBF 01EO1503), as well as Tanja Falter (BMBF 01EO1003), were supported by the Federal Ministry of Education and Research.

Institutional Review Board Statement: The study that was approved by German law (Landeskrankenhausgesetz §36 and §37) in accordance with the Declaration of Helsinki and by the local Ethics Committee of "Landesärztekammer Rheinland-Pfalz" (837.265.14 (9504-F)).

Informed Consent Statement: Informed consent was obtained from all subjects involved in the study.

Data Availability Statement: The data presented in this study are available on request from the corresponding author. The data are not publicly available due to data privacy act.

Conflicts of Interest: The authors state that they have no conflict of interest with this publication. Inge Scharrer is a member of the Data Safety Monitoring Board in the BAX 930 study (investigating recombi-nant ADAMTS13 infusion in hereditary TTP). Bernhard Lämmle is chairman of the Data Safety Monitoring Committee of the BAXALTA 281102 and the SHP655201 studies (now both run by TAKEDA), investigating recombinant ADAMTS13 in congenital and acquired TTP, respectively. He is on the Advisory Board of Sanofi for Caplacizumab, and received travel and accommodation support for participating at scientific meetings and/or lecture fees from Ablynx, Alexion, Siemens, Bayer, Roche, and Sanofi.

References

1. Tsai, H.M. Pathophysiology of thrombotic thrombocytopenic purpura. *Int. J. Hematol.* **2010**, *91*, 1–19. [CrossRef] [PubMed]
2. Crawley, J.T.; Scully, M.A. Thrombotic thrombocytopenic purpura: Basic pathophysiology and therapeutic strategies. *Hematol. Am. Soc. Hematol. Educ. Program.* **2013**, *2013*, 292–299. [CrossRef] [PubMed]
3. Hovinga, J.A.K.; Vesely, S.K.; Terrell, D.R.; Lammle, B.; George, J.N. Survival and relapse in patients with thrombotic thrombocytopenic purpura. *Blood* **2010**, *115*, 1500–1511. [CrossRef] [PubMed]
4. Kennedy, A.S.; Lewis, Q.F.; Scott, J.G.; Hovinga, J.A.K.; Lammle, B.; Terrell, D.R.; Vesely, S.K.; George, J.N. Cognitive deficits after recovery from thrombotic thrombocytopenic purpura. *Transfusion* **2009**, *49*, 1092–1101. [CrossRef]
5. Cataland, S.R.; Scully, M.A.; Paskavitz, J.; Maruff, P.; Witkoff, L.; Jin, M.; Uva, N.; Gilbert, J.C.; Wu, H.M. Evidence of persistent neurologic injury following thrombotic thrombocytopenic purpura. *Am. J. Hematol.* **2011**, *86*, 87–89. [CrossRef]
6. Han, B.; Page, E.E.; Stewart, L.M.; Deford, C.C.; Scott, J.G.; Schwartz, L.H.; Perdue, J.J.; Terrell, D.R.; Vesely, S.K.; George, J.N. Depression and cognitive impairment following recovery from thrombotic thrombocytopenic purpura. *Am. J. Hematol.* **2015**, *90*, 709–714. [CrossRef]
7. Riva, S.; Mancini, I.; Maino, A.; Ferrari, B.; Artoni, A.; Agosti, P.; Peyvandi, F. Long-term neuropsychological sequelae, emotional wellbeing and quality of life in patients with acquired thrombotic thrombocytopenic purpura. *Haematologica* **2020**, *105*, 1957–1962. [CrossRef]
8. Deford, C.C.; Reese, J.A.; Schwartz, L.H.; Perdue, J.J.; Hovinga, J.A.K.; Lammle, B.; Terrell, D.R.; Vesely, S.K.; George, J.N. Multiple major morbidities and increased mortality during long-term follow-up after recovery from thrombotic thrombocytopenic purpura. *Blood* **2013**, *122*, 2023–2029. [CrossRef]
9. Chaturvedi, S.; Oluwole, O.; Cataland, S.; McCrae, K.R. Post-traumatic stress disorder and depression in survivors of thrombotic thrombocytopenic purpura. *Thromb Res.* **2017**, *151*, 51–56. [CrossRef]
10. Falter, T.; Schmitt, V.; Herold, S.; Weyer, V.; von Auer, C.; Wagner, S.; Hefner, G.; Beutel, M.; Lackner, K.; Lammle, B.; et al. Depression and cognitive deficits as long-term consequences of thrombotic thrombocytopenic purpura. *Transfusion* **2017**, *57*, 1152–1162. [CrossRef]
11. Kauhanen, M.; Korpelainen, J.T.; Hiltunen, P.; Brusin, E.; Mononen, H.; Maatta, R.; Nieminen, P.; Sotaniemi, K.A.; Myllyla, V.V. Poststroke depression correlates with cognitive impairment and neurological deficits. *Stroke* **1999**, *30*, 1875–1880. [CrossRef] [PubMed]
12. Robinson, R.G.; Spalletta, G. Poststroke depression: A review. *Can. J. Psychiatry* **2010**, *55*, 341–349. [CrossRef] [PubMed]
13. Siegert, R.J.; Abernethy, D.A. Depression in multiple sclerosis: A review. *J. Neurol. Neurosurg. Psychiatry* **2005**, *76*, 469–475. [CrossRef]

14. Jones, K.H.; Ford, D.V.; Jones, P.A.; John, A.; Middleton, R.M.; Lockhart-Jones, H.; Osborne, L.A.; Noble, J.G. A large-scale study of anxiety and depression in people with Multiple Sclerosis: A survey via the web portal of the UK MS Register. *PLoS ONE* **2012**, *7*, e41910. [CrossRef] [PubMed]
15. Clarke, D.M.; Currie, K.C. Depression, anxiety and their relationship with chronic diseases: A review of the epidemiology, risk and treatment evidence. *Med. J. Aust.* **2009**, *190*, S54–S60. [CrossRef] [PubMed]
16. Van der Kooy, K.; van Hout, H.; Marwijk, H.; Marten, H.; Stehouwer, C.; Beekman, A. Depression and the risk for cardiovascular diseases: Systematic review and meta analysis. *Int. J. Geriatr. Psychiatry* **2007**, *22*, 613–626. [CrossRef]
17. Cuijpers, P.; Smit, F. Excess mortality in depression: A meta-analysis of community studies. *J. Affect Disord.* **2002**, *72*, 227–236. [CrossRef]
18. Schiele, M.A.; Domschke, K. Epigenetics at the crossroads between genes, environment and resilience in anxiety disorders. *Genes Brain Behav.* **2018**, *17*, e12423. [CrossRef]
19. De Berardis, D.; Fornaro, M.; Valchera, A.; Rapini, G.; Di Natale, S.; De Lauretis, I.; Serroni, N.; Orsolini, L.; Tomasetti, C.; Bustini, M.; et al. Alexithymia, resilience, somatic sensations and their relationships with suicide ideation in drug naive patients with first-episode major depression: An exploratory study in the "real world" everyday clinical practice. *Early Interv. Psychiatry* **2020**, *14*, 336–342. [CrossRef]
20. George, J.N.; Vesely, S.K.; Terrell, D.R.; Deford, C.C.; Reese, J.A.; Al-Nouri, Z.L.; Stewart, L.M.; Lu, K.H.; Muthurajah, D.S. The Oklahoma Thrombotic Thrombocytopenic Purpura-haemolytic Uraemic Syndrome Registry. A model for clinical research, education and patient care. *Hamostaseologie* **2013**, *33*, 105–112. [CrossRef]
21. Kroenke, K.; Spitzer, R.L.; Williams, J.B. The PHQ-9: Validity of a brief depression severity measure. *J. Gen. Intern. Med.* **2001**, *16*, 606–613. [CrossRef]
22. Spitzer, R.L.; Kroenke, K.; Williams, J.B.; Lowe, B. A brief measure for assessing generalized anxiety disorder: The GAD-7. *Arch. Intern. Med.* **2006**, *166*, 1092–1097. [CrossRef] [PubMed]
23. Beblo, T.; Kunz, M.; Brokate, B.; Scheurich, A.; Weber, B.; Albert, A.; Richter, P.; Lautenbacher, S. Construction of a Questionnaire for Complaints of Cognitive Disturbances in Patients with Mental Disorders. *Z. Neuropsychol.* **2010**, *21*, 143–151. [CrossRef]
24. Wagnild, G.M.; Young, H.M. Development and psychometric evaluation of the Resilience Scale. *J. Nurs. Meas* **1993**, *1*, 165–178. [PubMed]
25. Scheier, M.F.; Carver, C.S.; Bridges, M.W. Distinguishing optimism from neuroticism (and trait anxiety, self-mastery, and self-esteem): A reevaluation of the Life Orientation Test. *J. Personal. Soc. Psychol.* **1994**, *67*, 1063–1078. [CrossRef]
26. Aaronson, N.K.; Ahmedzai, S.; Bergman, B.; Bullinger, M.; Cull, A.; Duez, N.J.; Filiberti, A.; Flechtner, H.; Fleishman, S.B.; de Haes, J.C.; et al. The European Organization for Research and Treatment of Cancer QLQ-C30: A quality-of-life instrument for use in international clinical trials in oncology. *J. Natl. Cancer Inst.* **1993**, *85*, 365–376. [CrossRef]
27. Schwarz, R.; Hinz, A. Reference data for the quality of life questionnaire EORTC QLQ-C30 in the general German population. *Eur. J. Cancer* **2001**, *37*, 1345–1351. [CrossRef]
28. Jacobi, F.; Hofler, M.; Strehle, J.; Mack, S.; Gerschler, A.; Scholl, L.; Busch, M.A.; Maske, U.; Hapke, U.; Gaebel, W.; et al. Mental disorders in the general population: Study on the health of adults in Germany and the additional module mental health (DEGS1-MH). *Nervenarzt* **2014**, *85*, 77–87. [CrossRef]
29. Terrell, D.R.; Tolma, E.L.; Stewart, L.M.; Shirley, E.A. Thrombotic thrombocytopenic purpura patients' attitudes toward depression management: A qualitative study. *Health Sci. Rep.* **2019**, *2*, e136. [CrossRef]
30. George, J.N. TTP: Long-term outcomes following recovery. *Hematol. Am. Soc. Hematol. Educ. Program.* **2018**, *2018*, 548–552. [CrossRef]
31. Harter, M.; Baumeister, H.; Reuter, K.; Jacobi, F.; Hofler, M.; Bengel, J.; Wittchen, H.U. Increased 12-month prevalence rates of mental disorders in patients with chronic somatic diseases. *Psychother. Psychosom.* **2007**, *76*, 354–360. [CrossRef] [PubMed]
32. Alwan, F.; Mahdi, D.; Tayabali, S.; Cipolotti, L.; Lakey, G.; Hyare, H.; Scully, M. Cerebral MRI findings predict the risk of cognitive impairment in thrombotic thrombocytopenic purpura. *Br. J. Haematol.* **2020**, *191*, 868–874. [CrossRef] [PubMed]
33. Jacobi, F.; Hofler, M.; Siegert, J.; Mack, S.; Gerschler, A.; Scholl, L.; Busch, M.A.; Hapke, U.; Maske, U.; Seiffert, I.; et al. Twelve-month prevalence, comorbidity and correlates of mental disorders in Germany: The Mental Health Module of the German Health Interview and Examination Survey for Adults (DEGS1-MH). *Int. J. Methods Psychiatr. Res.* **2014**, *23*, 304–319. [CrossRef] [PubMed]
34. Martin-Subero, M.; Kroenke, K.; Diez-Quevedo, C.; Rangil, T.; de Antonio, M.; Morillas, R.M.; Loran, M.E.; Mateu, C.; Lupon, J.; Planas, R.; et al. Depression as Measured by PHQ-9 Versus Clinical Diagnosis as an Independent Predictor of Long-Term Mortality in a Prospective Cohort of Medical Inpatients. *Psychosom. Med.* **2017**, *79*, 273–282. [CrossRef] [PubMed]
35. Lewis, Q.F.; Lanneau, M.S.; Mathias, S.D.; Terrell, D.R.; Vesely, S.K.; George, J.N. Long-term deficits in health-related quality of life after recovery from thrombotic thrombocytopenic purpura. *Transfusion* **2009**, *49*, 118–124. [CrossRef]
36. Kaiser, T.; Janssen, B.; Schrader, S.; Geerling, G. Depressive symptoms, resilience, and personality traits in dry eye disease. *Graefes Arch. Clin. Exp. Ophthalmol.* **2019**, *257*, 591–599. [CrossRef]
37. Toukhsati, S.R.; Jovanovic, A.; Dehghani, S.; Tran, T.; Tran, A.; Hare, D.L. Low psychological resilience is associated with depression in patients with cardiovascular disease. *Eur. J. Cardiovasc. Nurs.* **2017**, *16*, 64–69. [CrossRef]
38. Avila, M.P.W.; Lucchetti, A.L.; Lucchetti, G. Association between depression and resilience in older adults: A systematic review and meta-analysis. *Int. J. Geriatr. Psychiatry* **2017**, *32*, 237–246. [CrossRef]

39. Hu, T.; Xiao, J.; Peng, J.; Kuang, X.; He, B. Relationship between resilience, social support as well as anxiety/depression of lung cancer patients: A cross-sectional observation study. *J. Cancer Res. Ther.* **2018**, *14*, 72–77. [CrossRef]
40. Choi, Y.; Choi, S.H.; Yun, J.Y.; Lim, J.A.; Kwon, Y.; Lee, H.Y.; Jang, J.H. The relationship between levels of self-esteem and the development of depression in young adults with mild depressive symptoms. *Medicine (Baltim.)* **2019**, *98*, e17518. [CrossRef]
41. Southwick, S.M.; Charney, D.S. The science of resilience: Implications for the prevention and treatment of depression. *Science* **2012**, *338*, 79–82. [CrossRef] [PubMed]
42. Knoebl, P.; Cataland, S.; Peyvandi, F.; Coppo, P.; Scully, M.; Hovinga, J.A.K.; Metjian, A.; de la Rubia, J.; Pavenski, K.; Edou, J.M.M.; et al. Efficacy and safety of open-label caplacizumab in patients with exacerbations of acquired thrombotic thrombocytopenic purpura in the HERCULES study. *J. Thromb. Haemost.* **2020**, *18*, 479–484. [CrossRef] [PubMed]

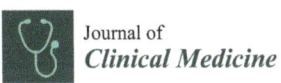

Review

Learning the Ropes of Platelet Count Regulation: Inherited Thrombocytopenias

Loredana Bury, Emanuela Falcinelli and Paolo Gresele *

Department of Medicine and Surgery, Section of Internal and Cardiovascular Medicine, University of Perugia, Centro Didattico, Edificio B Piano 1, 06132 Perugia, Italy; loredana.bury@unipg.it (L.B.); emanuelafalcinelli@gmail.com (E.F.)
* Correspondence: paolo.gresele@unipg.it; Tel.: +39-075-578-3989; Fax: +39-075-571-6083

Abstract: Inherited thrombocytopenias (IT) are a group of hereditary disorders characterized by a reduced platelet count sometimes associated with abnormal platelet function, which can lead to bleeding but also to syndromic manifestations and predispositions to other disorders. Currently at least 41 disorders caused by mutations in 42 different genes have been described. The pathogenic mechanisms of many forms of IT have been identified as well as the gene variants implicated in megakaryocyte maturation or platelet formation and clearance, while for several of them the pathogenic mechanism is still unknown. A range of therapeutic approaches are now available to improve survival and quality of life of patients with IT; it is thus important to recognize an IT and establish a precise diagnosis. ITs may be difficult to diagnose and an initial accurate clinical evaluation is mandatory. A combination of clinical and traditional laboratory approaches together with advanced sequencing techniques provide the highest rate of diagnostic success. Despite advancement in the diagnosis of IT, around 50% of patients still do not receive a diagnosis, therefore further research in the field of ITs is warranted to further improve patient care.

Keywords: inherited thrombocytopenias; platelets; bleeding

Citation: Bury, L.; Falcinelli, E.; Gresele, P. Learning the Ropes of Platelet Count Regulation: Inherited Thrombocytopenias. *J. Clin. Med.* **2021**, *10*, 533. https://doi.org/10.3390/jcm10030533

Academic Editor: Hugo ten Cate
Received: 30 December 2020
Accepted: 25 January 2021
Published: 2 February 2021

Publisher's Note: MDPI stays neutral with regard to jurisdictional claims in published maps and institutional affiliations.

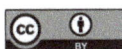

Copyright: © 2021 by the authors. Licensee MDPI, Basel, Switzerland. This article is an open access article distributed under the terms and conditions of the Creative Commons Attribution (CC BY) license (https://creativecommons.org/licenses/by/4.0/).

1. Introduction

Platelets, or thrombocytes, are small and anuclear blood cells with discoid shape and a size of 1.5–3.0 µm which play a crucial function in primary hemostasis. Their normal life span is 9–10 days and total circulating mass 10^{12}, thus about 10^{11} platelets are released each day from their bone marrow precursors, megakaryocytes, to maintain a normal circulating platelet count of 1.5 to 4×10^9/L.

Inherited thrombocytopenias (ITs) are a heterogeneous group of congenital disorders characterized by a reduction of platelet number, a widely-variable bleeding diathesis, sometimes aggravated by associated impairment of platelet function, and frequently associated with additional defects, which may heavily impact patient lives.

ITs are rare diseases, with an estimated prevalence of 2.7 in 100,000 [1] although this figure is probably underestimated because they are often misdiagnosed as immune thrombocytopenia (ITP). A recent study on the assessment of the frequency of naturally occurring loss-of-function variants in genes associated with platelet disorders (52% of which were associated with ITs) from a large genome aggregation database showed that 0.329% of subjects in the general population have a clinically meaningful loss-of-function variant in a platelet-associated gene [2].

The first IT, Bernard Soulier syndrome, was described in 1948 and subsequently only few additional forms were reported until Sanger sequencing first, and next generation sequencing later became widely applied rapidly bringing the known ITs from less than a dozen to currently at least 41 disorders caused by mutations in 42 different genes [3,4].

Despite these advancements however, it is estimated that genetic etiology of nearly 50% of patients with IT still remains undefined [5].

2. Megakaryocytopoiesis and Platelet Production

Platelets are produced by megakaryocytes (MKs), their giant bone marrow polyploid precursors, through a complex and highly regulated process. During maturation megakaryocytes become polyploid and accumulate massive amounts of proteins and membranes. Then, through a cytoskeletal-driven process, they extend long branching protrusions called proplatelets into sinusoidal blood vessels to release platelets [6]. However, under special conditions associated with strongly increased platelet turnover, platelets can be released through megakaryocyte rupture [7]. More recently, based on the calculation of the rate of proplatelet formation required for physiological platelet replacement, it has been suggested that membrane budding, rather than proplatelet formation, supplies the majority of the platelet biomass in vivo [8]. The release of platelets in lungs by megakaryocytes entered in blood and disintegrated by the impact with the pulmonary microcirculation has also been shown, but its relevance for platelet production is a matter of controversy [9].

The process of megakaryopoiesis involves multiple genes, coding for transcription factors, cytoskeletal proteins, membrane receptors and signaling proteins, which regulate megakaryocyte differentiation and platelet formation and release. Variants in any of these genes may cause IT.

3. Hereditary Disorders of Platelet Number

Given the wide heterogeneity of IT, there is no consensus on their classification, and several criteria have been proposed, such as on clinical features (e.g., age at presentation, severity, associated developmental abnormalities), platelet size or inheritance pattern (e.g., autosomal dominant, autosomal recessive and X-linked) [4,10,11].

Here we have grouped them according to the pathogenic mechanisms of thrombocytopenia.

ITs are primarily caused by mutations in genes involved in megakaryocyte differentiation, maturation and platelet production [12] (Table 1, Figure 1).

Table 1. IT classified based on the defective step of platelet count regulation involved.

Defective Step of Thrombopoiesis	Affected Gene	Disorder	Pathogenic Mechanism (Reference)	Additional Features (e.g., Syndromic Manifestations, Predisposition)
Defective megakaryocyte maturation	ANKRD26	ANKRD26-related thrombocytopenia	Loss of ANKRD26 silencing during the last phases of megakaryocytopoiesis causes ERK1/2 phosphorylation that interferes with megakaryocyte maturation [13]	Predisposition to hematological malignancies
	ETV6	ETV6-related thrombocytopenia	ETV6 is a transcriptional repressor that promotes the late phases of megakaryopoiesis. Mutations in ETV6 cause defective megakaryocyte maturation and impaired proplatelet formation [14]	Predisposition to hematological malignancies
	FLI1	FLI1-related thrombocytopenia	FLI1 is a transcription factor regulating many genes associated with megakaryocyte development. Therefore, FLI1 mutations promote defective megakaryocyte maturation [15]	Not reported
	FLI1 deletion	Paris-Trousseau syndrome/Jacobsen syndrome		Abnormalities of heart and face, intellectual disabilities
	FYB	FYB-related thrombocytopenia	ADAP is a protein involved in the remodeling of cytoskeleton. Mutations in ADAP cause defective maturation of megakaryocytes and clearance of platelets [16]	Mild iron deficiency anemia
	GATA1	GATA1-relate disease	GATA1 is a transcription factor regulating many genes associated with megakaryocyte development therefore GATA1 defects cause alterations of megakaryocyte maturation [17]	Dyserythropoietic anemia, beta-thalassemia, congenital erythropoietic porphyria, splenomegaly
	GFI1B	GFI1B-related thrombocytopenia	GFI1B is a transcription factor involved in homeostasis of hematopoietic stem cells and development of megakaryocytes therefore GFI1B defects cause alterations of megakaryocyte maturation [18]	Mild myelofibrosis

Table 1. Cont.

Defective Step of Thrombopoiesis	Affected Gene	Disorder	Pathogenic Mechanism (Reference)	Additional Features (e.g., Syndromic Manifestations, Predisposition)
	HOXA11	Amegakaryocytic thrombocytopenia with radio-ulnar synostosis	HOXA11 is a transcription factor involved in the regulation of early hematopoiesis, its defect causes reduced number of megakaryocytes [19]	Bilateral radioulnar synostosis, severe bone marrow failure culminating in aplastic anemia in majority of cases, cardiac and renal malformations, hearing loss, clinodactyly, skeletal abnormalities, pancytopenia
	MECOM		MECOM is a transcription factor involved in the regulation of early hematopoiesis, its defect causes reduced number of megakaryocytes [20]	
	IKZF5	IKZF5-related thrombocytopenia	IKZF5 is a previously unknown transcriptional regulator of megakaryopoiesis [21]	Not reported
	MPL	Congenital amegakaryocytic thrombocytopenia	MPL is the receptor for thrombopoietin. MPL defects cause impaired thrombopoietin binding and thus impaired megakaryocyte maturation [22]	Acquired bone marrow aplasia
	NBEAL2	Gray platelet syndrome	Mutations in NBEAL2 cause impaired megakaryocyte maturation however its role in megakaryocytopoiesis is not clear [23]	Myelofibrosis, immune dysregulation (autoimmune diseases, positive autoantibodies, reduced leukocyte counts), proinflammatory profile
	RBM8A	Thrombocytopenia-absent radius	RBM8A is a protein of the exon-junction complex involved in RNA processing. It has been hypothesized that RBM8A defects cause wrong mRNA processing of unknown components of the TPO-MPL pathway impairing megakaryocyte maturation [24]	Bilateral radial aplasia, anemia, skeletal, urogenital, kidney, heart defects
	RUNX1	Familial platelet disorder with predisposition to hematological malignancies	RUNX1 is a transcription factor regulating many genes associated with megakaryocyte development therefore RUNX1 mutations promote defective megakaryocyte maturation [25]	Predisposition to hematological malignancies
	THPO	THPO-related disease	THPO is the gene for thrombopoietin, essential for hematopoietic stem cell survival and megakaryocyte maturation [26]	Bone marrow aplasia
Defective platelet production/increased clearance	ACTB	Baraitser–Winter syndrome 1 with macrothrombocytopenia	Mutations in β-cytoplasmic actin inhibit the final stages of platelet maturation by compromising microtubule organization [27]	Microcephaly, facial anomalies, mild intellectual disability, developmental delay
	ACTN1	ACTN1-related thrombocytopenia	ACTN-1 is involved in cytoskeletal remodeling, defects in ACTN-1 cause defective proplatelet formation [28]	Not reported
	ARPC1B	Platelet abnormalities with eosinophilia and immune-mediated inflammatory disease	The actin-related protein 2/3 complex (Arp2/3) is a regulator of the actin cytoskeleton and its mutation causes impaired proplatelet formation [29]	Immunodeficiency, systemic inflammation, vasculitis, inflammatory colitis, eosinophilia, eczema, lymphadenomegaly, hepato-splenomegaly, growth failure
	CYCS	CYCS-related thrombocytopenia	CYCS is a mitochondrial protein with a role in respiration and apoptosis. Mutations in CYCS cause ectopic premature proplatelet formation with an unknown mechanism [30]	Not reported
	DIAPH1	DIAPH1-related thrombocytopenia	DIAPH1 is involved in cytoskeletal remodeling, defects in DIAPH1 cause defective proplatelet formation [31]	Hearing loss
	FLNA	FLNA-related thrombocytopenia	Filamin A is involved in cytoskeletal remodeling, defects in FLNA cause defective proplatelet formation [32]	Periventricular nodular heterotopia and otopalatodigital syndrome spectrum of disorders

Table 1. Cont.

Defective Step of Thrombopoiesis	Affected Gene	Disorder	Pathogenic Mechanism (Reference)	Additional Features (e.g., Syndromic Manifestations, Predisposition)
	GP1BA, GP1BB, GP9 (loss of function)	Bernard–Soulier syndrome monoallelic	The intracellular portion of the GPIb/IX/V complex links the receptor to the cytoskeleton. Disruption of this link causes impaired proplatelet formation [33]	Not reported
		Bernard–Soulier syndrome biallelic		
	GP1BA (gain of function)	Platelet-type von Willebrand disease	The extracellular portion of the GPIb/IX/V complex binds VWF. Constitutive binding of VWF to its receptor triggers the Src kinases pathway causing impaired proplatelet formation, ectopic platelet production and increased platelet clearance [34]	Not reported
	ITGA2B, ITGB3	ITGA2B/ITGB3-related thrombocytopenia	Constitutive activation of $\alpha_{IIb}\beta_3$ causes cytoskeletal perturbation leading to impaired proplatelet formation [35,36]	Not reported
	KDSR	Thrombocytopenia and erythrokeraderma	KDSR is an essential enzyme for de novo sphingolipid synthesis, this suggests an important role for sphingolipids as regulators of cytoskeletal organization during megakaryopoiesis and proplatelet formation [37]	Dermatologic involvement ranging from hyperkeratosis/erythema to ichthyosis. One family with no or very mild skin lesions but associated anemia has been reported
	MYH9	MYH9-related disorder	MYH9 regulates cytoskeleton remodeling and mediates signal transduction pathways involved in proplatelet formation. Abnormalities of MYH9 cause hyperactivation of the Rho/ROCK pathway causing ectopic platelet formation [38]	Kidney disease, cataract, deafness, elevated liver enzymes
	MPIG6B	Thrombocytopenia, anemia and myelofibrosis	G6b-B is a transmembrane receptor with an ITIM motif with a not well defined role in proplatelet formation [39]	Microcitic anemia, myelofibrosis, leukocytosis may be present
	PRKACG	PRKACG-related thrombocytopenia	PKA activates many proteins involved in megakaryocyte and platelet function, among them FLNa and GPIbβ therefore its dysfunction causes impaired proplatelet formation [40]	Not reported
	STIM1	Stormorken syndrome	STIM1 mutations cause a constitutively active store operated Ca^{2+} release-activated Ca^{2+} (CRAC) channel which triggers Ca^{2+} entry with consequent increased clearance of activated platelets [41]	Tubular myopathy and congenital myosis. Severe immune dysfunction
	TRPM7	TRPM7-related thrombocytopenia	Defects of the Mg^{2+} channel TRPM7, a regulator of embryonic development and cell survival, cause cytoskeletal alterations resulting in impaired proplatelet formation [42]	Atrial fibrillation
	TPM4	TPM4-related thrombocytopenia	Tropomyosin 4 is an actin cytoskeletal regulator. Insufficient TPM4 expression in human and mouse megakaryocytes resulted in a defect in the terminal stages of platelet production [43]	Not reported
	TUBB1	TUBB1-related thrombocytopenia	Tubulin beta1 is a major component of microtubules therefore defects in TUBB1 cause impaired proplatelet formation [44]	Not reported

Table 1. Cont.

Defective Step of Thrombopoiesis	Affected Gene	Disorder	Pathogenic Mechanism (Reference)	Additional Features (e.g., Syndromic Manifestations, Predisposition)
Other/unknown pathogenic mechanism	WAS	Wiskott–Aldrich syndrome	The WASP protein is a regulator of the actin cytoskeleton and its defect causes ectopic platelet formation and increased platelet clearance [45]	Immunodeficiency, hematopoietic malignancies, eczema, autoimmune hemolytic anemia.
		X-linked thrombocytopenia		Not reported
	ABCG5, ABCG8	Thrombocytopenia associated with sitosterolemia	ABCG5 and ABCG8 regulate plant sterol and cholesterol absorption. It is supposed that sterol-enriched platelets are more rapidly cleared [46]	Xanthomas and pre-mature coronary atherosclerosis due to hypercholesterolemia
	CDC42	Takenouchi-Kosaki syndrome with macrothrombocytopenia	CDC42 is a critical molecule in various biological processes including the cell cycle, cell division, and the formation of the actin cytoskeleton [47]	Defective growth and psychomotor development, intellectual disability, facial abnormalities, brain malformation, muscle tone abnormalities, immunodeficiency, eczema, hearing/visual disability, lymphedema, cardiac, genitourinary, and/or skeletal malformations
	GNE	GNE-related thrombocytopenia	GNE encodes an enzyme involved in the sialic acid biosynthesis pathway and it is known that thrombocytopenia is associated with increased platelet desialylation [48]	Some patients presented myopathy with rimmed vacuoles with onset in early adulthood
	SLNF14	SLNF14-related thrombocytopenia	SLNF14 is an endoribonuclease and its role in the generation of thrombocytopenia is unknown [49]	Not reported
	SRC	SRC-related thrombocytopenia	Src-family kinase regulates multiple signaling pathways, its role in the generation of thrombocytopenia is unknown [50]	Myelofibrosis, bone pathologies, bone marrow dysplasia, splenomegaly, congenital facial dysmorphism
	PTPRJ	PTPRJ-related thrombocytopenia	PTPRJ is a protein tyrosine phosphatase expressed abundantly in platelets and megakaryocytes, its role in the generation of thrombocytopenia is unknown [51]	None

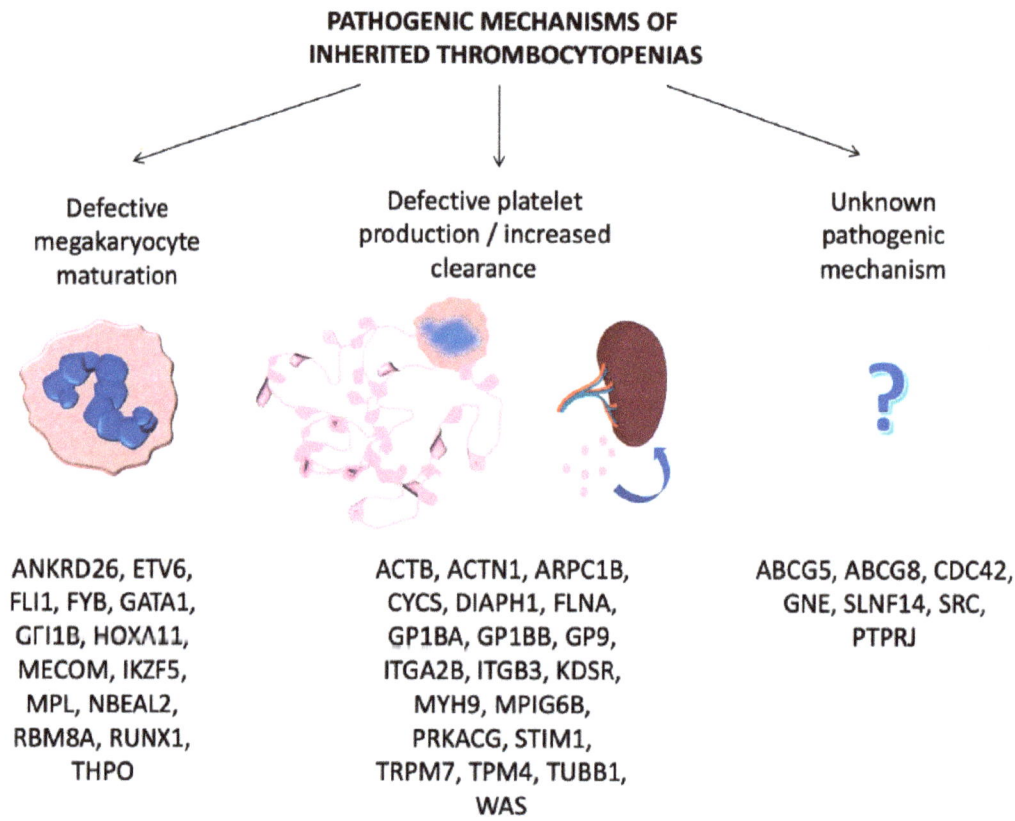

Figure 1. Genes involved in inherited thrombocytopenias classified according to the pathogenic mechanisms.

3.1. ITs Caused by Defective Megakaryocyte Maturation and Differentiation

ITs due to defective differentiation of hematopoietic stem cells (HSCs) into MKs are characterized by the absence or severe reduction in the number of bone marrow MKs.

ITs caused by altered MK maturation are characterized by a normal or increased number of bone marrow MKs which however are immature, dysmorphic and dysfunctional and include at least 14 different forms. Eight of these are caused by mutations of transcription factors with a key role in megakaryopoiesis, i.e., RUNX1, FLI1, GATA1, GFI1b, ETV6, HOXA11, MECOM, IKZF5. These transcription factors regulate, as activator or repressor, the expression of numerous genes, therefore these disorders are characterized by the concurrent alterations of multiple steps in MK and platelet development. For instance, RUNX1 transactivates transcription factors involved in MK maturation, proteins of the MK cytoskeleton (MYH9, MYL9, MYH10) or implicated in α and dense granule development (RAB1B, PLDN, NFE2) and members of the MK/platelet signaling pathways (ANKRD26, MPL, PRKCQ, ALOX12, PCTP) [17]. FLI1 activates the transcription of several genes associated with the production of mature MKs, including *MPL, ITGA2B, GP9, GPIBA* and *PF4* [52]. Thrombocytopenia of TCPT/JBS, caused by deletions of the long arm of chromosome 11q, is due to reduced expression of *FLI1* which is included in the deleted region.

Disorders caused by GATA1 and GFI1B mutations are associated with erythrocyte abnormalities showing the essential role of these transcription factors in controlling also red cell production. Moreover, the predisposition to haematological neoplasms of patients with *RUNX1* and *ETV6* variants highlights how these pathogenic variants also disrupt the homeostasis of myeloid and multipotent progenitors, respectively. Amegakaryocytic thrombocytopenia with radio-ulnar synostosis (ATRUS), a rare IT which often evolves in trilinear bone marrow failure, is due to variants in HOXA11 and MECOM, members of a family of genes encoding for DNA-binding proteins involved in the regulation of early hematopoiesis [53]. IKZF5 is a transcription factor with a non-clear role in hematopoiesis and is involved in IKZF5-RT [21].

Variants in THPO, the gene coding for thrombopoietin, a growth factor essential for hematopoietic stem cell survival and megakaryocyte maturation, and in *MPL*, coding for the thrombopoietin receptor, cause *THPO*-related thrombocytopenia (*THPO*-RT) and congenital amegakaryocytic thrombocytopenia (CAMT), respectively. FYB-RT is caused by variants in the FYB gene, coding for a cytoskeletal protein [16], and thrombocytopenia-absent radius is caused by variants in RBM8A, a protein of the exon-junction complex [24]. Finally, ANKRD26 and NBEAL2, proteins with an unknown role, are involved in *ANKRD26*-RT [13] and Gray platelet syndrome (GPS) [23], respectively.

3.2. ITs Caused by Defective Platelet Production/Clearance

ITs derived from defects of the generation of proplatelets from mature MKs and/or of the conversion of proplatelets to platelets in the bloodstream are characterized by normal MK differentiation and maturation but by ectopic release of platelets in the bone marrow and/or increased clearance of platelets from the circulation. Most of these forms are associated with enlarged platelets and derive from mutations in genes encoding for components of the acto-myosin or microtubular cytoskeletal system, such as *MYH9*, *ACTN1*, *FLNA*, *TPM4*, *TRPM7* or *TUBB1*, or from mutations of genes for the major membrane glycoprotein (GP) complexes GPIb/IX/V and GPIIb/IIIa that indirectly affect cytoskeletal structure or reorganization, i.e., like biallelic and monoallelic Bernard Soulier syndrome (BSS) and *ITGA2B/ITGB3*-RT. In the latter case macrothrombocytopenia results from the disruption of the interactions of integrins with the actomyosin cytoskeleton which is essential for preserving MK cytoskeletal structure and organization. For instance, *ITGA2B/ITGB3*-RT is due to gain-of-function variants resulting in the constitutive, inappropriate activation of GPIIb/IIIa triggering outside-in signaling with consequent altered remodeling of the actin cytoskeleton [35,54,55]. Another example is platelet type VWD, or pseudo von Willebrand, due to gain-of-function mutations that increase the affinity of GPIbα for VWF with the consequent triggering of the Src kinases pathway downstream of activated GPIbα [34].

Wiskott–Aldrich syndrome (WAS) is a syndromic IT and X-linked thrombocytopenia (XLT) is a milder variant with only isolated thrombocytopenia which derive from mutations in the WAS gene leading to defective expression or activity of its product WASp. WASp is expressed exclusively in hematopoietic cells and has a key role in actin polymerization and cytoskeleton rearrangement. Studies in mice have shown ineffective platelet production with ectopic proplatelet formation (PPF) within the bone marrow and impaired SDF1-driven MK migration to the vascular niche [56]. The observation that splenectomy enhances the platelet count in WAS and XLT patients however, suggests that increased platelet clearance is also an important mechanism of thrombocytopenia in these disorders.

An additional group of IT belonging to those caused by impaired platelet production is due to variants in genes not directly involved in proplatelet formation, such as *CYCS*-RT, caused by dysfunction of a mitochondrial protein that causes thrombocytopenia by enhancing an apoptotic pathway [30], or *PRKACG*-RT, leading to dysfunction of PKA, which activates many proteins involved in megakaryocyte and platelet function such as FLNa and GPIbβ [40]. The Stormorken syndrome is due to gain of function mutations of STIM1 [57]. In these patients platelets circulate in an activated state due to a constitutively active store operated Ca^{2+} release-activated Ca^{2+} (CRAC) channel which triggers Ca^{2+} entry with consequent increased clearance of activated platelets by the spleen which causes a reduction in the number of circulating platelets [58].

Ectopic proplatelet formation in bone marrow is a peculiar mechanism causing thrombocytopenia in *FYB*, *GP1BA* (gain-of-function variants) and *MYH9*.

3.3. ITs Caused by Unknown Pathogenic Mechanisms

One last group of ITs is caused by variants in genes not known to be involved in megakaryocyte maturation or platelet production, and that cause thrombocytopenia by still unknown mechanisms.

An interesting IT is thrombocytopenia associated with sitosterolemia, a rare autosomal recessive disorder caused by mutations in two adjacent ATP-binding cassette transport genes (*ABCG5* and *ABCG8*) encoding proteins (sterolins-1 and -2) that pump sterols out of cells [59]. Among the manifestations of this complex disorder due to the accumulation of sterols in plasma and cell membranes are haematological abnormalities, including thrombocytopenia, provoked by the increased stiffness of sterol-enriched membranes with possible enhanced susceptibility to lysis and rupture [60].

Another recently discovered gene causing IT is *SLFN14*, an endoribonuclease degrading mRNA [49,61,62]. Alongside reduced platelet number, these patients show increased platelet clearance and platelet dysfunction. However, the mechanism through which mutations in *SLFN14* induce enhanced platelet turnover and abnormal platelet function is unknown. Similarly, the pathogenic mechanisms of one of the most recently reported causative genes of IT, GNE, are unknown. Mutations of *GNE*, the gene encoding Glucosamine (UDP-NAcetyl)-2-Epimerase/N-Acetylmannosamine kinase, cause sialuria and hereditary inclusion body myopathy [63] but are also associated with severe thrombocytopenia characterized by shortened platelet lifespan, but the exact mechanisms have not been clarified [48].

4. Diagnostic Approach

4.1. Introduction

Patients referred for investigation of bleeding symptoms should undergo preliminary laboratory investigations including full blood count, prothrombin time, activated partial thromboplastin time and von Willebrand factor (VWF) screening tests (VWF antigen, ristocetin cofactor activity and factor VIII coagulant activity). If from full blood count thrombocytopenia is identified, a diagnostic work-up for IT should be pursued. If these are normal the presence of an inherited platelet function disorder (IPFD) should be explored. IPFD are listed under Table 2.

Table 2. Inherited platelet function disorders: disorders in which platelet dysfunction is the dominant phenotypic feature independent of platelet count.

Disease	Inheritance	Gene	Bleeding Diathesis
Arthrogryposis, renal dysfunction and cholestasis	AR	VPS33B VIPAS39	Severe
CalDAG-GEFI related platelet disorder	AR	RASGRP2	Moderate-severe
Cediak-Higashi Syndrome	AR	CHS1	Moderate-severe
Combined alpha-delta granule deficiency	AR/AD	Unknown	Mild-moderate
COX-1 deficiency	AR/AD	PTGSA	Moderate-severe
Delta granule deficiency	AR/AD	Unknown	Mild-moderate
Glanzmann thrombasthenia	AR	ITGA2B, ITGB3	Moderate-severe
Glycoprotein IV (GPIV) deficiency	AR	GP4	Mild
Glycoprotein VI (GPVI) deficiency	AR	GP6	Mild
G_s platelet defect	AD (if paternally inherited)	GNAS	Mild

Table 2. Cont.

Disease	Inheritance	Gene	Bleeding Diathesis
Hermansky–Pudlak syndrome	AR	HPS1, ADTB3A, HPS3, HPS4, HPS5, HPS6, DTNBP1, BLOC1S3, AP3D1, BLOC1S6	Moderate-severe
Leukocyte adhesion deficiency, type III	AR	FERMT3	Moderate-severe
P2Y12 deficiency	AR	P2RY12	Moderate-severe
Phospholipase A_2 ($cPLA_2$) deficiency	not determined	PLA2G4A	Moderate-severe
PKCδ deficiency	AR	PRKCD	Absent
Primary secretion defect	AR/AD	Unknown	Mild-moderate
Quebec platelet disorder	AD	PLAU	Moderate-severe
Scott syndrome	AR	TMEM16F	Mild-moderate
Thromboxane A2 receptor defect	AD	TBXA2R	Mild
T_x synthase deficiency	AD/AR	TBXAS1	Moderate

The diagnostic approach to ITs can be divided into two steps. The first is the recognition of the hereditary nature of thrombocytopenia, the second is the diagnosis of a specific disorder. In fact, ITs are often confused with acquired thrombocytopenias, leading many patients to receive futile and often dangerous treatments. Careful medical history and accurate evaluation of some simple laboratory parameters help to avoid misdiagnosis [64,65]. A diagnostic algorithm for inherited thrombocytopenias was proposed several years ago and it is still valid to orient towards specific disorders [66,67]. History and clinical examination are crucial for patients with syndromic forms, whereas cell counting and the examination of peripheral blood films may guide diagnosis in non-syndromic forms [68]. However, in most cases genetic studies are required to confirm the diagnostic suspicion [3,69]. Here we propose a diagnostic flow chart for diagnosis of IT.

4.2. Clinical Examination

The first step for IT diagnosis is a careful clinical evaluation of the proband, including the personal and family bleeding history. Treatment with drugs (continuous or intermittent), recent infection, previously diagnosed haematologic disease, nonhaematologic diseases known to decrease platelet counts (e.g., eclampsia, sepsis, DIC, anaphylactic shock, hypothermia, massive transfusions), recent live virus vaccination, poor nutritional status, pregnancy, recent organ transplantation from a donor sensitized to platelet alloantigens and recent transfusion of a platelet-containing product in an allosensitized recipient should be excluded. Thrombocytopenia and/or bleeding history in other family members support the hypothesis of an IT, however a negative family history does not exclude it because some forms are recessive or derive from de novo mutations.

The most severe ITs, such as congenital amegakaryocytic thrombocytopenia or biallelic BSS, are typically identified early in infancy because of bleeding diathesis, while for several ITs spontaneous bleeding is absent or very mild explaining why they are often recognized in adult life.

Besides hemorrhagic manifestations, physical examination should also explore other organs/systems abnormalities for syndromic ITs.

In most syndromic forms the associated manifestations are present since the first months of life, such as in CAMT, Jacobsen and Wiskott–Aldrich syndrome and thrombocytopenia with absent radii, while in others they may become apparent later in life, such as renal failure in MYH9-RD, and in the latter case their genetic origin may be missed.

4.3. Laboratory Tests

At the first identification of thrombocytopenia, "pseudothrombocytopenia", a relatively common artifactual phenomenon caused by platelet clumping in the test tube due to the presence of EDTA (ethylenediaminetetraacetic acid) as anticoagulant accounting for 0.07% to 0.27% of all cases of isolated thrombocytopenia, should be excluded [70].

Evaluation of peripheral blood smears can guide the diagnostic workup because 29 of the 41 forms that have been identified so far display morphological abnormalities of platelets, granulocytes, and/or erythrocytes [68].

When platelet size is reduced, X-linked thrombocytopenia (XLT), WAS and ITs associated with variants in FYB and PTPRJ should be considered [71]. When platelet size is enhanced MYH9-RD, BSS, GPS, thrombocytopenia linked to DIAPH1, FLNA, GATA-1, GNE, TUBB-1, GFI1b, PRKACG, SLF14, TRPM7, TPM4 and ACTN1, Paris-Trousseau thrombocytopenia, PT-VWD, ITGA2B/ITGB3-RT or thrombocytopenia associated with sitosterolemia should be considered. Among these, giant platelets characterize MYH9-RD, bBSS and TUBB1-RT. ITs associated with a normal platelet size instead are ATRUS, SRC-RT, TAR, thrombocytopenia and erythrokeraderma, CYCS-RT, FLI1-RT, IKZF5-RT, THPO-RT, ANKRD26-RT, CAMT, ETV6-RT and FPD/AML.

Abnormality of platelet granules may be observed in some ITs, with reduced or absent granules with enlarged platelets in GPS and GFI1b-RT and with reduced granules with normal-sized platelets in ANKRD26-RT [13,23,72].

Immunofluorescence performed on blood smears has recently been proposed as a method to identify defective membrane protein expression, disturbed distribution of cytoskeletal proteins, and reduction of α or delta granules, however this method requires interlaboratory validation [68].

Classic tests of platelet function, such as aggregometry (light transmission or impedance aggregometry), flow cytometry, secretion assays, electron microscopy and western blotting, may help for some ITs as subsequent steps in the diagnostic algorithm (Table 3) [18,73–75].

Table 3. Main features of inherited thrombocytopenias.

Form	Disease	Inheritance	Degree of Thrombocytopenia	Key Laboratory Features	References
	Amegakaryocytic thrombocytopenia with radio-ulnar synostosis (ATRUS)	AD	severe	Normal platelet size and morphology	[19,20]
	Baraitser–Winter syndrome 1 with macrothrombocytopenia	AD	absent	Macrothrombocytopenia; leukocytosis with eosinophilia, leukopenia	[27]
	FLNA-related thrombocytopenia	XL	moderate	Macrothrombocytopenia; impaired platelet aggregation GPVI-triggered; heterogeneous α-granules, occasionally giant; abnormal distribution of FLNa	[32]
	GATA-1-related disease	XL	severe	Macrothrombocytopenia; reduced platelet aggregation by collagen and ristocetin; reduced α-granule content and release	[17]
	GNE-related thrombocytopenia	AR	from mild to severe	Macrothrombocytopenia	[48]
Syndromic	Gray platelet syndrome	AR	moderate/severe	Macrothrombocytopenia; grey or pale platelets; dyserytropoiesis; absence of α-granules; defective TRAP-induced platelet aggregation	[23]

Table 3. Cont.

Form	Disease	Inheritance	Degree of Thrombocytopenia	Key Laboratory Features	References
	Paris-Trousseau thrombocytopenia, Jacobsen syndrome	AD	severe	Macrothrombocytopenia; defective platelet aggregation by thrombin; giant α-granules	[15]
	Platelet abnormalities with eosinophilia and immune-mediated inflammatory disease	AR	moderate	Small platelets; eosinophilia; reduced platelet spreading; decreased platelet dense granules	[29]
	PTPRJ-related thrombocytopenia	AR	moderate/severe	Microthrombocytopenia; impaired activation by the GPVI-specific agonist convulxin and the thrombin receptor-activating peptide but normal response to ADP	[51]
	SRC-related thrombocytopenia	AD	moderate/severe	Platelets deficient in granules and rich in vacuoles	[50]
	Stormorken syndrome	AD	moderate/severe	Howell-Jolly bodies in red blood cells; enhanced annexin V binding, defective GPIIb/IIIa activation (PAC-1)	[41]
	Takenouchi-Kosaki syndrome with macrothrombocytopenia	AD	absent	Macrothrombocytopenia, abnormal platelet spreading and filopodia formation	[47]
	Thrombocytopenia-absent radius syndrome (TAR)	AR	severe	Normal platelet size and morphology, thrombocytopenia	[24]
	Thrombocytopenia and erythrokeraderma	AR	moderate	Thrombocytopenia and presence of 3-keto-dihydrosphingosine in plasma	[37]
	Thrombocytopenia, anemia and myelofibrosis	AR	mild/moderate	Macrothrombocytopenia, anemia	[39]
	Wiskott–Aldrich syndrome	XL	severe	Microthrombocytopenia; Reduced α/δ granules release	[45]
	X-linked thrombocytopenia	XL	mild/moderate	Microthrombocytopenia; Reduced α/δ granules release	[45]
Non-syndromic	ACTN1-related thrombocytopenia	AD	mild	Macrothrombocytopenia	[28]
	Bernard Soulier syndrome monoallelic biallelic	AD AR	mild moderate/severe	Macrothrombocytopenia; lack of platelet agglutination to ristocetin with normal aggregation to other agonists; severe reduction or complete lack of GPIb/IX/V	[33]
	CYCS-related thrombocytopenia	AD	mild	Normal platelet size and morphology	[30]
	FLI1-related thrombocytopenia	AD/AR	moderate	Reduced platelet aggregation in response to collagen and PAR-1 agonists; δ-granule deficiency	[15]
	FYB-related thrombocytopenia	AR	moderate/severe	Microthrombocytopenia; increased expression of P-selectin and PAC-1 by resting platelets but impaired upon stimulation with ADP	[16]

Table 3. Cont.

Form	Disease	Inheritance	Degree of Thrombocytopenia	Key Laboratory Features	References
	GFI1b-related thrombocytopenia	AD/AR	mild/moderate	Macrothrombocytopenia; dyserytropoiesis; reduced α-granule content and release; diminished expression of GPIbα, red cell anisocytosis	[18]
	IKZF5-related thrombocytopenia	AD	absent	Thrombocytopenia; deficiency of platelet alpha granules.	[21]
	ITGA2B/ITGB3-related thrombocytopenia	AD	mild/moderate	Macrothrombocytopenia; reduced GPIIb/IIIa; defective GPIIb/IIIa activation (PAC-1)	[35,36,54]
	PT-VWD	AD	mild/moderate	Macrothrombocytopenia; increased response to ristocetin and decreased VWF-ristocetin cofactor activity (VWF:RCo) Mixing tests discriminate the plasmatic (VWD type2B) from platelet (PT-VWD) origin of hyperreactivity to ristocetin	[36,76,77]
	PRKACG-related thrombocytopenia	AR	severe	Macrothrombocytopenia; defective platelet $\alpha_{IIb}\beta_3$ activation and P-selectin exposure in response to TRAP6; defective Ca^{2+} mobilization in response to thrombin	[40]
	THPO-related thrombocytopenia	AD	mild	Normal or slightly increased platelet size	[26]
	TRPM7-related thrombocytopenia	AD	mild/moderate	Macrothrombocytopenia; aberrant distribution of granules	[42]
	Tropomyosin 4 (TPM)-related thrombocytopenia	AD	mild	Macrothrombocytopenia	[43]
	TUBB-1-related thrombocytopenia	AD	mild	Macrothrombocytopenia; platelet anisocytosis	[44]
	SLFN14-related thrombocytopenia	AD	mild/moderate	Macrothrombocytopenia; δ-granule deficiency with decreased ATP secretion in response to ADP, collagen and TRAP-6	[49]
Forms predisposing to additional diseases	ANKRD26-related thrombocytopenia	AD	mild/moderate	Reduced α-granules in some patients	[13]
	Congenital amegakaryocytic thrombocytopenia (CAMT)	AR	severe	Elevated serum levels of TPO	[22]
	DIAPH1-related thrombocytopenia	AD	mild/severe	Macrothrombocytopenia	[31]
	ETV6-related thrombocytopenia	AD	mild/moderate	Decreased ability of platelets to spread on fibrinogen covered surfaces; abnormal clot retraction	[14]

Table 3. *Cont.*

Form	Disease	Inheritance	Degree of Thrombocytopenia	Key Laboratory Features	References
	Familial platelet disorder with predisposition to hematological malignancies (FPD/AML)	AD	moderate	Abnormal aggregation in response to multiple agonists; δ (occasionally α)-granule deficiency	[25]
	MYH9-related disease	AD	mild/severe	Macrothrombocytopenia; Döhl-like body cytoplasmic leukocyte inclusions	[38]
	Thrombocytopenia associated with sitosterolemia		moderate/severe	Macrothrombocytopenia; hyperactivatable platelets with constitutive binding of fibrinogen to $\alpha_{IIb}\beta_3$ integrin; shedding of GPIbα; impaired platelet adhesion to von Willebrand factor	[46]

The platelet aggregation pattern may be typical of some ITs like biallelic BSS, associated with no response to ristocetin but normal aggregation to all other agonists, or PT-VWD, with increased response to ristocetin.

Measurement of platelet glycoproteins by flow cytometry, using a well-defined set of antibodies, is the gold standard for the diagnosis of biallelic and monoallelic BSS, *ITGA2B/ITGB3*-RT and *GFI1B*-RT.

The measurement of platelet granule content and secretion can reveal alterations, e.g., in WAS and thrombocytopenia with absent radii (TAR) a reduced number of densegranules has been reported, GPS is characterized by absent or reduced α-granules [78], Paris-Trousseau (PTS) and Jacobsen syndromes show abnormally large α-granules, while patients with *FLNA*-RT show some platelets having a reduced number of α-granules and others with enlarged α-granules [15,79].

Other structural abnormalities, like membranous inclusions, platelet organelle abnormalities, endoplasmic reticulum (ER)-derived inclusion bodies or particulate cytoplasmic structures with immunoreactivity for polyubiquitinated proteins and proteasome (PaCSs) [32], can be detected by electron microscopy in platelets from some specific ITs (Table 3) [18].

Additional tests may be required for complex cases, including the measurement of platelet phosphatidylserine expression, by flow cytometry, to detect enhanced procoagulant activity (Stormorken syndrome), spreading or adhesion assays to detect increased spreading in *FLNA*-RT, or western blotting for detection of specific proteins usually absent from platelets (e.g., MYH10 in FPD/AML and FLI1-RT).

Some additional non platelet-related laboratory tests may complement physical examination in the search for syndromic manifestations, like urinalysis, to detect proteinuria as the first sign of renal impairment in *MYH9*-RD, or the liver enzymes, which are elevated in approximately 50% of patients with this disease [80].

4.4. Genetic Analysis

While genotyping has mainly been used as a confirmatory test in the past, it is now playing an increasing role in the initial diagnostic approach to IT.

Until a few years ago, in fact, when the inherited nature of thrombocytopenia was suspected, a series of laboratory tests (e.g., flow cytometry for platelet surface GPs, examination of peripheral blood smear and immunofluorescence assay for MYH9 protein aggregates in neutrophils, platelet aggregometry) were performed to orient towards the candidate gene/genes to be sequenced by Sanger sequencing [66]. The application of high throughput sequencing (HTS) techniques to platelet disorders has allowed for the discovery of several novel genes associated with IT in a few years and has opened the possibility of approaching IT diagnosis by a single-step strategy. In fact, the simultaneous screening of several genes by targeted sequencing platforms, whole exome sequencing (WES) or whole genome sequencing (WGS) has been shown to provide diagnosis in 30% to 50% of patients with suspected IT [81–83]. Indeed, HTS is being proposed as a first line diagnostic investigation by an increasing number of authors [82–85]. However, the interpretation of genetic variants is challenging and requires a careful expert team evaluation in light of a well characterized patient phenotype [84] and when new variants in diagnostic-grade (TIER1) genes are found by targeted sequencing, WES or WGS or new genes are identified by WES or WGS it is essential that rigorous guidelines (i.e., the ACMG guidelines [86]) are applied to confirm their pathogenicity [84]. No guidelines are available yet regarding which suspected IT patients should undergo genetic testing. Some ITs with pathognonomic laboratory or clinical features, such as BSS, TAR, *GATA1*-RD, ATRUS, Stormorken syndrome and WAS, can be clearly diagnosed without the need of genetic testing. For other ITs, for which a strong genotype–phenotype correlation has been described, e.g., *MYH9*-RD, genotyping may be advisable for prognostic evaluation and possible preventive intervention. Other forms that do not have any specific diagnostic, clinical or laboratory features would require genetic testing for definite diagnosis. However, for some of these, e.g., *ACTN1*-RT or *TUBB1*-RT, a genetic diagnosis does not have any significant impact on patient management, while for others it may inform patients monitoring and treatment. Among these there are thrombocytopenias with normal platelet volume, including forms like FPD/AML, *ANKRD26*-RT and *ETV6*-RT which are predisposed to hematological malignancies (Figure 2). There are ethical implications of detecting variants in these genes and other unexpected genetic defects, such as a carrier status of a recessive gene. It is thus recommended to strictly follow an informed consent protocol ensuring that patients comprehend the possible implications of unsolicited genetic findings [85].

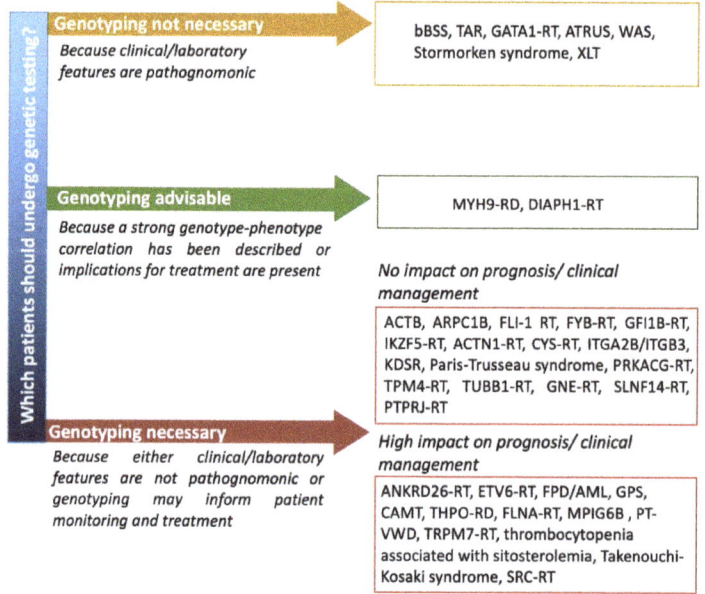

Figure 2. Proposal of a flow chart guiding the use of genetic testing for patients with suspected IT. ACTB = Baraitser–Winter syndrome 1 with macrothrombocytopenia, ARPC1B = Platelet abnormalities with eosinophilia and immune-mediated inflammatory disease, ATRUS = amegakaryocytic thrombocytopenia with radio-ulnar synostosis, bBSS = biallelic Bernard Soulier syndrome, CAMT = congenital amegakaryocytic thrombocytopenia, MPIG6B = thrombocytopenia, anemia and myelofibrosis, PT-VWD = platelet-type von Willebrand disease, RD = related disorder, RT = related thrombocytopenia, TAR = thrombocytopenia with absent radii, XLT = X-linked thrombocytopenia, WAS = Wiskott–Aldrich syndrome.

In summary, the optimal diagnostic approach to ITs is still being debated and a combination of clinical/traditional laboratory approach with advanced gene sequencing techniques may provide the highest rate of diagnostic success [69], and the best patient management.

4.5. Undefined Aspects and Possible Future Research Lines

A consensus on the classification of ITs has not been reached yet, but it would be highly advisable to avoid, for example, ambiguity on disease nomenclature.

A guidance flow chart about which suspected IT patients should undergo genetic testing is not yet available and the generation of consensus documents promoted by the relevant international scientific societies (ISTH, EHA, ASH) is highly warranted.

Moreover, development of guidelines on informed consent documents, reporting of new variants in variant databases to improve variant classification, development of user-friendly interpretation softwares of HTS results, promotion of research for discovery of new genes causing IT and development of advanced cell-based models to study platelet formation and function are valuable future perspectives.

5. Bleeding and Other Manifestations

Bleeding manifestations of IT are of variable severity, ranging from severe in rare cases, recognized within a few weeks from birth, to mild or absent [87]. They are characterized by mucocutaneous symptoms, including epistaxis, easy bruising, petechiae, prolonged bleeding from cuts, gum bleeding, hematuria and menorrhagia in women but also by excessive bleeding after surgery or post-partum hemorrhages [5,88,89].

A recent large systematic investigation on the diagnostic utility of the ISTH bleeding assessment tool (ISTH-BAT) in patients with inherited platelet disorders showed that the bleeding history of most patients with IT without associated platelet function defect is not severe, with a median ISTH-BAT bleeding score (BS) of 2, quite comparable to that of healthy subjects [65]. Usually, the bleeding risk is negligible in subjects with more than 100×10^9 platelets/L, mild/moderate in subjects with $50-100 \times 10^9$ platelets/L (risk of hemorrhages on the occasion of major hemostatic challenges) and significant when platelets are lower than 50×10^9/L, especially when below 20×10^9/L [90].

On the other hand, in ITs associated with defective platelet function (Table 2) the bleeding history shows a moderate/severe hemorrhagic tendency, with high BS, like in patients with biallelic-BSS (median BS 8.5), GPS (median BS 12) and ITGA2B/ITGB3-RT (median BS 8) [65]. For other rare and/or underdiagnosed ITs, such as PT-VWD, GATA-1 RD or CYCS-RT [65,91], the hemorrhagic risk is still poorly defined.

Pregnancy and delivery are a major concern for patients with ITs because both the mother and the affected newborn may be at risk of bleeding. A large multicentric, retrospective study evaluated 339 pregnancies in 181 women with 13 different forms of IT and showed that neither the degree of thrombocytopenia nor the severity of the bleeding tendency worsened during pregnancy and that, in general, the course of pregnancy did not differ from that of healthy subjects. However, post-partum hemorrhage was more frequent in ITs, ranging from 6.8% to 14.2% vs. 3% to 7% in control women, with the degree of thrombocytopenia (platelet count at delivery below 50×10^9/L) and previous history of severe bleeding being predictive of delivery-associated hemorrhage. Patients with MYH9-RD, ANKRD26-RT, biallelic and monoallelic BSS, FPD/AML, GPS and PT-VWD showed the highest frequency of post-partum bleeding [72].

Delivery-related neonatal hemorrhages were instead quite rare (4.5% of affected newborns), although two fatal cerebral hemorrhages out of 278 childbirths were reported [72]. Recently, pregnancy and delivery in a woman with DIAPH1-RD were reported with no changes in platelet count and no bleeding at delivery or postpartum [92].

Another feared complication in patients with IT is excessive bleeding after surgery and a multicentric, retrospective worldwide study recently assessed the bleeding complications of surgery, the preventive and therapeutic approaches adopted and their efficacy in patients with inherited platelet disorders. The study showed that the frequency of surgical bleeding was higher in patients than in healthy controls (19.7% vs. 1.4%–6%), however in patients with IT and normal platelet function bleeding incidence was relatively low (13.4%) with 68×10^9/L platelets being the threshold below which bleeding rate increased significantly, while in IT patients with associated platelet dysfunction post-surgical hemorrhage was frequent, in particular in those with bBSS (44.4%), FPD/AML (30.8%), GPS (23.5%) and ITGA2B/ITGB3-RT (22.7%) [93].

Although bleeding is conventionally considered the main clinical complication in patients with IT, some ITs have the propensity to develop other disorders, including hematological malignancies or bone marrow aplasia [82,94], while others have associated syndromic manifestations, like skeletal malformations, liver and kidney malfunction and deafness. For instance, 40% of subjects with FDP/AML develop acute myelogenous leukemia (AML) or myelodysplastic syndromes (MDS) with a median age of onset of 33 years old, 8% of subjects with *ANRD26*-RT develop MDS or AML and 25% of subjects with ETV6-RT develop hematologic malignancies [95]. Moreover, genotype–phenotype correlation studies in MYH9-RD patients have reported that variants in the head domain of MYH9 are associated with more severe thrombocytopenia and a higher frequency and/or rapid progression of deafness and nephropathy than variants in the tail domain, with the amino acid substitution p.Arg702Cys being associated with the most severe phenotype [96,97].

6. Prophylaxis and Treatment Options

The management of patients with IT should aim to prevent bleeding and treat hemorrhages but also to arrest or slowdown the development of systemic complications or treat them [98,99].

6.1. General Prophylactic Measures

Patients should avoid drugs interfering with platelet function, such as aspirin and non-steroidal anti-inflammatory drugs, perform accurate dental hygiene, and, for the most serious forms, avoid contact sports. Given the possibility that these patients will be exposed to blood transfusions during their life, it is important that they receive immunization against hepatitis A and B and annual liver function tests [99]. Correction of iron deficiency is often required, especially in children and young women [100]. Prenatal diagnosis can be carried out for the most serious forms when the familial mutation is known. Moreover, mutational screening of potential sibling donors is highly warranted for patients with risk of developing hematological malignancy who may therefore require future hematopoietic stem cells transplantation, such as in FPD/AML, ANKRD26-RT and ETV6-RD [101]. Screening for renal failure and cataract in MYH9-RT, for deafness in MYH9-RD and DIAPH1-RT, and for myelofibrosis and immune disorders in GPS is warranted. In fact, immune derangement in GPS has been recently shown, with more than one-half of patients having detectable autoantibodies and one-quarter clinically evident autoimmune disorders, including Hashimoto's thyroiditis, rheumatoid arthritis, alopecia, discoid lupus erythematosus, vitiligo and atypical autoimmune lymphoproliferative syndrome usually associated with cytopenia of at least one leukocyte type [79].

6.2. Female Hormones

Menarche, particularly in patients with BSS, may be associated with excessive bleeding [89]. This can be treated by intravenous (IV) infusion of high-dose conjugated estrogen for 24–48 h followed by high doses of oral estrogen–progestin. Thereafter, a combined oral contraceptive can be given continuously for 2–3 months. In women in whom antifibrinolytic agents fail to decrease menorrhagia, long term oral contraceptives can be given, especially when iron deficiency anemia develops [102].

6.3. Local Hemostatic Measures

Electrocautery and nasal packing are used for epistaxis, while compression, suturing, and application of gelatin sponges or gauzes soaked in tranexamic acid for accidental or surgical wound bleedings. Mouthwashes with tranexamic acid, application of fibrin sealant or absorbable gelatin sponge with topical thrombin may be useful for gingival bleeding. Non-conventional hemostatic agents, such as Ankaferd Blood Stopper has been used in some patients in cases of inefficacy of the classical measures [103]. A relatively new method proposed for the acceleration of wound healing are platelet-rich clots, due to the release of several growth factors from platelets, although it still requires standardization and validation [104]. Autologous platelet-rich clots were used with success, in conjunction with tranexamic acid given orally, to prevent bleeding during dental extraction for a patient with PT-VWD [105].

6.4. Platelet Transfusions

Given the risk of alloimmunization, allergic reactions and infections, platelet transfusion should be used only for severe bleeding which cannot be managed by local measures. Moreover, to prevent HLA-alloimmunization and reactions, HLA-matched and leukodepleted concentrates should be used. In case alloimmune antibodies develop, e.g., against GPIb/IX/V in BSS, immunosuppression and/or plasmapheresis can restore platelet transfusion efficacy.

Of note, the use of pre-operative antihemorrhagic prophylaxis was associated with a lower bleeding frequency in patients with inherited platelet function disorders but not with IT, indeed in the latter group bleeding was reported in 12.7% of the procedures carried out without preparation and in 14.9% of the procedures carried out with pre-operative antihemorrhagic prophylaxis. On the other hand, the choice of the preventive measures did not appear to be always appropriate, in fact platelet transfusions, the most frequently used prophylactic treatment, revealed to be poorly effective, suggesting that either other treatments are required, or that the way platelet transfusions are employed (amount, type, timing) is inappropriate [93].

6.5. Antifibrinolytic Agents

Antifibrinolytic agents (AF), such as ε-aminocaproic acid or tranexamic acid, used as single drugs or in association with other treatments, have been shown to be useful for covering minor surgery in patients with IT or in arresting epistaxis, gingival bleeding or menorrhagia [93,96]. However, no specific prospective clinical study on the effectiveness of these drugs in ITs has been performed, and should therefore be considered empirical. AFs are usually contraindicated for hematuria given the risk of clot formation in the urinary tract [106], however exceptions have been reported [107] and the evidence of AF-associated clot risk is weak and based on old, uncontrolled data [108].

6.6. Desmopressin

Desmopressin (1-deamino-8-D-arginine vasopressin, DDAVP) is an approved treatment for mild hemophilia A and type 1 von Willebrand disease, but is also used for congenital and acquired defects of platelet function because it has a general prohemostatic effect and it enhances the procoagulant activity of platelets [109]. Clinical studies on the efficacy of DDAVP in ITs are lacking, however DDAVP has been shown to successfully cover minor surgery in some IT patients, such as MYH9-RD, ANKRD26-RT and Paris-Trousseau syndrome [92,110,111]. In elderly patients and in patients with a history of cardiovascular disease DDAVP should be used with caution for increased risk of thrombosis as well as in infants below two years of age for the risk of fluid retention.

6.7. VWF-Rich Concentrates

VWF-rich concentrates are the most effective treatments, together with platelet transfusions, for major bleeding in PT-VWD. The dose of VWF-rich concentrates depends on the level of VWF:RCo and can be adjusted on demand. A target of 50–60% VWF:RCo/VWF activity in major surgery and 30–50% in minor ones is advisable (typically from 10 to 30 U/kg at 12 h intervals) [76].

6.8. Activated Recombinant Factor VIIa (rFVIIa)

rFVIIa is currently approved for treating hemophiliacs with inhibitors and patients with Glanzmann thrombasthenia [112]. In the setting of ITs, rFVIIa has been successfully used as prophylactic measure for invasive procedures in biallelic BSS, PT-VWD and TAR [113]. Severe adverse events, including myocardial infarction, ischemic stroke and venous thromboembolism have occasionally been reported.

6.9. Eltrombopag

Eltrombopag is an oral TPO-mimetic indicated for chronic refractory immune thrombocytopenic purpura (ITP), severe aplastic anemia and HCV-related thrombocytopenia. It has been shown to be effective in increasing transiently the platelet count in ITs. In two phase 2 clinical trials, eltrombopag given for three to six weeks was shown to be safe and effective in increasing platelet count and reducing bleeding symptoms in 10 out of 11 patients with *MYH9*-RD [114] and in 21 out of 23 patients with *MYH9*-RD, *ANKRD26*-RD, XLT/WAS, monoallelic BSS and *ITGA2B/ITGB3*-RT [115].

Long-term eltrombopag (i.e., eltrombopag administration for more than six months) to maintain stable safe platelet counts has been used in eight patients with WAS/XLT and severe thrombocytopenia. Five responded well, obtaining a stable increase of platelet count and reduction of spontaneous bleeding without major adverse events [116]. However, potential side effects of a life-long treatment (such as bone marrow fibrosis) need to be carefully considered.

Moreover, eltrombopag has been successfully used for preparation to surgery in patients with MYH9-RD and severe thrombocytopenia [117–119]. Recently, treatment with eltrombopag allowed to attain a safe and stable platelet count to allow chemotherapy in a patient with MHY9-related disorder and pancreatic cancer and permitted to perform endoscopic placement of a biliary stent with no bleeding complications [120].

6.10. Hematopoietic Stem Cell Transplantation (HSCT) and Gene Therapy

HSCT has become the treatment of choice for patients with WAS, with a 5-year overall survival rate of 90%–100% [121], and with CAMT, with a long-term survival rate of 80% [122], patients who have, without this treatment, a life expectancy of 15 years and a few months, respectively [122,123]. Bone marrow transplantation from HLA-identical donors has also been used with success in some cases of BSS with severe hemorrhage and/or alloantibodies [124] and in patients with XLT [125]. However, a careful evaluation of the risk-benefit ratio must always be made.

In humans, the feasibility of gene therapy has been proven in patients with WAS with sustained clinical benefit, normalization of platelet volume and partial increase of platelet count [126–128]. Research is ongoing for gene therapy of BSS in a mouse model [129] and of CAMT in induced pluripotent stem cells [22].

6.11. Splenectomy

Splenectomy is effective in patients with WAS/XLT, increasing platelet count and reducing the incidence of serious bleedings, however it significantly increases the incidence of subsequent severe infectious events and it does not increase overall survival [130]. Thus, the risk–benefit balance should be carefully weighed in each patient and vaccination and anti-infective prophylaxis should always be performed [131].

7. Conclusions

Thrombocytopenia is a frequent condition for the internist and the hematologist, and its differential diagnosis is frequently complex and cumbersome. Among the various possible etiologies of thrombocytopenias, inherited forms should be promptly recognized to avoid unnecessary, and frequently potentially dangerous treatments, and to allow the precise formulation of prognostic expectations.

Recent advances in the understanding of the pathogenic mechanisms of gene variants provoking thrombocytopenia, of the phenotypic manifestations of specific IT-associated gene variants, in the diagnostic approach to ITs and in the therapeutic opportunities have yielded improvements in patient care and deeper insight into the physiologic regulation of circulating platelet levels.

Future challenges are the identification of the genetic cause of the remaining 50% of so far unclassified ITs, the unraveling of the precise phenotypic features of several IT forms, the understanding of the role in megakaryopoiesis of some mutated genes found to be associated with ITs, the development of new therapeutic approaches and of the best use of those currently available and the identification of sophisticated in vitro models of megakaryopoiesis to allow better modelling studies with patient derived MK or induced pluripotent stem cells.

Only continued research and the creation of a wide international collaborative network among investigators and clinicians in the field will allow to respond to these.

Author Contributions: E.F. and L.B. prepared the original draft; P.G. supervised the manuscript preparation and reviewed the manuscript. All authors have read and agreed to the published version of the manuscript.

Funding: This work was supported by a fellowship by Fondazione Umberto Veronesi to LB and EF.

Conflicts of Interest: The authors declare no conflict of interest.

References

1. Balduini, C.L.; Pecci, A.; Noris, P. Inherited thrombocytopenias: The evolving spectrum. *Hamostaseologie* **2012**, *32*, 259–270. [PubMed]
2. Oved, J.H.; Lambert, M.P.; Kowalska, M.A.; Poncz, M.; Karczewski, K.J. Population based frequency of naturally occurring loss-of-function variants in genes associated with platelet disorders. *J. Thromb. Haemost.* **2021**, *19*, 248–254. [CrossRef] [PubMed]
3. Bury, L.; Falcinelli, E.; Gresele, P. Qualitative Disorders of Platelet Function. In *Wintrobe's Clinical Hematology*, 14th ed.; Greer, J.P., Appelbaum, F., Arber, D.A., Dispenzieri, A., Fehniger, T., Glader, B., List, A.F., Eds.; Lippincott Williams & Wilkins: Philadelphia, PA, USA, 2018; pp. 3482–3527.
4. Pecci, A.; Balduini, C.L. Inherited thrombocytopenias: An updated guide for clinicians. *Blood Rev.* **2020**, 100784. [CrossRef] [PubMed]
5. Johnson, B.; Doak, R.; Allsup, D.; Astwood, E.; Evans, G.; Grimley, C.; James, B.; Myers, B.; Stokley, S.; Thachil, J.; et al. A comprehensive targeted next-generation sequencing panel for genetic diagnosis of patients with suspected inherited thrombocytopenia. *Res. Pract. Thromb. Haemost.* **2018**, *2*, 640–652. [CrossRef]
6. Machlus, K.R.; Italiano, J.E. The incredible journey: From megakaryocyte development to platelet formation. *J. Cell Biol.* **2013**, *201*, 785–796. [CrossRef]
7. Nishimura, S.; Nagasaki, M.; Kunishima, S.; Sawaguchi, A.; Sakata, A.; Sakaguchi, H.; Ohmori, T.; Manabe, I.; Italiano, J.E.; Ryu, T.; et al. IL-1α induces thrombopoiesis through megakaryocyte rupture in response to acute platelet needs. *J. Cell Biol.* **2015**, *209*, 453–466. [CrossRef]
8. Potts, K.S.; Farley, A.; Dawson, C.A.; Rimes, J.S.; Biben, C.; De Graaf, C.A.; Potts, M.A.; Stonehouse, O.J.; Carmagnac, A.; Gangatirkar, P.; et al. Membrane budding is a major mechanism of in vivo platelet biogenesis. *J. Exp. Med.* **2020**, *217*. [CrossRef]
9. Looney, M.R. The incomparable platelet: Holy alveoli. *Blood* **2018**, *132*, 1088–1089. [CrossRef]
10. AlMazni, I.; Stapley, R.; Morgan, N.V. Inherited Thrombocytopenia: Update on Genes and Genetic Variants Which may be Associated with Bleeding. *Front. Cardiovasc. Med.* **2019**, *6*, 80. [CrossRef]
11. Nurden, A.T.; Nurden, P. Inherited thrombocytopenias: History, advances and perspectives. *Haematologica* **2020**, *105*, 2004–2019. [CrossRef]
12. Balduini, C.L.; Melazzini, F.; Pecci, A. Inherited thrombocytopenias—recent advances in clinical and molecular aspects. *Platelets* **2017**, *28*, 3–13. [CrossRef] [PubMed]
13. Bluteau, D.; Balduini, A.; Balayn, N.; Currao, M.; Nurden, P.; Deswarte, C.; Leverger, G.; Noris, P.; Perrotta, S.; Solary, E.; et al. Thrombocytopenia associated mutations in the ANKRD26 regulatory region induce MAPK hyperactivation. *J. Clin. Investig.* **2014**, *124*, 580–591. [CrossRef] [PubMed]
14. Noetzli, L.; Lo, R.W.; Lee-Sherick, A.B.; Callaghan, M.; Noris, P.; Savoia, A.; Rajpurkar, M.; Jones, K.; Gowan, K.; Balduini, C.L.; et al. Germline mutations in ETV6 are associated with thrombocytopenia, red cell macrocytosis and predisposition to lymphoblastic leukemia. *Nat. Genet.* **2015**, *47*, 535–553. [CrossRef] [PubMed]

15. Nurden, P.; Debili, N.; Coupry, I.; Bryckaert, M.; Youlyouz-Marfak, I.; Sole´, G.; Pons, A.C.; Berrou, E.; Adam, F.; Kauskot, A.; et al. Thrombocytopenia resulting from mutations in filamin A can be expressed as an isolated syndrome. *Blood* **2011**, *118*, 5928–5937. [CrossRef] [PubMed]
16. Levin, C.; Koren, A.; Pretorius, E.; Rosenberg, N.; Shenkman, B.; Hauschner, H.; Zalman, L.; Khayat, M.; Salama, I.; Elpeleg, O.; et al. Deleterious mutation in the FYB gene is associated with congenital autosomal recessive small-platelet thrombocytopenia. *J. Thromb. Haemost.* **2015**, *13*, 1285–1292. [CrossRef]
17. Songdej, N.; Rao, A.K. Hematopoietic transcription factor mutations and inherited platelet dysfunction. *F1000Prime Rep.* **2015**, *7*, 66. [CrossRef]
18. Gresele, P. Subcommittee on Platelet Physiology of the International Society on Thrombosis and Haemostasis. Diagnosis of inherited platelet function disorders: Guidance from the SSC of the ISTH. *J. Thromb. Haemost.* **2015**, *13*, 314–322. [CrossRef]
19. Horvat-Switzer, R.D.; Thompson, A.A. HOXA11 mutation in amegakaryocytic thrombocytopenia with radio-ulnar synostosis syndrome inhibits megakaryocytic differentiation in vitro. *Blood Cells Mol. Dis.* **2006**, *37*, 55–63. [CrossRef]
20. Germeshausen, M.; Ancliff, P.; Estrada, J.; Metzler, M.; Ponstingl, E.; Rütschle, H.; Schwabe, D.; Scott, R.H.; Unal, S.; Wawer, A.; et al. MECOM-associated syndrome: A heterogeneous inherited bone marrow failure syndrome with amegakaryocytic thrombocytopenia. *Blood Adv.* **2018**, *2*, 586–596. [CrossRef]
21. Lentaigne, C.; Greene, D.; Sivapalaratnam, S.; Favier, R.; Seyres, D.; Thys, C.; Grassi, L.; Mangles, S.; Sibson, K.; Stubbs, M.J.; et al. Germline mutations in the transcription factor IKZF5 cause thrombocytopenia. *Blood* **2019**, *134*, 2070–2081. [CrossRef]
22. Hirata, S.; Takayama, N.; Jono-Ohnishi, R.; Endo, H.; Nakamura, S.; Dohda, T.; Nishi, M.; Hamazaki, Y.; Ishii, E.; Kaneko, S.; et al. Congenital amegakaryocytic thrombocytopenia iPS cells exhibit defective MPL-mediated signaling. *J. Clin. Investig.* **2013**, *123*, 3802–3814. [CrossRef] [PubMed]
23. Pluthero, F.G.; Di Paola, J.; Carcao, M.D.; Kahr, W.H.A. NBEAL2 mutations and bleeding in patients with gray platelet syndrome. *Platelets* **2018**, *29*, 632–635. [CrossRef] [PubMed]
24. Albers, C.A.; Newbury-Ecob, R.; Ouwehand, W.H.; Ghevaert, C. New insights into the genetic basis of TAR (thrombocytopenia-absent radii) syndrome. *Curr. Opin. Genet. Dev.* **2013**, *23*, 316–323. [CrossRef] [PubMed]
25. Sakurai, M.; Kunimoto, H.; Watanabe, N.; Fukuchi, Y.; Yuasa, S.; Yamazaki, S.; Nishimura, T.; Sadahira, K.; Fukuda, K.; Okano, H.; et al. Impaired hematopoietic differentiation of RUNX1-mutated induced pluripotent stem cells derived from FPD/AML patients. *Leukemia* **2014**, *28*, 2344–2354. [CrossRef]
26. Dasouki, M.J.; Rafi, S.K.; Olm-Shipman, A.J.; Wilson, N.R.; Abhyankar, S.; Lanter, B.; Furness, L.M.; Fang, J.; Calado, R.T.; Saadi, I. Exome sequencing reveals a thrombopoietin ligand mutation in a Micronesian family with autosomal recessive aplastic anemia. *Blood* **2013**, *122*, 3440–3449. [CrossRef]
27. Latham, S.L.; Ehmke, N.; Reinke, P.Y.A.; Taft, M.H.; Eicke, D.; Reindl, T.; Stenzel, W.; Lyons, M.J.; Friez, M.J.; Lee, J.A.; et al. Variants in exons 5 and 6 of ACTB cause syndromic thrombocytopenia. *Nat. Commun.* **2018**, *9*, 4250. [CrossRef]
28. Kunishima, S.; Okuno, Y.; Yoshida, K.; Shiraishi, Y.; Sanada, M.; Muramatsu, H.; Chiba, K.; Tanaka, H.; Miyazaki, K.; Sakai, M.; et al. ACTN1 mutations cause congenital macrothrombocytopenia. *Am. J. Hum. Genet.* **2013**, *92*, 431–438. [CrossRef]
29. Kahr, W.H.; Pluthero, F.G.; Elkadri, A.; Warner, N.; Drobac, M.; Chen, C.H.; Lo, R.W.; Li, L.; Li, R.; Li, Q.; et al. Loss of the Arp2/3 complex component ARPC1B causes platelet abnormalities and predisposes to inflammatory disease. *Nat. Commun.* **2017**, *8*, 14816. [CrossRef]
30. Morison, I.M.; Cramer Borde, E.M.; Cheesman, E.J.; Cheong, P.L.; Holyoake, A.J.; Fichelson, S.; Weeks, R.J.; Lo, A.; Davies, S.M.; Wilbanks, S.M.; et al. A mutation of human cytochrome c enhances the intrinsic apoptotic pathway but causes only thrombocytopenia. *Nat. Genet.* **2008**, *40*, 387–389. [CrossRef]
31. Stritt, S.; Nurden, P.; Turro, E.; Greene, D.; Jansen, S.B.; Westbury, S.K.; Petersen, R.; Astle, W.J.; Marlin, S.; Bariana, T.K.; et al. A gain-of-function variant in DIAPH1 causes dominant macrothrombocytopenia and hearing loss. *Blood* **2016**, *127*, 2903–2914. [CrossRef]
32. Necchi, V.; Balduini, A.; Noris, P.; Barozzi, S.; Sommi, P.; di Buduo, C.; Balduini, C.L.; Solcia, E.; Pecci, A. Ubiqui-tin/proteasome-rich particulate cytoplasmic structures (PaCSs) in the platelets and megakaryocytes of ANKRD26-related thrombo-cytopenia. *Thromb. Haemost.* **2013**, *109*, 263–271. [CrossRef] [PubMed]
33. Balduini, A.; Malara, A.; Balduini, C.L.; Noris, P. Megakaryocytes derived from patients with the classical form of Bernard-Soulier syndrome show no ability to extend proplatelets in vitro. *Platelets* **2011**, *22*, 308–311. [CrossRef] [PubMed]
34. Bury, L.; Malara, A.; Momi, S.; Petito, E.; Balduini, A.; Gresele, P. Mechanisms of thrombocytopenia in platelet-type von Willebrand disease. *Haematologica* **2019**, *104*, 1473–1481. [CrossRef] [PubMed]
35. Bury, L.; Falcinelli, E.; Chiasserini, D.; Springer, T.A.; Italiano, J.E., Jr.; Gresele, P. Cytoskeletal perturbation leads to platelet dysfunction and thrombocytopenia in Glanzmann variants. *Haematologica* **2016**, *101*, 46–56. [CrossRef]
36. Bury, L.; Malara, A.; Gresele, P.; Balduini, A. Outside-in signalling generated by a constitutively activated integrin $\alpha IIb\beta 3$ impairs proplatelet formation in human megakaryocytes. *PLoS ONE* **2012**, *7*, e34449. [CrossRef]
37. Bariana, T.K.; Labarque, V.; Heremans, J.; Thys, C.; De Reys, M.; Greene, D.; Jenkins, B.; Grassi, L.; Seyres, D.; Burden, F.; et al. Sphingolipid dysregulation due to lack of functional KDSR impairs proplatelet formation causing thrombocytopenia. *Haematologica* **2019**, *104*, 1036–1045. [CrossRef]
38. Pecci, A.; Malara, A.; Badalucco, S.; Bozzi, V.; Torti, M.; Balduini, C.L.; Balduini, A. Megakaryocytes of patients with MYH9-related thrombocytopenia present an altered proplatelet formation. *Thromb. Haemost.* **2009**, *102*, 90–96.

39. Hofmann, I.; Geer, M.J.; Vögtle, T.; Crispin, A.; Campagna, D.R.; Barr, A.; Calicchio, M.L.; Heising, S.; van Geffen, J.P.; Kuijpers, M.J.E.; et al. Congenital macrothrombocytopenia with focal myelofibrosis due to mutations in human G6b-B is rescued in humanized mice. *Blood* **2018**, *132*, 1399–1412. [CrossRef]
40. Manchev, V.T.; Hilpert, M.; Berrou, E.; Elaib, Z.; Aouba, A.; Boukour, S.; Souquere, S.; Pierron, G.; Rameau, P.; Andrews, R.; et al. A new form of macro-thrombocytopenia induced by germ-line mutation in the PRKACG gene. *Blood* **2014**, *124*, 2554–2563. [CrossRef]
41. Morin, G.; Bruechle, N.O.; Singh, A.R.; Knopp, C.; Jedraszak, G.; Elbracht, M.; Bre´mond-Gignac, D.; Hartmann, K.; Sevestre, H.; Deutz, P.; et al. Gain-of-function mutation in STIM1 (P.R304W) is associated with Stormorken syndrome. *Hum. Mutat.* **2014**, *35*, 1221–1232. [CrossRef]
42. Stritt, S.; Nurden, P.; Favier, R.; Favier, M.; Ferioli, S.; Gotru, S.K.; van Eeuwijk, J.M.M.; Schulze, H.; Nurden, A.T.; Lambert, M.P.; et al. Defects in TRPM7 channel function deregulate thrombopoiesis through altered cellular Mg(2+) homeostasis and cytoskeletal architecture. *Nat. Commun.* **2016**, *7*, 11097. [CrossRef] [PubMed]
43. Pleines, I.; Woods, J.; Chappaz, S.; Kew, V.; Foad, N.; Ballester-Beltrán, J.; Aurbach, K.; Lincetto, C.; Lane, R.M.; Schevzov, G.; et al. Mutations in tropomyosin 4 underlie a rare form of human macrothrombocytopenia. *J. Clin. Investig.* **2017**, *127*, 814–829. [CrossRef] [PubMed]
44. Kunishima, S.; Kobayashi, R.; Itoh, T.J.; Hamaguchi, M.; Saito, H. Mutation of the beta1-tubulin gene associated with congenital macrothrombocytopenia affecting microtubule assembly. *Blood* **2009**, *113*, 458–461. [CrossRef] [PubMed]
45. Massaad, M.J.; Ramesh, N.; Geha, R.S. Wiskott-Aldrich syndrome: A comprehensive review. *Ann. N. Y. Acad. Sci.* **2013**, *1285*, 26–43. [CrossRef] [PubMed]
46. Rees, D.C.; Iolascon, A.; Carella, M.; O'marcaigh, A.S.; Kendra, J.R.; Jowitt, S.N.; Wales, J.K.; Vora, A.; Makris, M.; Manning, N.; et al. Stomatocytic haemolysis and macrothrombocytopenia (Mediterranean stomatocytosis/macrothrombocytopenia) is the haematological presentation of phytosterolaemia. *Br. J. Haematol.* **2005**, *130*, 297–309. [CrossRef] [PubMed]
47. Takenouchi, T.; Okamoto, N.; Ida, S.; Uehara, T.; Kosaki, K. Further evidence of a mutation in CDC42 as a cause of a recognizable syndromic form of thrombocytopenia. *Am. J. Med. Genet. A* **2016**, *170*, 852–855. [CrossRef]
48. Futterer, J.; Dalby, A.; Lowe, G.C.; Johnson, B.; Simpson, M.A.; Motwani, J.; Williams, S.P.; Morgan, N.V. Mutation in GNE is associated with severe congenital thrombocytopenia. *Blood* **2018**, *132*, 1855–1858. [CrossRef]
49. Fletcher, S.J.; Johnson, B.; Lowe, G.C.; Bem, D.; Drake, S.; Lordkipanidzé, M. SLFN14 mutations underlie thrombocytopenia with excessive bleeding and platelet secretion defects. *J. Clin. Investig.* **2015**, *125*, 3600–3605. [CrossRef] [PubMed]
50. Turro, E.; Greene, D.; Wijgaerts, A.; Thys, C.; Lentaigne, C.; Bariana, T.K.; Westbury, S.K.; Kelly, A.M.; Sellesag, D.; Stephens, J.C.; et al. A dominant gain-of-function mutation in universal tyrosine kinase SRC causes thrombocytopenia, myelofibrosis, bleeding, and bone pathologies. *Sci. Transl. Med.* **2016**, *8*, 328ra30. [CrossRef] [PubMed]
51. Marconi, C.; Di Buduo, C.A.; LeVine, K.; Barozzi, S.; Faleschini, M.; Bozzi, V.; Palombo, F.; McKinstry, S.; Lassandro, G.; Giordano, P.; et al. Loss-of-function mutations in PTPRJ cause a new form of inherited thrombocytopenia. *Blood* **2019**, *133*, 1346–1357. [CrossRef] [PubMed]
52. Raslova, H.; Komura, E.; Le Couédic, J.P.; Larbret, F.; Debili, N.; Feunteun, J.; Danos, O.; Albagli, O.; Vainchenker, W.; Favier, R. FLI1 monoallelic expression combined with its hemizygous loss underlies Paris-Trousseau/Jacobsen thrombopenia. *J. Clin. Investig.* **2004**, *114*, 77–84. [CrossRef] [PubMed]
53. Thompson, A.A.; Woodruff, K.; Feig, S.A.; Nguyen, L.T.; Schanen, N.C. Congenital thrombocytopenia and radio-ulnar synostosis: A new familial syndrome. *Br. J. Haematol.* **2001**, *113*, 866–870. [CrossRef] [PubMed]
54. Gresele, P.; Falcinelli, E.; Giannini, S.; D'Adamo, P.; D'Eustacchio, A.; Corazzi, T.; Mezzasoma, A.M.; Di Bari, F.; Guglielmini, G.; Cecchetti, L.; et al. Dominant inheritance of a novel integrin beta3 mutation associated with a hereditary macrothrombocytopenia and platelet dysfunction in two Italian families. *Haematologica* **2009**, *94*, 663–669. [CrossRef] [PubMed]
55. Bury, L.; Zetterberg, E.; Leinøe, E.B.; Falcinelli, E.; Marturano, A.; Manni, G.; Nurden, A.T.; Gresele, P. A novel variant Glanzmann thrombasthenia due to co-inheritance of a loss- and a gain-of-function mutation of ITGB3: Evidence of a dominant effect of gain-of-function mutations. *Haematologica* **2018**, *103*, e259–e263. [CrossRef]
56. Sabri, S.; Foudi, A.; Boukour, S.; Franc, B.; Charrier, S.; Jandrot-Perrus, M.; Farndale, R.W.; Jalil, A.; Blundell, M.P.; Cramer, E.M.; et al. Deficiency in the Wiskott-Aldrich protein induces premature proplatelet formation and platelet production in the bone marrow compartment. *Blood* **2006**, *108*, 134–140. [CrossRef]
57. Nesin, V.; Wiley, G.; Kousi, M.; Ong, E.-C.; Lehmann, T.; Nicholl, D.J.; Suri, M.; Shahrizaila, N.; Katsanis, N.; Gaffney, P.M.; et al. Activating mutations in STIM1 and ORAI1 cause overlapping syndromes of tubular myopathy and congenital miosis. *Proc. Natl. Acad. Sci. USA* **2014**, *111*, 4197–4202. [CrossRef]
58. Grosse, J.; Braun, A.; Varga-Szabo, D.; Beyersdorf, N.; Schneider, B.; Zeitlmann, L.; Hanke, P.; Schropp, P.; Mühlstedt, S.; Zorn, C.; et al. An EF hand mu-tation in Stim1 causes premature platelet activation and bleeding in mice. *J. Clin. Investig.* **2007**, *117*, 3540–3550. [CrossRef]
59. Berge, K.E.; Tian, H.; Graf, G.A.; Yu, L.; Grishin, N.V.; Schultz, J.; Kwiterovich, P.; Shan, B.; Barnes, R.; Hobbs, H.H. Accu-mulation of dietary cholesterol in sitosterolemia caused by mutations in adjacent ABC transporters. *Science* **2000**, *290*, 1771–1775. [CrossRef]
60. Su, Y.; Wang, Z.; Yang, H.; Cao, L.; Liu, F.; Bai, X.; Ruan, C. Clinical and molecular genetic analysis of a family with sitosterolemia and co-existing erythrocyte and platelet abnormalities. *Haematologica* **2006**, *91*, 1392–1395.

61. Pisareva, V.P.; Muslimov, I.A.; Tcherepanov, A.; Pisarev, A.V. Characterization of novel ribosome-associated endoribonuclease SLFN14 from rabbit reticulocytes. *Biochemistry* **2015**, *54*, 3286–3301. [CrossRef]
62. Marconi, C.; Di Buduo, C.A.; Barozzi, S.; Palombo, F.; Pardini, S.; Zaninetti, C.; Pippucci, T.; Noris, P.; Balduini, A.; Marconi, C.; et al. SLFN14-related thrombocytopenia: Identification within a large series of patients with inherited thrombocytopenia. *Thromb. Haemost.* **2016**, *115*, 1076–1079. [CrossRef] [PubMed]
63. Eisenberg, I.; Avidan, N.; Potikha, T.; Hochner, H.; Chen, M.; Olender, T.; Barash, M.; Shemesh, M.; Sadeh, M.; Grabov-Nardini, G.; et al. The UDP-N-acetylglucosamine 2-epimerase/N-acetylmannosamine kinase gene is mutated in recessive hereditary inclusion body myopathy. *Nat. Genet.* **2001**, *29*, 83–87. [CrossRef] [PubMed]
64. Rodeghiero, F.; Pabinger, I.; Ragni, M.; Abdul-Kadir, R.; Berntorp, E.; Blanchette, V.; Bodó, I.; Casini, A.; Gresele, P.; Lassila, R.; et al. Fundamentals for a systematic approach to mild and moderate inherited bleeding disorders: A EHA consensus report. *Hemasphere* **2019**, *3*, e286. [CrossRef] [PubMed]
65. Gresele, P.; Orsini, S.; Noris, P.; Falcinelli, E.; Alessi, M.C.; Bury, L.; Borhany, M.; Santoro, C.; Glembotsky, A.C.; Cid, A.R.; et al. BAT-VAL study investigators. Validation of the ISTH/SSC bleeding assessment tool for inherited platelet disorders: A communication from the Platelet Physiology SSC. *J. Thromb. Haemost.* **2020**, *18*, 732–739. [CrossRef] [PubMed]
66. Balduini, C.L.; Cattaneo, M.; Fabris, F.; Gresele, P.; Iolascon, A.; Pulcinelli, F.M.; Savoia, A. Inherited thrombocytopenias: A proposed diagnostic algorithm from the Italian Gruppo di Studio delle Piastrine. *Haematologica* **2003**, *88*, 582–592. [PubMed]
67. Noris, P.; Pecci, A.; Di Bari, F.; Di Stazio, M.T.; Di Pumpo, M.; Ceresa, I.F.; Arezzi, N.; Ambaglio, C.; Savoia, A.; Balduini, C.L. Application of a diagnostic algorithm for inherited thrombocytopenias to 46 consecutive patients. *Haematologica* **2004**, *89*, 1219–1225. [PubMed]
68. Zaninetti, C.; Greinacher, A. Diagnosis of Inherited Platelet Disorders on a Blood Smear. *J. Clin. Med.* **2020**, *9*, 539. [CrossRef]
69. Bury, L.; Falcinelli, E.; Gresele, P. Inherited Platelet Function Disorders: Algorithms for Phenotypic and Genetic Investigation. *Semin. Thromb. Hemost.* **2016**, *42*, 292–305. [CrossRef]
70. Podda, G.M.; Pugliano, M.; Femia, E.A.; Mezzasoma, A.M.; Gresele, P.; Carpani, G.; Cattaneo, M. The platelet count in EDTA-anticoagulated blood from patients with thrombocytopenia may be underestimated when measured in routine laboratories. *Am. J. Hematol.* **2012**, *87*, 727–728. [CrossRef]
71. Noris, P.; Biino, G.; Pecci, A.; Civaschi, E.; Savoia, A.; Seri, M.; Melazzini, F.; Loffredo, G.; Russo, G.; Bozzi, V.; et al. Platelet diameters in inherited thrombocytopenias: Analysis of 376 patients with all known disorders. *Blood* **2014**, *124*, e4–e10. [CrossRef]
72. Monteferrario, D.; Bolar, N.A.; Marneth, A.E.; Hebeda, K.M.; Bergevoet, S.M.; Veenstra, H.; Laros-van Gorkom, B.A.; MacKenzie, M.A.; Khandanpour, C.; Botezatu, L.; et al. A dominant-negative GFI1B mutation in the gray platelet syndrome. *N. Engl. J. Med.* **2014**, *370*, 245–253. [CrossRef] [PubMed]
73. Gresele, P.; Bury, L.; Mezzasoma, A.M.; Falcinelli, E. Platelet function assays in diagnosis: An update. *Expert Rev. Hematol.* **2019**, *12*, 29–46. [CrossRef] [PubMed]
74. Gresele, P.; Falcinelli, E.; Bury, L. Laboratory diagnosis of clinically relevant platelet function disorders. *Int. J. Lab. Hematol.* **2018**, *40*, 34–45. [CrossRef] [PubMed]
75. Mumford, A.D.; Frelinger, A.L., 3rd; Gachet, C.; Gresele, P.; Noris, P.; Harrison, P.; Mezzano, D. A review of platelet secretion assays for the diagnosis of inherited platelet secretion disorders. *Thromb. Haemost.* **2015**, *114*, 14–25. [CrossRef] [PubMed]
76. Othman, M.; Gresele, P. Guidance on the diagnosis and management of platelet-type von Willebrand disease: A communication from the Platelet Physiology Subcommittee of the ISTH. *J. Thromb. Haemost.* **2020**, *18*, 1855–1858. [CrossRef] [PubMed]
77. Giannini, S.; Cecchetti, L.; Mezzasoma, A.M.; Gresele, P. Diagnosis of platelet-type von Willebrand disease by flow cytometry. *Haematologica* **2010**, *95*, 1021–1024. [CrossRef] [PubMed]
78. Sims, M.C.; Mayer, L.; Collins, J.H.; Bariana, T.K.; Megy, K.; Lavenu-Bombled, C.; Seyres, D.; Kollipara, L.; Burden, F.S.; Greene, D.; et al. Novel manifestations of immune dysregulation and granule defects in gray platelet syndrome. *Blood* **2020**, *136*, 1956–1967. [CrossRef] [PubMed]
79. Stevenson, W.S.; Rabbolini, D.J.; Beutler, L.; Chen, Q.; Gabrielli, S.; Mackay, J.P.; Brighton, T.A.; Ward, C.M.; Morel-Kopp, M.C. Paris-Trousseau thrombocytopenia is phenocopied by the autosomal recessive inheritance of a DNA-binding domain mutation in FLI1. *Blood* **2015**, *126*, 2027–2030. [CrossRef]
80. Pecci, A.; Biino, G.; Fierro, T.; Bozzi, V.; Mezzasoma, A.; Noris, P.; Ramenghi, U.; Loffredo, G.; Fabris, F.; Momi, S.; et al. Alteration of Liver Enzymes Is a Feature of the Myh9-Related Disease Syndrome. *PLoS ONE* **2012**, *7*, e35986. [CrossRef]
81. Noris, P.; Pecci, A. Hereditary thrombocytopenias: A growing list of disorders. *Hematology* **2017**, *2017*, 385–399. [CrossRef]
82. Simeoni, I.; Stephens, J.C.; Hu, F.; Deevi, S.V.V.; Megy, K.; Bariana, T.K.; Lentaigne, C.; Schulman, S.; Sivapalaratnam, S.; Vries, M.J.A.; et al. A high-throughput sequencing test for diagnosing inherited bleeding, thrombotic, and platelet disorders. *Blood* **2016**, *127*, 2791–2803. [CrossRef] [PubMed]
83. Downes, K.; Megy, K.; Duarte, D.; Vries, M.; Gebhart, J.; Hofer, S.; Shamardina, O.; Deevi, S.V.V.; Stephens, J.; Mapeta, R.; et al. Diagnostic high-throughput sequencing of 2396 patients with bleeding, thrombotic, and platelet disorders. *Blood* **2019**, *134*, 2082–2091. [CrossRef] [PubMed]
84. Megy, K.; Downes, K.; Simeoni, I.; Bury, L.; Morales, J.; Mapeta, R.; Bellissimo, D.B.; Bray, P.F.; Goodeve, A.C.; Gresele, P.; et al. Subcommittee on Genomics in Thrombosis and Hemostasis. Cu-rated disease-causing genes for bleeding, thrombotic, and platelet disorders: Communication from the SSC of the ISTH. *J. Thromb. Haemost.* **2019**, *17*, 1253–1260. [CrossRef] [PubMed]

85. Downes, K.; Borry, P.; Ericson, K.; Gomez, K.; Greinacher, A.; Lambert, M.; Leinoe, E.; Noris, P.; Van Geet, C.; Freson, K. Subcommittee on Genomics in Thrombosis, Hemostasis. Clinical management, ethics and informed consent related to multi-gene panel-based high throughput sequencing testing for platelet disorders: Communication from the SSC of the ISTH. *J. Thromb. Haemost.* **2020**, *18*, 2751–2758. [CrossRef] [PubMed]
86. Richards, S.; Aziz, N.; Bale, S.; Bick, D.; Das, S.; Gastier-Foster, J.; Grody, W.W.; Hegde, M.; Lyon, E.; Spector, E.; et al. ACMG Laboratory Quality Assurance Committee. Standards and guidelines for the interpretation of sequence variants: A joint consensus recommendation of the American College of Medical Genetics and Genomics and the Association for Molecular Pathology. *Genet. Med.* **2015**, *17*, 405–424. [CrossRef] [PubMed]
87. Drachman, J.G. Inherited thrombocytopenia: When a low platelet count does not mean ITP. *Blood* **2004**, *103*, 390–398. [CrossRef]
88. Johnson, B.; Lowe, G.C.; Futterer, J.; Lordkipanidzé, M.; Macdonald, D.; Simpson, M.A.; Guiú, I.S.; Drake, S.; Bem, D.; Leo, V.; et al. Whole exome sequencing identifies genetic variants in inherited thrombocytopenia with secondary qualitative function defects. *Haematologica* **2016**, *101*, 1170–1179. [CrossRef]
89. Gresele, P.; Falcinelli, E.; Bury, L. Inherited platelet disorders in women. *Thromb. Res.* **2019**, *181*, S54–S59. [CrossRef]
90. Balduini, C.L.; Melazzini, F.; Pecci, A. Inherited Thrombocytopenias. In *Platelets in Thrombotic and Non Thrombotic Disorders*; Gresele, P., Kleiman, N.S., Lopez, J.A., Page, C.P., Eds.; Springer Gmbh: Cambridge, UK, 2017; pp. 727–747.
91. Kaur, H.; Ozelo, M.; Scovil, S.; James, P.D.; Othman, M. Systematic analysis of bleeding phenotype in PT-VWD compared to type 2B VWD using an electronic bleeding questionnaire. *Clin. Appl. Thromb. Hemost.* **2014**, *20*, 765–771. [CrossRef]
92. Nurden, P.; Nurden, A.; Favier, R.; Gleyze, M. Management of pregnancy for a patient with the new syndromic macrothrombocytopenia, DIAPH1-related disease. *Platelets* **2018**, *29*, 737–738. [CrossRef]
93. Orsini, S.; Noris, P.; Bury, L.; Heller, P.G.; Santoro, C.; Kadir, R.A.; Butta, N.C.; Falcinelli, E.; Cid, A.R.; Fabris, F.; et al. European Hematology Association—Scientific Working Group (EHA-SWG) on thrombocytopenias and platelet function disorders. Bleeding risk of surgery and its pre-vention in patients with inherited platelet disorders. *Haematologica* **2017**, *102*, 1192–1203. [CrossRef] [PubMed]
94. Morgan, N.V.; Daly, M.E. Gene of the issue: RUNX1 mutations and inherited bleeding. *Platelets* **2017**, *28*, 208–210. [CrossRef] [PubMed]
95. Melazzini, F.; Zaninetti, C.; Balduini, C.L. Bleeding is not the main clinical issue in many patients with inherited thrombocytopaenias. *Haemophilia* **2017**, *23*, 673–681. [CrossRef] [PubMed]
96. Pecci, A.; Klersy, C.; Gresele, P.; Lee, K.J.; De Rocco, D.; Bozzi, V.; Russo, G.; Heller, P.G.; Loffredo, G.; Ballmaier, M.; et al. MYH9-related disease: A novel prognostic model to predict the clinical evolution of the disease based on genotype-phenotype correlations. *Hum. Mutat.* **2014**, *35*, 236–247. [CrossRef]
97. Bury, L.; Megy, K.; Stephens, J.C.; Grassi, L.; Greene, D.; Gleadall, N.; Althaus, K.; Allsup, D.; Bariana, T.K.; Bonduel, M.; et al. Next-generation sequencing for the diagnosis of MYH9 -RD: Predicting pathogenic variants. *Hum. Mutat.* **2019**, *41*, 277–290. [CrossRef]
98. Falcinelli, E.; Bury, L.; Gresele, P. Inherited platelet function disorders. *Hämostaseologie* **2016**, *36*, 265–278. [CrossRef]
99. Makris, M.; Conlon, C.P.; Watson, H.G. Immunization of patients with bleeding disorders. *Haemophilia* **2003**, *9*, 541–546. [CrossRef]
100. Bolton-Maggs, P.; Chalmers, E.A.; Collins, P.W.; Harrison, P.; Kitchen, S.; Liesner, R.J.; Minford, A.; Mumford, A.D.; Parapia, L.A.; Perry, D.J.; et al. A review of inherited platelet disorders with guidelines for their management on behalf of the UKHCDO. *Br. J. Haematol.* **2006**, *135*, 603–633. [CrossRef]
101. Buijs, A.; Poddighe, P.; van Wijk, R.; van Solinge, W.; Borst, E.; Verdonck, L.; Hagenbeek, A.; Pearson, P.; Lokhorst, H. A novel CBFA2 single-nucleotide mutation in familial platelet disorder with propensity to develop myeloid malig-nancies. *Blood* **2001**, *98*, 2856–2858. [CrossRef]
102. Demers, C.; Derzko, C.; David, M.; Douglas, J. Gynaecological and obstetrical management of women with inherited bleeding disorders. *Int. J. Gynaecol. Obstet.* **2006**, *95*, 75–87. [CrossRef]
103. Sogut, O.; Erdogan, M.O.; Kose, R.; Boleken, M.E.; Kaya, H.; Gokdemir, M.T.; Ozgonul, A.; Iynen, I.; Albayrak, L.; Dokuzoglu, M.A. Hemostatic Efficacy of a Traditional Medicinal Plant Extract (Ankaferd Blood Stopper) in Bleeding Control. *Clin. Appl. Thromb. Hemost.* **2015**, *21*, 348–353. [CrossRef] [PubMed]
104. Harrison, P. Subcommittee on Platelet Physiology. The use of platelets in regenerative medicine and proposal for a new classification system: Guidance from the SSC of the ISTH. *J. Thromb. Haemost.* **2018**, *16*, 1895–1900. [CrossRef] [PubMed]
105. Nurden, P.; Youlouz-Marfak, I.; Siberchicot, F.; Kostrzewa, E.; Andia, I.; Anitua, E.; Nurden, A.T. Use of autologous platelet-rich clots for the prevention of local injury bleeding in patients with severe inherited mucocutaneous bleeding disorders. *Haemophilia* **2011**, *17*, 620–624. [CrossRef] [PubMed]
106. Kumar, S.; Randhawa, M.S.; Ganesamoni, R.; Singh, S.K. Tranexamic Acid Reduces Blood Loss During Percutaneous Nephrolithotomy: A Prospective Randomized Controlled Study. *J. Urol.* **2013**, *189*, 1757–1761. [CrossRef] [PubMed]
107. Vujkovac, B.; Sabovic, M. A successful treatment of life-threatening bleeding from polycystic kidneys with anti-fibrinolytic agent tranexamic acid. *Blood Coagul. Fibrinolysis* **2006**, *17*, 589–591. [CrossRef]
108. Dunn, C.J.; Goa, K.L. Tranexamic acid: A review of its use in surgery and other indications. *Drugs* **1999**, *57*, 1005–1032. [CrossRef]
109. Colucci, G.; Stutz, M.; Rochat, S.; Conte, T.; Pavicic, M.; Reusser, M.; Giabbani, E.; Huynh, A.; Thürlemann, C.; Keller, P.; et al. The effect of desmopressin on platelet function: A selective enhancement of procoagulant COAT platelets in patients with primary platelet function defects. *Blood* **2014**, *123*, 1905–1916. [CrossRef]

110. Tosetto, A.; Balduini, C.L.; Cattaneo, M.; De Candia, E.; Mariani, G.; Molinari, A.C.; Rossi, E.; Siragusa, S. Italian Society for Haemostasis and Thrombosis. Management of bleeding and of invasive procedures in patients with platelet disorders and/or thrombocytopenia: Guidelines of the Italian Society for Haemostasis and Thrombosis (SISET). *Thromb. Res.* **2009**, *124*, 13–18. [CrossRef]
111. Sehbai, A.S.; Abraham, J.; Brown, V.K. Perioperative management of a patient with May-Hegglin anomaly requiring craniotomy. *Am. J. Hematol.* **2005**, *79*, 303–308. [CrossRef]
112. Poon, M.C. The evidence for the use of recombinant human activated factor VII in the treatment of bleeding patients with quantitative and qualitative platelet disorders. *Transfus. Med. Rev.* **2007**, *21*, 223–236. [CrossRef]
113. Franchini, M. The use of recombinant activated factor VII in the treatment of bleeding patients with quantitative and qualitative platelet disorders. *Blood Transfus.* **2009**, *7*, 24–28. [PubMed]
114. Pecci, A.; Gresele, P.; Klersy, C.; Savoia, A.; Noris, P.; Fierro, T.; Bozzi, V.; Mezzasoma, A.M.; Melazzini, F.; Balduini, C.L. Eltrombopag for the treatment of the inherited thrombocytopenia deriving from MYH9 mutations. *Blood* **2010**, *116*, 5832–5837. [CrossRef] [PubMed]
115. Zaninetti, C.; Gresele, P.; Bertomoro, A.; Klersy, C.; De Candia, E.; Veneri, D.; Barozzi, S.; Fierro, T.; Alberelli, M.A.; Musella, V.; et al. Eltrombopag for the treatment of inherited thrombocytopenias: A phase 2 clinical trial. *Haematologica* **2020**, *105*, 820–828. [CrossRef]
116. Gerrits, A.J.; Leven, E.A.; Frelinger, A.L.; Brigstocke, S.L.; Berny-Lang, M.A.; Mitchell, W.B.; Revel-Vilk, S.; Tamary, H.; Carmichael, S.L.; Barnard, M.R.; et al. Effects of eltrombopag on platelet count and platelet activation in Wiskott-Aldrich syndrome/X-linked thrombocytopenia. *Blood* **2015**, *126*, 1367–1378. [CrossRef] [PubMed]
117. Pecci, A.; Verver, E.J.; Schlegel, N.; Canzi, P.; Boccio, C.M.; Platokouki, H.; Krause, E.; Benazzo, M.; Topsakal, V.; Greinacher, A. Cochlear implantation is safe and effective in patients with MYH9-related disease. *Orphanet. J. Rare Dis.* **2014**, *9*, 100. [CrossRef]
118. Favier, R.; Feriel, J.; Favier, M.; Denoyelle, F.; Martignetti, J.A. First Successful Use of Eltrombopag Before Surgery in a Child With MYH9-Related Thrombocytopenia. *Pediatrics* **2013**, *132*, e793–e795. [CrossRef]
119. Zaninetti, C.; Barozzi, S.; Bozzi, V.; Gresele, P.; Balduini, C.L.; Pecci, A. Eltrombopag in preparation for surgery in patients with severe MYH9-related thrombocytopenia. *Am. J. Hematol.* **2019**, *94*, e199–e201. [CrossRef]
120. Paciullo, F.; Bury, L.; Gresele, P. Eltrombopag to allow chemotherapy in a patient with MYH9-related inherited thrombocytopenia and pancreatic cancer. *Int. J. Hematol.* **2020**, *112*, 1–3. [CrossRef]
121. Moratto, D.; Giliani, S.; Bonfim, C.; Mazzolari, E.; Fischer, A.; Ochs, H.D.; Cant, A.J.; Thrasher, A.J.; Cowan, M.J.; Albert, M.H.; et al. Long-term outcome and lineage-specific chimerism in 194 patients with Wiskott-Aldrich syndrome treated by hematopoietic cell transplantation in the period 1980–2009: An international collaborative study. *Blood* **2011**, *118*, 1675–1684. [CrossRef]
122. Ballmaier, M.; Germeshausen, M. Congenital Amegakaryocytic Thrombocytopenia: Clinical Presentation, Diagnosis, and Treatment. *Semin. Thromb. Hemost.* **2011**, *37*, 673–681. [CrossRef]
123. Bosticardo, M.; Marangoni, F.; Aiuti, A.; Villa, A.; Grazia Roncarolo, M. Recent advances in understanding the pathophysiology of Wiskott-Aldrich syndrome. *Blood* **2009**, *113*, 6288–6295. [CrossRef] [PubMed]
124. Locatelli, F.; Rossi, G.; Balduini, C. Hematopoietic stem-cell transplantation for the Bernard-Soulier syndrome. *Ann. Intern. Med.* **2003**, *138*, 79. [CrossRef] [PubMed]
125. Oshima, K.; Imai, K.; Albert, M.H.; Bittner, T.C.; Strauss, G.; Filipovich, A.H.; Morio, T.; Kapoor, N.; Dalal, J.; Schultz, K.R.; et al. Hematopoietic stem cell transplantation for X-linked thrombo-cytopenia with mutations in the WAS gene. *J. Clin. Immunol.* **2015**, *35*, 15–21. [CrossRef] [PubMed]
126. Aiuti, A.; Biasco, L.; Scaramuzza, S.; Ferrua, F.; Cicalese, M.P.; Baricordi, C.; Dionisio, F.; Calabria, A.; Giannelli, S.; Castiello, M.C.; et al. Lentiviral Hematopoietic Stem Cell Gene Therapy in Patients with Wiskott-Aldrich Syndrome. *Science* **2013**, *341*, 1233151. [CrossRef] [PubMed]
127. Hacein-Bey Abina, S.; Gaspar, H.B.; Blondeau, J.; Caccavelli, L.; Charrier, S.; Buckland, K.; Picard, C.; Six, E.; Himoudi, N.; Gilmour, K.; et al. Outcomes following gene therapy in patients with severe Wiskott-Aldrich syndrome. *JAMA* **2015**, *313*, 1550–1563. [CrossRef]
128. Pala, F.; Morbach, H.; Castiello, M.C.; Schickel, J.N.; Scaramuzza, S.; Chamberlain, N.; Cassani, B.; Glauzy, S.; Romberg, N.; Candotti, F.; et al. Lentiviral mediated gene therapy restores B cell tolerance in Wiskott-Aldrich syndrome patients. *J. Clin. Investig.* **2015**, *125*, 3941–3951. [CrossRef]
129. Kanaji, S.; Kuether, E.L.; Fahs, S.A.; Schroeder, J.A.; Ware, J.; Montgomery, R.R.; Shi, Q. Correction of murine Bernard-Soulier syndrome by lentivirus-mediated gene therapy. *Mol. Ther.* **2012**, *20*, 625–632. [CrossRef]
130. Albert, M.H.; Bittner, T.C.; Nonoyama, S.; Notarangelo, L.D.; Burns, S.; Imai, K.; Espanol, T.; Fasth, A.; Pellier, I.; Strauss, G.; et al. X-linked thrombocytopenia (XLT) due to WAS mutations: Clinical characteristics, long-term outcome, and treatment options. *Blood* **2010**, *115*, 3231–3238. [CrossRef]
131. Mullen, C.A.; Anderson, K.D.; Blaese, R.M. Splenectomy and/or bone marrow transplantation in the management of the Wiskott-Aldrich syndrome: Long-term follow-up of 62 cases. *Blood* **1993**, *82*, 2961–2966. [CrossRef]

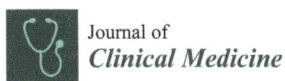

Review

Thrombotic Thrombocytopenic Purpura: Pathophysiology, Diagnosis, and Management

Senthil Sukumar [1], Bernhard Lämmle [2,3,4] and Spero R. Cataland [1,*]

1. Division of Hematology, Department of Medicine, The Ohio State University, Columbus, OH 43210, USA; senthil.sukumar@osumc.edu
2. Department of Hematology and Central Hematology Laboratory, Inselspital, Bern University Hospital, University of Bern, CH 3010 Bern, Switzerland; bernhard.laemmle@uni-mainz.de
3. Center for Thrombosis and Hemostasis, University Medical Center, Johannes Gutenberg University, 55131 Mainz, Germany
4. Haemostasis Research Unit, University College London, London WC1E 6BT, UK
* Correspondence: spero.cataland@osumc.edu

Abstract: Thrombotic thrombocytopenic purpura (TTP) is a rare thrombotic microangiopathy characterized by microangiopathic hemolytic anemia, severe thrombocytopenia, and ischemic end organ injury due to microvascular platelet-rich thrombi. TTP results from a severe deficiency of the specific von Willebrand factor (VWF)-cleaving protease, ADAMTS13 (a disintegrin and metalloprotease with thrombospondin type 1 repeats, member 13). ADAMTS13 deficiency is most commonly acquired due to anti-ADAMTS13 autoantibodies. It can also be inherited in the congenital form as a result of biallelic mutations in the *ADAMTS13* gene. In adults, the condition is most often immune-mediated (iTTP) whereas congenital TTP (cTTP) is often detected in childhood or during pregnancy. iTTP occurs more often in women and is potentially lethal without prompt recognition and treatment. Front-line therapy includes daily plasma exchange with fresh frozen plasma replacement and immunosuppression with corticosteroids. Immunosuppression targeting ADAMTS13 autoantibodies with the humanized anti-CD20 monoclonal antibody rituximab is frequently added to the initial therapy. If available, anti-VWF therapy with caplacizumab is also added to the front-line setting. While it is hypothesized that refractory TTP will be less common in the era of caplacizumab, in relapsed or refractory cases cyclosporine A, N-acetylcysteine, bortezomib, cyclophosphamide, vincristine, or splenectomy can be considered. Novel agents, such as recombinant ADAMTS13, are also currently under investigation and show promise for the treatment of TTP. Long-term follow-up after the acute episode is critical to monitor for relapse and to diagnose and manage chronic sequelae of this disease.

Keywords: thrombotic thrombocytopenic purpura; TTP; ADAMTS13; treatment; diagnosis; follow-up; review; caplacizumab

Citation: Sukumar, S.; Lämmle, B.; Cataland, S.R. Thrombotic Thrombocytopenic Purpura: Pathophysiology, Diagnosis, and Management. *J. Clin. Med.* **2021**, *10*, 536. https://doi.org/10.3390/jcm10030536

Academic Editor: Michael Callaghan
Received: 30 December 2020
Accepted: 27 January 2021
Published: 2 February 2021

Publisher's Note: MDPI stays neutral with regard to jurisdictional claims in published maps and institutional affiliations.

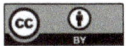

Copyright: © 2021 by the authors. Licensee MDPI, Basel, Switzerland. This article is an open access article distributed under the terms and conditions of the Creative Commons Attribution (CC BY) license (https://creativecommons.org/licenses/by/4.0/).

1. Introduction

1.1. History of Thrombotic Thrombocytopenic Purpura

In 1924, Dr. Eli Moschcowitz described a previously healthy 16-year-old girl who became acutely ill with fever, weakness, focal neurological symptoms, and severe thrombocytopenia. Ultimately, she became comatose and died after one week. Autopsy revealed widely disseminated thrombi in the terminal arterioles and capillaries of various organs but the underlying etiology of this mysterious illness was unknown [1,2]. This poorly understood condition was named thrombotic thrombocytopenic purpura (TTP) by Singer in 1947 [3]. Two decades later, Amorosi and Ultmann introduced the classic diagnostic pentad of TTP consisting of fever, thrombocytopenia, hemolytic anemia, renal injury, and neurological manifestations. Their case series and review of the literature also highlighted the >90% mortality rate of this devastating condition [4]. Shortly thereafter, case reports detailing the successful treatment of congenital TTP (cTTP) patients with infusions of plasma led to the conclusion that a deficiency of an unknown plasma factor contributed to the disease [5,6]. In 1982, Moake et al. first identified "unusually large" von Willebrand factor (VWF) multimers in the plasma of four chronic relapsing TTP patients—similar to the large multimers synthesized and secreted by human endothelial cells in culture. They hypothesized that these hyperadhesive ultralarge VWF (ULVWF) multimers were due to a suspected deficiency of a VWF depolymerase present in normal plasma [7]. Their hypothesis was reinforced when a highly effective therapy for TTP, plasma exchange, was described in 1991. The treatment of immune-mediated TTP (iTTP) was revolutionized and the mortality rate was improved from >90% to 10–20% with prompt therapy [8]. Five years later, a novel metalloprotease which specifically cleaved ULVWF was purified from human plasma [9,10]. A severe deficiency of this protease was noted in TTP patients, both through acquired autoantibodies and through an inherited deficiency [11,12]. In 2001, this was subsequently identified as ADAMTS13 (a disintegrin and metalloprotease with thrombospondin type 1 motifs, member 13), the only known function of which is to cleave VWF [13–17]. As of 2020, the improved molecular understanding of TTP along with study of survivors have allowed for marked advancements in diagnosis [18], treatment [19–22], and the long-term management [23–25] of these patients.

1.2. Definitions and Terminology

Thrombotic microangiopathy (TMA) is a broad term which has both pathologic (occlusive microvascular or macrovascular disease commonly with intraluminal thrombus formation) and clinical (microangiopathic hemolytic anemia (MAHA) with thrombocytopenia) definitions [26,27]. The different entities presenting with TMA findings have historically been difficult to distinguish from one another, but elucidating the pathophysiology of TTP has allowed for more accurate differentiation. As a result, standard definitions and terminology have been adopted [27,28].

TTP is characterized by MAHA with severe thrombocytopenia and variable organ ischemia, most commonly neurologic, cardiac, or renal [3,4,23,29]. The diagnosis is confirmed by a severe deficiency (<10%) of ADAMTS13 activity [11,12,27]. TTP is further divided into two categories based on the mechanism of ADAMTS13 deficiency: congenital (inherited) vs. immune-mediated (acquired). Congenital TTP, also known as Upshaw–Schulman syndrome or hereditary TTP, is defined by a persistent severe deficiency (<10%) in ADAMTS13 caused by biallelic pathogenic mutations in the *ADAMTS13* gene [27]. Immune-mediated TTP, sometimes referred to as acquired TTP, is caused by ADAMTS13 deficiency mediated by autoantibodies [12,27]. iTTP is further subdivided into primary iTTP, when there is no obvious associated disorder, and secondary iTTP, when an associated condition can be identified [27].

2. Epidemiology

iTTP typically presents in adulthood, accounting for 90% of cases [29]. The annual incidence is 1.5–6 cases per million per year in adults [29–32]. Discrepancies in annual incidence rate are likely due to demographic factors in the country of origin. In France and Germany, which are predominantly Caucasian, the incidence is ~1.5 cases per million per year [29,32]. The annual incidence in the U.S. is 2.99 cases per million per year, possibly a result of the higher proportion of African Americans, who have an approximately eightfold-increased incidence rate of TTP [31,33]. In a regional UK registry, the incidence rate was found to be six per million, though this could represent an overestimation as TTP was diagnosed clinically and did not rely on ADAMTS13 measurement in all cases [30].

Childhood-onset iTTP is considerably less common, comprising approximately 10% of all cases [34]. There is a scarcity of data regarding the incidence and prevalence of child and adolescent onset iTTP. The French National TMA Registry estimates the yearly incidence of childhood-onset iTTP to be 0.2 new cases per million with a prevalence of 1 case per million as of December 2015 [34]. This is consistent with the childhood iTTP incidence rate found in the Oklahoma (U.S.) registry of 0.1 cases per million [31].

Women are two to three times more likely to develop iTTP, which is consistent across registries globally [29–32,34–37]. ADAMTS13 deficiency is caused by an acquired autoimmune mechanism for the vast majority of TTP cases.

An inherited deficiency of ADAMTS13 due to mutations in the *ADAMTS13* gene occurs in approximately 3–5% of patients with TTP [29–31,36]. The exact prevalence of cTTP is uncertain, though some experts estimate this to be 0.5–2 cases per million; further investigation is needed [38]. cTTP often presents in childhood prior to 10 years of age [39–42] but large registries have reported that 10% of cases occur after the age of 40 [40–42]. cTTP accounts for a significant proportion of TTP cases in children and obstetrical TTP patients, consisting of 33% and 34% of all cases in those cohorts respectively [29,34].

3. Pathophysiology

3.1. Role of ADAMTS13 and VWF in TTP

ADAMTS13 is a critically important enzyme, synthesized in hepatic stellate cells [43,44], whose only known function is to regulate VWF multimers [9,10]. In physiologic conditions, ADAMTS13 is in a latent, closed conformation and VWF, secreted by platelets and endothelial cells, is in a globular state (Figure 1a) [45,46]. Proteolytic activity of ADAMTS13 on VWF is dependent on the conformational change of both proteins [45–50]. Under shear forces VWF unravels and exposes its A1 domain allowing for interaction with platelets through the GpIb/IX/V complex (Figure 1b) [51–53]. In this unraveled state, the A2 domain of VWF is elongated and exposes the ADAMTS13 binding sites [48,50] and the cleavage site Tyr1605-Met1606 [9,10]. Initial interaction of CUB1-2 domains with VWF D4-CK domains allosterically activates ADAMTS13, inducing an open conformation (Figure 1c) [47,49]. Sequential exosite interactions and binding of the disintegrin-like domain of ADAMTS13 to VWF induces further allosteric activation of the metalloprotease domain which results in proteolysis (Figure 1d) [54]. When severe ADAMTS13 deficiency (<10%) is present, ULVWF multimers can accumulate leading to unregulated platelet adhesion and aggregation, resulting in TTP with disseminated microthrombi and organ ischemia [4,7,26].

Though a severe ADAMTS13 deficiency is necessary for the development of TTP, enzyme deficiency alone may not be sufficient to induce the clinical syndrome [40,55–58]. Activation of the complement system has also been suggested to play a role in acute TTP [59–62]. In fact, ULVWF multimers serve as a scaffold for the assembly and activation of the alternative pathway of the complement system [61]. VWF acts as a cofactor for complement factor I mediated cleavage and inactivation of complement C3b, thereby regulating alternative pathway activation. This regulatory process is dependent on VWF multimer size with the smaller, physiologic VWF multimers enhancing cleavage of C3b and the ULVWF multimers losing this function [62]. Further studies have demonstrated a correlation between the presence of ULVWF multimers and higher levels of sC5b-9, C3a, and C5a [63]. Experimental mouse models have recently demonstrated a synergistic effect of ADAMTS13 deficiency and complement dysregulation. Mice with Adamts13$^{-/-}$ or heterozygous complement factor H (CFH) hyperfunctional mutation (cfh$^{W/R}$) alone remained asymptomatic. However, mice that were both Adamts13$^{-/-}$ and cfh$^{W/R}$ went on to develop clinical TMA findings [64]. Clinically, complement activation has also been reported to be associated with increased mortality from an acute TTP episode [60]. These and other findings have led to a "second hit" hypothesis, suggesting that another stressor in conjunction with severe deficiency of ADAMTS13 activity is usually required to develop clinical TTP [65,66].

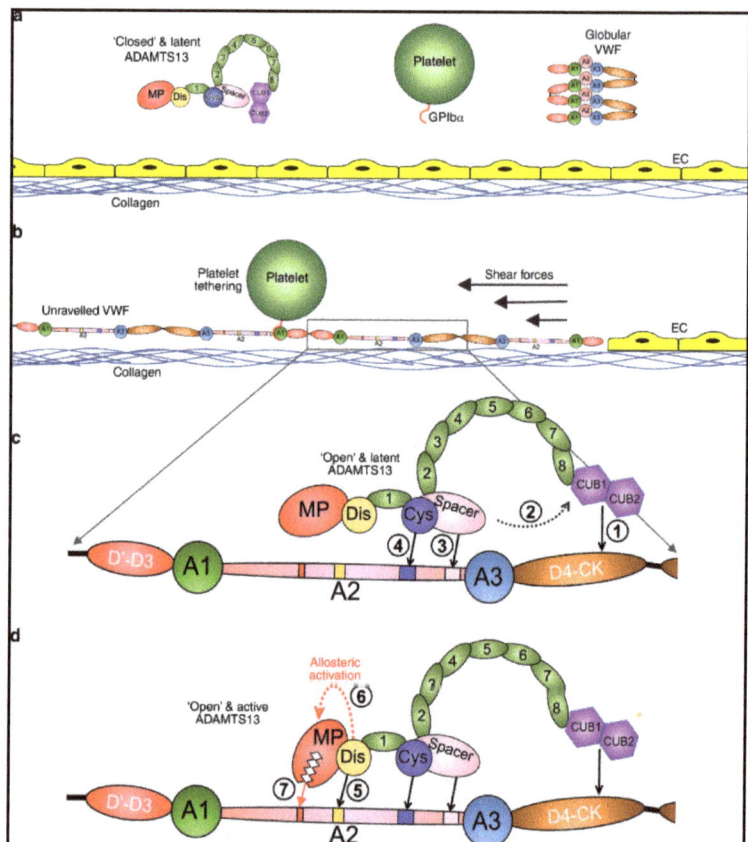

Figure 1. Mode of action of ADAMTS13. (**a**) Under normal circumstances, multimeric von Willebrand factor (VWF) circulates in the plasma in a globular conformation, in which its A1 domains are concealed, and so does not interact with platelets. ADAMTS13 circulates in a "closed" conformation stabilized through the interaction of the C-terminal CUB domains with the central Spacer domain. The MP domain of ADAMTS13 also has a latent conformation in which the active site cleft is occluded by the Ca2+-binding loop. This prevents ADAMTS13 from proteolyzing off-target substrates and confers resistance to plasma inhibitors. (**b**) Following vessel damage, the endothelium (EC) is disrupted to reveal subendothelial collagen. Globular VWF binds to this surface via its A3 domain and unravels into an elongated conformation in response to the shear forces exerted by the flowing blood. This reveals the A1 domain that can then capture platelets via the GPIbα receptor on the platelet surface. Unravelling of VWF also unravels the VWF A2 domain into a linear polypeptide conformation that reveals the binding sites for ADAMTS13 and the Tyr1605-Met1606 cleavage site, making it susceptible to proteolysis by ADAMTS13. (**c**) ADAMTS13 recognizes unfolded VWF through multiple interactions. (1) The CUB domains bind the VWF D4-CK domains, which (2) induces their dissociation from the Spacer domain. (3) The Spacer and (4) cysteine (Cys)-rich domain exosites recognize the C-terminal region of the unfolded A2 domain to bring the enzyme and substrate into proximity. (**d**) Once bound, (5) the disintegrin-like (Dis) domain exosite engages VWF residues Asp1614–Asp1622. This interaction (6) induces an allosteric change in the MP domain. This causes a conformational change, disrupting the "gatekeepertriad" that otherwise occludes the active site cleft, to reveal the S1′ pocket. Once allosterically activated, (7) the MP domain proteolyzes the scissile bond. Petri et al. [54], pp. 1–16. The corresponding author, James Crawley agreed to use of the Figure. No changes were made to the original figure. Creative Commons License: http://creativecommons.org/liceses/by/4.0/.

3.2. Congenital ADAMTS13 Deficiency

cTTP (also known as Upshaw–Schulman syndrome OMIM 274150) is an autosomal recessive condition caused by biallelic mutations in the *ADAMTS13* gene located on chromosome 9q34 [14]. Approximately 200 causative mutations have been identified in more than 150 patients, which span the entire *ADAMTS13* gene [14,39–42,67,68]. The majority of ADAMTS13 mutations are confined to single families [40,42]. Missense mutations are most common (59%), followed by nonsense mutations (13%), deletions (13%), splice site mutations (9%), and insertions (6%) [67]. There is some geographic variability and certain mutations have increased frequency in different regions. Two mutations in particular, p.R1060W [39,41,42,68–72] and insertion c.4143_4144dupA [42,68,69,73] are more prominent in cTTP patients with European ancestry. The p.R1060W mutation, a single nucleotide variant located on exon 24, also occurred in a high proportion (75–80%) of cTTP patients that presented during pregnancy in the French and UK cohorts [70,71]. Though no definite genotype–phenotype relationships have been established [41,67], earlier onset of disease appears to be related to earlier sequence mutations in the prespacer region of ADAMTS13 [41,72,74]. Often, mutations in *ADAMTS13* result in secretion deficiencies but they can also affect ADAMTS13 activity [67,74–76]. Indeed, in an effort to explain the variance of clinical phenotype, residual ADAMTS13 activity of different genotypes was measured and the results showed that residual ADAMTS13 activity <3% was correlated with earlier age of disease onset, need for prophylactic plasma infusions, and an annual event rate >1 [42,74]. However, this does not fully explain the phenotypic differences in cTTP as studies have demonstrated that many patients homozygous for the c.4143_4144dupA mutation had ADAMTS13 activity <1% but widely varying clinical courses [42,69,73].

3.3. Acquired ADAMTS13 Deficiency

3.3.1. Risk Factors

iTTP is due to acquired anti-ADAMTS13 autoantibodies [11,12]. Certain factors, such as African ancestry and female sex, predispose to the development of these antibodies [29–33]. Human leukocyte antigen (HLA)-DRB1*11 and HLA-DQB1*03:01 alleles are also overrepresented in white iTTP patients, with HLA-DRB1*04 having a protective effect [77–80]. The frequency of the HLA-DRB1*04 allele is dramatically decreased in iTTP patients with African ancestry, indicating that a low natural frequency of this allele may contribute to the greater risk in this population. However, there does not appear to be an increased risk of mortality in these patients [33]. An analysis of Japanese patients identified HLA-DRB1*08:03, HLA-DRB3/4/5*blank, HLA-DQA1*01:03, and HLA-DQB1*06:01 as predisposing factors for iTTP, with HLA-DRB1*15:01 and HLA-DRB5*01:01 being identified as weakly protective [81]. In contrast to white iTTP patients, HLA-DRB1*11 and HLA-DRB1*04 were not associated with iTTP in the Japanese [81].

3.3.2. Anti-ADAMTS13 Autoantibodies

Anti-ADAMTS13 autoantibodies are largely divided into two categories: inhibitory and non-inhibitory. Inhibitory antibodies neutralize the proteolytic activity of ADAMTS13 and non-inhibitory antibodies bind to the protease, accelerating its clearance from plasma [11,12,82–84]. It was previously widely held that inhibitory antibodies were the main cause of ADAMTS13 deficiency, but recent studies have demonstrated that antigen depletion also significantly contributes to deficiency [85]. Even a small amount of anti-ADAMTS13 autoantibodies can induce ADAMTS13 deficiency [86]. Anti-ADAMTS13 autoantibodies have been found against all domains of ADAMTS13, indicating a polyclonal immune response. However, the spacer domain of ADAMTS13 has been identified as an immunogenic region, as anti-spacer antibodies are present in most iTTP patients [85–92]. Recently, anti-ADAMTS13 autoantibodies that induce the open conformation of ADAMTS13 have been identified [18,93]. The role these conformation-changing antibodies play in the pathophysiology of TTP and their clinical significance is still being explored.

The most common isotype class of anti-ADAMT13 autoantibodies are IgG, followed by IgA and IgM (20% of cases). Among the IgG isotype, the IgG4 subclass is most common, followed by IgG1 [83,91,94–98]. During acute episodes of iTTP, approximately 75% of cases have detectable free anti-ADAMTS13 IgG [29]. The anti-ADAMTS13 autoantibody isotype may contribute to the severity of the disease phenotype. High IgA antibody titers were suggested to be associated with lower platelet counts, increased mortality, and a worse prognosis [94–96]. Though no bacterial or viral infections are known to directly lead to iTTP, molecular mimicry between ADAMTS13 and certain pathogens such as influenza A [99], *Helicobacter pylori* [100], *Legionella* [101], hepatitis C virus [102], and HIV [103] may evoke an immune response [91,104].

3.3.3. Immune Complexes

In addition to free anti-ADAMTS13 autoantibodies, immune complexes containing ADAMTS13 have also been found in 39–93% of patients during acute iTTP [105–107]. Given that C3a and C5a are elevated during the acute iTTP episode, this could suggest that the complement is activated through the classic pathway, via ADAMTS13 antigen-antibody immune complexes; the elevated levels of factor Bb, however, suggest activation of the alternative pathway [60,63,104,105,108]. The clinical significance of complement activation in TTP is still unclear, though it further supports the "second hit" hypothesis that another physiologic stressor in conjunction with severe ADAMTS13 deficiency is required to induce the clinical syndrome [65,66].

3.3.4. Primary and Secondary iTTP

iTTP is classified as primary when no obvious underlying associated disease can be determined and as secondary when a defined underlying disorder is identified [27]. The majority of iTTP cases are primary. Secondary iTTP can be associated with infections as mentioned previously, though the best evidence is its association with HIV [103,109,110]. Acute stressors, such as pancreatitis, may induce secondary iTTP [111]. Many drugs have also been implicated in secondary TMA but are only rarely accompanied by ADAMTS13 deficiency, indicating that they mostly represent a separate drug-induced TMA (DI-TMA) and not TTP [112]. One exception is ticlopidine, which has been associated with severely deficient ADAMTS13 and this condition may be considered as secondary iTTP [113]. Notably, not all thienopyridine-derivatives (ticlopidine, clopidogrel, and prasugrel) are associated with TTP. Of 97 cases of TMA associated with ticlopidine, 80% had severely deficient ADAMT13 activity confirming the diagnosis of TTP. A clear causal relationship, however, has not been confirmed between the use of ticlopidine and the development of anti-ADAMTS13 antibodies. In 197 patients with clopidogrel associated TMA, 0% had severely deficient ADAMTS13 [114], which is consistent with DI-TMA, not TTP. Secondary iTTP can also be associated with various autoimmune conditions, though it is most commonly associated with systemic lupus erythematosus (SLE) [23,24,115–117]. In either primary or secondary iTTP, prompt therapy is essential. Secondary iTTP typically also requires treatment of the underlying condition in addition to standard TTP therapies.

4. Diagnosis

4.1. Clinical Presentation

Previously, TTP was defined by a clinical "pentad" consisting of fever, microangiopathic hemolytic anemia, thrombocytopenia, neurological deficits, and renal insufficiency [4]. However, the pentad was reported at a time before the effectiveness of plasma-based therapy in treating TTP was firmly established. Today, the presence of thrombocytopenia and MAHA alone, without an alternative explanation, should prompt serious consideration of the diagnosis of TTP or another TMA. Large cohort studies from various registries worldwide indicate that less than 10% of patients with acute TTP present with all five symptoms [29–31,35–37]. In fact, the clinical features of acute TTP can be extraordinarily diverse and a high degree of suspicion is required to diagnose TTP and promptly initiate appropriate management [118]. The differential diagnosis for patients with possible TTP is broad and described in Table 1. In obstetric patients with TMA, hemolysis, elevated liver enzyme, and low platelet (HELLP) syndrome and preeclampsia should be ruled out prior to evaluating for other conditions such as iTTP, cTTP, or complement-mediated hemolytic-uremic syndrome (CM-HUS) [27,112,119].

Table 1. Differential diagnosis for patients presenting with MAHA-T [27,112].

Disease	Comment
TTP	Defined by ADAMTS13 activity <10%
IA-HUS	TMA presenting 5–7 days after infection, often hemorrhagic colitis caused by enteropathogenic *Escherichia* coli, or *Shigella*.
CM-HUS	Triggered by infections, vaccination, pregnancy, or surgeries. Diagnosis may be confirmed by complement mutations
DI-TMA	May occur with gemcitabine, bleomycin, mitomycin, quinine, cyclosporine, simvastatin, and others. VEGF inhibitors have also been implicated.
TA-TMA	May occur with hematopoietic stem cell transplantation or solid organ transplantation. Often associated with immunosuppressive therapy (tacrolimus or cyclosporine A), GVHD, or underlying opportunistic infections
Malignant HTN TMA	TMA precipitated by chronic, severe uncontrolled HTN. Acute but not chronic end-organ injury may improve with control of blood pressure
DIC	Coagulopathy with TMA caused by underlying condition, most often sepsis, malignancy, trauma, obstetric complications, or hematologic disorder
APLS	TMA in context of underlying autoimmune disease and meeting positive diagnostic criteria for APLS
Pregnancy-associated TMA (HELLP syndrome, preeclampsia)	TMA associated with obstetrical complications. Presence of significant proteinuria and de novo HTN are concerning for preeclampsia. Treatments can include control of BP and delivery

APLS, antiphospholipid syndrome; BP, blood pressure; CM-HUS, complement-mediated hemolytic-uremic syndrome; DIC, disseminated intravascular coagulation; DI-TMA, drug-induced thrombotic microangiopathy; GVHD, graft versus host disease; HELLP, hemolysis, elevated liver enzyme, and low platelet syndrome; HTN, hypertension; IA-HUS, infection-associated hemolytic-uremic syndrome; MAHA-T, microangiopathic hemolytic anemia with thrombocytopenia; TA-TMA, transplant-associated thrombotic microangiopathy; TMA, thrombotic microangiopathy; TTP, thrombotic thrombocytopenic purpura; VEGF, vascular endothelial growth factor.

Acute TTP almost uniformly presents with severe thrombocytopenia (typically <30 × 10^9/L) and microangiopathic hemolytic anemia, often with evidence of erythrocyte fragmentation on the peripheral blood smear [119]. Frequently, other classical parameters of hemolysis are also present, including an undetectable haptoglobin concentration accompanied by an elevated reticulocyte count, elevated total bilirubin (predominantly unconjugated), and an elevated lactate dehydrogenase (LDH) level, a marker for both red cell destruction and organ ischemia [120]. Coombs' testing is usually negative and coagulation parameters are not severely deranged in TTP.

Signs and symptoms of organ ischemia due to microthrombi formation are variable at presentation. More than 60% of patients have neurological manifestations which range broadly from mild confusion or altered sensorium to stroke, seizures, or coma [25,29,30,36,37]. Gastrointestinal ischemia is present in 35% of patients and can result in abdominal pain, nausea, and diarrhea [29]. Evidence of myocardial ischemia is present in a quarter of acute TTP patients and can be characterized by an abnormal electrocardiogram, or more commonly, elevated cardiac troponin-I measurements. Cardiac symptoms consistent with congestive heart failure or myocardial infarction can also be seen [121]. Renal injury is not uncommon in TTP, though acute renal failure requiring renal replacement therapy is quite rare in iTTP. Hematuria and proteinuria are the most commonly seen renal manifestations. Though modest renal insufficiency may occur, most patients present with a creatinine below 2 mg/dL [122–125]. Severely deficient ADAMTS13 activity serves to confirm the diagnosis of TTP [11,12,27].

4.2. ADAMTS13 Investigation

4.2.1. ADAMTS13 Activity

Assaying the ADAMTS13 activity is the first test which should be undertaken in patients with a suspected TMA. Severe ADAMTS13 deficiency, which is defined by an activity level <10%, is required to confirm the diagnosis of TTP (Figure 2) [119]. ADAMTS13 activity assays are based on degradation of either full-length VWF or synthetic peptides of VWF by ADAMTS13 in the plasma sample being tested. VWF cleavage products are detected by fluorescence resonance energy transfer (FRETS), enzyme-linked immunosorbent assays (ELISAs), surface-enhanced laser desorption/ionization time-of-flight (SELDI-TOF)-mass spectrometry, electrophoresis, reduced collagen binding, or reduced ristocetin-induced platelet agglutination [11,12,126–133]. Though multiple assays have been developed, the FRETS-VWF73-based assay [128,134] is most commonly used in clinical settings [135] and is considered as the reference method for ADAMTS13 activity, typically calibrated against the World Health Organization International Standard ADAMTS13 plasma (normal 100%) [136]. However, ADAMTS13 activity testing is labor intensive, time consuming, and limited to reference laboratories typically. Though the FRETS assay can be completed quickly, the turnaround time for results can be three to six days as it is typically performed only in reference centers. Given the variability in ADAMTS13 testing turnaround time for any individual center, point-based scoring systems which predict the probability of severely deficient ADAMTS13 have been developed to avoid delays in prompt treatment initiation [122,137,138]. Importantly, these scores are not meant to replace ADAMTS13 testing but to aid decision making until test results are available. Recently, fully automated chemiluminescence immunoassays have been developed with drastically reduced analytical times of approximately 30 min [139,140]. In addition, a semiquantitative ADAMTS13 activity assay has also been developed which provides an easily interpreted four-level indicator of ADAMTS13 activity, allowing identification of activity levels < 10% [141]. A potential advantage of such an assay is rapid screening for severely deficient ADAMTS13 activity which can be utilized at non-specialized centers to facilitate referral to tertiary centers for additional testing and management.

4.2.2. Anti-ADAMTS13 Autoantibodies

When severely deficient ADAMTS13 activity is confirmed, the next step of investigation is to determine if an antibody inhibitor to ADAMTS13 is present [11,12]. Understanding the mechanism of ADAMTS13 deficiency is critical in differentiating iTTP from cTTP and has important treatment implications. This distinction is also especially important in children and obstetrical patients, owing to higher rates of cTTP in these cohorts [29,34,71]. ADAMTS13 autoantibodies, predominantly anti-ADAMTS13 IgG, can be readily detected using in-house or commercial ELISA kits by laboratories [83,94]. A Bethesda assay can only detect ADAMTS13 autoantibodies which functionally inhibit ADAMTS13 (inhibitory antibodies), unlike the anti-ADAMTS13 IgG ELISA which can detect both inhibitory and non-inhibitory antibodies [25,142]. For both inhibitory and non-inhibitory anti-ADAMTS13 autoantibodies, assays only detect free autoantibodies whereas those bound to ADAMTS13 (immune complexes) are not detected by standard assays. In patients who have persistent severe ADAMTS13 deficiency during periods of remission and in whom no inhibitory autoantibody is detected, *ADAMTS13* gene analysis should be pursued to confirm a diagnosis of cTTP [38].

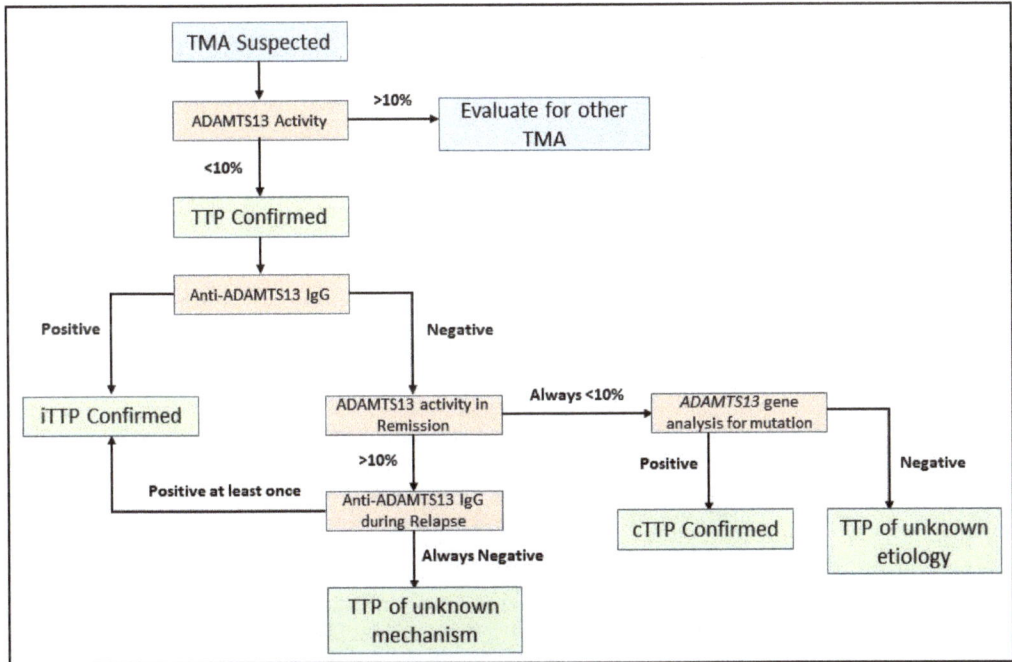

Figure 2. Flowchart for ADAMTS13 investigation in TTP. Severely deficient ADAMTS13 activity of <10% is required to establish a diagnosis of TTP. Further investigation of anti-ADAMTS13 IgG inhibitory autoantibodies are required to document the mechanism of ADAMTS13 deficiency. *ADAMTS13* gene analysis for biallelic mutations is reserved for selected situations to confirm a diagnosis of cTTP. In some cases, the underlying mechanism of ADAMTS13 activity deficiency is not immediately clear and repeated measurements of ADAMTS13 activity in remission and anti-ADAMTS13 IgG during relapse events can help establish a diagnosis.

4.2.3. ADAMTS13 Antigen

ADAMTS13 antigen can be measured by ELISA but this is not yet part of routine clinical practice. A recent study evaluated the prognostic value of anti-ADAMTS13 autoantibody titers and antigen levels in patients with iTTP [143]. Patients in the lowest quartile, with an antigen level <1.5%, had a mortality rate of 18% compared with a mortality rate of ~4% for those in the highest quartile, with an antigen level >11%. Those in the lowest antigen quartile and the highest antibody quartile had the highest mortality rate of 27%. This suggests that there could be some prognostic value for this test and that it has the potential to be incorporated in clinical practice in the future.

4.3. Emerging Biomarkers

It has previously been demonstrated that ADAMTS13 circulates in the "open" conformation in iTTP patients during the acute phase [93]. Recently, anti-ADAMT13 autoantibodies were revealed to induce the open ADAMTS13 conformation. Additionally, the open ADAMTS13 conformation preceded significant decrement in ADAMTS13 activity in one patient followed longitudinally [18]. While these findings warrant further study, there are many potentially important implications with regard to treatment and long term follow-up. As discussed previously, though it is a major risk factor, not all patients who have undetectable ADAMTS13 activity in remission uniformly go on to relapse [55,56,58,144]. However, being able to identify the open versus closed conformation of ADAMTS13 may potentially be useful to decide on the necessity of prophylactic therapy in select iTTP patients during remission.

5. Acute Management

TTP is a clinical emergency and in patients with suspected TTP treatment should be initiated promptly as delays in therapy may result in significant morbidity and mortality. Often therapy decisions are required prior to the availability of confirmatory ADAMTS13 testing. A blood sample for ADAMTS13 activity testing should immediately be obtained from a patient with TMA and frontline therapy can then commence based on clinical presentation alone. Severe ADAMTS13 deficiency is still required to confirm the diagnosis but should not delay the initiation of treatment [145]. Below are definitions of treatment response from the International Working Group for Thrombotic Thrombocytopenic Purpura [27]:

- Clinical response—a normalization of the platelet count to a level greater than the lower limit of the established reference range (150×10^9/L) and the LDH level to <1.5× the upper limit of normal (ULN). If initial presentation is severe with evidence of significant end-organ damage, stabilization of these parameters with improvement in function should also be required to qualify for a clinical response.
- Clinical remission—a sustained clinical response which is maintained for >30 days after the cessation of plasma exchange.
- Exacerbation—a decreasing platelet count with rising LDH and the need to restart plasma exchange therapy within 30 days of cessation after an initial clinical response is noted.
- Relapse—a fall in platelet count below the lower limit of the established reference range (~150×10^9/L), with or without clinical symptoms, during a clinical remission that requires reinitiating therapy. ADAMTS13 activity will most likely be <10%.
- Refractory TTP—persistent thrombocytopenia (platelet count <50×10^9/L, without increment) and persistently elevated LDH (>1.5 × ULN) despite five plasma exchange treatments in conjunction with adequate steroid treatment. If platelet count remains <30×10^9/L, this is classified as severe refractory TTP.

5.1. iTTP

Patients with both primary and secondary iTTP should be treated similarly in the acute inpatient setting. Importantly, patients with secondary iTTP should also have the underlying etiology managed appropriately in addition to the acute iTTP event. For example, in a patient with secondary iTTP due to underlying HIV infection, appropriate antiretroviral therapy would also be warranted in addition to management of TTP.

5.1.1. Plasma Exchange

Therapeutic plasma exchange (TPE) with fresh frozen plasma (FFP) replacement is the foundation of front-line therapy for TTP [8]. The proposed mechanism of TPE is that it supplies adequate levels of ADAMTS13 while removing circulating anti-ADAMTS13 autoantibodies. Delays in therapy can lead to early mortality, which may be preventable with prompt initiation of TPE [146]. Typically 1–1.5× plasma volume exchange is performed for the first three days, followed by 1× plasma volume exchange each day thereafter [8]. While there is no optimal duration of therapy or pre-specified number of procedures required, therapy should be continued daily until clinical response is achieved and sustained for two days. In patients with refractory TTP or evidence of progressive end organ damage, more intensive therapy, such as twice daily TPE, may be considered [147]. The efficacy of this approach is difficult to determine as it is usually accompanied by the addition or intensification of concurrent therapies. Generally, there are no significant differences between readily available therapeutic plasma replacement products [148,149]. Previously, cryosupernatant plasma devoid of ULVWF multimers was suggested to be more efficacious than fresh frozen plasma [150], but equivalency of these plasma products was demonstrated in a small randomized controlled trial [151].

5.1.2. Immune Suppression

In conjunction with TPE, immunosuppressive therapy is a cornerstone of acute iTTP management. The general principle of therapy is to target antibody production to allow for recovery of circulating levels of ADAMTS13. Therapy is typically started concurrently with TPE.

Glucocorticoids: steroids are widely used in conjunction with TPE at the initiation of therapy for acute iTTP. Though there are no randomized clinical trials comparing TPE with steroids vs. TPE alone, there is high biological plausibility for concurrent immunosuppression given the autoimmune nature of the condition. A small prospective randomized controlled trial comparing prednisone with cyclosporine A as an adjunct to TPE demonstrated that prednisone was superior in the initial treatment of iTTP [152]. This is also the only prospective randomized trial confirming the efficacy of steroids in the acute setting in decreasing anti-ADAMTS13 IgG and thereby increasing ADAMTS13 activity. No optimal dose or route of administration has been identified. High dose pulse steroids with methylprednisolone 10 mg/kg/day for three days followed by 2.5 mg/kg/day thereafter may be more efficacious than 1 mg/kg/day dosing [153]. Most standards of practice recommend oral prednisone 1 mg/kg/day or equivalent [149], gradually tapered over 3–4 weeks after clinical response is achieved. In patients with severe presentations or neurological symptoms, intravenous methylprednisolone 1 g/day for three days can be considered.

Rituximab: rituximab is a monoclonal antibody against CD20, specifically targeting B-cells. Rituximab is given most commonly during the acute phase of iTTP, typically during the first days of hospitalization or shortly thereafter. A non-randomized prospective phase 2 trial has shown its safety and efficacy in the front-line setting [154]. Additionally, this trial and many observational cohort studies suggest that rituximab given in the acute phase results in fewer relapses [20,154–157]. While a lower relapse rate did not reach statistical significance in all studies [158,159], a recent meta-analysis shows that rituximab administered during an acute iTTP episode not only lowers the relapse rate vs. control, but also reduces mortality [160]. Rituximab also appears to be effective in patients with refractory TTP or poor response to TPE [20,157,158]. The standard dosing for rituximab is 375 mg/m^2 given weekly for a total of four doses, which is recommended for both initial iTTP episodes and the acute phase of relapsing episodes. Emerging evidence for the efficacy of low dose rituximab (100 mg–200 mg/per dose) comes from a small prospective trial [161] and retrospective studies [162] but it has not yet been widely incorporated into standard practice.

Alternative immunosuppressive therapies: in patients with contraindications to steroids or with refractory disease, cyclosporine A can be effective [19,163]. Mycophenolate mofetil has also been used with success in some case reports [164,165]. Prior to the use of rituximab, vincristine was used for refractory disease, but this is no longer preferred [166]. Bortezomib, a proteasome inhibitor targeting plasma cells, has been used successfully as an alternative agent to rituximab [167,168]. Cyclophosphamide and/or splenectomy are also options for refractory or chronically relapsing cases [169].

5.1.3. Anti-VWF Strategy

Caplacizumab: caplacizumab, a humanized immunoglobulin originally from llamas, targeting the A1 domain of VWF and thereby preventing its interaction with platelets is the first medication approved specifically to treat TTP. In the recent phase 2 TITAN [21] and phase 3 HERCULES [22] trials, caplacizumab along with TPE and immunosuppression significantly reduced time to platelet count normalization and the exacerbation rate when compared with placebo. The initial dose is 10 mg given intravenously prior to the first TPE, followed by 10 mg daily and subcutaneously thereafter. Caplacizumab is well tolerated and has a good safety profile with the most common side effect being minor bleeding, which is often easily managed [170]. By blocking microvascular thrombi formation it is hypothesized that tissue ischemia can be decreased. Caplacizumab effectively blocks the end-organ damage caused by TTP; however, concomitant immunosuppression is required as the underlying deficient ADAMTS13 function is not addressed by this therapy. It is unsurprising then that exacerbations and early relapses can occur when the drug is discontinued while ADAMTS13 activity remains severely deficient. As a result, treatment is typically continued until the recovery of ADAMTS13 activity. As a novel agent, one limitation of incorporating caplacizumab into current standard practice is its high cost. At its current price level (in the United States) as of 2020, a recent analysis suggested that the addition of caplacizumab to the front line treatment for all patients with iTTP would not be cost-effective [171]. As caplacizumab is increasingly utilized, treatment response definitions may need to be revisited in the future as platelet count alone may not be an accurate measure of disease activity.

N-acetylcysteine: N-acetylcysteine (NAC) is a mucolytic approved by the Food and Drug Administration which is predominantly used to treat lung diseases. Its efficacy in TTP has been examined given that VWF multimers polymerize in a similar manner to mucins. NAC was found to degrade ULVWF multimer strings and inhibited VWF-dependent platelet aggregation and collagen binding in vitro [172,173]. NAC has been effective in some cases of severe and refractory iTTP but only a few case reports exist to date [174,175]. Animal models examining NAC have produced mixed results. NAC was able to prevent iTTP in mice but NAC administration was not successful in resolving TTP in either mice or baboons [176].

Emerging anti-VWF therapies: in 2012, ARC1779, a nucleic acid macromolecule, or aptamer, that blocks platelet binding by the A1 domain of VWF, was evaluated in TTP patients in a small trial [177]. Nine patients were recruited to the study, seven of whom received ARC1779. The study was halted for financial reasons before sufficient patients could be enrolled to ascertain the efficacy but there were no bleeding complications, despite ARC1779 suppression of VWF function in patients with severe thrombocytopenia. Development of ARC1779 has not been continued, but the safety profile from this trial encouraged the development of second generation anti-VWF aptamers. A novel DNA aptamer, TAGX-0004, showed a stronger ability to inhibit ristocetin- or botrocetin-induced platelet agglutination/aggregation than ARC1779 and a similar inhibitory effect to caplacizumab [178]. Another synthetic aptamer, BT200, has shown inhibition of human VWF in vitro and prevented arterial thrombosis in non-human primates [179]. Further studies incorporating this approach are in development.

5.2. cTTP

Acute episodes in patients with known cTTP can be successfully treated with plasma infusions (FFP, 10–15 mL/kg/day). Treatment is continued until clinical response is achieved [38,41,42]. In patients with a recurring cTTP phenotype, prophylactic plasma infusions may be required. Prophylactic plasma infusions have also been shown to improve chronic symptoms not related to an acute episode [39,41]. In patients who receive chronic plasma infusions, the ADAMTS13 activity half-life has been reported to be 2.5–5.4 days [180–182]. Consequently, ADAMTS13 activity is expected to return to baseline activity after approximately 5–10 days. Treatments are usually given every 2–3 weeks, depending on clinical symptoms, platelet counts, and patient preferences [38,41,42,181,182].

5.3. Emerging Therapies

Upfront therapy of TTP has seen innovative strategies in the last five years. Recombinant ADAMTS13 (BAX 930, rADAMTS13) has shown promise in a recent phase 1/2 study in cTTP patients [183]. A phase 3 clinical trial to assess the efficacy of rADAMTS13 for prophylactic and on-demand treatment of cTTP compared to plasma infusion therapy is ongoing (https://www.clinicaltrials.gov/ct2/show/study/NCT03393975). There is also evidence that rADAMTS13 may be effective in patients with iTTP, a hypothesis that is presently being prospectively studied as well (https://www.clinicaltrials.gov/ct2/show/NCT03922308) [184].

With ever growing treatment options for the acute phase of TTP, the classic treatment paradigm is constantly being re-examined. Though TPE is the cornerstone of acute therapy, there are not insignificant risks associated with the procedures required and replacement plasma products [23]. There are an increasing number of case reports detailing treatment of acute iTTP with caplacizumab and immunosuppression, without TPE, in the context of religious beliefs prohibiting blood products [185], shared decision making [186,187], and anaphylaxis to plasma [188]. As novel treatments become readily available, acute TTP management may soon enter an era without obligatory reliance on plasma exchange.

6. Special Populations

6.1. Pregnancy

TTP in the pregnant patient presents many difficulties and challenges. These patients should be managed by a multidisciplinary team typically including hematologists, high-risk obstetricians, and, occasionally, neonatologists. Prompt recognition and differentiation from preeclampsia or HELLP syndrome followed by appropriate treatment is critical, as maternal/fetal morbidity and mortality are high if unrecognized [70]. Pregnancy can trigger acute episodes in cTTP patients who have previously been asymptomatic. Approximately 25–30% of all obstetrical TTP cases were due to cTTP in some cohorts [29,34,71]. Thus, a high suspicion for cTTP is warranted in pregnant patients and appropriate diagnostic workup should be pursued if there is no evidence of an inhibitor or anti-ADAMTS13 autoantibodies. Acute management of cTTP in pregnancy includes plasma infusions but more severe cases may require TPE [38].

In pregnant patients with iTTP, the acute phase should be managed with TPE with the addition of corticosteroids if tolerated [70]. Though corticosteroids may confer some risks if given during the first trimester, these are largely outweighed by the potential benefits in this clinical context. Further immunosuppression with rituximab has not been studied in pregnant iTTP patients and its use is not standard. Routine use of caplacizumab is not recommended given the theoretical risk of fetal hemorrhage.

In remission after an episode during pregnancy, cTTP patients may require prophylactic therapy prior to and during their next pregnancy. The recently published International Society of Thrombosis and Haemostasis (ISTH) guidelines for management of TTP state that pregnant cTTP patients should receive prophylactic plasma infusions to prevent relapse [189].

In remission after any acute episode, iTTP patients who are pregnant or could become pregnant should have ADAMTS13 monitored periodically. Severely deficient ADAMTS13 activity in pregnancy appears to uniformly predict relapse of iTTP [190]. Though there is currently a lack of strong evidence, prophylactic therapy for pregnant patients with a history of iTTP and severely deficient ADAMTS13 activity in remission is suggested due to the risk of mortality to both mother and fetus associated with relapse [191]. No standard prophylactic regimen has yet been determined for this indication.

6.2. Jehovah's Witnesses/Contraindication to Blood Products

Certain groups, including Jehovah's Witnesses, may not accept exogenous blood products on the basis of religious or other beliefs. As TPE is the foundation of management of acute episodes, this presents a unique challenge in the management of these patients. Various regimens have previously been tried, including vincristine [192] and plasma exchange with albumin [193] or cryosupernatant [194] replacement. With the use of caplacizumab alongside improved immunosuppressive therapy, successful treatment without TPE has been described not only in this patient population [185] but also in other selected patients, including one with anaphylaxis to plasma [186–188].

7. Long-Term Follow-Up and Remission Management

TTP was previously thought to only be an acute illness but long-term follow-up of TTP survivors reveals many potential chronic complications and morbidity in addition to the risk of relapse [23,24,195–197]. Severely deficient ADAMTS13 activity (<10–20%) in remission suggests an increased risk of relapse and maintaining activity above this level appears adequate to prevent relapse [55,56,198]. Therefore, serial ADAMTS13 activity should be monitored in patients after remission. This is routinely accompanied by a chemistry panel, complete blood count, and measurement of LDH level. After resolution of an acute episode, ADAMTS13 activity can be measured monthly for 3 months, then every 3 months for 1 year, then every 6–12 months if stable. If ADAMTS13 activity consistently decreases, then more frequent monitoring may be appropriate [191]. However, ADAMTS13 activity is not a perfect predictive biomarker and not all patients with severely deficient activity go on to relapse [58]. Further studies highlighting the role of complement activation in the presence of ULVWF multimers suggest that the addition of other biomarkers may more accurately predict relapse in asymptomatic patients [63]. Emerging biomarkers such as the "open" vs. "closed" conformation of ADAMTS13 may also help to better predict which patients with severely deficient activity will ultimately progress to another episode [18,93].

In asymptomatic patients with ADAMTS13 activity persistently <10%, preemptive therapy with rituximab can effectively prevent relapse [144,160,198]. Cyclosporine has also been used for prophylaxis [199] and can be an option for patients who do not respond to rituximab. For the chronically relapsing patient, splenectomy is a viable option. Though falling out of favor with the development of improved immunomodulatory therapy, splenectomy has both a high and a durable response rate in some case series with a 10-year relapse-free survival of 70% [200]. Splenectomy is usually efficacious, with a nonresponse rate as low as 8% in some reports [201]. It has also been shown to induce durable remissions and reduce relapse rate in some of these challenging patients [200,202]. Though previously splenectomy had increased risk for adverse events, especially when used in refractory TTP [203], improvements in surgical technique have decreased complications considerably, especially when laparoscopic technique is utilized [201].

Long-term complications are prevalent in both iTTP and cTTP patients. Many adverse health sequelae are seen in TTP survivors, including higher rates of obesity, stroke, hypertension, mood disorders, cognitive impairment, and reduced quality of life [42,195,196,204–206]. TTP survivors also appear to have a higher all-cause mortality than reference populations [24,197]. Low-normal levels of ADAMTS13 activity have recently been implicated as a risk factor for coronary artery disease [207,208], stroke [209], and all-cause/cardiovascular mortality [210] in the general population. While the mechanism for the development of these complications is not known, reduced ADAMTS13 activity may contribute to cardiovascular risk. Further studies investigating this relationship as well as other potential mechanisms leading to the development of these chronic complications are warranted.

8. Conclusions/Summary

TTP is a life-threatening illness which requires prompt recognition and management given its high mortality if left untreated. Acute management and long-term follow-up are evolving as new therapies and potential biomarkers emerge. Given the rarity of this disease, TTP registries and multicenter cohort studies are critical to continue advancing the field.

Author Contributions: S.S. conducted the literature review and drafted the manuscript. B.L. critically reviewed and edited the manuscript. S.R.C. critically reviewed and edited the manuscript. All authors have read and agreed to the published version of the manuscript.

Funding: This review article received no external funding.

Institutional Review Board Statement: Not applicable.

Informed Consent Statement: Not applicable.

Data Availability Statement: Not applicable.

Conflicts of Interest: S.S. has no conflict of interest; B.L. is chairman of the Data Safety Monitoring Committees for studies on recombinant ADAMTS13 in congenital and acquired TTP (now run by Takeda); he is on the Advisory Board of Sanofi for the development of caplacizumab for acquired TTP; he received congress travel support and/or lecture fees from Ablynx, Alexion, Siemens, Bayer, Roche, and Sanofi; S.R.C. has received research funding and consulting/speaking fees from Sanofi-Genzyme and Takeda.

References

1. Moschcowitz, E. Hyaline Thrombosis of the Terminal Arterioles and Capillaries: A Hitherto Undescribed Disease. *Proc. N. Y. Pathol. Soc.* **1924**, *24*, 21–24.
2. Moschowitz, E. An acute febrile pleiochromic anemia with hyaline thrombosis of the terminal arterioles and capillaries: An undescribed disease. *Arch. Intern. Med.* **1925**, *36*, 89–93. [CrossRef]
3. Singer, K.; Bornstein, F.P.; Wile, S.A. Thrombotic thrombocytopenic purpura; hemorrhagic diathesis with generalized platelet thromboses. *Blood* **1947**, *2*, 542–554. [CrossRef] [PubMed]
4. Amorosi, E.L.; Ultmann, J.E. Thrombotic Thrombocytopenic Pupura: Report of 16 cases and Review of the Literature. *Medicine* **1966**, *45*, 139–159. [CrossRef]
5. Byrnes, J.J.; Khurana, M. Treatment of thrombotic thrombocytopenic purpura with plasma. *N. Engl. J. Med.* **1977**, *297*, 1386–1389. [CrossRef] [PubMed]
6. Upshaw, J.D. Congenital deficiency of a factor in normal plasma that reverses microangiopathic hemolysis and thrombocytopenia. *N. Engl. J. Med.* **1978**, *298*, 1350–1352. [CrossRef]
7. Moake, J.L.; Rudy, C.K.; Troll, J.H.; Weinstein, M.J.; Colannino, N.M.; Azocar, J.; Seder, R.H.; Hong, S.L.; Deykin, D. Unusually large plasma factor VIII:von Willebrand factor multimers in chronic relapsing thrombotic thrombocytopenic purpura. *N. Engl. J. Med.* **1982**, *307*, 1432–1435. [CrossRef]
8. Rock, G.A.; Shumak, K.H.; Buskard, N.A.; Blanchette, V.S.; Kelton, J.G.; Nair, R.C.; Spasoff, R.A. Comparison of plasma exchange with plasma infusion in the treatment of thrombotic thrombocytopenic purpura. Canadian Apheresis Study Group. *N. Engl. J. Med.* **1991**, *325*, 393–397. [CrossRef]
9. Furlan, M.; Robles, R.; Lämmle, B. Partial purification and characterization of a protease from human plasma cleaving von Willebrand factor to fragments produced by in vivo proteolysis. *Blood* **1996**, *87*, 4223–4234. [CrossRef]
10. Tsai, H.M. Physiologic cleavage of von Willebrand factor by a plasma protease is dependent on its conformation and requires calcium ion. *Blood* **1996**, *87*, 4235–4244. [CrossRef]
11. Furlan, M.; Robles, R.; Galbusera, M.; Remuzzi, G.; Kyrle, P.A.; Brenner, B.; Krause, M.; Scharrer, I.; Aumann, V.; Mittler, U.; et al. von Willebrand factor-cleaving protease in thrombotic thrombocytopenic purpura and the hemolytic-uremic syndrome. *N. Engl. J. Med.* **1998**, *339*, 1578–1584. [CrossRef] [PubMed]
12. Tsai, H.M.; Lian, E.C. Antibodies to von Willebrand factor-cleaving protease in acute thrombotic thrombocytopenic purpura. *N. Engl. J. Med.* **1998**, *339*, 1585–1594. [CrossRef] [PubMed]
13. Soejima, K.; Mimura, N.; Hirashima, M.; Maeda, H.; Hamamoto, T.; Nakagaki, T.; Nozaki, C. A novel human metalloprotease synthesized in the liver and secreted into the blood: Possibly, the von Willebrand factor-cleaving protease? *J. Biochem.* **2001**, *130*, 475–480. [CrossRef] [PubMed]
14. Levy, G.G.; Nichols, W.C.; Lian, E.C.; Foroud, T.; McClintick, J.N.; McGee, B.M.; Yang, A.Y.; Siemieniak, D.R.; Stark, K.R.; Gruppo, R.; et al. Mutations in a member of the ADAMTS gene family cause thrombotic thrombocytopenic purpura. *Nature* **2001**, *413*, 488–494. [CrossRef] [PubMed]
15. Gerritsen, H.E.; Robles, R.; Lämmle, B.; Furlan, M. Partial amino acid sequence of purified von Willebrand factor-cleaving protease. *Blood* **2001**, *98*, 1654–1661. [CrossRef]
16. Fujikawa, K.; Suzuki, H.; McMullen, B.; Chung, D. Purification of human von Willebrand factor-cleaving protease and its identification as a new member of the metalloproteinase family. *Blood* **2001**, *98*, 1662–1666. [CrossRef]
17. Zheng, X.; Chung, D.; Takayama, T.K.; Majerus, E.M.; Sadler, J.E.; Fujikawa, K. Structure of von Willebrand factor-cleaving protease (ADAMTS13), a metalloprotease involved in thrombotic thrombocytopenic purpura. *J. Biol. Chem.* **2001**, *276*, 41059–41063. [CrossRef]
18. Roose, E.; Schelpe, A.S.; Tellier, E.; Sinkovits, G.; Joly, B.S.; Dekimpe, C.; Kaplanski, G.; Le Besnerais, M.; Mancini, I.; Falter, T.; et al. Open ADAMTS13, induced by antibodies, is a biomarker for subclinical immune-mediated thrombotic thrombocytopenic purpura. *Blood* **2020**, *136*, 353–361. [CrossRef]
19. Cataland, S.R.; Jin, M.; Ferketich, A.K.; Kennedy, M.S.; Kraut, E.H.; George, J.N.; Wu, H.M. An evaluation of cyclosporin and corticosteroids individually as adjuncts to plasma exchange in the treatment of thrombotic thrombocytopenic purpura. *Br. J. Haematol.* **2007**, *136*, 146–149. [CrossRef]

20. Froissart, A.; Buffet, M.; Veyradier, A.; Poullin, P.; Provôt, F.; Malot, S.; Schwarzinger, M.; Galicier, L.; Vanhille, P.; Vernant, J.P.; et al. Efficacy and safety of first-line rituximab in severe, acquired thrombotic thrombocytopenic purpura with a suboptimal response to plasma exchange. Experience of the French Thrombotic Microangiopathies Reference Center. *Crit. Care Med.* **2012**, *40*, 104–111. [CrossRef]
21. Peyvandi, F.; Scully, M.; Kremer Hovinga, J.A.; Cataland, S.; Knöbl, P.; Wu, H.; Artoni, A.; Westwood, J.P.; Mansouri Taleghani, M.; Jilma, B.; et al. Caplacizumab for Acquired Thrombotic Thrombocytopenic Purpura. *N. Engl. J. Med.* **2016**, *374*, 511–522. [CrossRef] [PubMed]
22. Scully, M.; Cataland, S.R.; Peyvandi, F.; Coppo, P.; Knöbl, P.; Kremer Hovinga, J.A.; Metjian, A.; de la Rubia, J.; Pavenski, K.; Callewaert, F.; et al. Caplacizumab Treatment for Acquired Thrombotic Thrombocytopenic Purpura. *N. Engl. J. Med.* **2019**, *380*, 335–346. [CrossRef] [PubMed]
23. Page, E.E.; Kremer Hovinga, J.A.; Terrell, D.R.; Vesely, S.K.; George, J.N. Thrombotic thrombocytopenic purpura: Diagnostic criteria, clinical features, and long-term outcomes from 1995 through 2015. *Blood Adv.* **2017**, *1*, 590–600. [CrossRef] [PubMed]
24. Deford, C.C.; Reese, J.A.; Schwartz, L.H.; Perdue, J.J.; Kremer Hovinga, J.A.; Lämmle, B.; Terrell, D.R.; Vesely, S.K.; George, J.N. Multiple major morbidities and increased mortality during long-term follow-up after recovery from thrombotic thrombocytopenic purpura. *Blood* **2013**, *122*, 2023–2029. [CrossRef] [PubMed]
25. Kremer Hovinga, J.A.; Vesely, S.K.; Terrell, D.R.; Lämmle, B.; George, J.N. Survival and relapse in patients with thrombotic thrombocytopenic purpura. *Blood* **2010**, *115*, 1500–1511. [CrossRef]
26. Moake, J.L. Thrombotic microangiopathies. *N. Engl. J. Med.* **2002**, *347*, 589–600. [CrossRef]
27. Scully, M.; Cataland, S.; Coppo, P.; de la Rubia, J.; Friedman, K.D.; Kremer Hovinga, J.; Lämmle, B.; Matsumoto, M.; Pavenski, K.; Sadler, E.; et al. Consensus on the standardization of terminology in thrombotic thrombocytopenic purpura and related thrombotic microangiopathies. *J. Thromb. Haemost.* **2017**, *15*, 312–322. [CrossRef]
28. Sarode, R.; Bandarenko, N.; Brecher, M.E.; Kiss, J.E.; Marques, M.B.; Szczepiorkowski, Z.M.; Winters, J.L. Thrombotic thrombocytopenic purpura: 2012 American Society for Apheresis (ASFA) consensus conference on classification, diagnosis, management, and future research. *J. Clin. Apher.* **2014**, *29*, 148–167. [CrossRef]
29. Mariotte, E.; Azoulay, E.; Galicier, L.; Rondeau, E.; Zouiti, F.; Boisseau, P.; Poullin, P.; de Maistre, E.; Provôt, F.; Delmas, Y.; et al. Epidemiology and pathophysiology of adulthood-onset thrombotic microangiopathy with severe ADAMTS13 deficiency (thrombotic thrombocytopenic purpura): A cross-sectional analysis of the French national registry for thrombotic microangiopathy. *Lancet Haematol.* **2016**, *3*, e237–e245. [CrossRef]
30. Scully, M.; Yarranton, H.; Liesner, R.; Cavenagh, J.; Hunt, B.; Benjamin, S.; Bevan, D.; Mackie, I.; Machin, S. Regional UK TTP registry: Correlation with laboratory ADAMTS 13 analysis and clinical features. *Br. J. Haematol.* **2008**, *142*, 819–826. [CrossRef]
31. Reese, J.A.; Muthurajah, D.S.; Kremer Hovinga, J.A.; Vesely, S.K.; Terrell, D.R.; George, J.N. Children and adults with thrombotic thrombocytopenic purpura associated with severe, acquired Adamts13 deficiency: Comparison of incidence, demographic and clinical features. *Pediatr. Blood Cancer* **2013**, *60*, 1676–1682. [CrossRef] [PubMed]
32. Miesbach, W.; Menne, J.; Bommer, M.; Schönermarck, U.; Feldkamp, T.; Nitschke, M.; Westhoff, T.H.; Seibert, F.S.; Woitas, R.; Sousa, R.; et al. Incidence of acquired thrombotic thrombocytopenic purpura in Germany: A hospital level study. *Orphanet. J. Rare Dis.* **2019**, *14*, 260. [CrossRef] [PubMed]
33. Martino, S.; Jamme, M.; Deligny, C.; Busson, M.; Loiseau, P.; Azoulay, E.; Galicier, L.; Pène, F.; Provôt, F.; Dossier, A.; et al. Thrombotic Thrombocytopenic Purpura in Black People: Impact of Ethnicity on Survival and Genetic Risk Factors. *PLoS ONE* **2016**, *11*, e0156679. [CrossRef] [PubMed]
34. Joly, B.S.; Stepanian, A.; Leblanc, T.; Hajage, D.; Chambost, H.; Harambat, J.; Fouyssac, F.; Guigonis, V.; Leverger, G.; Ulinski, T.; et al. Child-onset and adolescent-onset acquired thrombotic thrombocytopenic purpura with severe ADAMTS13 deficiency: A cohort study of the French national registry for thrombotic microangiopathy. *Lancet Haematol.* **2016**, *3*, e537–e546. [CrossRef]
35. Blombery, P.; Kivivali, L.; Pepperell, D.; McQuilten, Z.; Engelbrecht, S.; Polizzotto, M.N.; Phillips, L.E.; Wood, E.; Cohney, S. Diagnosis and management of thrombotic thrombocytopenic purpura (TTP) in Australia: Findings from the first 5 years of the Australian TTP/thrombotic microangiopathy registry. *Intern. Med. J.* **2016**, *46*, 71–79. [CrossRef]
36. Fujimura, Y.; Matsumoto, M. Registry of 919 patients with thrombotic microangiopathies across Japan: Database of Nara Medical University during 1998–2008. *Intern. Med.* **2010**, *49*, 7–15. [CrossRef]
37. Jang, M.J.; Chong, S.Y.; Kim, I.H.; Kim, J.H.; Jung, C.W.; Kim, J.Y.; Park, J.C.; Lee, S.M.; Kim, Y.K.; Lee, J.E.; et al. Clinical features of severe acquired ADAMTS13 deficiency in thrombotic thrombocytopenic purpura: The Korean TTP registry experience. *Int. J. Hematol.* **2011**, *93*, 163–169. [CrossRef]
38. Kremer Hovinga, J.A.; George, J.N. Hereditary Thrombotic Thrombocytopenic Purpura. *N. Engl. J. Med.* **2019**, *381*, 1653–1662. [CrossRef]
39. Joly, B.S.; Boisseau, P.; Roose, E.; Stepanian, A.; Biebuyck, N.; Hogan, J.; Provot, F.; Delmas, Y.; Garrec, C.; Vanhoorelbeke, K.; et al. ADAMTS13 Gene Mutations Influence ADAMTS13 Conformation and Disease Age-Onset in the French Cohort of Upshaw-Schulman Syndrome. *Thromb. Haemost.* **2018**, *118*, 1902–1917. [CrossRef]
40. Fujimura, Y.; Matsumoto, M.; Isonishi, A.; Yagi, H.; Kokame, K.; Soejima, K.; Murata, M.; Miyata, T. Natural history of Upshaw-Schulman syndrome based on ADAMTS13 gene analysis in Japan. *J. Thromb. Haemost.* **2011**, *9* (Suppl. 1), 283–301. [CrossRef]

41. Alwan, F.; Vendramin, C.; Liesner, R.; Clark, A.; Lester, W.; Dutt, T.; Thomas, W.; Gooding, R.; Biss, T.; Watson, H.G.; et al. Characterization and treatment of congenital thrombotic thrombocytopenic purpura. *Blood* **2019**, *133*, 1644–1651. [CrossRef] [PubMed]
42. van Dorland, H.A.; Taleghani, M.M.; Sakai, K.; Friedman, K.D.; George, J.N.; Hrachovinova, I.; Knöbl, P.N.; von Krogh, A.S.; Schneppenheim, R.; Aebi-Huber, I.; et al. The International Hereditary Thrombotic Thrombocytopenic Purpura Registry: Key findings at enrollment until 2017. *Haematologica* **2019**, *104*, 2107–2115. [CrossRef] [PubMed]
43. Zhou, W.; Inada, M.; Lee, T.P.; Benten, D.; Lyubsky, S.; Bouhassira, E.E.; Gupta, S.; Tsai, H.M. ADAMTS13 is expressed in hepatic stellate cells. *Lab. Investig.* **2005**, *85*, 780–788. [CrossRef] [PubMed]
44. Uemura, M.; Tatsumi, K.; Matsumoto, M.; Fujimoto, M.; Matsuyama, T.; Ishikawa, M.; Iwamoto, T.A.; Mori, T.; Wanaka, A.; Fukui, H.; et al. Localization of ADAMTS13 to the stellate cells of human liver. *Blood* **2005**, *106*, 922–924. [CrossRef] [PubMed]
45. South, K.; Luken, B.M.; Crawley, J.T.; Phillips, R.; Thomas, M.; Collins, R.F.; Deforche, L.; Vanhoorelbeke, K.; Lane, D.A. Conformational activation of ADAMTS13. *Proc. Natl. Acad. Sci. USA* **2014**, *111*, 18578–18583. [CrossRef] [PubMed]
46. Deforche, L.; Roose, E.; Vandenbulcke, A.; Vandeputte, N.; Feys, H.B.; Springer, T.A.; Mi, L.Z.; Muia, J.; Sadler, J.E.; Soejima, K.; et al. Linker regions and flexibility around the metalloprotease domain account for conformational activation of ADAMTS-13. *J. Thromb. Haemost.* **2015**, *13*, 2063–2075. [CrossRef] [PubMed]
47. Muia, J.; Zhu, J.; Gupta, G.; Haberichter, S.L.; Friedman, K.D.; Feys, H.B.; Deforche, L.; Vanhoorelbeke, K.; Westfield, L.A.; Roth, R.; et al. Allosteric activation of ADAMTS13 by von Willebrand factor. *Proc. Natl. Acad. Sci. USA* **2014**, *111*, 18584–18589. [CrossRef]
48. Dong, J.F.; Moake, J.L.; Nolasco, L.; Bernardo, A.; Arceneaux, W.; Shrimpton, C.N.; Schade, A.J.; McIntire, L.V.; Fujikawa, K.; López, J.A. ADAMTS-13 rapidly cleaves newly secreted ultralarge von Willebrand factor multimers on the endothelial surface under flowing conditions. *Blood* **2002**, *100*, 4033–4039. [CrossRef]
49. Zanardelli, S.; Chion, A.C.; Groot, E.; Lenting, P.J.; McKinnon, T.A.; Laffan, M.A.; Tseng, M.; Lane, D.A. A novel binding site for ADAMTS13 constitutively exposed on the surface of globular VWF. *Blood* **2009**, *114*, 2819–2828. [CrossRef]
50. Zhang, X.; Halvorsen, K.; Zhang, C.Z.; Wong, W.P.; Springer, T.A. Mechanoenzymatic cleavage of the ultralarge vascular protein von Willebrand factor. *Science* **2009**, *324*, 1330–1334. [CrossRef]
51. Sixma, J.J.; van Zanten, G.H.; Huizinga, E.G.; van der Plas, R.M.; Verkley, M.; Wu, Y.P.; Gros, P.; de Groot, P.G. Platelet adhesion to collagen: An update. *Thromb. Haemost.* **1997**, *78*, 434–438. [CrossRef] [PubMed]
52. Savage, B.; Almus-Jacobs, F.; Ruggeri, Z.M. Specific synergy of multiple substrate-receptor interactions in platelet thrombus formation under flow. *Cell* **1998**, *94*, 657–666. [CrossRef]
53. Moroi, M.; Jung, S.M.; Nomura, S.; Sekiguchi, S.; Ordinas, A.; Diaz-Ricart, M. Analysis of the involvement of the von Willebrand factor-glycoprotein Ib interaction in platelet adhesion to a collagen-coated surface under flow conditions. *Blood* **1997**, *90*, 4413–4424. [CrossRef] [PubMed]
54. Petri, A.; Kim, H.J.; Xu, Y.; de Groot, R.; Li, C.; Vandenbulcke, A.; Vanhoorelbeke, K.; Emsley, J.; Crawley, J.T.B. Crystal structure and substrate-induced activation of ADAMTS13. *Nat. Commun.* **2019**, *10*, 3781. [CrossRef] [PubMed]
55. Jin, M.; Casper, T.C.; Cataland, S.R.; Kennedy, M.S.; Lin, S.; Li, Y.J.; Wu, H.M. Relationship between ADAMTS13 activity in clinical remission and the risk of TTP relapse. *Br. J. Haematol.* **2008**, *141*, 651–658. [CrossRef] [PubMed]
56. Peyvandi, F.; Lavoretano, S.; Palla, R.; Feys, H.B.; Vanhoorelbeke, K.; Battaglioli, T.; Valsecchi, C.; Canciani, M.T.; Fabris, F.; Zver, S.; et al. ADAMTS13 and anti-ADAMTS13 antibodies as markers for recurrence of acquired thrombotic thrombocytopenic purpura during remission. *Haematologica* **2008**, *93*, 232–239. [CrossRef]
57. Furlan, M.; Lämmle, B. Aetiology and pathogenesis of thrombotic thrombocytopenic purpura and haemolytic uraemic syndrome: The role of von Willebrand factor-cleaving protease. *Best Pract. Res. Clin. Haematol.* **2001**, *14*, 437–454. [CrossRef]
58. Page, E.E.; Kremer Hovinga, J.A.; Terrell, D.R.; Vesely, S.K.; George, J.N. Clinical importance of ADAMTS13 activity during remission in patients with acquired thrombotic thrombocytopenic purpura. *Blood* **2016**, *128*, 2175–2178. [CrossRef]
59. Réti, M.; Farkas, P.; Csuka, D.; Rázsó, K.; Schlammadinger, Á.; Udvardy, M.L.; Madách, K.; Domján, G.; Bereczki, C.; Reusz, G.S.; et al. Complement activation in thrombotic thrombocytopenic purpura. *J. Thromb. Haemost.* **2012**, *10*, 791–798. [CrossRef]
60. Wu, T.C.; Yang, S.; Haven, S.; Holers, V.M.; Lundberg, A.S.; Wu, H.; Cataland, S.R. Complement activation and mortality during an acute episode of thrombotic thrombocytopenic purpura. *J. Thromb. Haemost.* **2013**, *11*, 1925–1927. [CrossRef]
61. Turner, N.; Sartain, S.; Moake, J. Ultralarge von Willebrand factor-induced platelet clumping and activation of the alternative complement pathway in thrombotic thrombocytopenic purpura and the hemolytic-uremic syndromes. *Hematol. Oncol. Clin. N. Am.* **2015**, *29*, 509–524. [CrossRef] [PubMed]
62. Feng, S.; Liang, X.; Kroll, M.H.; Chung, D.W.; Afshar-Kharghan, V. von Willebrand factor is a cofactor in complement regulation. *Blood* **2015**, *125*, 1034–1037. [CrossRef] [PubMed]
63. Wu, H.; Jay, L.; Lin, S.; Han, C.; Yang, S.; Cataland, S.R.; Masias, C. Interrelationship between ADAMTS13 activity, von Willebrand factor, and complement activation in remission from immune-mediated trhrombotic thrombocytopenic purpura. *Br. J. Haematol.* **2020**, *189*, e18–e20. [CrossRef] [PubMed]
64. Zheng, L.; Zhang, D.; Cao, W.; Song, W.C.; Zheng, X.L. Synergistic effects of ADAMTS13 deficiency and complement activation in pathogenesis of thrombotic microangiopathy. *Blood* **2019**, *134*, 1095–1105. [CrossRef] [PubMed]
65. Miyata, T.; Fan, X. A second hit for TMA. *Blood* **2012**, *120*, 1152–1154. [CrossRef]

66. Fuchs, T.A.; Kremer Hovinga, J.A.; Schatzberg, D.; Wagner, D.D.; Lämmle, B. Circulating DNA and myeloperoxidase indicate disease activity in patients with thrombotic microangiopathies. *Blood* **2012**, *120*, 1157–1164. [CrossRef]
67. Lotta, L.A.; Garagiola, I.; Palla, R.; Cairo, A.; Peyvandi, F. ADAMTS13 mutations and polymorphisms in congenital thrombotic thrombocytopenic purpura. *Hum. Mutat.* **2010**, *31*, 11–19. [CrossRef]
68. Kremer Hovinga, J.A.; Heeb, S.R.; Skowronska, M.; Schaller, M. Pathophysiology of thrombotic thrombocytopenic purpura and hemolytic uremic syndrome. *J. Thromb. Haemost.* **2018**, *16*, 618–629. [CrossRef]
69. von Krogh, A.S.; Quist-Paulsen, P.; Waage, A.; Langseth, Ø.; Thorstensen, K.; Brudevold, R.; Tjønnfjord, G.E.; Largiadèr, C.R.; Lämmle, B.; Kremer Hovinga, J.A. High prevalence of hereditary thrombotic thrombocytopenic purpura in central Norway: From clinical observation to evidence. *J. Thromb. Haemost.* **2016**, *14*, 73–82. [CrossRef]
70. Scully, M.; Thomas, M.; Underwood, M.; Watson, H.; Langley, K.; Camilleri, R.S.; Clark, A.; Creagh, D.; Rayment, R.; Mcdonald, V.; et al. Thrombotic thrombocytopenic purpura and pregnancy: Presentation, management, and subsequent pregnancy outcomes. *Blood* **2014**, *124*, 211–219. [CrossRef]
71. Moatti-Cohen, M.; Garrec, C.; Wolf, M.; Boisseau, P.; Galicier, L.; Azoulay, E.; Stepanian, A.; Delmas, Y.; Rondeau, E.; Bezieau, S.; et al. Unexpected frequency of Upshaw-Schulman syndrome in pregnancy-onset thrombotic thrombocytopenic purpura. *Blood* **2012**, *119*, 5888–5897. [CrossRef] [PubMed]
72. Camilleri, R.S.; Cohen, H.; Mackie, I.J.; Scully, M.; Starke, R.D.; Crawley, J.T.; Lane, D.A.; Machin, S.J. Prevalence of the ADAMTS-13 missense mutation R1060W in late onset adult thrombotic thrombocytopenic purpura. *J. Thromb. Haemost.* **2008**, *6*, 331–338. [CrossRef] [PubMed]
73. Schneppenheim, R.; Kremer Hovinga, J.A.; Becker, T.; Budde, U.; Karpman, D.; Brockhaus, W.; Hrachovinová, I.; Korczowski, B.; Oyen, F.; Rittich, S.; et al. A common origin of the 4143insA ADAMTS13 mutation. *Thromb. Haemost.* **2006**, *96*, 3–6. [CrossRef] [PubMed]
74. Lotta, L.A.; Wu, H.M.; Mackie, I.J.; Noris, M.; Veyradier, A.; Scully, M.A.; Remuzzi, G.; Coppo, P.; Liesner, R.; Donadelli, R.; et al. Residual plasmatic activity of ADAMTS13 is correlated with phenotype severity in congenital thrombotic thrombocytopenic purpura. *Blood* **2012**, *120*, 440–448. [CrossRef]
75. Kokame, K.; Matsumoto, M.; Soejima, K.; Yagi, H.; Ishizashi, H.; Funato, M.; Tamai, H.; Konno, M.; Kamide, K.; Kawano, Y.; et al. Mutations and common polymorphisms in ADAMTS13 gene responsible for von Willebrand factor-cleaving protease activity. *Proc. Natl. Acad. Sci. USA* **2002**, *99*, 11902–11907. [CrossRef]
76. Plaimauer, B.; Fuhrmann, J.; Mohr, G.; Wernhart, W.; Bruno, K.; Ferrari, S.; Konetschny, C.; Antoine, G.; Rieger, M.; Scheiflinger, F. Modulation of ADAMTS13 secretion and specific activity by a combination of common amino acid polymorphisms and a missense mutation. *Blood* **2006**, *107*, 118–125. [CrossRef]
77. Coppo, P.; Busson, M.; Veyradier, A.; Wynckel, A.; Poullin, P.; Azoulay, E.; Galicier, L.; Loiseau, P.; Microangiopathies, F.R.C.F.T. HLA-DRB1*11: A strong risk factor for acquired severe ADAMTS13 deficiency-related idiopathic thrombotic thrombocytopenic purpura in Caucasians. *J. Thromb. Haemost.* **2010**, *8*, 856–859. [CrossRef]
78. Scully, M.; Brown, J.; Patel, R.; McDonald, V.; Brown, C.J.; Machin, S. Human leukocyte antigen association in idiopathic thrombotic thrombocytopenic purpura: Evidence for an immunogenetic link. *J. Thromb. Haemost.* **2010**, *8*, 257–262. [CrossRef]
79. John, M.L.; Hitzler, W.; Scharrer, I. The role of human leukocyte antigens as predisposing and/or protective factors in patients with idiopathic thrombotic thrombocytopenic purpura. *Ann. Hematol.* **2012**, *91*, 507–510. [CrossRef]
80. Mancini, I.; Giacomini, E.; Pontiggia, S.; Artoni, A.; Ferrari, B.; Pappalardo, E.; Gualtierotti, R.; Trisolini, S.M.; Capria, S.; Facchini, L.; et al. The HLA Variant rs6903608 Is Associated with Disease Onset and Relapse of Immune-Mediated Thrombotic Thrombocytopenic Purpura in Caucasians. *J. Clin. Med.* **2020**, *9*, 3379. [CrossRef]
81. Sakai, K.; Kuwana, M.; Tanaka, H.; Hosomichi, K.; Hasegawa, A.; Uyama, H.; Nishio, K.; Omae, T.; Hishizawa, M.; Matsui, M.; et al. HLA loci predisposing to immune TTP in Japanese: Potential role of the shared ADAMTS13 peptide bound to different HLA-DR. *Blood* **2020**, *135*, 2413–2419. [CrossRef] [PubMed]
82. Scheiflinger, F.; Knöbl, P.; Trattner, B.; Plaimauer, B.; Mohr, G.; Dockal, M.; Dorner, F.; Rieger, M. Nonneutralizing IgM and IgG antibodies to von Willebrand factor-cleaving protease (ADAMTS-13) in a patient with thrombotic thrombocytopenic purpura. *Blood* **2003**, *102*, 3241–3243. [CrossRef] [PubMed]
83. Rieger, M.; Mannucci, P.M.; Kremer Hovinga, J.A.; Herzog, A.; Gerstenbauer, G.; Konetschny, C.; Zimmermann, K.; Scharrer, I.; Peyvandi, F.; Galbusera, M.; et al. ADAMTS13 autoantibodies in patients with thrombotic microangiopathies and other immunomediated diseases. *Blood* **2005**, *106*, 1262–1267. [CrossRef] [PubMed]
84. Feys, H.B.; Liu, F.; Dong, N.; Pareyn, I.; Vauterin, S.; Vandeputte, N.; Noppe, W.; Ruan, C.; Deckmyn, H.; Vanhoorelbeke, K. ADAMTS-13 plasma level determination uncovers antigen absence in acquired thrombotic thrombocytopenic purpura and ethnic differences. *J. Thromb. Haemost.* **2006**, *4*, 955–962. [CrossRef]
85. Thomas, M.R.; de Groot, R.; Scully, M.A.; Crawley, J.T. Pathogenicity of Anti-ADAMTS13 Autoantibodies in Acquired Thrombotic Thrombocytopenic Purpura. *EBioMedicine* **2015**, *2*, 942–952. [CrossRef] [PubMed]
86. Luken, B.M.; Turenhout, E.A.; Hulstein, J.J.; Van Mourik, J.A.; Fijnheer, R.; Voorberg, J. The spacer domain of ADAMTS13 contains a major binding site for antibodies in patients with thrombotic thrombocytopenic purpura. *Thromb. Haemost.* **2005**, *93*, 267–274. [CrossRef]

87. Soejima, K.; Matsumoto, M.; Kokame, K.; Yagi, H.; Ishizashi, H.; Maeda, H.; Nozaki, C.; Miyata, T.; Fujimura, Y.; Nakagaki, T. ADAMTS-13 cysteine-rich/spacer domains are functionally essential for von Willebrand factor cleavage. *Blood* **2003**, *102*, 3232–3237. [CrossRef]
88. Klaus, C.; Plaimauer, B.; Studt, J.D.; Dorner, F.; Lämmle, B.; Mannucci, P.M.; Scheiflinger, F. Epitope mapping of ADAMTS13 autoantibodies in acquired thrombotic thrombocytopenic purpura. *Blood* **2004**, *103*, 4514–4519. [CrossRef]
89. Zheng, X.L.; Wu, H.M.; Shang, D.; Falls, E.; Skipwith, C.G.; Cataland, S.R.; Bennett, C.L.; Kwaan, H.C. Multiple domains of ADAMTS13 are targeted by autoantibodies against ADAMTS13 in patients with acquired idiopathic thrombotic thrombocytopenic purpura. *Haematologica* **2010**, *95*, 1555–1562. [CrossRef]
90. Yamaguchi, Y.; Moriki, T.; Igari, A.; Nakagawa, T.; Wada, H.; Matsumoto, M.; Fujimura, Y.; Murata, M. Epitope analysis of autoantibodies to ADAMTS13 in patients with acquired thrombotic thrombocytopenic purpura. *Thromb. Res.* **2011**, *128*, 169–173. [CrossRef]
91. Pos, W.; Sorvillo, N.; Fijnheer, R.; Feys, H.B.; Kaijen, P.H.; Vidarsson, G.; Voorberg, J. Residues Arg568 and Phe592 contribute to an antigenic surface for anti-ADAMTS13 antibodies in the spacer domain. *Haematologica* **2011**, *96*, 1670–1677. [CrossRef] [PubMed]
92. Grillberger, R.; Casina, V.C.; Turecek, P.L.; Zheng, X.L.; Rottensteiner, H.; Scheiflinger, F. Anti-ADAMTS13 IgG autoantibodies present in healthy individuals share linear epitopes with those in patients with thrombotic thrombocytopenic purpura. *Haematologica* **2014**, *99*, e58–e60. [CrossRef] [PubMed]
93. Roose, E.; Schelpe, A.S.; Joly, B.S.; Peetermans, M.; Verhamme, P.; Voorberg, J.; Greinacher, A.; Deckmyn, H.; De Meyer, S.F.; Coppo, P.; et al. An open conformation of ADAMTS-13 is a hallmark of acute acquired thrombotic thrombocytopenic purpura. *J. Thromb. Haemost.* **2018**, *16*, 378–388. [CrossRef] [PubMed]
94. Ferrari, S.; Scheiflinger, F.; Rieger, M.; Mudde, G.; Wolf, M.; Coppo, P.; Girma, J.P.; Azoulay, E.; Brun-Buisson, C.; Fakhouri, F.; et al. Prognostic value of anti-ADAMTS 13 antibody features (Ig isotype, titer, and inhibitory effect) in a cohort of 35 adult French patients undergoing a first episode of thrombotic microangiopathy with undetectable ADAMTS 13 activity. *Blood* **2007**, *109*, 2815–2822. [CrossRef] [PubMed]
95. Ferrari, S.; Mudde, G.C.; Rieger, M.; Veyradier, A.; Kremer Hovinga, J.A.; Scheiflinger, F. IgG subclass distribution of anti-ADAMTS13 antibodies in patients with acquired thrombotic thrombocytopenic purpura. *J. Thromb. Haemost.* **2009**, *7*, 1703–1710. [CrossRef]
96. Bettoni, G.; Palla, R.; Valsecchi, C.; Consonni, D.; Lotta, L.A.; Trisolini, S.M.; Mancini, I.; Musallam, K.M.; Rosendaal, F.R.; Peyvandi, F. ADAMTS-13 activity and autoantibodies classes and subclasses as prognostic predictors in acquired thrombotic thrombocytopenic purpura. *J. Thromb. Haemost.* **2012**, *10*, 1556–1565. [CrossRef]
97. Hrdinová, J.; D'Angelo, S.; Graça, N.A.G.; Ercig, B.; Vanhoorelbeke, K.; Veyradier, A.; Voorberg, J.; Coppo, P. Dissecting the pathophysiology of immune thrombotic thrombocytopenic purpura: Interplay between genes and environmental triggers. *Haematologica* **2018**, *103*, 1099–1109. [CrossRef]
98. Luken, B.M.; Kaijen, P.H.; Turenhout, E.A.; Kremer Hovinga, J.A.; van Mourik, J.A.; Fijnheer, R.; Voorberg, J. Multiple B-cell clones producing antibodies directed to the spacer and disintegrin/thrombospondin type-1 repeat 1 (TSP1) of ADAMTS13 in a patient with acquired thrombotic thrombocytopenic purpura. *J. Thromb. Haemost.* **2006**, *4*, 2355–2364. [CrossRef]
99. Kosugi, N.; Tsurutani, Y.; Isonishi, A.; Hori, Y.; Matsumoto, M.; Fujimura, Y. Influenza A infection triggers thrombotic thrombocytopenic purpura by producing the anti-ADAMTS13 IgG inhibitor. *Intern. Med.* **2010**, *49*, 689–693. [CrossRef]
100. Franchini, M. Thrombotic thrombocytopenic purpura: Proposal of a new pathogenic mechanism involving Helicobacter pylori infection. *Med. Hypotheses* **2005**, *65*, 1128–1131. [CrossRef]
101. Talebi, T.; Fernandez-Castro, G.; Montero, A.J.; Stefanovic, A.; Lian, E. A case of severe thrombotic thrombocytopenic purpura with concomitant Legionella pneumonia: Review of pathogenesis and treatment. *Am. J. Ther.* **2011**, *18*, e180–e185. [CrossRef] [PubMed]
102. Yagita, M.; Uemura, M.; Nakamura, T.; Kunitomi, A.; Matsumoto, M.; Fujimura, Y. Development of ADAMTS13 inhibitor in a patient with hepatitis C virus-related liver cirrhosis causes thrombotic thrombocytopenic purpura. *J. Hepatol.* **2005**, *42*, 420–421. [CrossRef] [PubMed]
103. Gunther, K.; Garizio, D.; Nesara, P. ADAMTS13 activity and the presence of acquired inhibitors in human immunodeficiency virus-related thrombotic thrombocytopenic purpura. *Transfusion* **2007**, *47*, 1710–1716. [CrossRef] [PubMed]
104. Verbij, F.C.; Fijnheer, R.; Voorberg, J.; Sorvillo, N. Acquired TTP: ADAMTS13 meets the immune system. *Blood Rev.* **2014**, *28*, 227–234. [CrossRef] [PubMed]
105. Lotta, L.A.; Valsecchi, C.; Pontiggia, S.; Mancini, I.; Cannavò, A.; Artoni, A.; Mikovic, D.; Meloni, G.; Peyvandi, F. Measurement and prevalence of circulating ADAMTS13-specific immune complexes in autoimmune thrombotic thrombocytopenic purpura. *J. Thromb. Haemost.* **2014**, *12*, 329–336. [CrossRef]
106. Ferrari, S.; Palavra, K.; Gruber, B.; Kremer Hovinga, J.A.; Knöbl, P.; Caron, C.; Cromwell, C.; Aledort, L.; Plaimauer, B.; Turecek, P.L.; et al. Persistence of circulating ADAMTS13-specific immune complexes in patients with acquired thrombotic thrombocytopenic purpura. *Haematologica* **2014**, *99*, 779–787. [CrossRef]
107. Mancini, I.; Ferrari, B.; Valsecchi, C.; Pontiggia, S.; Fornili, M.; Biganzoli, E.; Peyvandi, F.; Investigators, I.G.o.T. ADAMTS13-specific circulating immune complexes as potential predictors of relapse in patients with acquired thrombotic thrombocytopenic purpura. *Eur. J. Intern. Med.* **2017**, *39*, 79–83. [CrossRef]

108. Westwood, J.P.; Langley, K.; Heelas, E.; Machin, S.J.; Scully, M. Complement and cytokine response in acute Thrombotic Thrombocytopenic Purpura. *Br. J. Haematol.* **2014**, *164*, 858–866. [CrossRef]
109. Hart, D.; Sayer, R.; Miller, R.; Edwards, S.; Kelly, A.; Baglin, T.; Hunt, B.; Benjamin, S.; Patel, R.; Machin, S.; et al. Human immunodeficiency virus associated thrombotic thrombocytopenic purpura–favourable outcome with plasma exchange and prompt initiation of highly active antiretroviral therapy. *Br. J. Haematol.* **2011**, *153*, 515–519. [CrossRef]
110. Malak, S.; Wolf, M.; Millot, G.A.; Mariotte, E.; Veyradier, A.; Meynard, J.L.; Korach, J.M.; Malot, S.; Bussel, A.; Azoulay, E.; et al. Human immunodeficiency virus-associated thrombotic microangiopathies: Clinical characteristics and outcome according to ADAMTS13 activity. *Scand. J. Immunol.* **2008**, *68*, 337–344. [CrossRef]
111. Swisher, K.K.; Doan, J.T.; Vesely, S.K.; Kwaan, H.C.; Kim, B.; Lämmle, B.; Kremer Hovinga, J.A.; George, J.N. Pancreatitis preceding acute episodes of thrombotic thrombocytopenic purpura-hemolytic uremic syndrome: Report of five patients with a systematic review of published reports. *Haematologica* **2007**, *92*, 936–943. [CrossRef] [PubMed]
112. Masias, C.; Vasu, S.; Cataland, S.R. None of the above: Thrombotic microangiopathy beyond TTP and HUS. *Blood* **2017**, *129*, 2857–2863. [CrossRef]
113. Tsai, H.M.; Rice, L.; Sarode, R.; Chow, T.W.; Moake, J.L. Antibody inhibitors to von Willebrand factor metalloproteinase and increased binding of von Willebrand factor to platelets in ticlopidine-associated thrombotic thrombocytopenic purpura. *Ann. Intern. Med.* **2000**, *132*, 794–799. [CrossRef] [PubMed]
114. Jacob, S.; Dunn, B.L.; Qureshi, Z.P.; Bandarenko, N.; Kwaan, H.C.; Pandey, D.K.; McKoy, J.M.; Barnato, S.E.; Winters, J.L.; Cursio, J.F.; et al. Ticlopidine-, clopidogrel-, and prasugrel-associated thrombotic thrombocytopenic purpura: A 20-year review from the Southern Network on Adverse Reactions (SONAR). *Semin. Thromb. Hemost.* **2012**, *38*, 845–853. [CrossRef] [PubMed]
115. Roriz, M.; Landais, M.; Desprez, J.; Barbet, C.; Azoulay, E.; Galicier, L.; Wynckel, A.; Baudel, J.L.; Provôt, F.; Pène, F.; et al. Risk Factors for Autoimmune Diseases Development After Thrombotic Thrombocytopenic Purpura. *Medicine* **2015**, *94*, e1598. [CrossRef]
116. Schattner, A.; Friedman, J.; Klepfish, A. Thrombotic thrombocytopenic purpura as an initial presentation of primary Sjögren's syndrome. *Clin. Rheumatol.* **2002**, *21*, 57–59. [CrossRef]
117. Matsuyama, T.; Kuwana, M.; Matsumoto, M.; Isonishi, A.; Inokuma, S.; Fujimura, Y. Heterogeneous pathogenic processes of thrombotic microangiopathies in patients with connective tissue diseases. *Thromb. Haemost.* **2009**, *102*, 371–378. [CrossRef]
118. George, J.N.; Chen, Q.; Deford, C.C.; Al-Nouri, Z. Ten patient stories illustrating the extraordinarily diverse clinical features of patients with thrombotic thrombocytopenic purpura and severe ADAMTS13 deficiency. *J. Clin. Apher.* **2012**, *27*, 302–311. [CrossRef]
119. George, J.N.; Nester, C.M. Syndromes of thrombotic microangiopathy. *N. Engl. J. Med.* **2014**, *371*, 1847–1848. [CrossRef]
120. Veyradier, A.; Meyer, D. Thrombotic thrombocytopenic purpura and its diagnosis. *J. Thromb. Haemost.* **2005**, *3*, 2420–2427. [CrossRef]
121. Benhamou, Y.; Boelle, P.Y.; Baudin, B.; Ederhy, S.; Gras, J.; Galicier, L.; Azoulay, E.; Provôt, F.; Maury, E.; Pène, F.; et al. Cardiac troponin-I on diagnosis predicts early death and refractoriness in acquired thrombotic thrombocytopenic purpura. Experience of the French Thrombotic Microangiopathies Reference Center. *J. Thromb. Haemost.* **2015**, *13*, 293–302. [CrossRef] [PubMed]
122. Coppo, P.; Schwarzinger, M.; Buffet, M.; Wynckel, A.; Clabault, K.; Presne, C.; Poullin, P.; Malot, S.; Vanhille, P.; Azoulay, E.; et al. Predictive features of severe acquired ADAMTS13 deficiency in idiopathic thrombotic microangiopathies: The French TMA reference center experience. *PLoS ONE* **2010**, *5*, e10208. [CrossRef] [PubMed]
123. Vesely, S.K.; George, J.N.; Lämmle, B.; Studt, J.D.; Alberio, L.; El-Harake, M.A.; Raskob, G.E. ADAMTS13 activity in thrombotic thrombocytopenic purpura-hemolytic uremic syndrome: Relation to presenting features and clinical outcomes in a prospective cohort of 142 patients. *Blood* **2003**, *102*, 60–68. [CrossRef] [PubMed]
124. Hassan, S.; Westwood, J.P.; Ellis, D.; Laing, C.; Mc Guckin, S.; Benjamin, S.; Scully, M. The utility of ADAMTS13 in differentiating TTP from other acute thrombotic microangiopathies: Results from the UK TTP Registry. *Br. J. Haematol.* **2015**, *171*, 830–835. [CrossRef]
125. Zafrani, L.; Mariotte, E.; Darmon, M.; Canet, E.; Merceron, S.; Boutboul, D.; Veyradier, A.; Galicier, L.; Azoulay, E. Acute renal failure is prevalent in patients with thrombotic thrombocytopenic purpura associated with low plasma ADAMTS13 activity. *J. Thromb. Haemost.* **2015**, *13*, 380–389. [CrossRef]
126. Obert, B.; Tout, H.; Veyradier, A.; Fressinaud, E.; Meyer, D.; Girma, J.P. Estimation of the von Willebrand factor-cleaving protease in plasma using monoclonal antibodies to vWF. *Thromb. Haemost.* **1999**, *82*, 1382–1385. [CrossRef]
127. Gerritsen, H.E.; Turecek, P.L.; Schwarz, H.P.; Lämmle, B.; Furlan, M. Assay of von Willebrand factor (vWF)-cleaving protease based on decreased collagen binding affinity of degraded vWF: A tool for the diagnosis of thrombotic thrombocytopenic purpura (TTP). *Thromb. Haemost.* **1999**, *82*, 1386–1389. [CrossRef]
128. Kokame, K.; Nobe, Y.; Kokubo, Y.; Okayama, A.; Miyata, T. FRETS-VWF73, a first fluorogenic substrate for ADAMTS13 assay. *Br. J. Haematol.* **2005**, *129*, 93–100. [CrossRef]
129. Thouzeau, S.; Capdenat, S.; Stépanian, A.; Coppo, P.; Veyradier, A. Evaluation of a commercial assay for ADAMTS13 activity measurement. *Thromb. Haemost.* **2013**, *110*, 852–853. [CrossRef]
130. Joly, B.; Stepanian, A.; Hajage, D.; Thouzeau, S.; Capdenat, S.; Coppo, P.; Veyradier, A. Evaluation of a chromogenic commercial assay using VWF-73 peptide for ADAMTS13 activity measurement. *Thromb. Res.* **2014**, *134*, 1074–1080. [CrossRef]

131. Jin, M.; Cataland, S.; Bissell, M.; Wu, H.M. A rapid test for the diagnosis of thrombotic thrombocytopenic purpura using surface enhanced laser desorption/ionization time-of-flight (SELDI-TOF)-mass spectrometry. *J. Thromb. Haemost.* **2006**, *4*, 333–338. [CrossRef] [PubMed]
132. Kato, S.; Matsumoto, M.; Matsuyama, T.; Isonishi, A.; Hiura, H.; Fujimura, Y. Novel monoclonal antibody-based enzyme immunoassay for determining plasma levels of ADAMTS13 activity. *Transfusion* **2006**, *46*, 1444–1452. [CrossRef] [PubMed]
133. Böhm, M.; Vigh, T.; Scharrer, I. Evaluation and clinical application of a new method for measuring activity of von Willebrand factor-cleaving metalloprotease (ADAMTS13). *Ann. Hematol.* **2002**, *81*, 430–435. [CrossRef] [PubMed]
134. Tripodi, A.; Peyvandi, F.; Chantarangkul, V.; Palla, R.; Afrasiabi, A.; Canciani, M.T.; Chung, D.W.; Ferrari, S.; Fujimura, Y.; Karimi, M.; et al. Second international collaborative study evaluating performance characteristics of methods measuring the von Willebrand factor cleaving protease (ADAMTS-13). *J. Thromb. Haemost.* **2008**, *6*, 1534–1541. [CrossRef]
135. Masias, C.; Cataland, S.R. The role of ADAMTS13 testing in the diagnosis and management of thrombotic microangiopathies and thrombosis. *Blood* **2018**, *132*, 903–910. [CrossRef]
136. Hubbard, A.R.; Heath, A.B.; Kremer Hovinga, J.A.; Factor, S.o.v.W. Establishment of the WHO 1st International Standard ADAMTS13, plasma (12/252): Communication from the SSC of the ISTH. *J. Thromb. Haemost.* **2015**, *13*, 1151–1153. [CrossRef]
137. Bentley, M.J.; Wilson, A.R.; Rodgers, G.M. Performance of a clinical prediction score for thrombotic thrombocytopenic purpura in an independent cohort. *Vox Sang* **2013**, *105*, 313–318. [CrossRef]
138. Bendapudi, P.K.; Hurwitz, S.; Fry, A.; Marques, M.B.; Waldo, S.W.; Li, A.; Sun, L.; Upadhyay, V.; Hamdan, A.; Brunner, A.M.; et al. Derivation and external validation of the PLASMIC score for rapid assessment of adults with thrombotic microangiopathies: A cohort study. *Lancet Haematol.* **2017**, *4*, e157–e164. [CrossRef]
139. Favresse, J.; Lardinois, B.; Chatelain, B.; Jacqmin, H.; Mullier, F. Evaluation of the Fully Automated HemosIL Acustar ADAMTS13 Activity Assay. *Thromb. Haemost.* **2018**, *118*, 942–944. [CrossRef]
140. Valsecchi, C.; Mirabet, M.; Mancini, I.; Biganzoli, M.; Schiavone, L.; Faraudo, S.; Mane-Padros, D.; Giles, D.; Serra-Domenech, J.; Blanch, S.; et al. Evaluation of a New, Rapid, Fully Automated Assay for the Measurement of ADAMTS13 Activity. *Thromb. Haemost.* **2019**, *119*, 1767–1772. [CrossRef] [PubMed]
141. Moore, G.W.; Meijer, D.; Griffiths, M.; Rushen, L.; Brown, A.; Budde, U.; Dittmer, R.; Schocke, B.; Leyte, A.; Geiter, S.; et al. A multi-center evaluation of TECHNOSCREEN. *J. Thromb. Haemost.* **2020**, *18*, 1686–1694. [CrossRef] [PubMed]
142. Vendramin, C.; Thomas, M.; Westwood, J.P.; Scully, M. Bethesda Assay for Detecting Inhibitory Anti-ADAMTS13 Antibodies in Immune-Mediated Thrombotic Thrombocytopenic Purpura. *TH Open* **2018**, *2*, e329–e333. [CrossRef] [PubMed]
143. Alwan, F.; Vendramin, C.; Vanhoorelbeke, K.; Langley, K.; McDonald, V.; Austin, S.; Clark, A.; Lester, W.; Gooding, R.; Biss, T.; et al. Presenting ADAMTS13 antibody and antigen levels predict prognosis in immune-mediated thrombotic thrombocytopenic purpura. *Blood* **2017**, *130*, 466–471. [CrossRef] [PubMed]
144. Hie, M.; Gay, J.; Galicier, L.; Provôt, F.; Presne, C.; Poullin, P.; Bonmarchand, G.; Wynckel, A.; Benhamou, Y.; Vanhille, P.; et al. Preemptive rituximab infusions after remission efficiently prevent relapses in acquired thrombotic thrombocytopenic purpura. *Blood* **2014**, *124*, 204–210. [CrossRef] [PubMed]
145. Sadler, J.E.; Moake, J.L.; Miyata, T.; George, J.N. Recent advances in thrombotic thrombocytopenic purpura. *Hematol. Am. Soc. Hematol. Educ. Program.* **2004**, 407–423. [CrossRef]
146. Pereira, A.; Mazzara, R.; Monteagudo, J.; Sanz, C.; Puig, L.; Martínez, A.; Ordinas, A.; Castillo, R. Thrombotic thrombocytopenic purpura/hemolytic uremic syndrome: A multivariate analysis of factors predicting the response to plasma exchange. *Ann. Hematol.* **1995**, *70*, 319–323. [CrossRef] [PubMed]
147. Nguyen, L.; Li, X.; Duvall, D.; Terrell, D.R.; Vesely, S.K.; George, J.N. Twice-daily plasma exchange for patients with refractory thrombotic thrombocytopenic purpura: The experience of the Oklahoma Registry, 1989 through 2006. *Transfusion* **2008**, *48*, 349–357. [CrossRef]
148. Toussaint-Hacquard, M.; Coppo, P.; Soudant, M.; Chevreux, L.; Mathieu-Nafissi, S.; Lecompte, T.; Gross, S.; Guillemin, F.; Schneider, T. Type of plasma preparation used for plasma exchange and clinical outcome of adult patients with acquired idiopathic thrombotic thrombocytopenic purpura: A French retrospective multicenter cohort study. *Transfusion* **2015**, *55*, 2445–2451. [CrossRef] [PubMed]
149. Scully, M.; Hunt, B.J.; Benjamin, S.; Liesner, R.; Rose, P.; Peyvandi, F.; Cheung, B.; Machin, S.J. Guidelines on the diagnosis and management of thrombotic thrombocytopenic purpura and other thrombotic microangiopathies. *Br. J. Haematol.* **2012**, *158*, 323–335. [CrossRef]
150. Rock, G.; Shumak, K.H.; Sutton, D.M.; Buskard, N.A.; Nair, R.C. Cryosupernatant as replacement fluid for plasma exchange in thrombotic thrombocytopenic purpura. Members of the Canadian Apheresis Group. *Br. J. Haematol.* **1996**, *94*, 383–386. [CrossRef]
151. Zeigler, Z.R.; Shadduck, R.K.; Gryn, J.F.; Rintels, P.B.; George, J.N.; Besa, E.C.; Bodensteiner, D.; Silver, B.; Kramer, R.E. Cryoprecipitate poor plasma does not improve early response in primary adult thrombotic thrombocytopenic purpura (TTP). *J. Clin. Apher.* **2001**, *16*, 19–22. [CrossRef] [PubMed]
152. Cataland, S.R.; Kourlas, P.J.; Yang, S.; Geyer, S.; Witkoff, L.; Wu, H.; Masias, C.; George, J.N.; Wu, H.M. Cyclosporine or steroids as an adjunct to plasma exchange in the treatment of immune-mediated thrombotic thrombocytopenic purpura. *Blood Adv.* **2017**, *1*, 2075–2082. [CrossRef] [PubMed]

153. Balduini, C.L.; Gugliotta, L.; Luppi, M.; Laurenti, L.; Klersy, C.; Pieresca, C.; Quintini, G.; Iuliano, F.; Re, R.; Spedini, P.; et al. High versus standard dose methylprednisolone in the acute phase of idiopathic thrombotic thrombocytopenic purpura: A randomized study. *Ann. Hematol.* **2010**, *89*, 591–596. [CrossRef] [PubMed]
154. Scully, M.; McDonald, V.; Cavenagh, J.; Hunt, B.J.; Longair, I.; Cohen, H.; Machin, S.J. A phase 2 study of the safety and efficacy of rituximab with plasma exchange in acute acquired thrombotic thrombocytopenic purpura. *Blood* **2011**, *118*, 1746–1753. [CrossRef] [PubMed]
155. Page, E.E.; Kremer Hovinga, J.A.; Terrell, D.R.; Vesely, S.K.; George, J.N. Rituximab reduces risk for relapse in patients with thrombotic thrombocytopenic purpura. *Blood* **2016**, *127*, 3092–3094. [CrossRef] [PubMed]
156. Abdel Karim, N.; Haider, S.; Siegrist, C.; Ahmad, N.; Zarzour, A.; Ying, J.; Yasin, Z.; Sacher, R. Approach to management of thrombotic thrombocytopenic purpura at university of cincinnati. *Adv. Hematol.* **2013**, *2013*, 195746. [CrossRef]
157. Rinott, N.; Mashiach, T.; Horowitz, N.A.; Schliamser, L.; Sarig, G.; Keren-Politansky, A.; Dann, E.J. A 14-Year Experience in the Management of Patients with Acquired Immune Thrombotic Thrombocytopenic Purpura in Northern Israel. *Acta Haematol.* **2015**, *134*, 170–176. [CrossRef]
158. Uhl, L.; Kiss, J.E.; Malynn, E.; Terrell, D.R.; Vesely, S.K.; George, J.N. Rituximab for thrombotic thrombocytopenic purpura: Lessons from the STAR trial. *Transfusion* **2017**, *57*, 2532–2538. [CrossRef]
159. Falter, T.; Herold, S.; Weyer-Elberich, V.; Scheiner, C.; Schmitt, V.; von Auer, C.; Messmer, X.; Wild, P.; Lackner, K.J.; Lämmle, B.; et al. Relapse Rate in Survivors of Acute Autoimmune Thrombotic Thrombocytopenic Purpura Treated with or without Rituximab. *Thromb. Haemost.* **2018**, *118*, 1743–1751. [CrossRef]
160. Owattanapanich, W.; Wongprasert, C.; Rotchanapanya, W.; Owattanapanich, N.; Ruchutrakool, T. Comparison of the Long-Term Remission of Rituximab and Conventional Treatment for Acquired Thrombotic Thrombocytopenic Purpura: A Systematic Review and Meta-Analysis. *Clin. Appl. Thromb. Hemost.* **2019**, *25*. [CrossRef]
161. Zwicker, J.I.; Muia, J.; Dolatshahi, L.; Westfield, L.A.; Nieters, P.; Rodrigues, A.; Hamdan, A.; Antun, A.G.; Metjian, A.; Sadler, J.E.; et al. Adjuvant low-dose rituximab and plasma exchange for acquired TTP. *Blood* **2019**, *134*, 1106–1109. [CrossRef] [PubMed]
162. Reddy, M.S.; Hofmann, S.; Shen, Y.M.; Nagalla, S.; Rambally, S.; Usmani, A.; Sarode, R. Comparison of low fixed dose versus standard-dose rituximab to treat thrombotic thrombocytopenic purpura in the acute phase and preemptively during remission. *Transfus. Apher. Sci.* **2020**, 102805. [CrossRef] [PubMed]
163. Nosari, A.; Redaelli, R.; Caimi, T.M.; Mostarda, G.; Morra, E. Cyclosporine therapy in refractory/relapsed patients with thrombotic thrombocytopenic purpura. *Am. J. Hematol.* **2009**, *84*, 313–314. [CrossRef] [PubMed]
164. Ahmad, H.N.; Thomas-Dewing, R.R.; Hunt, B.J. Mycophenolate mofetil in a case of relapsed, refractory thrombotic thrombocytopenic purpura. *Eur. J. Haematol.* **2007**, *78*, 449–452. [CrossRef]
165. Fioredda, F.; Cappelli, E.; Mariani, A.; Beccaria, A.; Palmisani, E.; Grossi, A.; Ceccherini, I.; Venè, R.; Micalizzi, C.; Calvillo, M.; et al. Thrombotic thrombocytopenic purpura and defective apoptosis due to CASP8/10 mutations: The role of mycophenolate mofetil. *Blood Adv.* **2019**, *3*, 3432–3435. [CrossRef]
166. Ziman, A.; Mitri, M.; Klapper, E.; Pepkowitz, S.H.; Goldfinger, D. Combination vincristine and plasma exchange as initial therapy in patients with thrombotic thrombocytopenic purpura: One institution's experience and review of the literature. *Transfusion* **2005**, *45*, 41–49. [CrossRef]
167. Shortt, J.; Oh, D.H.; Opat, S.S. ADAMTS13 antibody depletion by bortezomib in thrombotic thrombocytopenic purpura. *N. Engl. J. Med.* **2013**, *368*, 90–92. [CrossRef]
168. Patriquin, C.J.; Thomas, M.R.; Dutt, T.; McGuckin, S.; Blombery, P.A.; Cranfield, T.; Westwood, J.P.; Scully, M. Bortezomib in the treatment of refractory thrombotic thrombocytopenic purpura. *Br. J. Haematol.* **2016**, *173*, 779–785. [CrossRef]
169. Beloncle, F.; Buffet, M.; Coindre, J.P.; Munoz-Bongrand, N.; Malot, S.; Pène, F.; Mira, J.P.; Galicier, L.; Guidet, B.; Baudel, J.L.; et al. Splenectomy and/or cyclophosphamide as salvage therapies in thrombotic thrombocytopenic purpura: The French TMA Reference Center experience. *Transfusion* **2012**, *52*, 2436–2444. [CrossRef]
170. Knoebl, P.; Cataland, S.; Peyvandi, F.; Coppo, P.; Scully, M.; Kremer Hovinga, J.A.; Metjian, A.; de la Rubia, J.; Pavenski, K.; Minkue Mi Edou, J.; et al. Efficacy and safety of open-label caplacizumab in patients with exacerbations of acquired thrombotic thrombocytopenic purpura in the HERCULES study. *J. Thromb. Haemost.* **2020**, *18*, 479–484. [CrossRef]
171. Goshua, G.; Sinha, P.; Hendrickson, J.E.; Tormey, C.A.; Bendapudi, P.; Lee, A.I. Cost effectiveness of caplacizumab in acquired thrombotic thrombocytopenic purpura. *Blood* **2020**. [CrossRef]
172. Chen, J.; Reheman, A.; Gushiken, F.C.; Nolasco, L.; Fu, X.; Moake, J.L.; Ni, H.; López, J.A. N-acetylcysteine reduces the size and activity of von Willebrand factor in human plasma and mice. *J. Clin. Invest.* **2011**, *121*, 593–603. [CrossRef] [PubMed]
173. Turner, N.; Nolasco, L.; Moake, J. Generation and breakdown of soluble ultralarge von Willebrand factor multimers. *Semin. Thromb. Hemost.* **2012**, *38*, 38–46. [CrossRef] [PubMed]
174. Rottenstreich, A.; Hochberg-Klein, S.; Rund, D.; Kalish, Y. The role of N-acetylcysteine in the treatment of thrombotic thrombocytopenic purpura. *J. Thromb. Thrombolysis* **2016**, *41*, 678–683. [CrossRef] [PubMed]
175. Li, G.W.; Rambally, S.; Kamboj, J.; Reilly, S.; Moake, J.L.; Udden, M.M.; Mims, M.P. Treatment of refractory thrombotic thrombocytopenic purpura with N-acetylcysteine: A case report. *Transfusion* **2014**, *54*, 1221–1224. [CrossRef]

176. Tersteeg, C.; Roodt, J.; Van Rensburg, W.J.; Dekimpe, C.; Vandeputte, N.; Pareyn, I.; Vandenbulcke, A.; Plaimauer, B.; Lamprecht, S.; Deckmyn, H.; et al. N-acetylcysteine in preclinical mouse and baboon models of thrombotic thrombocytopenic purpura. *Blood* **2017**, *129*, 1030–1038. [CrossRef]
177. Cataland, S.R.; Peyvandi, F.; Mannucci, P.M.; Lämmle, B.; Kremer Hovinga, J.A.; Machin, S.J.; Scully, M.; Rock, G.; Gilbert, J.C.; Yang, S.; et al. Initial experience from a double-blind, placebo-controlled, clinical outcome study of ARC1779 in patients with thrombotic thrombocytopenic purpura. *Am. J. Hematol.* **2012**, *87*, 430–432. [CrossRef]
178. Sakai, K.; Someya, T.; Harada, K.; Yagi, H.; Matsui, T.; Matsumoto, M. Novel aptamer to von Willebrand factor A1 domain (TAGX-0004) shows total inhibition of thrombus formation superior to ARC1779 and comparable to caplacizumab. *Haematologica* **2019**. [CrossRef]
179. Zhu, S.; Gilbert, J.C.; Hatala, P.; Harvey, W.; Liang, Z.; Gao, S.; Kang, D.; Jilma, B. The development and characterization of a long acting anti-thrombotic von Willebrand factor (VWF) aptamer. *J. Thromb. Haemost.* **2020**, *18*, 1113–1123. [CrossRef]
180. Furlan, M.; Robles, R.; Morselli, B.; Sandoz, P.; Lämmle, B. Recovery and half-life of von Willebrand factor-cleaving protease after plasma therapy in patients with thrombotic thrombocytopenic purpura. *Thromb. Haemost.* **1999**, *81*, 8–13.
181. Kovarova, P.; Hrdlickova, R.; Blahutova, S.; Cermakova, Z. ADAMTS13 kinetics after therapeutic plasma exchange and plasma infusion in patients with Upshaw-Schulman syndrome. *J. Clin. Apher.* **2019**, *34*, 13–20. [CrossRef] [PubMed]
182. Taylor, A.; Vendramin, C.; Oosterholt, S.; Della Pasqua, O.; Scully, M. Pharmacokinetics of plasma infusion in congenital thrombotic thrombocytopenic purpura. *J. Thromb. Haemost.* **2019**, *17*, 88–98. [CrossRef] [PubMed]
183. Scully, M.; Knöbl, P.; Kentouche, K.; Rice, L.; Windyga, J.; Schneppenheim, R.; Kremer Hovinga, J.A.; Kajiwara, M.; Fujimura, Y.; Maggiore, C.; et al. Recombinant ADAMTS-13: First-in-human pharmacokinetics and safety in congenital thrombotic thrombocytopenic purpura. *Blood* **2017**, *130*, 2055–2063. [CrossRef] [PubMed]
184. Plaimauer, B.; Kremer Hovinga, J.A.; Juno, C.; Wolfsegger, M.J.; Skalicky, S.; Schmidt, M.; Grillberger, L.; Hasslacher, M.; Knöbl, P.; Ehrlich, H.; et al. Recombinant ADAMTS13 normalizes von Willebrand factor-cleaving activity in plasma of acquired TTP patients by overriding inhibitory antibodies. *J. Thromb. Haemost.* **2011**, *9*, 936–944. [CrossRef] [PubMed]
185. Chander, D.P.; Loch, M.M.; Cataland, S.R.; George, J.N. Caplacizumab Therapy without Plasma Exchange for Acquired Thrombotic Thrombocytopenic Purpura. *N. Engl. J. Med.* **2019**, *381*, 92–94. [CrossRef]
186. Sukumar, S.; George, J.N.; Cataland, S.R. Shared decision making, thrombotic thrombocytopenic purpura, and caplacizumab. *Am. J. Hematol.* **2020**. [CrossRef]
187. Völker, L.A.; Brinkkoetter, P.T.; Knöbl, P.N.; Krstic, M.; Kaufeld, J.; Menne, J.; Buxhofer-Ausch, V.; Miesbach, W. Treatment of acquired thrombotic thrombocytopenic purpura without plasma exchange in selected patients under caplacizumab. *J. Thromb. Haemost.* **2020**. [CrossRef]
188. Irani, M.S.; Sanchez, F.; Friedman, K. Caplacizumab for treatment of thrombotic thrombocytopenic purpura in a patient with anaphylaxis to fresh-frozen plasma. *Transfusion* **2020**. [CrossRef]
189. Zheng, X.L.; Vesely, S.K.; Cataland, S.R.; Coppo, P.; Geldziler, B.; Iorio, A.; Matsumoto, M.; Mustafa, R.A.; Pai, M.; Rock, G.; et al. ISTH guidelines for treatment of thrombotic thrombocytopenic purpura. *J. Thromb. Haemost.* **2020**. [CrossRef]
190. Masias, C.; Carter, K.; Wu, H.; Yang, S.; Flowers, A.; Cataland, S. Severely Deficient ADAMTS13 Activity Predicts Relapse of Immune-Mediated Thrombotic Thrombocytopenic Purpura in Pregnancy. *Blood* **2019**, *134*, 1098. [CrossRef]
191. Zheng, X.L.; Vesely, S.K.; Cataland, S.R.; Coppo, P.; Geldziler, B.; Iorio, A.; Matsumoto, M.; Mustafa, R.A.; Pai, M.; Rock, G.; et al. Good practice statements (GPS) for the clinical care of patients with thrombotic thrombocytopenic purpura. *J. Thromb. Haemost.* **2020**. [CrossRef] [PubMed]
192. Walia, S.S.; Walia, M.S.; Walia, H.S. Thrombotic thrombocytopenic purpura treated with vincristine in a Jehovah's witness. *Asian J. Transfus. Sci.* **2011**, *5*, 180–181. [CrossRef] [PubMed]
193. George, J.N.; Sandler, S.A.; Stankiewicz, J. Management of thrombotic thrombocytopenic purpura without plasma exchange: The Jehovah's Witness experience. *Blood Adv.* **2017**, *1*, 2161–2165. [CrossRef]
194. Lim, M.Y.; Greenberg, C.S. Successful Management of Thrombotic Thrombocytopenic Purpura in a Jehovah's Witness: An Individualized Approach With Joint Decision-Making. *J. Patient Exp.* **2020**, *7*, 8–11. [CrossRef] [PubMed]
195. Cataland, S.R.; Scully, M.A.; Paskavitz, J.; Maruff, P.; Witkoff, L.; Jin, M.; Uva, N.; Gilbert, J.C.; Wu, H.M. Evidence of persistent neurologic injury following thrombotic thrombocytopenic purpura. *Am. J. Hematol.* **2011**, *86*, 87–89. [CrossRef] [PubMed]
196. Chaturvedi, S.; Abbas, H.; McCrae, K.R. Increased morbidity during long-term follow-up of survivors of thrombotic thrombocytopenic purpura. *Am. J. Hematol.* **2015**, *90*, E208. [CrossRef]
197. George, J.N. TTP: Long-term outcomes following recovery. *Hematol. Am. Soc. Hematol. Educ. Program* **2018**, *2018*, 548–552. [CrossRef]
198. Jestin, M.; Benhamou, Y.; Schelpe, A.S.; Roose, E.; Provôt, F.; Galicier, L.; Hié, M.; Presne, C.; Poullin, P.; Wynckel, A.; et al. Preemptive rituximab prevents long-term relapses in immune-mediated thrombotic thrombocytopenic purpura. *Blood* **2018**, *132*, 2143–2153. [CrossRef]
199. Cataland, S.R.; Jin, M.; Lin, S.; Kraut, E.H.; George, J.N.; Wu, H.M. Effect of prophylactic cyclosporine therapy on ADAMTS13 biomarkers in patients with idiopathic thrombotic thrombocytopenic purpura. *Am. J. Hematol.* **2008**, *83*, 911–915. [CrossRef]
200. Kappers-Klunne, M.C.; Wijermans, P.; Fijnheer, R.; Croockewit, A.J.; van der Holt, B.; de Wolf, J.T.; Löwenberg, B.; Brand, A. Splenectomy for the treatment of thrombotic thrombocytopenic purpura. *Br. J. Haematol.* **2005**, *130*, 768–776. [CrossRef]

201. Dubois, L.; Gray, D.K. Case series: Splenectomy: Does it still play a role in the management of thrombotic thrombocytopenic purpura? *Can. J. Surg.* **2010**, *53*, 349–355.
202. Kremer Hovinga, J.A.; Studt, J.D.; Demarmels Biasiutti, F.; Solenthaler, M.; Alberio, L.; Zwicky, C.; Fontana, S.; Taleghani, B.M.; Tobler, A.; Lämmle, B. Splenectomy in relapsing and plasma-refractory acquired thrombotic thrombocytopenic purpura. *Haematologica* **2004**, *89*, 320–324. [PubMed]
203. Bell, W.R.; Braine, H.G.; Ness, P.M.; Kickler, T.S. Improved survival in thrombotic thrombocytopenic purpura-hemolytic uremic syndrome. Clinical experience in 108 patients. *N. Engl. J. Med.* **1991**, *325*, 398–403. [CrossRef] [PubMed]
204. Chaturvedi, S.; Oluwole, O.; Cataland, S.; McCrae, K.R. Post-traumatic stress disorder and depression in survivors of thrombotic thrombocytopenic purpura. *Thromb. Res.* **2017**, *151*, 51–56. [CrossRef]
205. Upreti, H.; Kasmani, J.; Dane, K.; Braunstein, E.M.; Streiff, M.B.; Shanbhag, S.; Moliterno, A.R.; Sperati, C.J.; Gottesman, R.F.; Brodsky, R.A.; et al. Reduced ADAMTS13 activity during TTP remission is associated with stroke in TTP survivors. *Blood* **2019**, *134*, 1037–1045. [CrossRef] [PubMed]
206. Falter, T.; Schmitt, V.; Herold, S.; Weyer, V.; von Auer, C.; Wagner, S.; Hefner, G.; Beutel, M.; Lackner, K.; Lämmle, B.; et al. Depression and cognitive deficits as long-term consequences of thrombotic thrombocytopenic purpura. *Transfusion* **2017**, *57*, 1152–1162. [CrossRef]
207. Sonneveld, M.A.; Kavousi, M.; Ikram, M.A.; Hofman, A.; Rueda Ochoa, O.L.; Turecek, P.L.; Franco, O.H.; Leebeek, F.W.; de Maat, M.P. Low ADAMTS-13 activity and the risk of coronary heart disease—A prospective cohort study: The Rotterdam Study. *J. Thromb. Haemost.* **2016**, *14*, 2114–2120. [CrossRef]
208. Bongers, T.N.; de Bruijne, E.L.; Dippel, D.W.; de Jong, A.J.; Deckers, J.W.; Poldermans, D.; de Maat, M.P.; Leebeek, F.W. Lower levels of ADAMTS13 are associated with cardiovascular disease in young patients. *Atherosclerosis* **2009**, *207*, 250–254. [CrossRef]
209. Sonneveld, M.A.; de Maat, M.P.; Portegies, M.L.; Kavousi, M.; Hofman, A.; Turecek, P.L.; Rottensteiner, H.; Scheiflinger, F.; Koudstaal, P.J.; Ikram, M.A.; et al. Low ADAMTS13 activity is associated with an increased risk of ischemic stroke. *Blood* **2015**, *126*, 2739–2746. [CrossRef]
210. Sonneveld, M.A.; Franco, O.H.; Ikram, M.A.; Hofman, A.; Kavousi, M.; de Maat, M.P.; Leebeek, F.W. Von Willebrand Factor, ADAMTS13, and the Risk of Mortality: The Rotterdam Study. *Arter. Thromb. Vasc. Biol.* **2016**, *36*, 2446–2451. [CrossRef]

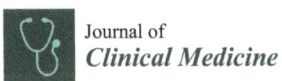

Review

Pseudothrombocytopenia—A Review on Causes, Occurrence and Clinical Implications

Benjamin Lardinois [1], Julien Favresse [1], Bernard Chatelain [1], Giuseppe Lippi [2] and François Mullier [1,*]

1. Namur Thrombosis and Hemostasis Center (NTHC), CHU UCL Namur, Université Catholique de Louvain, 5530 Yvoir, Belgium; benjamin.lardinois@uclouvain.be (B.L.); j.favresse@labstluc.be (J.F.); bernard.chatelain@gmail.com (B.C.)
2. Section of Clinical Biochemistry, University of Verona, 37134 Verona, Italy; giuseppe.lippi@univr.it
* Correspondence: francois.mullier@uclouvain.be; Tel.: +32-(0)8-1424-986

Citation: Lardinois, B.; Favresse, J.; Chatelain, B.; Lippi, G.; Mullier, F. Pseudothrombocytopenia—A Review on Causes, Occurrence and Clinical Implications. *J. Clin. Med.* **2021**, *10*, 594. https://doi.org/10.3390/jcm10040594

Academic Editor: Hugo ten Cate
Received: 31 December 2020
Accepted: 1 February 2021
Published: 4 February 2021

Publisher's Note: MDPI stays neutral with regard to jurisdictional claims in published maps and institutional affiliations.

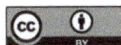

Copyright: © 2021 by the authors. Licensee MDPI, Basel, Switzerland. This article is an open access article distributed under the terms and conditions of the Creative Commons Attribution (CC BY) license (https://creativecommons.org/licenses/by/4.0/).

Abstract: Pseudothrombocytopenia (PTCP), a relative common finding in clinical laboratories, can lead to diagnostic errors, overtreatment, and further (even invasive) unnecessary testing. Clinical consequences with potential life-threatening events (e.g., unnecessary platelet transfusion, inappropriate treatment including splenectomy or corticosteroids) are still observed when PTCP is not readily detected. The phenomenon is even more complex when occurring with different anticoagulants. In this review we present a case of multi-anticoagulant PTCP, where we studied different parameters including temperature, amikacin supplementation, measurement methods, and type of anticoagulant. Prevalence, clinical risk factors, pre-analytical and analytical factors, along with clinical implications, will be discussed. The detection of an anticoagulant-dependent PTCP does not necessarily imply the presence of specific disorders. Conversely, the incidence of PTCP seems higher in patients receiving low molecular weight heparin, during hospitalization, or in men aged 50 years or older. New analytical technologies, such as fluorescence or optical platelet counting, will be soon overturning traditional algorithms and represent valuable diagnostic aids. A practical laboratory approach, based on current knowledge of PTCP, is finally proposed for overcoming spuriously low platelet counts.

Keywords: pseudothrombocytopenia; platelets; hematimetry; fluorescence; amikacin; anticoagulants; COVID-19

1. Introduction

Reported for the first time in 1969 [1], pseudothrombocytopenia (PTCP) has been increasingly described in patients suffering from various disorders and more recently even in patients with coronavirus disease 2019 (COVID-19) [2,3].

This well-known in vitro phenomenon but still underrecognized may lead to misdiagnosis of thrombocytopenia, overtreatment, and further, even invasive, unnecessary testing. This phenomenon can typically be identified by reviewing the peripheral blood smear (PBS), using a different anticoagulant than dipotassium ethylenediaminetetraacetic acid (EDTA) for blood collection, or maintaining the sample at around 37 °C before testing [4]. The prevalence of this phenomenon in EDTA is estimated to be 0.03–0.27% of the general population [5–7], though multiple anticoagulant PTCPs with citrate, heparin, or sodium fluoride have also been described [8]. Some parameters can positively influence platelet counting in presence of PTCP. These include the following:

(i) In vitro amikacin supplementation can prevent and dissociate platelet clumps due to EDTA, citrate [4], or heparin-PTCP [9] although controversially discussed [10];
(ii) Maintaining blood samples to 37 °C could lead to a more accurate platelet count (PC) or prevent EDTA-dependent PTCP [11,12];
(iii) A rapid analysis of EDTA blood specimen is advocated, due to time-dependent fall in PC from 1 min after blood collection to 4 h afterwards [4,12,13];

(iv) Fluorescence platelet counting can be effective in correcting spurious low PC [14];
(v) Capillary blood is prone to platelet clumping [15], but it has been described as less rich in aggregates [16];
(vi) Alternative anticoagulants such as magnesium sulfate [5,8,17] and acid citrate dextrose (ACD) [18] are interesting tools to overcome platelets clumps. Hirudin has been studied in few reports only [8,19,20].

Despite the many case studies and the different approaches described, there are few specific expert recommendations on detection and management of PTCP. In this review we discuss the cause, occurrence, and clinical implication of this condition, specifically anticoagulant-dependent PTCP. We start this review by presenting a case study of multi-anticoagulant PTCP, in whom we established a study protocol to assess the PC. A laboratory management algorithm, based on current knowledge, is finally proposed.

2. Case Study

A 47-year-old woman was referred to the local laboratory of Namur Thrombosis and Hemostasis Center (Yvoir, Belgium), for performing a preoperative hemostasis assessment before radical cancer hysterectomy. She did not have any bleeding problems during the delivery of her two children, though her medical history revealed two severe postoperative hemorrhages and menorrhagia. The patient had autoimmune background, as evidenced by high antinuclear antibodies titer (>1:1280) and platelet-bound GPIIbIIIa antibodies. In another laboratory, PTCP with numerous platelet clumps on blood smear had previously been observed using three different anticoagulants: K2-EDTA, sodium citrate, and citrate-theophylline-adenosine-dipyridamole (CTAD).

According to this information and patient's multi-anticoagulant PTCP, we established a study protocol to find the most convenient way to assess PC (Figure 1).

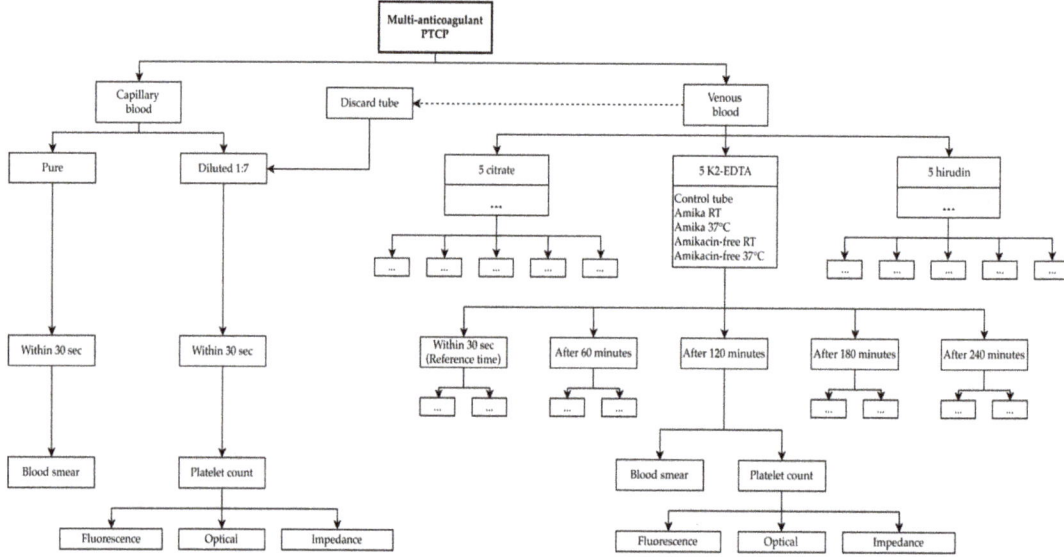

Figure 1. Study protocol. Empty boxes just repeat the same elements as adjacent boxes. The time is expressed in seconds or minutes after blood collection. Abbreviations: PTCP, Pseudothrombocytopenia; RT, room temperature; EDTA, ethylenediaminetetraacetic acid.

After a 30 min rest, a capillary blood drop from the pulp of index was obtained by a lancing device (Accu-Chek, Roche, Switzerland), which was then used to immediately prepare a blood smear and perform PC. Due to the small volume of sample, the manufacturer's diluent (DCL-pack, Sysmex Corporation, Kobe, Japan) was used to obtain a blood to diluent ratio of 1:7 for platelet counting in fluorescent (PLT-F), impedance (PLT-I), and optical (PLT-O) channels of a Sysmex XN-1000 blood count analyzer (Sysmex Corporation, Kobe, Japan). Thereafter, a venepuncture in the median cubital vein with 21 gauge needle (Greiner Bio-One, Courtaboeuf, France) was carried out according to recommended venous blood collection practices [21]. Five vacuum blood tubes containing K2-EDTA, five containing 109 mmol/L buffered sodium citrate with blood to anticoagulant ratio of 9:1 (Vacuette®, Greiner Bio-One, Courtaboeuf, France), and five containing hirudin 525 ATU/mL (Monovette®, Sarstedt, Nümbrecht, Germany) were collected. Each set of anticoagulant tubes was used to study the effect of temperature and in vitro amikacin supplementation (5 mg/mL) [22] on PC at 0.5, 60, 120, 180, and 240 min after blood collection. No significant clinical changes were considered when PC remained over time within the reference change value (RCV) calculated for each channel (14% for PLT-F and PLT-O, 25% for PLT-I) according to the following formula: RCV = $2^{1/2} * Z * (CV_A^2 + CV_I^2)^{1/2}$ [23] assuming Z-score of 1.96 used (95% probability) and CV_I of 5.6% obtained from the European Federation of Clinical Chemistry and Laboratory Medicine biological variation database [24]. The analysis of blood smear was performed, with special focus on peripheral film (as recommended) [25], and platelet clump was defined as a minimum of five attached platelets [4].

Amikacin-free specimens were diluted with manufacturer's diluent, for achieving the same dilution as in tubes containing amikacin; the dilution effect of sodium citrate, amikacin, or diluent were calculated. A patient control sample without amikacin or diluent was maintained at room temperature (RT) for each set. PC and platelet surface glycoproteins expression levels by flow cytometry (FCM), platelet function, fibrinolysis, fibrin formation, mixing studies, and serum anti-platelet antibodies were also assessed.

Platelet clumping was observed irrespective of the types of tube used and until the last measurement at 240 min (Figure 2). PCs according to different anticoagulants, conditions, and measuring channels on XN-1000 hematology analyzer are shown in Figure 3.

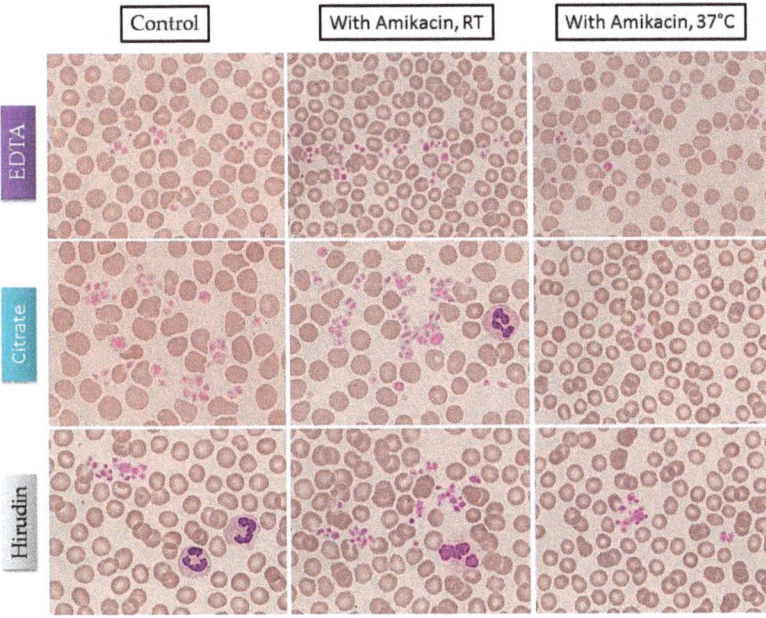

Figure 2. Platelet clumps observed on blood smears from samples obtained at baseline according to different anticoagulants tubes and conditions. Clumps were observed until the last observation at 240 min. Although not illustrated, amikacin-free specimens also displayed several clumps. Abbreviations: EDTA, ethylenediaminetetraacetic acid.; RT, room temperature.

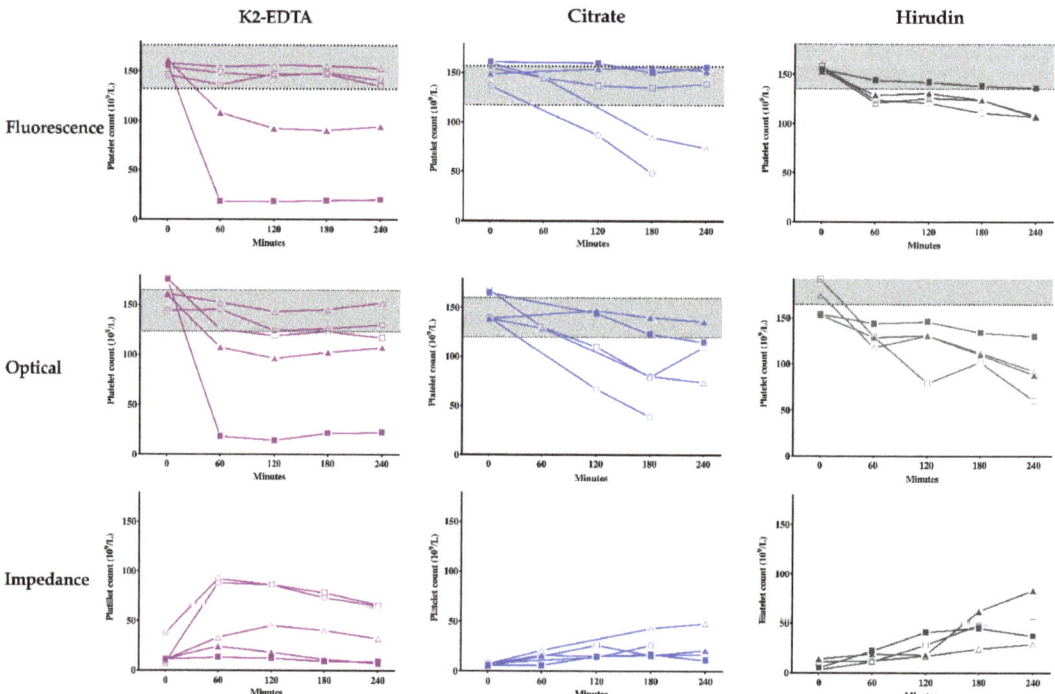

Figure 3. Changes of platelet counts over time according to different anticoagulants (K_2-EDTA, Na-citrate, hirudin), measurement methods and conditions (control, amikacin or not, room temperature or 37 °C). The grey zone corresponds to the RCV based on the control tube at baseline for K_2-EDTA, sodium citrate and on amikacin-free tube at room temperature for hirudin. Control hirudin tube was excluded since a blood clot was found. ○ Control, RT, △ Amikacin, RT, ▲ Amikacin, 37 °C, □ No amikacin, RT, ■ No amikacin, 37 °C.

The PC obtained with capillary blood in fluorescent and optical channels were 214×10^9/L and 141×10^9/L, respectively. The impedance method generated no data. In venous blood, the PCs with the PLT-F channel at baseline were approximately 150×10^9/L regardless of type of tube and storing condition. The PLT-O showed higher variability than PLT-F, both at baseline and at different time points. The impedance method generated low PC for each set. Mean platelet volume (MPV), platelet larger cell ratio, and platelet distribution width obtained at baseline in patient control EDTA sample were 13.3 fL, 54.0%, and 18.7%, respectively.

Tubes containing citrate, kept at 37 °C, displayed the greatest stability, independent of amikacin, as did K_2-EDTA stored at RT, with the entire range of values remaining within the RCV. Maintenance of EDTA tubes at 37 °C rather than at RT had negative impact on PC, with all analytical techniques used. This was particularly observed for amikacin-free specimens at 37 °C, with many clumps observed on the blood smear. Hirudin specimens displayed the worst stability over time, in all conditions.

The PC obtained with the reference method in FCM on K_2-EDTA (145×10^9/L) was quite similar to that obtained at baseline in fluorescence and optical channels. Platelet surface glycoproteins, platelet function, fibrinolysis, and fibrin formation were normal. In addition, mixing studies and serum anti-platelet antibody test were reported as normal. A Von Willebrand disease (VWD), including type 2B VWD and platelet type VWD was also ruled out. Thus we concluded that there was multi-anticoagulant PTCP and the actual PC was 145×10^9/L.

This single person experimental approach had some limitations. First, control measurements with blood from individuals without PTCP were not carried out. This would have assessed the in vitro cell shrinking or swelling, thus resulting in additionally measurable platelets, observed in the EDTA control tube by the increase of PLT-I and MPV from 13.3 to 15.1 fL within the first hour. This phenomenon does not interfere with PLT-F or PLT-O. Secondly, no control tube at 37 °C was obtained; therefore, a general effect of temperature on platelet clumps could not be excluded. Thirdly, no data were available to explain the decreasing PC in citrated sample, though the hypothesis of calcium release from reversible citrate binding could be suggested. Fourthly, other anticoagulants, including magnesium sulfate, could have been studied, but these were not available in our laboratory when the case study was carried out.

3. Mechanisms, Prevalence and Risk Factors

3.1. Mechanisms

First described by Gowland et al. in 1969 in a patient with a malignant non-Hodgkin's lymphoma [1], PTCP was rapidly identified as being in vitro phenomenon with many further observations in healthy subjects, without a significant bleeding phenotype. EDTA-dependent PTCP has also been described in animals such as cats, minipigs, dogs, and horses [26–30].

Manthorpe et al. in 1981 first reported anti-platelet antibody activity based on immunofluorescence experiments using Fab'2-fragments of isolated IgG [31]. Then, Pegels et al. confirmed the existence of an immunologically-mediated phenomenon caused by presence of IgG, IgM, or IgA directed against platelet antigens, manifesting mostly at 0–4 °C in EDTA samples [32]. Other immunological studies proved the varied origin of antibodies, belonging to different classes of immunoglobulins, mainly IgG (and especially IgG1), sometimes concomitantly with IgA and IgM. These could be either acquired or naturally occurring autoantibodies [33–36]. Bizzaro et al. identified the presence of anticardiolipin antibodies in up to two-thirds of samples containing antiplatelet antibodies [37]. However, a recent study showed that there was no significant difference in anticardiolipin antibody titers between individuals with PTCP and a control group of healthy patients [38]. Unlike these previous observations, PTCP in a patient with clinical anti-phospholipid syndrome was only reported in 2018 for the first time [39]. Cold agglutinins and antinuclear antibodies were found to be significantly more frequent in individuals with PTCP compared to healthy volunteers [38,40–42]. To the best of our knowledge, no other immunological studies have been carried out since the beginning of this century.

Although the phenomenon has not been fully elucidated, it has been suggested that these autoantibodies may be directed against cryptic exposed epitopes of the GpIIbIIIa complex (fibrinogen receptor), a calcium dependent heterodimer, and/or negatively charged phospholipids, therefore responsible for in vitro platelet agglutination after activation via tyrosine kinase [4,12]. It could hence be considered as aggregation rather than agglutination. Interestingly, platelets from patients with Glanzmann's thrombasthenia (absence of or minimal residual amounts of GPIIbIIIa or abnormal fibrinogen receptor) fail to bind these autoantibodies [42]. Recently, an IgM class agglutinin against collagen receptor GPVI and triggering platelet activation has been identified in citrate anticoagulated blood of a patient suffering from moderate bleeding diathesis [43]. These cryptic epitopes are mostly exposed when platelets react with EDTA [44,45], which irreversibly chelates calcium [46], leading to remarkable conformational changes of these neoantigens [37,47]. This phenomenon may be observed with any EDTA formulation [12], and has also been described for molecules resembling EDTA such as ethylenetriamine tetraacetic acid [48]. Interestingly, this conformational change is not observed with alternative anticoagulants such as citrate [10], although a recent report suggested that conformational changes could also appear with this latter anticoagulant or even with heparin [49]. Other immune complexes interacting with Fc receptors on platelet surface could be implicated in the PTCP process, with varying degrees of specificity [7].

The PTCP spectrum may involve other additives, thus describing a new, rarer entity, which can be conventionally called multi-anticoagulant PTCP [3,8,49–52]. It has even led some authors to mention an "Anticoagulant-induced" PTCP rather than "anticoagulant-dependent" PTCP.

This phenomenon can be persistent or transient, sometimes showing alternating periods without aggregates generation [10]. A recent case of transient PTCP has been described in a COVID-19 patient during viral immunization [2].

Transplacental transmission of maternal IgG leading to PTCP in newborns has been described [53–55]. This condition should be considered in neonates with prolonged thrombocytopenia [56]. Pediatrics is therefore not safe from this phenomenon, though the majority of cases were children suffering with infectious diseases [57–61]. Nonetheless, a case of healthy children has been described [62].

Spurious thrombocytopenia could also be related to platelet satellitism around white blood cells. Classically observed as an in vitro phenomenon with platelet rosetting around the cytoplasm of neutrophils, it has been less frequently observed around lymphocytes [7,63]. The underlying mechanism has not been fully elucidated so far, though IgG autoantibodies targeting GpIIbIIIa would be involved in binding to neutrophil Fc Gamma receptor [64]. Other non-immune hypotheses pinpoint that proteins from alpha granules or thrombospondin would be expressed on platelet membrane, thus leading to adhesion to neutrophils [65]. This in vitro process would then evolve towards a more generalized agglutination of platelets and neutrophils in large aggregates containing over 100 cells. The latter phenomenon can be more rarely detected, and seems to be especially EDTA-dependent.

3.2. Prevalence

Several studies, most retrospective, have been conducted for assessing the prevalence of PTCP in different populations. The prevalence in K2-EDTA has been estimated at around 0.03–0.27% in an outpatient population [6,7,35,66–72], increasing to 15.3% in patients referred to an outpatient clinic for isolated thrombocytopenia [73,74]. Up to 17% of patients with EDTA-dependent PTCP display also a low PC in citrate samples [35]. Three studies evaluated the prevalence of PTCP in blood and platelet apheresis donors, with frequency ranging from 0.01% to 0.2% [75–77]. Although the prevalence of EDTA-PTCP did not appear to be significantly influenced by age or gender [12], a recent retrospective Chinese study of 190,940 individuals with regular hospital checkups showed that this condition was significantly higher in males aged 50 years or older [72]. Platelet satellitism is even rarer, approximately 1 every 12,000 blood counts [7,78].

3.3. Clinical Risk Factors

Since the discovery in 1969, numerous hypotheses on the origin of anti-platelet antibody production have been formulated, and many studies have attempted to identify some putative risk factors.

The commonly accepted hypothesis entails antibody production due to cross-reactivity, as recently described in two COVID-19 patients during viral immunization [2,3], or in autoimmune antibodies as described here. The presence of platelet-bound GpIIbIIIa antibodies, found in 80% of cases (as well as in our patient), reinforced this hypothesis.

Figure 4 summarizes the relationship between PTCP and clinical conditions. No particular disease is strongly associated with presence of PTCP, or show significant differences from a control population of healthy individuals. However, the incidence of EDTA-PTCP seems increased with hospitalization or in patients with some specific disorders, such as autoimmune diseases. Infection, pregnancy, and use of medication such as low-molecular-weight heparin (LMWH) have also been identified as significant risk factors [12,38,41]. As earlier mentioned, males >50 years could be at higher risk [72]. Additional conditions found to be especially associated with PTCP are reported in the scientific literature as case reports. These basically include viral infections [3,59,79], sepsis [80], thrombotic and cardiovascular disorder, heparin-induced thrombocytopenia (HIT) [41,81,82], auto-immune disorders [39,83], liver diseases [51,84], cancer [85,86], surgical settings [87–89], post stem cell transplantation [90,91], treatment with valproic acid [51], insulin, antibiotics [92], or chemotherapeutic agents such as sunitinib [52]. Some authors prefer to use the term "coincidental PTCP" or "concomitant PTCP" rather than expressly associating this condition with a particular disease [43,81]. Several recent cases with therapy based on monoclonal antibodies have also been described, encompassing GpIIbIIIa [93] or immune checkpoint inhibitor such as pembrolizumab [94].

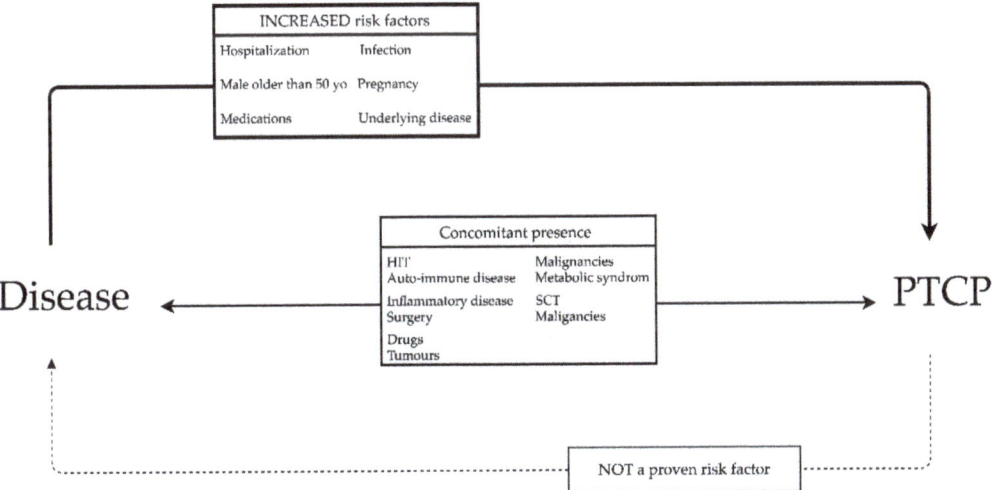

Figure 4. Relationship between anticoagulant-dependent pseudothrombocytopenia and disease. Increased prevalence of PTCP has been described in populations in the upper box. Concomitant presence of PTCP and a disease have been observed without proving an increased risk for one or the other. The presence of a PTCP does not increase the risk of developing a specific disorder. Abbreviations: HIT, heparin-induced thrombocytopenia; LMWH, low-molecular-weight heparin; SCT, stem cell transplantation.

Notably, the identification of PTCP does not seem to enhance the risk of developing a certain disorder [43]. Some individuals have persistent PTCP for decades, without reporting any relevant pathological state. More data are hence necessary to evaluate PTCP as a clinical condition for possible diseases. However, it has already been suggested that it may be advisable to investigate the presence of an autoimmune disease when observing PTCP [38]. In addition, platelet satellitism has been found both in healthy people and in patients with cancer, infections, or autoimmune disorders [78,95]. Critical recognition of PTCP in situation at higher bleeding risk, including patients undergoing cardiac surgery [89,96,97] or with life-threatening disorders such as disseminated intravascular coagulation (DIC) and HIT [12], could prove advantageous. PTCP shall also be accurately ruled out in patients undergoing treatment with GPIIbIIIa antagonists, due to the high risk of stent thrombosis that would result from discontinuation of such therapy [98].

4. Pre-Analytical and Analytical Influencing Factors
4.1. Collection

Laborious venipuncture, overfilled blood specimens, or blood draws from indwelling lines may trigger platelet clumps by spurious activation of coagulation in vitro [7]. Capillary venous blood seems also more vulnerable to platelet clumping [15], though it has been described as having a lower number of aggregates [16].

Although capillary blood displayed the highest PC in our case report, uncertainty remains concerning buffer dilution and a possible matrix effect, since the analyzer is calibrated for using venous blood.

4.2. Aminoglycosides and Other Compounds

Aminoglycoside supplementation in EDTA blood sample has been extensively investigated [5,9,13,50,69,99,100], maybe for its wider hospital availability compared to other compounds.

In our case, the presence of a stabilizer in the preparation of the aminoglycoside (e.g., sodium citrate) [101] may explain why the addition of amikacin in citrated tubes did not resolve the issue. In contrast, K2-EDTA supplemented with amikacin displayed greater stability of platelet values, thus revealing a possible benefit from dual anticoagulation. However, the package insert does not specify the concentration of sodium citrate in solution [22], so that the role of stabilizers in PTCP needs to be further elucidated.

More importantly, amikacin is not always effective in correcting PCs in vitro [13], since its activity is dependent on the type of anticoagulants to which it is added [9]. The mechanism of aminoglycosides activity in PTCP remains hypothetical [9,11], and its use controversial [10].

Other aminosides including kanamycin can be added in EDTA-samples to prevent or even dissociate platelet aggregates, though displaying variable outcomes [13,50,69]. Supplementation with other pharmaceutical drugs in blood samples such as potassium azide, calcium chloride, antiplatelet agents including GpIIbIIIa inhibitors, thromboxane inhibitors, irreversible cyclooxygenase inhibitors, or apyrase have also been described [4,12]. However, no single additive has been shown to be reproducibly effective against platelet clumping. Moreover, these laboratory procedures are time-consuming, and must be hence reserved to specific cases.

4.3. Temperature

Alternative strategies, such as maintaining the whole blood sample at 37 °C until analysis, can be seen as reliable means for preventing platelet clumping, though will not be effective to solve the interference when already present, as in our case. Interestingly, the reticulocyte channels for PLT-O and PLT-F on Sysmex XN® instrumentation are pre-warmed before platelet enumeration, which has plausibly influenced the counting. Future evaluations should also consider comparing PC at lower temperatures, given the observation of higher PCs obtained at RT than at 37 °C in K2-EDTA specimens in our case.

Indeed, heating EDTA-blood samples to 37 °C does not guarantee an accurate PC in 20–35% of reported cases [11,35,99], either because this phenomenon is sometimes temperature-independent, or some autoantibodies (especially IgM) have best clumping activity at 37 °C, thus resulting in instant aggregation in any anticoagulated blood sample [10,102]. When performed, incubation at 37 °C should be initiated as early as possible after phlebotomy [103].

The broad spectrum of described case reports, even for similar conditions (e.g., anticoagulants, temperature) is perhaps attributable to different physico-chemical properties of the antibodies, as well as to confounding variables (time after sampling, pH, medications, and so forth).

4.4. Time

The need for rapid analysis of an EDTA blood tube has been suggested by French guidelines [4] and others [10]. This is due to the time-dependent fall in PC, from 1 min after blood collection to 4 h afterwards [12,13,101,104,105]. Citrate-anticoagulated specimen also evidence underestimated PC when analyzed over 3 h after phlebotomy [106]. This may be explained by the reversible calcium-chelation, which triggers progressive aggregates generation. However, time was not a substantial parameter in our case report, as the PC remained stable in K2-EDTA stored at RT.

4.5. Analytical Techniques

The detection of PTCP is highly dependent on the analytical technique, each showing its own sensitivity and/or vulnerability to the presence of platelet aggregates.

The analytical technique has been a cornerstone for partially avoiding interference due to clumps for this patient. Indeed, PLT-F, PLT-O, and FCM displayed the highest PC, thus suggesting partial dissociation of aggregates using these techniques, as opposed to the impedance method, which was the most vulnerable to platelet clumping. This dissociation effect, independent of manufacturer's fluorescent dye staining, has been assumed in a recent Chinese study [14]. However, sample treatment with hematology or flow cytometry analyzer reagents could not be carried out in our case.

The majority of clinical laboratories are currently using impedance technique for platelet counting, as a consequence of larger availability of instruments based on this standard technology in the market. This method, encompassing variation in electric current intensity when a blood particle passes through two electrodes, does not discriminate platelets from other blood elements with similar same size range [4,107,108]. This technique hence displays high inaccuracy in several clinical situations, despite implementation of computerized algorithms ("moving threshold" and "curve fitting") [107], and remains vulnerable to platelet clumps, as highlighted in this case report. Depending on size, platelet clumps are then enumerated as single large platelets, or as small lymphocytes, resulting in spuriously low PC, and sometimes leading to falsely elevated leukocyte count [4]. Interestingly, the impedance histogram is a useful tool to detect PTCP, as it may display sawtooth irregularities in the curve and serrated tail, sometimes with no return to the baseline at 20 fL, along with the inability of the analyzer to determine a cut-off between platelets and red blood cell fragments or microcytic red blood cells [4,14,108,109].

Under these measurement conditions, the presence of large platelets (e.g., macroplatelets or giant platelets) as observed in constitutional thrombocytopenias, myeloproliferative neoplasms, or immune thrombocytopenias, may also lead to underestimation of PC, whether or not in vivo thrombocytopenia is present. This less known phenomenon could hence lead to PTCP, not related to the EDTA, but to limitations of current instrumentation when analyzing large platelets.

The impedance method is usually used in routine settings for PC, though laboratory technicians could switch to optical-based or fluorescence-based methods using the reticulocyte mode on demand [110,111]. In our laboratory, these methods are set up as "reflex test", when abnormal histograms of RBC or platelet size are encountered.

The optical platelet-counting method identifies platelets with laser light scatter technique. It uses bi-parametric analysis, based on size and RNA content of particles (except for ADVIA counters). This method overcomes some of impedance drawbacks [107], though obtaining an accurate PC remains challenging in some cases. In our case, PLT-O at baseline showed PC close to FCM reference method.

The fluorescence-based technology is currently marketed by two manufacturers, Sysmex (Kobe, Japan) and Mindray (Shenzhen, China), respectively. On Sysmex XE and XN instruments, this technique combines scattered light and side fluorescence detectors. A fluorescent dye (oxazine) is used beforehand to stain platelets and reticulocytes. It has been shown as a reliable method for accurate platelet counting in thrombocytopenic patients, and one of the most reliable for taking clinical decisions on platelet concentrate transfusions [112–117]. Compared to PLT-O, PLT-F can more clearly distinguish PLT from other blood cells, and is also more accurate for analysis of giant thrombocytes [4,115]. More importantly, it has recently been described as effective in correcting spurious low PC on the two platforms Sysmex XN 9000 and Mindray SF-cube, even suggesting that an alternative anticoagulant will probably no longer be necessary in case of EDTA-PTCP [14,108]. Limitations of this enumeration technique are longer turnaround time, increased reagent costs due fluorescent dye, and need of larger sample volume [113]. Additional studies with large number of patients are still needed to demonstrate that Sysmex XN 9000 and Mindray SF-cube are actually correcting spuriously low platelet counts.

Although the immuno-platelet counting using monoclonal CD41 and CD61 antibodies by FCM is the reference assay for accurate PC [118], this approach requires specific skills, is time consuming, and not applicable in practice when dealing with PTCP. It has been poorly investigated in case of PTCP, and our results show that PLT-F and PLT-O were quite similar. This led us to suggest that even this method does not allow optimal thrombocyte counting in presence of PTCP, despite a possible partial aggregates dissociation.

Based on the available literature and this report, we hence suggest fluorescence-based counting as the most useful second-line technique given the nature of FCM and the larger variability observed with PLT-O.

Alternative microscopic methods in case of multi-anticoagulant PTCP should also be considered, such as manual counting on native whole blood sample [4] (i.e., capillary blood or venous blood from discard tube) or on PBS, the latter being able to benefit from double platform counting [119] by multiplying the platelet to red blood cell ratio by the concentration of red blood cells counted on the analyzer. The accuracy and efficiency of this counting method can be improved by using digital microscopy. However, this has been shown on normal samples but has never been evaluated in the presence of platelet clumps.

4.6. Alternative Anticoagulants

Sodium citrate is the most widely used alternative anticoagulant to EDTA due to its wider availability on the market and its lower risk of clump formation. However, PTCP has been described with EDTA and citrate concomitantly, and even with more than two anticoagulants [3,8,49–52], including in this case report. The major disadvantage of citrate is the introduction of a dilution factor, since the anticoagulant is only available in liquid form. The most commonly used correction of 110% may not be sufficient, because the PC is underestimated compared to EDTA [106]. Two reports showed the need for a higher corrective factor; one suggested 117% and the other 125%, respectively [11,120]. However, French guidelines still recommend the 110% correction factor, and caution is advised for citrate samples processed more than 3 h after collection. The PC on citrate therefore remains slightly insufficient when correcting EDTA-PTCP, albeit to a lower extent than in the presence of aggregates.

Heparin is another commonly used alternative anticoagulant, though is currently no longer recommended by the French guidelines. Its weak staining properties make interpretation of blood smears challenging due to the presence of halos around cellular elements, while it seems also not always efficient to prevent PTCP [4].

Sodium fluoride [109,121], CPT (Trisodium citrate, pyridoxal-5′ phosphate and Tris) [122,123] and CTAD (citrate, theophylline, adenosine, and dipyridamole) can also be used. No cases of PTCP have been reported for the last two additives. Although the latter also suffers from a dilutional effect due to anticoagulant availability in liquid form, several studies including some on animals showed its benefit in resolving EDTA-PTCP [124–126].

Two anticoagulants especially useful in PTCP should also be considered, although they have not been studied here. One of these, based on magnesium sulfate, is effective to prevent PTCP and hence recommended for PC once PTCP has been documented [10,17,101,127,128]. Magnesium inhibits platelet aggregation through its ability to prevent intracellular calcium influx and by inhibiting thromboxane A2 formation. In addition, it interferes with fibrinogen binding to stimulated thrombocytes [17,101]. Historically used for platelet counting, it has been offset by automation in hematology, which has propelled EDTA as the reference additive. Its effectiveness has even been proven in multi-anticoagulant PTCP, as the most effective compound to prevent platelet clumps among the five anticoagulants [8]. No case report of PTCP with this additive has yet been published to the best of our knowledge. The other additive, acid citrate dextrose (ACD), may almost invariably prevent platelet aggregation [18], even more effectively than using sodium citrate, due to the more acidic content along with a lower aggregation.

Before being replaced by EDTA, the ACD was the most widely used additive for routine platelet enumeration [31].

Given the few hirudin-PTCP reports described and its increasing use in clinical laboratories, especially for multiple electrode aggregometry [129], the hirudin tube was also studied in this experimental protocol. This study can be added to the previous reports that showed that hirudin specimens had no advantage in correcting PTCP [8,19,20], in addition to being expensive.

5. Clinical Implications

Although laboratory awareness of this PTCP has led to a proactive attitude towards clinicians, this phenomenon continues to have clinical consequences. Recent published cases of PTCP, leading to undesirable clinical implications, are summarized in Table 1.

Table 1. PTCPs with clinical impact reported in the literature since 2015.

Author (Ref.)	Anticoagulant-Induced Ptcp	Medical Condition	Clinical Implication	Confirmation on Alternative Anticoagulants
Akyol et al., 2015 [130]	EDTA	SLE & Lupus nephritis	Unnecessary platelet transfusion	Citrate
Kohlschein et al., 2015 [128]	EDTA, Citrate	Paroxysmal atrial fibrillation	Delayed cardiological intervention	Magnesium sulfate
Greinacher et al., 2016 [98]	EDTA, Citrate	ACS under GpIIb/IIIa antagonist (Eptifibatide)	Therapeutic management issues and wrongly transferred in ICU	ND
Shi et al., 2017 [80]	EDTA	Sepsis	Unnecessary platelet transfusion	Citrate
Li et al., 2020 [2]	EDTA	Viral infection (COVID 19)	Unnecessary platelet transfusion	Citrate
Kuhlman et al., 2020 [3]	EDTA, Citrate, Heparin	Viral infection (COVID 19)	Associated with an arterial occlusive stent (STEMI)	None
Zhong et al., 2020 [49]	EDTA, Citrate, Heparin	Viral infection (gastroenteritis)	Treated with dexamethasone due to misdiagnosis of ITP	None

Abbreviations: ACS, Acute coronary syndrome; ICU, Intensive care unit; ITP, immune thrombocytopenia; ND, not determined; SLE, Systemic lupus erythematosus; STEMI, ST-Elevation myocardial infarction.

The PTCP may have only minor pathophysiologic significance. However, this situation must be distinguished from true in vivo platelet clumps detected by chance during a blood test. Some reports have mentioned this possibility. One described in vivo platelets clumps due to arterial occlusive stent [3]. The pathogenesis of clump formation in arterial thrombosis has no strict relationship with the dynamics of aggregates formation in PTCP. Other cases described in vivo platelet clumping in patients with type 2B VWD, who were misdiagnosed with EDTA-PTCP [131–133]. Interestingly, morphological features of clumps in this setting are different from the aggregates encountered in EDTA-dependent PTCP, being characterized by more heterogeneous and larger sizes [15,132]. Findings of platelet clumps on blood smears from whole blood (either finger prick or discard tubes) may suggest this pathology [131]. Although we did observe platelet clumps on whole blood samples, VWD including VWD 2B and platelet type VWD could be ruled out in our patient. A significant increasing of in vivo platelet clumps have also been described in healthy marathon runners, 30 min after the race [134].

As the in vitro phenomenon of PTCP could be misdiagnosed with thrombocytopenia, it does affect diagnostic, management, and therapeutic decisions. Inadequate treatments such as platelet transfusion [2,80,128,130,135] or high doses corticosteroids against immune thrombocytopenia [49,83,100] may be frequently used, hopefully with minor iatrogenic consequences. Nonetheless, other implications such as discontinuation of heparin therapy could be potentially life-threatening [81]. Detection of PTCP can even modify the decision to initiate heparin therapy, especially when managing acute coronary syndrome [96]. Unnecessary investigations such as a bone marrow biopsy and unwarranted surgical procedures such as splenectomy have also been described [7,96,136,137].

Given the potential life-threatening situations, some authors suggested that PTCP must be in the differential diagnosis, or even ruled out, before considering a diagnosis, for example in patients with cancer [94] or HIT [81]. Interestingly, a study observed that 88% of patients with EDTA and citrate dependent-PTCP had anti-platelet factor 4 (PF4)/heparin antibodies [82], thus potentially leading to diagnose HIT and discontinuing heparin therapy. However, larger clinical studies are needed to demonstrate the presence of these antibodies in PTCP [41]. In addition, laboratory tests used for HIT diagnosis must be integrated into a clinico-pathological approach. In a patient with positive pre-test score, the presence of anti-platelet factor 4 (PF4)/heparin antibodies should be confirmed by a functional assay, which measures heparin-dependent platelet activation/aggregation induced by HIT antibodies [138]. Finally, a B-cell lymphoproliferative disorder could be suspected in the presence of platelet satellitism around lymphocytes [63].

6. Management in the Laboratory and Practical Flowchart

A careful search in the literature about management of PTCP shows different approaches, though most of these generally follow a three step process: identification, confirmation, and prevention. Below, we propose a specific algorithm, based on the current knowledge of PTCP (Figure 5). This flowchart is based on the recent decision tree from the last recommendations of Groupe Francophone d'Hématologie Cellulaire (GFHC) for thrombocytopenia [4].

Once the presence of clots has been ruled out, inspection of histograms and scattergrams of RBCs, platelets, and white blood cells is carried out during the staining of the May–Grünwald–Giemsa smear. These may already suggest the presence of platelet satellitism, giant platelets, or aggregates, which must then be confirmed on PBS. If fluorescence or optical measurements are available, they should be considered either on the basis of histograms or on PBS. When these methods do not remove the interference, an alternative anticoagulant should be considered to differentiate between a preanalytical problem, an EDTA-dependent PTCP, or a multi-anticoagulant PTCP. In the latter case, third-line anticoagulants such as magnesium sulfate or ACD are recommended. Interestingly, these anticoagulants are already used as second-line anticoagulants instead of citrate in some laboratories. Manual counting or variation of physico-chemical parameters should be performed in a limited number of cases. Finally, the preferred counting technique should always be reported, at least within the laboratory information system (LIS), thus limiting further investigations and potential clinical repercussions.

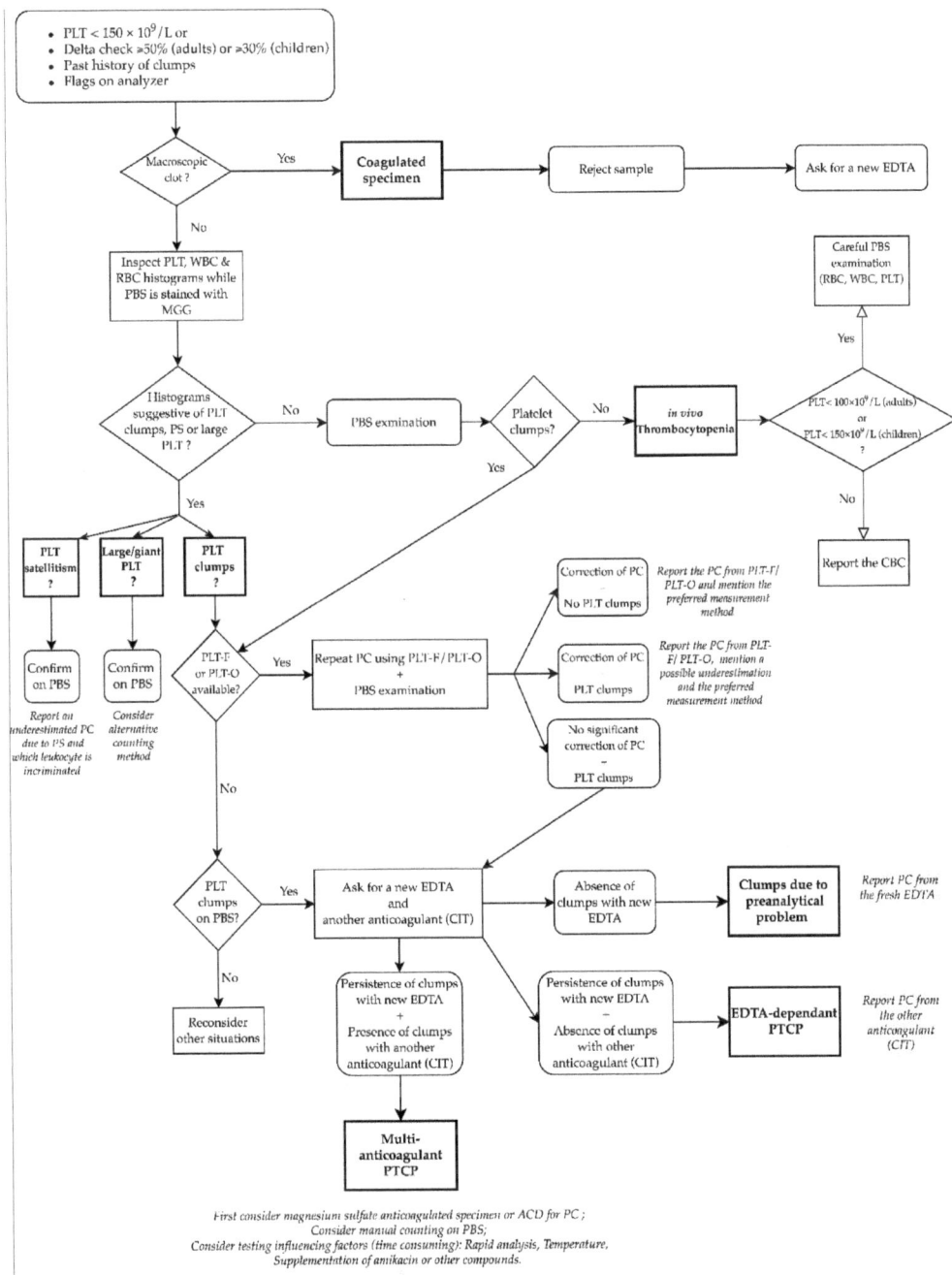

Figure 5. Modified flowchart diagram of EDTA thrombocytopenia based on the decision tree from Baccini et al., 2020 (GFHC, French Society of Haematology). This provides a practical approach for laboratory staff in the presence of thrombocytopenia. ACD: acid citrate dextrose; CBC: complete blood count; CIT: citrate; MGG: May–Grünwald–Giemsa staining; PBS: peripheral blood smear; PC: platelet count; PLT: platelet; PS: platelet satellitism; PLT-O: optical-based platelet count; PLT-F: fluorescence-based platelet count; PTCP: pseudothrombocytopenia; RBC: red blood cells; WBC: white blood cells.

7. Conclusions

PTCP is a complex phenomenon, influenced by the method used for counting thrombocytes and including also preanalytical issues. It seems that no particular disease may be specially associated with PTCP. This condition could still lead to misdiagnosis of thrombocytopenia, impairing diagnosis, management, and therapeutic decisions. Most cases of EDTA-dependent PTCP can be corrected by using different anticoagulants, whilst multiple anticoagulants PTCP is a less acknowledged laboratory phenomenon, resulting in more analytical challenges. Observing PTCP in individuals does not increase the risk of developing future disorder. Conversely, the incidence of PTCP is higher in patients with identified risk factors, including male sex, age over 50 years, underlying diseases, or therapy with drugs such as LMWH. New technologies such as fluorescence or optical platelet counting should be implemented in clinical laboratories, as they will provide a valuable and suitable support for correcting spuriously low PC. Heating the whole blood specimen at 37 °C, in vitro amikacin supplementation, or rapid sample analysis are more laborious strategies, which are not always effective to improve the accuracy of PC, as observed in this case report. Alternative anticoagulants to EDTA (e.g., magnesium sulfate or ACD) should now be reconsidered in sample with clear evidence of PTCP. Finally, the counting method should always be reported, at least in the LIS.

Author Contributions: B.L., J.F., B.C., and F.M. conceptualized and designed the methodology of the study. B.L. and J.F. carried out the experiment. B.L. wrote the manuscript. G.L revised the manuscript. All authors have read and agreed to the published version of the manuscript.

Funding: This research received no external funding.

Institutional Review Board Statement: Ethical review and approval were waived for this study, due to the case report with informed consent for the subject involved in the study.

Informed Consent Statement: Informed consent was obtained from the subject involved in the study.

Data Availability Statement: Please contact the corresponding author.

Acknowledgments: We thank the hematology laboratory technicians for their technical contribution to the experiment. The authors would like to thank Thomas Lecompte (Université de Genève) for providing very sound and helpful advice on the content of the manuscript.

Conflicts of Interest: The authors declare no conflict of interest.

References

1. Gowland, E.; Kay, H.E.M.; Spillman, J.C.; Williamson, J.R. Agglutination of platelets by a serum factor in the presence of EDTA. *J. Clin. Pathol.* **1969**, *22*, 460–464. [CrossRef]
2. Li, H.; Wang, B.; Ning, L.; Luo, Y.; Xiang, S. Transient appearance of EDTA dependent pseudothrombocytopenia in a patient with 2019 novel coronavirus pneumonia. *Platelets* **2020**, *31*, 825–826. [CrossRef]
3. Kuhlman, P.; Patrick, J.; Goodman, M. Pan-Pseudothrombocytopenia in COVID-19: A Harbinger for Lethal Arterial Thrombosis? *Fed. Pract.* **2020**, *37*, 354–368. [CrossRef]
4. Baccini, V.; Geneviève, F.; Jacqmin, H.; Chatelain, B.; Girard, S.; Wuilleme, S.; Vedrenne, A.; Guiheneuf, E.; Toussaint-Hacquard, M.; Everaere, F.; et al. Platelet Counting: Ugly Traps and Good Advice. Proposals from the French-Speaking Cellular Hematology Group (GFHC). *J. Clin. Med.* **2020**, *9*, 808. [CrossRef]
5. Chae, H.; Kim, M.; Lim, J.; Oh, E.-J.; Kim, Y.; Han, K. Novel method to dissociate platelet clumps in EDTA-dependent pseudothrombocytopenia based on the pathophysiological mechanism. *Clin. Chem. Lab. Med.* **2012**, *50*, 1387–1391. [CrossRef]
6. Froom, P.; Barak, M. Prevalence and course of pseudothrombocytopenia in outpatients. *Clin. Chem. Lab. Med.* **2011**, *49*, 111–114. [CrossRef]
7. Zandecki, M.; Genevieve, F.; Gerard, J.; Godon, A. Spurious counts and spurious results on haematology analysers: A review. Part I: Platelets. *Clin. Lab. Haematol.* **2007**, *29*, 4–20. [CrossRef] [PubMed]
8. Kovacs, F.; Varga, M.; Pataki, Z.; Rigo, E. Pseudothrombocytopenia with multiple anticoagulant sample collection tubes. *Interv. Med. Appl. Sci.* **2016**, *8*, 181–183. [CrossRef] [PubMed]
9. Bokaei, P.B.; Grabovsky, D.; Shehata, N.; Wang, C. Impact of Amikacin on Pseudothrombocytopenia. *Acta Haematol.* **2017**, *137*, 27–29. [CrossRef] [PubMed]
10. Schuff-Werner, P.; Mansour, J.; Gropp, A. Pseudo-thrombocytopenia (PTCP). A challenge in the daily laboratory routine? *LaboratoriumsMedizin* **2020**, *44*, 295–304. [CrossRef]

11. Ozcelik, F.; Oztosun, M.; Arslan, E.; Serdar, M.A.; Kurt, I.; Yiginer, O.; Kayadibi, H. A Useful Method for the Detection of Ethylenediaminetetraacetic Acid- and Cold Agglutinin-Dependent Pseudothrombocytopenia. *Am. J. Med. Sci.* **2012**, *344*, 357–362. [CrossRef] [PubMed]
12. Lippi, G.; Plebani, M. EDTA-dependent pseudothrombocytopenia: Further insights and recommendations for prevention of a clinically threatening artifact. *Clin. Chem. Lab. Med.* **2012**, *50*, 1281–1285. [CrossRef] [PubMed]
13. Lin, J.; Luo, Y.; Yao, S.; Yan, M.; Li, J.; Ouyang, W.; Kuang, M. Discovery and Correction of Spurious Low Platelet Counts due to EDTA-Dependent Pseudothrombocytopenia: In Vitro Blood Anticoagulants Associated Pseudothrombocytopenia. *J. Clin. Lab. Anal.* **2015**, *29*, 419–426. [CrossRef]
14. Bao, Y.; Wang, J.; Wang, A.; Bian, J.; Jin, Y. Correction of spurious low platelet counts by optical fluorescence platelet counting of BC-6800 hematology analyzer in EDTA-dependent pseudo thrombocytopenia patients. *Transl. Cancer Res.* **2020**, *9*, 166–172. [CrossRef]
15. Tan, G.C.; Stalling, M.; Dennis, G.; Nunez, M.; Kahwash, S.B. Pseudothrombocytopenia due to Platelet Clumping: A Case Report and Brief Review of the Literature. *Case Rep. Hematol.* **2016**, *2016*, 1–4. [CrossRef] [PubMed]
16. Robertson, W.O. Drug-Imprint Coding. *JAMA J. Am. Med. Assoc.* **1974**, *229*, 766. [CrossRef]
17. Mannuß, S.; Schuff-Werner, P.; Dreißiger, K.; Kohlschein, P. Magnesium Sulfate as an Alternative In Vitro Anticoagulant for the Measurement of Platelet Parameters? *Am. J. Clin. Pathol.* **2016**, *145*, 806–814. [CrossRef]
18. Lombarts, A.J.P.F.; de Kieviet, W. Recognition and Prevention of Pseudothrombocytopenia and Concomitant Pseudoleukocytosis. *Am. J. Clin. Pathol.* **1988**, *89*, 634–639. [CrossRef]
19. Robier, C.; Neubauer, M.; Sternad, H.; Rainer, F. Hirudin-induced pseudothrombocytopenia in a patient with EDTA-dependent platelet aggregation: Report of a new laboratory artefact. *Int. J. Lab. Hematol.* **2009**, *32*, 452–453. [CrossRef]
20. Nagler, M.; Keller, P.; Siegrist, D.; Alberio, L. A case of EDTA-dependent pseudothrombocytopenia: Simple recognition of an underdiagnosed and misleading phenomenon. *BMC Clin. Pathol.* **2014**, *14*, 19. [CrossRef]
21. Clinical and Laboratory Standards Institute. *Collection of Diagnostic Venous Blood Specimens*; Clinical and Laboratory Standards Institute: Wayne, PA, USA, 2017; ISBN 978-1-56238-812-6.
22. Notice: Information De L'utilisateur. Available online: bijsluiters.fagg-afmps.be/DownloadLeafletServlet?id=118724 (accessed on 1 December 2020).
23. Fraser, C.G. Reference change values. *Clin. Chem. Lab. Med.* **2012**, *50*, 807–812. [CrossRef]
24. Aarsand, A.K.; Fernandez-Calle, P.; Webster, C.; Coskun, A.; Gonzales-Lao, E.; Diaz-Garzon, J. The EFLM Biological Variation Data–Base. Available online: https://biologicalvariation.eu/ (accessed on 1 December 2020).
25. Bain, B.J. *Blood Cells: A Practical Guide*, 5th ed.; Wiley Blackwell: Hoboken, NJ, USA, 2015; ISBN 978-1-118-81729-2.
26. Wills, T.B.; Wardrop, K.J. Pseudothrombocytopenia Secondary to the Effects of EDTA in a Dog. *J. Am. Anim. Hosp. Assoc.* **2008**, *44*, 95–97. [CrossRef]
27. Riond, B.; Waßmuth, A.K.; Hartnack, S.; Hofmann-Lehmann, R.; Lutz, H. Effective prevention of pseudothrombocytopenia in feline blood samples with the prostaglandin I2 analogue Iloprost. *BMC Vet. Res.* **2015**, *11*, 183. [CrossRef]
28. Erkens, T.; Van den Sande, L.; Witters, J.; Verbraeken, F.; Looszova, A.; Feyen, B. Effect of time and temperature on anticoagulant-dependent pseudothrombocytopenia in Göttingen minipigs. *Vet. Clin. Pathol.* **2017**, *46*, 416–421. [CrossRef]
29. Paltrinieri, S.; Paciletti, V.; Zambarbieri, J. Analytical variability of estimated platelet counts on canine blood smears. *Vet. Clin. Pathol.* **2018**, *47*, 197–204. [CrossRef] [PubMed]
30. Hübers, E.; Bauer, N.; Fey, K.; Moritz, A.; Roscher, K. Thrombopenie beim Pferd. *Tierärztl. Prax. Ausg. G Großtiere Nutztiere* **2018**, *46*, 73–79. [PubMed]
31. Manthorpe, R.; Kofod, B.; Wiik, A.; Saxtrup, O.; Svehag, S.-E. Pseudothrombocytopenia: In Vitro Studies on the Underlying Mechanism. *Scand. J. Haematol.* **2009**, *26*, 385–392. [CrossRef]
32. Pegels, J.G.; Bruynes, E.C.; Engelfriet, C.P.; von dem Borne, A.E. Pseudothrombocytopenia: An immunologic study on platelet antibodies dependent on ethylene diamine tetra-acetate. *Blood* **1982**, *59*, 157–161. [CrossRef]
33. van Vliet, H.H.; Kappers-Klunne, M.C.; Abels, J. Pseudothrombocytopenia: A cold autoantibody against platelet glycoprotein GP IIb. *Br. J. Haematol.* **1986**, *62*, 501–511. [CrossRef]
34. Payne, B.A. EDTA-induced pseudothrombocytopenia. Recognizing a laboratory artifact. *Postgrad. Med.* **1985**, *77*, 75–76. [CrossRef]
35. Bizzaro, N. EDTA-dependent pseudothrombocytopenia: A clinical and epidemiological study of 112 cases, with 10-year follow-up. *Am. J. Hematol.* **1995**, *50*, 103–109. [CrossRef]
36. Casonato, A.; Bertomoro, A.; Pontara, E.; Dannhauser, D.; Lazzaro, A.R.; Girolami, A. EDTA dependent pseudothrombocytopenia caused by antibodies against the cytoadhesive receptor of platelet gpIIB-IIIA. *J. Clin. Pathol.* **1994**, *47*, 625–630. [CrossRef]
37. Bizzaro, N.; Brandalise, M. EDTA-dependent Pseudothrombocytopenia: Association with Antiplatelet and Antiphospholipid Antibodies. *Am. J. Clin. Pathol.* **1995**, *103*, 103–107. [CrossRef]
38. Isik, A.; Balcik, O.S.; Akdeniz, D.; Cipil, H.; Uysal, S.; Kosar, A. Relationship Between Some Clinical Situations, Autoantibodies, and Pseudothrombocytopenia. *Clin. Appl. Thromb.* **2012**, *18*, 645–649. [CrossRef]
39. Bai, M.; Feng, J.; Liang, G. Transient EDTA-Dependent Pseudothrombocytopenia Phenomenon in a Patient with Antiphospholipid Syndrome. *Clin. Lab.* **2018**, *64*, 1581–1583. [CrossRef]
40. Kurata, Y.; Hayashi, S.; Jouzaki, K.; Konishi, I.; Kashiwagi, H.; Tomiyama, Y. Four cases of pseudothrombocytopenia due to platelet cold agglutinins. *Rinsho Ketsueki* **2006**, *47*, 781–786.

41. Balcik, O.S.; Akdeniz, D.; Cipil, H.; Uysal, S.; Isik, A.; Kosar, A. Heparin Platelet Factor 4 Antibody Positivity in Pseudothrombocytopenia. *Clin. Appl. Thromb.* **2012**, *18*, 92–95. [CrossRef] [PubMed]
42. Veenhoven, W.A.; Van Der Schans, G.S.; Huiges, W.; Metting-Scherphuis, H.E.; Halie, M.R.; Nieweg, H.O. Pseudothrombocytopenia Due to Agglutinins. *Am. J. Clin. Pathol.* **1979**, *72*, 1005–1008. [CrossRef] [PubMed]
43. Sánchez Guiu, I.; Martínez-Martinez, I.; Martínez, C.; Navarro-Fernandez, J.; Garcia-Candel, F.; Ferrer-Marín, F.; Vicente, V.; Watson, S.; Andrews, R.; Gardiner, E.; et al. An atypical IgM class platelet cold agglutinin induces GPVI-dependent aggregation of human platelets. *Thromb. Haemost.* **2015**, *114*, 313–324. [CrossRef] [PubMed]
44. Banfi, G.; Salvagno, G.L.; Lippi, G. The role of ethylenediamine tetraacetic acid (EDTA) as in vitro anticoagulant for diagnostic purposes. *Clin. Chem. Lab. Med.* **2007**, *45*, 565–576. [CrossRef]
45. Dabadie, M.; Valli, N.; Jacobin, M.-J.; Laroche-Traineau, J.; Barat, J.-L.; Ducassou, D.; Nurden, A.T.; Clofent-Sanchez, G. Characterisation, cloning and sequencing of a conformation-dependent monoclonal antibody to the α IIb β 3 integrin: Interest for use in thrombus detection. *Platelets* **2001**, *12*, 395–405. [CrossRef]
46. Bowen, R.A.R.; Remaley, A.T. Interferences from blood collection tube components on clinical chemistry assays. *Biochem. Medica* **2014**, *24*, 31–44. [CrossRef]
47. Golański, J.; Pietrucha, T.; Baj, Z.; Greger, J.; Watala, C. A novel approach to inhibit the anticoagulant-induced spontaneous activation of blood platelets - effect of magnesium on platelet release reaction in whole blood. *Thromb. Res.* **1997**, *85*, 127–132. [CrossRef]
48. Onder, O.; Weinstein, A.; Hoyer, L.W. Pseudothrombocytopenia caused by platelet agglutinins that are reactive in blood anticoagulated with chelating agents. *Blood* **1980**, *56*, 177–182. [CrossRef] [PubMed]
49. Zhong, L.; Chadha, J.; Ameri, A. A Curious Case of Pseudothrombocytopenia due to In Vitro Agglutination. *Case Rep. Hematol.* **2020**, *2020*, 1–3. [CrossRef] [PubMed]
50. Zhou, X.; Wu, X.; Deng, W.; Li, J.; Luo, W. Amikacin Can Be Added to Blood to Reduce the Fall in Platelet Count. *Am. J. Clin. Pathol.* **2011**, *136*, 646–652. [CrossRef] [PubMed]
51. Yoshikawa, T.; Nakanishi, K.; Maruta, T.; Takenaka, D.; Hirota, S.; Matsumoto, S.; Saigo, K.; Ohno, Y.; Fujii, M.; Sugimura, K. Anticoagulant-Induced Pseudothrombocytopenia Occurring after Transcatheter Arterial Embolization for Hepatocellular Carcinoma. *Jpn. J. Clin. Oncol.* **2006**, *36*, 527–531. [CrossRef]
52. Albersen, A.; Porcelijn, L.; Schilders, J.; Zuetenhorst, H.; Njo, T.; Hamberg, P. Sunitinib-associated pseudothrombocytopenia induced by IgM antibody. *Platelets* **2013**, *24*, 566–570. [CrossRef]
53. Chiurazzi, F.; Villa, M.R.; Rotoli, B. Transplacental transmission of EDTA-dependent pseudothrombocytopenia. *Haematologica* **1999**, *84*, 664.
54. Korterink, J.J.; Boersma, B.; Schoorl, M.; Porcelijn, L.; Bartels, P.C.M. Pseudothrombocytopenia in a neonate due to mother? *Eur. J. Pediatr.* **2013**, *172*, 987–989. [CrossRef]
55. Ohno, N.; Kobayashi, M.; Hayakawa, S.; Utsunomiya, A.; Karakawa, S. Transient pseudothrombocytopenia in a neonate: Transmission of a maternal EDTA-dependent anticoagulant. *Platelets* **2012**, *23*, 399–400. [CrossRef]
56. Christensen, R.D. Pseudothrombocytopenia in a Preterm Neonate. *Pediatrics* **2004**, *114*, 273–275. [CrossRef]
57. Rajajee, S.; Subbiah, E.; Krishnamurthy, N.; Paranjothi, S.; Lohiya, N. Pseudothrombocytopenia and Usefulness of Platelet Aggregates in Peripheral Smear in the Diagnosis of Scrub Typhus. *Indian J. Pediatr.* **2019**, *86*, 93–94. [CrossRef] [PubMed]
58. Wong, V.K.; Robertson, R.; Nagaoka, E.; Ong, E.; Petz, L.; Stiehm, E.R. Pseudothrombocytopenia in a child with the acquired immunodeficiency syndrome. *West. J. Med.* **1992**, *157*, 668–670. [PubMed]
59. Hsieh, A.T.; Chao, T.Y.; Chen, Y.C. Pseudothrombocytopenia associated with infectious mononucleosis. *Arch. Pathol. Lab. Med.* **2003**, *127*, e17–e18. [CrossRef]
60. Vaidya, P.; Venkataraman, R. Pseudothrombocytopenia in a child with Dengue. *Indian J. Pediatr.* **2014**, *81*, 1395–1396. [CrossRef] [PubMed]
61. Igala, M.; Kouégnigan Rerambiah, L.; Ledaga Lentombo, L.E.; Ifoudji Makao, A.; Nto'o Eyene, S.; Mbiye Cheme, S.W.; Bouyou Akotet, M.; Boguikouma, J.B. Anticoagulant-induced pseudothrombocytopenia after a plasmodium falciparum infection in a five-year-old child. *Med. Sante Trop.* **2019**, *29*, 175–177.
62. Akbayram, S.; Dogan, M.; Akgun, C.; Caksen, H.; Oner, A.F. EDTA-Dependent Pseudothrombocytopenia in a Child. *Clin. Appl. Thromb.* **2011**, *17*, 494–496. [CrossRef]
63. Lopez-Molina, M.; Sorigue, M.; Martinez-Iribarren, A.; Orna Montero, E.; Tejedor Ganduxé, X.; Leis Sestayo, A.; Sala Sanjaume, M.A.; Llopis Díaz, M.-A.; Morales-Indiano, C. Platelet satellitism around lymphocytes: Case report and literature review. *Int. J. Lab. Hematol.* **2019**, *41*, e81–e83. [CrossRef]
64. Bizzaro, N.; Goldschmeding, R. Platelet Satellitism Is Fc Y RIII (CD 16) Receptor-Mediated. *Am. J. Clin. Pathol.* **1995**, *103*, 740–744. [CrossRef]
65. Christopoulos, C.; Mattock, C. Platelet satellitism and ox granule proteins. *J. Clin. Pathol.* **1991**, *44*, 788–789. [CrossRef]
66. Bartels, P.C.M.; Schoorl, M.; Lombarts, A.J.P.F. Screening for EDTA-dependent deviations in platelet counts and abnormalities in platelet distribution histograms in pseudothrombocytopenia. *Scand. J. Clin. Lab. Investig.* **1997**, *57*, 629–636. [CrossRef] [PubMed]
67. Vicari, A.; Banfi, G.; Bonini, P.A. EDTA-dependent pseudothrombocytopaenia: A 12-month epidemiological study. *Scand. J. Clin. Lab. Investig.* **1988**, *48*, 537–542. [CrossRef]
68. García Suárez, J.; Merino, J.L.; Rodríguez, M.; Velasco, A.; Moreno, M.C. Pseudothrombocytopenia: Incidence, causes and methods of detection. *Sangre* **1991**, *36*, 197–200. [PubMed]

69. Sakurai, S.; Shiojima, I.; Tanigawa, T.; Nakahara, K. Aminoglycosides prevent and dissociate the aggregation of platelets in patients with EDTA-dependent pseudothrombocytopenia. *Br. J. Haematol.* **1997**, *99*, 817–823. [CrossRef] [PubMed]
70. Fujii, H.; Watada, M.; Yamamoto, K.; Kanoh, T. [Seventeen cases of pseudothrombocytopenia, with special reference to the clinical problems, its pathogenesis and significance (author's transl)]. *Nihon Ketsueki Gakkai Zasshi J. Jpn. Haematol. Soc.* **1978**, *41*, 523–532.
71. Savage, R.A. Pseudoleukocytosis Due to EDTA-induced Platelet Clumping. *Am. J. Clin. Pathol.* **1984**, *81*, 317–322. [CrossRef]
72. Xiao, Y.; Yu, S.; Xu, Y. The Prevalence and Biochemical Profiles of EDTA-Dependent Pseudothrombocytopenia in a Generally Healthy Population. *Acta Haematol.* **2015**, *134*, 177–180. [CrossRef]
73. Lewinski, U.H.; Cycowitz, Z.; Cohen, A.M.; Gardyn, J.; Mittelman, M. The incidence of pseudothrombocytopenia in automatic blood analyzers. *Haematologia* **2000**, *30*, 117–121.
74. Silvestri, F.; Virgolini, L.; Savignano, C.; Zaja, F.; Velisig, M.; Baccarani, M. Incidence and Diagnosis of EDTA-Dependent Pseudothrombocytopenia in a Consecutive Outpatient Population Referred for Isolated Thrombocytopenia. *Vox Sang.* **1995**, *68*, 35–39. [CrossRef]
75. Tomicic, M.; Vuk, T.; Gulan-Harcet, J. Anticoagulant-induced pseudothrombocytopenia in blood donors: Letter to the Editor. *Transfus. Med.* **2015**, *25*, 47–48. [CrossRef] [PubMed]
76. Maslanka, K.; Marciniak-Bielak, D.; Szczepinski, A. Pseudothrombocytopenia in blood donors. *Vox Sang.* **2008**, *95*, 349. [CrossRef] [PubMed]
77. Sweeney, J.; Holme, S.; Heaton, W.; Campbell, D.; Bowen, M. Pseudothrombocytopenia in plateletpheresis donors. *Transfusion* **1995**, *35*, 46–49. [CrossRef] [PubMed]
78. Lazo-Langner, A.; Piedras, J.; Romero-Lagarza, P.; Lome-Maldonado, C.; Sánchez-Guerrero, J.; López-Karpovitch, X. Platelet satellitism, spurious neutropenia, and cutaneous vasculitis: Casual or causal association?: Case Report: Satellitism and Cutaneous Vasculitis. *Am. J. Hematol.* **2002**, *70*, 246–249. [CrossRef] [PubMed]
79. Choe, W.-H.; Cho, Y.-U.; Chae, J.-D.; Kim, S.-H. Pseudothrombocytopenia or platelet clumping as a possible cause of low platelet count in patients with viral infection: A case series from single institution focusing on hepatitis A virus infection. *Int. J. Lab. Hematol.* **2013**, *35*, 70–76. [CrossRef]
80. Shi, X.; Lin, Z.; He, L.; Li, W.; Mo, L.; Li, Y.; Yang, Z.; Mo, W.-N. Transient appearance of EDTA-dependent pseudothrombocytopenia in a postoperative patient with sepsis: A case report. *Medicine* **2017**, *96*, e6330. [CrossRef]
81. Zimrin, A.B.; Warkentin, T.E. Transient pseudothrombocytopenia associated with immune heparin-induced thrombocytopenia complicated by pulmonary embolism. *Thromb. Haemost.* **2013**, *109*, 971–973. [CrossRef]
82. Martin-Toutain, I.; Settegrana, C.; Ankri, A. High levels of heparin-platelet factor 4 antibodies in patients with pseudothrombocytopenia: Risk of misdiagnosis. *J. Thromb. Haemost.* **2009**, *7*, 1416–1418. [CrossRef]
83. Berkman, N.; Michaeli, Y.; Or, R.; Eldor, A. EDTA-dependent pseudothrombocytopenia: A clinical study of 18 patients and a review of the literature. *Am. J. Hematol.* **1991**, *36*, 195–201. [CrossRef]
84. Matarazzo, M.; Conturso, V.; Di Martino, M.; Chiurazzi, F.; Guida, G.; Morante, R. EDTA-dependent pseudothrombocytopenia in a case of liver cirrhosis. *Panminerva Med.* **2000**, *42*, 155–157.
85. Sahin, C.; Kırlı, I.; Sozen, H.; Canbek, T.D. EDTA-induced pseudothrombocytopenia in association with bladder cancer. *BMJ Case Rep.* **2014**, *2014*, bcr2014205130. [CrossRef]
86. Kim, H.J.; Moh, I.H.; Yoo, H.; Son, S.; Jung, D.H.; Lee, H.G.; Han, D.H.; Park, J.H.; Kim, H.S.; Kim, J.H. Ethylenediaminetetraacetic acid-dependent pseudothrombocytopenia associated with neuroendocrine carcinoma: A case report. *Oncol. Lett.* **2012**, *4*, 86–88. [CrossRef]
87. Dalamangas, C.; Slaughter, T.F. Ethylenediaminetetraacetic Acid-Dependent Pseudothrombocytopenia in a Cardiac Surgical Patient. *Anesth. Analg.* **1998**, *86*, 1210–1211.
88. Wenzel, F.; Lasshofer, R.; Rox, J.; Fischer, J.; Giers, G. Transient appearance of postoperative EDTA-dependent pseudothrombocytopenia in a patient after gastrectomy. *Platelets* **2011**, *22*, 72–74. [CrossRef] [PubMed]
89. Nair, S.K.; Shah, R.; Petko, M.; Keogh, B.E. Pseudothrombocytopenia in cardiac surgical practice. *Interact. Cardiovasc. Thorac. Surg.* **2007**, *6*, 565–566. [CrossRef] [PubMed]
90. Di Francesco, A.; Pasanisi, F.; Tsamesidis, I.; Podda, L.; Fozza, C. Pseudo-thrombocytopenia after autologous stem cell transplantation. *Blood Coagul. Fibrinolysis* **2019**, *30*, 66–67. [CrossRef] [PubMed]
91. Deeren, D.; Van Haute, I. Is pseudothrombocytopenia transmitted from hematopoietic stem cell donor to recipient?: Pseudothrombocytopenia in a Stem Cell Donor. *J. Clin. Apher.* **2014**, *29*, 290–291. [CrossRef] [PubMed]
92. Beyan, C.; Kaptan, K.; Ifran, A. Pseudothrombocytopenia after changing insulin therapy in a case with insulin-dependent diabetes mellitus: A first case report. *Am. J. Hematol.* **2010**, *85*, 909–910. [CrossRef] [PubMed]
93. Sane, D.C.; Damaraju, L.V.; Topol, E.J.; Cabot, C.F.; Mascelli, M.A.; Harrington, R.A.; Simoons, M.L.; Califf, R.M. Occurrence and clinical significance of pseudothrombocytopenia during abciximab therapy. *J. Am. Coll. Cardiol.* **2000**, *36*, 75–83. [CrossRef]
94. Krukowska, K.; Kieszko, R.; Kurek, K.; Chmielewska, I.; Krawczyk, P.; Milanowski, J. An Episode of Pseudothrombocytopenia during Pembrolizumab Therapy in NSCLC Patient. *Case Rep. Oncol. Med.* **2020**, *2020*, 1–4. [CrossRef]
95. Vidranski, V.; Laskaj, R.; Sikiric, D.; Skerk, V. Platelet satellitism in infectious disease? *Biochem. Medica* **2015**, *25*, 285–294. [CrossRef] [PubMed]
96. Kocum, T.H.; Katircibasi, T.M.; Sezgin, A.T.; Atalay, H. An unusual cause of mismanagement in an acute myocardial infarction case: Pseudothrombocytopenia. *Am. J. Emerg. Med.* **2008**, *26*, 740.e1–740.e2. [CrossRef] [PubMed]

97. Bizzaro, N. Platelet Cold Agglutinins and Cardiac Surgery Hypothermia. *Am. J. Hematol.* **1999**, *60*, 80–85. [CrossRef]
98. Greinacher, A.; Selleng, S. How I evaluate and treat thrombocytopenia in the intensive care unit patient. *Blood* **2016**, *128*, 3032–3042. [CrossRef]
99. Ahn, H.L.; Jo, Y.I.; Choi, Y.S.; Lee, J.Y.; Lee, H.W.; Kim, S.R.; Sim, J.; Lee, W.; Jin, C.J. EDTA—dependent Pseudothrombocytopenia Confirmed by Supplementation of Kanamycin; A Case Report. *Korean J. Intern. Med.* **2002**, *17*, 65–68. [CrossRef]
100. Lombarts, A.J.P.F.; Zijlstra, J.J.; Peters, R.H.M.; Thomasson, C.G.; Franck, P.F.H. Accurate Platelet Counting in an Insidious Case of Pseudothrombocytopenia. *Clin. Chem. Lab. Med.* **1999**, *37*, 1063–1066. [CrossRef]
101. Schuff-Werner, P.; Steiner, M.; Fenger, S.; Gross, H.-J.; Bierlich, A.; Dreissiger, K.; Mannuß, S.; Siegert, G.; Bachem, M.; Kohlschein, P. Effective estimation of correct platelet counts in pseudothrombocytopenia using an alternative anticoagulant based on magnesium salt. *Br. J. Haematol.* **2013**, *162*, 684–692. [CrossRef]
102. van der Meer, W.; Allebes, W.; Simon, A.; van Berkel, Y.; de Keijzer, M.H. Pseudothrombocytopenia: A report of a new method to count platelets in a patient with EDTA- and temperature-independent antibodies of the IgM type. *Eur. J. Haematol.* **2002**, *69*, 243–247. [CrossRef]
103. Asma, A.; Anissa, S.; Touhami, K. Aggregation kinetic and temperature optimum of an EDTA-dependent pseudothrombocytopenia. *Clin. Chem. Lab. Med. CCLM* **2020**, *59*, e31–e33. [CrossRef] [PubMed]
104. Salama, A. Autoimmune Thrombocytopenia Complicated by EDTA- and/or Citrate-Dependent Pseudothrombocytopenia. *Transfus. Med. Hemother.* **2015**, *42*, 345–348. [CrossRef] [PubMed]
105. Herb, A.; Maurer, M.; Alamome, I.; Bihl, P.-A.; Ghiura, C.; Hurstel, R. A case report of pseudo grey platelet syndrome with citrate-induced pseudothrombocytopenia: Those artifacts may interfere in the platelet numeration and lead to critical misdiagnosis. *Ann. Biol. Clin.* **2017**, *75*, 457–461. [CrossRef]
106. Védy, S.; Boom, B.; Perez, P.; Schillinger, S.; Ragot, C.; Bakkouch, S.; Puyhardy, J.-M. Automatic platelets numbering with citrate as anticoagulant: Is the result valid? *Ann. Biol. Clin.* **2011**, *69*, 453–458. [CrossRef]
107. Larsen, P.B.; Vikeså, J.; Friis-Hansen, L. EDTA-induced pseudothrombocytosis and citrate-induced platelet agglutination in a patient with Waldenstrom macroglobulinemia. *Clin. Case Rep.* **2017**, *5*, 1243–1247. [CrossRef]
108. Deng, J.; Chen, Y.; Zhang, S.; Li, L.; Shi, Q.; Liu, M.; Yu, X. Mindray SF-Cube technology: An effective way for correcting platelet count in individuals with EDTA dependent pseudo thrombocytopenia. *Clin. Chim. Acta* **2020**, *502*, 99–101. [CrossRef] [PubMed]
109. Lippi, G.; Guidi, G.; Nicoli, M. Platelet count in EDTA dependent pseudothrombocytopenia. *Eur. J. Haematol.* **1996**, *56*, 112–113. [CrossRef] [PubMed]
110. Briggs, C.; Harrison, P.; Grant, D.; Staves, J.; Machin, S.J. New quantitative parameters on a recently introduced automated blood cell counter—the XE 2100 TM: Automated blood cell counter quantitative parameters. *Clin. Lab. Haematol.* **2000**, *22*, 345–350. [CrossRef]
111. Sandhaus, L.M.; Osei, E.S.; Agrawal, N.N.; Dillman, C.A.; Meyerson, H.J. Platelet Counting by the Coulter LH 750, Sysmex XE 2100, and Advia 120: A Comparative Analysis Using the RBC/Platelet Ratio Reference Method. *Am. J. Clin. Pathol.* **2002**, *118*, 235–241. [CrossRef] [PubMed]
112. Briggs, C.; Longair, I.; Kumar, P.; Singh, D.; Machin, S.J. Performance evaluation of the Sysmex haematology XN modular system. *J. Clin. Pathol.* **2012**, *65*, 1024–1030. [CrossRef]
113. Kim, H.; Bang, S.; Cho, D.; Kim, H.; Kim, S. Performance evaluation of platelet counting of Abbott Alinity hq and Sysmex XN-9000 automated hematology analyzer compared with international reference method. *Int. J. Lab. Hematol.* **2020**, 13396. [CrossRef]
114. Sun, Y.; Hu, Z.; Huang, Z.; Chen, H.; Qin, S.; Jianing, Z.; Chen, S.; Qin, X.; Ye, Y.; Wang, C. Compare the accuracy and precision of Coulter LH780, Mindray BC-6000 Plus, and Sysmex XN-9000 with the international reference flow cytometric method in platelet counting. *PLoS ONE* **2019**, *14*, e0217298. [CrossRef]
115. Schoorl, M.; Schoorl, M.; Oomes, J.; van Pelt, J. New Fluorescent Method (PLT-F) on Sysmex XN2000 Hematology Analyzer Achieved Higher Accuracy in Low Platelet Counting. *Am. J. Clin. Pathol.* **2013**, *140*, 495–499. [CrossRef]
116. Park, S.H.; Park, C.-J.; Kim, M.-J.; Han, M.-Y.; Han, S.-H.; Cho, Y.-U.; Jang, S. The New Sysmex XN-2000 Automated Blood Cell Analyzer More Accurately Measures the Absolute Number and the Proportion of Hematopoietic Stem and Progenitor Cells Than XE-2100 When Compared to Flow Cytometric Enumeration of CD34^{+} Cells. *Ann. Lab. Med.* **2015**, *35*, 146–148. [CrossRef]
117. Hummel, K.; Sachse, M.; Hoffmann, J.J.M.L.; van Dun, L.P.J.M. Comparative evaluation of platelet counts in two hematology analyzers and potential effects on prophylactic platelet transfusion decisions: PLT COUNTS AND TRANSFUSION DECISIONS. *Transfusion* **2018**, *58*, 2301–2308. [CrossRef]
118. International Council for Standardization in Haematology Expert Panel on Cytometry; International Society of Laboratory Hematology Task Force on Platelet Counting. Platelet counting by the RBC/platelet ratio method: A reference method. *Am. J. Clin. Pathol.* **2001**, *115*, 460–464. [CrossRef]
119. Anchinmane, V.T.; Sankhe, S.V. Utility of peripheral blood smear in platelet count estimation. *Int. J. Res. Med. Sci.* **2019**, *7*, 434. [CrossRef]
120. Dumont, P.; Goussot, V.; David, A.; Lizard, S.; Riedinger, J.-M. Identification and validation of a factor of commutability between platelet counts performed on EDTA and citrate. *Ann. Biol. Clin.* **2017**, *75*, 61–66. [CrossRef] [PubMed]
121. Kabutomori, O.; Koh, T.; Amino, N.; Iwatani, Y. "Correct" platelet count in EDTA-dependent pseudothrombocytopenia. *Eur. J. Haematol.* **2009**, *55*, 67–68. [CrossRef] [PubMed]

122. Lippi, U.; Schinella, M.; Nicoli, M.; Modena, N.; Lippi, G. EDTA-induced platelet aggregation can be avoided by a new anticoagulant also suitable for automated complete blood count. *Haematologica* **1990**, *75*, 38–41.
123. Lippi, U.; Schinella, M.; Modena, N.; Nicoli, M.; Lippi, G. Advantages of a New Anticoagulant in Routine Hematology on the Coulter Counter®S-Plus STKR Analyzer. *Am. J. Clin. Pathol.* **1990**, *93*, 760–764. [CrossRef] [PubMed]
124. Granat, F.; Geffrè, A.; Braun, J.-P.; Trumel, C. Comparison of Platelet Clumping and Complete Blood Count Results with Sysmex XT-2000iV in Feline Blood Sampled on EDTA or EDTA plus CTAD (Citrate, Theophylline, Adenosine and Dipyridamole). *J. Feline Med. Surg.* **2011**, *13*, 953–958. [CrossRef]
125. Granat, F.A.; Geffré, A.; Lucarelli, L.A.; Braun, J.-P.D.; Trumel, C.; Bourgès-Abella, N.H. Evaluation of CTAD (citrate–theophylline–adenosine–dipyridamole) as a universal anticoagulant in dogs. *J. Vet. Diagn. Invest.* **2017**, *29*, 676–682. [CrossRef]
126. Yokota, M.; Tatsumi, N.; Tsuda, I.; Nishioka, T.; Takubo, T. CTAD as a universal anticoagulant. *J. Autom. Methods Manag. Chem.* **2003**, *25*, 17–20. [CrossRef] [PubMed]
127. François, D.; Masure, A.; Atallah, N.; Touil, L.; Vasse, M. Underestimation of platelet count on magnesium salt-anticoagulated samples. *Clin. Chem. Lab. Med.* **2014**, *52*, e95–e97. [CrossRef]
128. Kohlschein, P.; Bänsch, D.; Dreißiger, K.; Schuff-Werner, P. Exclusion of thrombocytopenia as a contraindication for invasive radiofrequency ablation in a patient with paroxysmal atrial fibrillation by using magnesium anticoagulation instead of EDTA: Another case of anticoagulant-induced pseudo-thrombocytopenia. *Heart Surg. Forum* **2015**, *18*, E90–E92. [CrossRef] [PubMed]
129. Hardy, M.; Lessire, S.; Kasikci, S.; Baudar, J.; Collard, A.; Dogn, J.-M.; Lecompte, T.; Mullier, F. Effects of Time-Interval since Blood Draw and of Anticoagulation on Platelet Testing (Count, Indices and Impedance Aggregometry): A Systematic Study with Blood from Healthy Volunteers. *J. Clin. Med.* **2020**, *9*, 2515. [CrossRef] [PubMed]
130. Akyol, L.; Onem, S.; Ozgen, M.; Sayarlioglu, M. Ethylenediaminetetraacetic acid-dependent pseudothrombocytopenia in a patient with systemic lupus erythematosus and lupus nephritis. *Eur. J. Rheumatol.* **2016**, *3*, 36–37. [CrossRef] [PubMed]
131. Hultin, M.B.; Sussman, I.I. Postoperative thrombocytopenia in type IIB von Willebrand disease. *Am. J. Hematol.* **1990**, *33*, 64–68. [CrossRef] [PubMed]
132. Kumar, R.; Creary, S.; Varga, E.A.; Kahwash, S.B. Thrombocytopenia Pitfalls: Misdiagnosing Type 2B von Willebrand Disease as Ethylenediaminetetraacetic Acid−Dependent Pseudothrombocytopenia. *J. Pediatr.* **2016**, *175*, 238–238.e1. [CrossRef] [PubMed]
133. Saba, H.I.; Saba, S.R.; Dent, J.; Ruggeri, Z.M.; Zimmerman, T.S. Type IIB Tampa: A variant of von Willebrand disease with chronic thrombocytopenia, circulating platelet aggregates, and spontaneous platelet aggregation. *Blood* **1985**, *66*, 282–286. [CrossRef]
134. Kratz, A.; Wood, M.J.; Siegel, A.J.; Hiers, J.R.; Van Cott, E.M. Effects of Marathon Running on Platelet Activation Markers: Direct Evidence for In Vivo Platelet Activation. *Am. J. Clin. Pathol.* **2006**, *125*, 296–300. [CrossRef] [PubMed]
135. Lau, L.G.; Chng, W.J.; Liu, T.C. Unnecessary transfusions due to pseudothrombocytopenia: TRANSFUSION MEDICINE ILLUSTRATED. *Transfusion* **2004**, *44*, 801. [CrossRef] [PubMed]
136. Yamada, E.J.; Souto, A.F.P.; Souza, E.D.E.O.D.; Nunes, C.A.; Dias, C.P. Pseudoplaquetopenia em paciente submetida à esplenectomia de baço acessório: Relato de caso. *Rev. Bras. Anestesiol.* **2008**, *58*, 485–491. [CrossRef] [PubMed]
137. Nilsson, T.; Norberg, B. Thrombocytopenia and pseudothrombocytopenia: A clinical and laboratory problem. *Eur. J. Haematol.* **1986**, *37*, 341–346. [CrossRef] [PubMed]
138. Tardy, B.; Lecompte, T.; Mullier, F.; Vayne, C.; Pouplard, C. Detection of Platelet-Activating Antibodies Associated with Heparin-Induced Thrombocytopenia. *J. Clin. Med.* **2020**, *9*, 1226. [CrossRef] [PubMed]

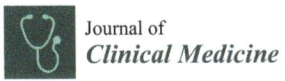

Review

Quantitative and Qualitative Platelet Derangements in Cardiac Surgery and Extracorporeal Life Support

Enrico Squiccimarro [1,2,3,†], Federica Jiritano [3,4,*,†], Giuseppe Filiberto Serraino [4], Hugo ten Cate [5,6,7], Domenico Paparella [8,9] and Roberto Lorusso [3,7]

1. Department of Cardiac Surgery, Mater Dei Hospital, 70125 Bari, Italy; e.squiccimarro@gmail.com
2. Department of Emergency and Organ Transplant (DETO), University of Bari, 70125 Bari, Italy
3. Cardio-Thoracic Surgery Department, Heart & Vascular Centre, Maastricht University Medical Centre (MUMC), 6229HX Maastricht, The Netherlands; robertolorussobs@gmail.com
4. Cardiac Surgery Unit, Department of Experimental and Clinical Medicine, University "Magna Graecia" of Catanzaro, 88100 Catanzaro, Italy; serraino@unicz.it
5. Center for Thrombosis and Hemostasis (CTH), University Medical Center of the Johannes Gutenberg-University Mainz, D-55131 Mainz, Germany; h.tencate@maastrichtuniversity.nl
6. Thrombosis Center Maastricht, Maastricht University Medical Center (MUMC), 6229HX Maastricht, The Netherlands
7. Cardiovascular Research Institute Maastricht (CARIM), 6229HX Maastricht, The Netherlands
8. Division of Cardiac Surgery, Santa Maria Hospital, GVM Care & Research, 70125 Bari, Italy; domenico.paparella@uniba.it
9. Department of Medical and Surgical Sciences, University of Foggia, 71122 Foggia, Italy
* Correspondence: fede.j@hotmail.it
† These authors equally contributed to this work.

Abstract: Thrombocytopenia and impaired platelet function are known as intrinsic drawbacks of cardiac surgery and extracorporeal life supports (ECLS). A number of different factors influence platelet count and function including the inflammatory response to a cardiopulmonary bypass (CPB) or to ECLS, hemodilution, hypothermia, mechanical damage and preoperative treatment with platelet-inhibiting agents. Moreover, although underestimated, heparin-induced thrombocytopenia is still a hiccup in the perioperative management of cardiac surgical and, above all, ECLS patients. Moreover, recent investigations have highlighted how platelet disorders also affect patients undergoing biological prosthesis implantation. Though many hypotheses have been suggested, the mechanism underlying thrombocytopenia and platelet disorders is still to be cleared. This narrative review aims to offer clinicians a summary of their major causes in the cardiac surgery setting.

Keywords: platelet; thrombocytopenia; cardiac surgery; inflammation; biological prosthesis; extracorporeal life support

1. Introduction

Platelets are anucleated blood components with a pivotal role in hemostasis and also other functions in the biology and pathophysiology of complex diseases [1]. Beyond hemostasis and thrombosis, contemporary knowledge ascribes to platelets a key role also in inflammation and innate immunity [2–5]. Therefore, platelets may be considered as immune cells [6]. Quantitative and qualitative platelet derangements represent a shortcoming in cardiac surgery and extracorporeal life supports (ECLS). Thrombocytopenia, indeed, is an intrinsic drawback of cardiac surgery with a prevalence > 30% [7,8]. It is not a trivial event but rather a clinically relevant entity independently associated with increased postoperative morbidity and mortality [7,8]. A conclusive knowledge about the causes of the phenomenon is lacking whereas certainty of its clinical implications exists [9].

Therefore, beyond the role of platelets in hemostasis and thrombosis, the present review aims to give a comprehensive analysis of platelet behavior in the cardiac surgery setting (Figure 1).

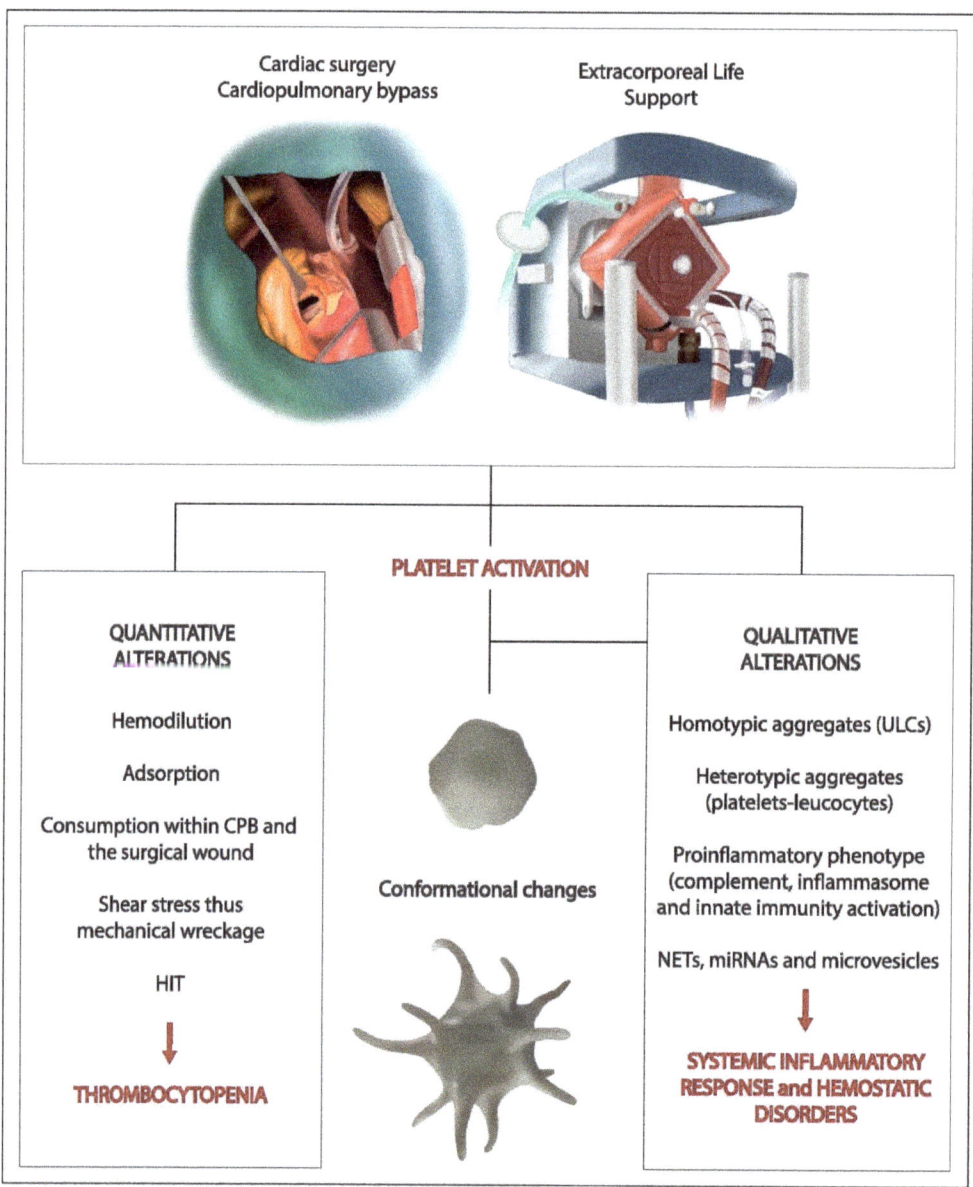

Figure 1. Platelet activation as a consequence of cardiopulmonary bypass-assisted cardiac surgery and extracorporeal life support. A summary of quantitative and qualitative platelet derangements. Abbreviations: cardiopulmonary bypass (CPB), heparin-induced thrombocytopenia (HIT), ultra-large antigenic complexes (ULCs), neutrophil extracellular traps (NETs), microRNAs (miRNAs).

2. Platelets, Cardiac Surgery and Extracorporeal Circulation: The Axis of Hemostasis, Inflammation and Innate Immunity

Multiple sides of platelet biology greatly impact on heart procedures because cardiac surgery enhances a systemic immuno-inflammation response, platelet activation and the coagulation cascade [10].

Platelets undergo both quantitative and qualitative alterations throughout a cardiopulmonary bypass (CPB), the extracorporeal circulation applied to cardiac surgery procedures. The interaction between blood and artificial surfaces of the CPB triggers damage to several cells, the release of various inflammatory cytokines and the activation of the complement and coagulation-fibrinolysis systems [11,12]. During a CPB, platelet changes are caused by hypothermia, shear stress, extensive exposure to artificial surfaces and the use of exogenous drugs (heparin and protamine) [11,12]. Moreover, the coagulation cascade also begins with the activation of factor XII. Clotting factor activation occurs and initiates the subsequent activation of kallikrein, the kinin-bradykinin system and the fibrinolytic and complement cascades [11,12]. All of these mechanisms lead to increased postoperative outcomes such as mortality, major complications (e.g., stroke, acute kidney injury, postoperative infections) and a prolonged in-hospital length of stay [7]. Moreover, the hemodilution related to a CPB contributes to increasing the rate of thrombocytopenia [10–12]. Therefore, cardiac surgery and a CPB lead to a complex homeostatic alteration that enhances the so-called "thromboinflammation", a complex mechanism involving inflammation, thrombosis and innate immunity [10,11]. The same scenario occurs also as a response to other triggers such as veno-arterial (V-A) and veno-venous (V-V) extracorporeal membrane oxygenation (ECMO) and cardiac prosthetic devices [1,13,14].

Moreover, a major role is attributed to the direct platelet-leucocyte interaction that bidirectionally boosts their reciprocal activation [15]. This cross-talk is fundamental in the multistep pathway of neutrophil extravasation (i.e., margination, rolling, extravasation and migration) that occurs in the systemic inflammatory response syndrome in patients on a CPB [16,17]. This process causes the activation of the endothelial cells and of several cellular adhesion molecules (CAMs) resulting lastly in tissue metabolic impairments and an ischemia-reperfusion injury (IRI) [16,17]. Moreover, the interplay between platelets and neutrophils was reported as a prerequisite for the release of neutrophil extracellular traps (NETs), which further triggers platelet activation and aggregation [18,19]. Furthermore, the binding of platelets' integrin αIIbβ3 to neutrophils' macrophage-1 antigen (Mac-1) stimulates the signaling leading to the formation of NETs. This interaction activates an inflammatory response mediated by the nuclear factor-kB (NF-kB) [20–23].

Platelets also modulate the immunoactivity of monocytes/macrophages by NF-kB activation. Moreover, the synthesis of proinflammatory mediators is stimulated. Platelets promote monocytes' chemokines synthesis via P-selectin/P-selectin glycoprotein ligand (PSGL)-1 axis mediated "regulated on activation, normal T cell expressed and secreted" (RANTES) activation [24]. Furthermore, platelet α-granules (their most abundant storage granules) contain a diverse range of cytokines and chemokines among which are CXCL1, platelet factor 4 (PF4; CXCL4), CXCL5, interleukin-8 (IL-8) and RANTES [25]. Platelets have also been shown to independently enhance the inflammatory cascade in innate immune cells in vivo, thus contributing to the release of IL-1 cytokines [26].

In addition to these direct and indirect biological mechanisms, platelets also interact with the classical and the alternative pathways of the complement system [27]. The release of chondroitin sulfate modulates complement activity promoting anaphylatoxins and membrane attack-complex (MAC) generation, thus inducing further platelet activation [28,29]. The interplay between platelets and the complement system seems to involve platelet microparticles containing complement components such as C5b-9 at their surface [30,31].

Furthermore, platelets are the main source of microparticles in the bloodstream [32]. Extracellular vesicles composition varies and includes chemokines, cytokines and CAMs as well as small non-coding RNAs called microRNA (miRNA) [33,34]. MiRNA are involved in gene expression via negative post-transcriptional regulation [33,34]. Circulating miRNAs (i.e., miR-223 and miR-499) were detected following thrombin stimulation [34,35]. Even if the underlying mechanism is still to be cleared, miRNAs could transfer genetic material to recipient cells (among which are endothelial and immune cells) impacting the biological functions of recipient cells (i.e., regulating CAMs expression) [34,35]. Indeed, plasma exosomal miR-223 concentration was found to increase after CPB onset and to downregulate the inflammatory response reducing IL-6 and NLRP3 expression in monocytes [36]. A few studies have suggested that platelet microparticles may also be a source of a circulating tissue factor, explaining the activation of the extrinsic coagulation cascade and again linking hemostasis with immuno-inflammation via platelet activity [37].

Therefore, platelets contain abundant RNAs even if they lack a nucleus. Intraplatelet miRNA alterations may influence platelet messenger RNAs and consequently their proteome. Platelet protein expression impairment may further contribute to postoperative platelet dysfunction. A platelet qualitative impairment such as a reduced surface GPIb expression was found to be associated with the overexpression of some miRNAs (i.e., mir-10b and mir-96) and also with enhanced platelet Bax apoptotic signaling in cardiac surgery cohorts [38,39]. Microcirculatory impairment is another factor associated with platelet dysfunction following heart procedures. It consists of the loss of capillary density and increased flow heterogeneity and reflects how endothelial activation and glycocalyx degradation are both a consequence and a determinant of the systemic inflammatory response [40–42]. Furthermore, a recent investigation showed how perivascular mast cells were activated through the release of the lipid mediator platelet activating factor (PAF) from gut microvascular endothelial-adherent platelets to explain the inflammatory mediated tissue damage and organ injury following a CPB [43]. This mechanism might highlight platelets as a direct determinant of IRI related tissue damage.

3. Platelets and Extracorporeal Membrane Oxygenation

ECMO is a temporary mechanical support for severe cardiac or respiratory failure or both [44,45]. Although the technology is almost identical, ECMO and a CPB differ in many aspects such as the setting of the application, the duration of the support and the rates of complications. Despite fifty years of continuous improvement in technology and management, ECMO has weaknesses to be overcome [46]. Thrombocytopenia and platelet dysfunction are ECMO shortcomings whose underlying mechanisms remain not fully understood.

First, the alteration in the phenotype and thrombocytopenia of platelets could be the result of a huge inflammatory response. As in CPB patients, activated platelets circulate in the bloodstream of patients on ECMO following contact with the circuit's artificial surfaces [47]. Blood exposure to non-physiological conditions promotes thrombotic events [47].

Secondly, the high-speed rotation of the centrifugal pump triggers a mechanical shear stress causing platelet dysfunction, rupture and the shedding of receptors [48]. In a recent ex vivo study, Sun and colleagues demonstrated the pivotal role of the oxygenator, pump and circuit in affecting platelet function [49]. Platelet receptor shedding and a persistent release in microparticles confirmed a deficient adhesion and platelet count reduction increasing over time [49]. Similarly, a decreased binding capacity of platelets was demonstrated by the loss of surface receptors [50–52]. Cannulation sites and components of the circuits have also been investigated to identify how they could alter platelet shape, function and count [53]. Fuchs and colleagues indicated the pump as the largest site risk for platelet activation followed by the reinfusion cannula and lastly the connectors [53].

Thirdly, as systemic anticoagulation is required, patients are likely to develop heparin-induced thrombocytopenia (HIT) [54]. The Extracorporeal Life Support Organization (ELSO) anticoagulation guideline recommends the administration of antithrombotic therapy during ECMO; unfractionated heparin (UFH) is widely administered [54,55]. The prevalence of HIT in adult ECMO patients is estimated at 3.7% with a similar prevalence between V-A and V-V ECMO [55,56]. However, this result could be biased by prompt HIT recognition and switching to alternative anticoagulants [56]. Frequently, physicians treat a patient by just thinking about HIT and without a solid diagnosis. Therefore, an agreed international protocol is strongly required for the early identification and univocal management of HIT patients in ECMO.

Other speculations have been advanced to justify thrombocytopenia during the ECMO run [57–59].

A few studies have focused attention on the duration of support and platelet count decrease [57–59]. Ang and colleagues showed how time on ECMO directly induced thrombocytopenia and the need for blood product transfusions, particularly platelets [60]. However, several factors such as a pre-existent disease (i.e., sepsis and postcardiotomy cardiogenic shock), antiplatelet drugs and bleeding events could have biased the authors' results. Panigada and co-workers observed similar outcomes in their cohort study [58]. Abrams first stated that platelet count reduction was mostly due to the severity of the disease of patients rather than related to the duration of ECMO support [57]. In a recent meta-regression, we confirmed that a worsening in thrombocytopenia was independent of the number of days on ECMO [56]. However, we speculated that after few days the inflammatory response induced by ECMO might not affect the freshly generated platelets due to the beginning of an endothelization mechanism of the circuit [56,61,62].

The ECMO mode also does not seem to influence the degree of thrombocytopenia [56]. After analyzing the available evidence in the literature, we estimated a comparable platelet count decrease in almost 25% and 23% of adult V-A and V-V ECMO subjects, respectively [56].

However, in addition to the causes, future research should focus on the possible clinical implications of platelet disorders (i.e., hemorrhagic or thrombotic events, blood product transfusions and mortality). Currently, the literature lacks trials that centrally address this issue. Researchers will have to face the multiple biases (i.e., pre-existing diseases, anticoagulation and antiplatelet drugs, sepsis) that make the investigation a real challenge.

4. Platelets and Aortic Biological Prosthesis

In the past years, physicians have had to cope with periprocedural thrombocytopenia in patients receiving an aortic biological prosthesis [63]. The discussion has focused on blood interaction with the artificial valves and the possible consequences [63]. An increased platelet turnover and destruction plays an important role [63]. Moreover, a major bleeding risk after an aortic valve replacement is not an uncommon event ranging from 4% for surgical tissue valves to 16% for the transcatheter prosthesis [63]. The shear stress through an artificial device has been suggested as a central mechanism of hemostatic dysfunction [64,65]. It can induce conflicting mechanisms at the same time; platelet activation, aggregation and generation of procoagulant microparticles as well as platelet dysfunction, loss of surface receptors and bleeding complications [64,65]. Furthermore, patients receiving surgical bioprostheses are exposed to the adverse effect of the CPB [54]. The CPB duration seems to be a major determinant for the development of postoperative thrombocytopenia [66]. However, this mechanism could change according to the different type of valve prosthesis implanted.

In 2006, Le Guyader and colleagues observed platelet activation after aortic valve replacements with two kinds of mechanical valves and three kinds of tissue valves [67]. They found platelet activation in all of the prostheses on the eighth postoperative day (POD) and was still present in the bioprosthesis group at the two month follow-up [67]. Ravenni and co-workers reported a decrease in platelet counts in different bioprosthesis types on the first POD; a stentless bioprosthesis showed a significant decrease in the postoperative platelet count compared with stented tissue valves [68]. Similarly, in 2016 Stanger and colleagues reported a significant decrease in the postoperative platelet count in three types of bioprostheses [69]. Nevertheless, those tissue valves were not associated with bleeding complications [69].

Several investigators have reported stentless bioprostheses as risk factors for postoperative thrombocytopenia [70–73]. Although showing a good hemodynamic performance, stentless bioprosthesis implantation has been associated with postoperative thrombocytopenia [63]. However, a decreased postoperative platelet count did not affect the postoperative outcomes compared with stented bioprostheses except for an increased rate of red blood cell transfusions [63]. The postoperative platelet count decreased from 60% to 77% after a stentless bioprosthesis implantation [63]. Likewise, the platelet count fell from 53% to 60% after the implantation of rapid deployment valves (RDVs) [63]. Like the stentless valves, thrombocytopenia after RDV implantation seemed to occur in the first PODs before a slow recovery within 7 to 10 days after surgery [69,74–76]. The origin of thrombocytopenia after RDV implantation is still unknown. To explain the phenomenon in RDVs, investigators have advanced analogous hypotheses to those for thrombocytopenia after the implantation of stentless bioprostheses [74–77].

Interestingly, thrombocytopenia and platelet disorders do not only occur after the implantation of surgical bioprostheses [63]. Several papers have reported that transcatheter aortic valve implantation (TAVI) patients have also experienced a temporary platelet count decrease following the procedure [63,78–90]. The platelet count drop ranged from 21% to 72% after TAVI with associated adverse outcomes [63,89,91]. The cause was most likely multifactorial; the valve design, the shear stress, the valve size, the length and type of the procedure and the amount of low-osmolar contrast agents used can interact together and elicit platelet destruction and increase the coagulation cascade and the inflammatory process leading to thrombocytopenia [63,89,90]. Moreover, mispositioning and TAVI migration are predictors of a platelet count decrease supporting the hypothesis of shear stress in the origin of thrombocytopenia [12]. Furthermore, thrombocytopenia occurs more frequently in patients with balloon-expandable valves (BEVs) [63,85,87,90]. Considering the prosthesis shape, the use of large sheaths, pre-dilatation and surgical cut-down for femoral access, a BEV was identified as a new predictor of TAVI related thrombocytopenia [63,85,87,90]. Furthermore, TAVI related thrombocytopenia has been found to be associated with increased early and overall mortality after TAVI [63,89].

Future investigations should focus on defining thrombocytopenia and platelet disorders after the implantation of biological prosthesis to improve patient management and to reduce adverse events.

5. Heparin-Induced Thrombocytopenia

Heparin-induced thrombocytopenia (HIT) is a rare drawback after the exposure to either unfractionated heparin (UFH) or low molecular weight heparin (LMWH). Heparin is a worldwide used anticoagulant because of its efficiency, accessibility, reversibility and costs beyond compare.

HIT is characterized by a decreased platelet count of about 30–50% leading to severe thrombocytopenia (<100×10^9/L). However, typical factors such as hemodilution must be ruled out in the diagnostic phase. Hemorrhagic complications are rare whereas thromboembolic events occur more frequently (up to ~ 50% if not diagnosed/treated) and might jeopardize the patient's outcome [92]. HIT is estimated to occur once in 1500 hospitalizations in the United States with high-risk cardiac surgery patients [92]. Furthermore, HIT is associated with a four-fold higher in-hospital mortality, three-fold longer median hospitalization time and four-fold higher costs of hospitalization compared with thrombocytopenia from other etiologies [93].

HIT's risk factors are both host and drug related; the female gender has been linked to a doubled risk of developing HIT [94] while a younger age (<40 years) seems to entail a milder risk [95]. Furthermore, recent genome-wide association studies (GWAS) have highlighted candidate gene variants (i.e., the HLA-DRB3*01:01 allele) associated with a risk of HIT [96–98]. Among the drug related factors, the duration of heparin exposure plays a major role with a shorter span carrying a lower risk [99]. UFH therapy is more likely to lead to HIT compared with LMWH [100–103]. Platelet factor 4 (PF4), indeed, forms oligomers binding multiple UFH oligosaccharides that further share several PF4 tetramers, leading to the assembly of ultra-large antigenic complexes (ULCs) [60,104,105]. Bovine heparin may carry a higher risk for HIT compared with porcine heparin [106,107].

HIT is a serious immune mediated adverse reaction to heparin polyanions caused by pathogenic immunoglobulin G (IgG) antibodies. IgGs bind to complexes of heparin and PF4, a cationic chemokine stored within platelet alpha granules characterized by a high affinity for anionic molecules. These complexes are optimally formed at a stoichiometric concentration (molar ratio 1:1). Noxae such as major surgery, a CPB and mechanical circulatory supports (MCSs) (e.g., ECMO and ventricular assist devices (VADs)) can trigger massive platelet activation and subsequent additional PF4 release [108]. ULCs consequently cross-link the surface receptors of platelets (FCγIIa) leading to a switch toward a hyper-aggregative phenotype [19,109,110]. The process promotes a complex cascade of events involving endothelial cells, immune cells and NETs and coagulation factors and other circulating molecules [19,109,110].

The mutual effect of pre-existent vascular stress, incessant platelet activation and the need of profound heparinization make adult cardiac surgery the most prone setting for HIT occurrence (50% to 70%) [111–114]. Conversely, pediatric patients show lower rates of seroconversions (0–2%) most likely due to the absence of chronic vascular insults [91]. Despite the recurrence of anti-PF4/heparin antibodies in heart surgery patients, only 2–3% develop HIT [115]. The detection of antibodies is required to diagnose HIT. In addition to the low platelet count, the "4 Ts" score is a bedside tool used to estimate the probability of HIT that improves the specificity of antibody tests in cardiac patients (Table 1) [116].

Table 1. Estimating the pre-test probability of HIT: the "4 Ts".

"4 Ts" Category	2 Points	1 Point	0 Points
Thrombocytopenia	Platelet count fall > 50% AND platelet nadir ≥ 20×10^9/L	Platelet count fall 30–50% OR platelet nadir $10–19 \times 10^9$/L	Platelet count fall < 30% OR platelet nadir < 10×10^9/L
Timing of platelet count fall	Clear onset between days 5–10 OR platelet fall ≤ 1 day (prior heparin exposure within 30 days)	Consistent with days 5–10 fall but not clear; onset after day 10 OR fall ≤ 1 day (prior heparin exposure 30–100 days ago)	Platelet count fall < 4 days without recent exposure
Thrombosis or other sequelae	New thrombosis OR skin necrosis; acute systemic reaction postintravenous heparin bolus	Progressive or recurrent thrombosis or non-necrotizing (erythematous) skin lesions or suspected thrombosis (not proven)	None
Other causes for thrombocytopenia	None apparent	Possible	Definite

Moreover, preoperative evidence of anti-PF4/heparin antibodies is reported in 5% to 22% of cardiac patients [117]. However, an uncertain prognostic value is attributed to this finding because of the controversial data about the preoperative positivity to anti-PF4/heparin antibodies and postoperative HIT, thrombosis and an adverse outcome [19,118–121]. Therefore, routine screening for such antibodies is discouraged (unless clinically evident HIT signs are manifested or in cases of a history of HIT).

HIT occurrence makes heart surgery a challenging event that can counteract the results of even the most successful operation. This eventuality should imply the deferral of any elective procedure until the results of laboratory tests are available. However, cardiac surgery is a practice in which deferring a procedure is not always a feasible option. Hence, several alternative strategies exist; pharmacological agents such as direct thrombin inhibitors (DTIs), factor Xa inhibitors (i.e., fondaparinux) and platelet inhibitors (i.e., prostaglandins) are plausible options.

Among DTIs, bivalirudin is the most used alternative agent in cardiac surgery showing a comparable efficiency and similar perioperative morbidity rates with heparin [122,123]. Furthermore, while DTIs are usually monitored by activated partial thromboplastin time (aPTT), the activated clotting time (ACT) appeared to be reliable in monitoring anticoagulation with bivalirudin during a CPB [121]. Other DTIs such as argatroban and danaparoid are not recommended as alternative therapies during a CPB [124,125]. Several studies have reported bleeding after therapy discontinuation and unexpected thrombosis (ACT > 500 s) [124,125]. While HIT treatment with either fondaparinux or other molecules (i.e., epoprostenol, iloprost) is almost anecdotal [126], off-pump procedures and a plasma exchange represent other controversial approaches to minimizing heparin exposure [127–130].

6. Conclusions

Platelet functional or structural alterations are not epiphenomena of the acute reaction to CPB-assisted cardiac surgery, biological bioprosthesis and ECMO but rather have a major role in the thread linking hemostasis, inflammation and innate immunity. The multiple direct/indirect mechanisms that regulate this connection are still partially unclear. However, further studies addressing the pathobiological dynamics concurring to the abovementioned quantitative (i.e., thrombocytopenia) and qualitative (i.e., platelet activation and a shift towards a proinflammatory phenotype) platelet derangements in a cardiac surgery setting and ECLS may provide new insights possibly leading to improved patient outcomes.

Author Contributions: Conceptualization E.S., F.J.; methodology, G.F.S., D.P.; validation, H.t.C.; investigation, E.S., F.J.; resources, E.S., F.J.; data curation, R.L.; writing—original draft preparation, E.S., F.J.; final review and editing, G.F.S., H.t.C., D.P., R.L.; visualization, E.S., F.J. All authors have read and agreed to the published version of the manuscript.

Funding: This research received no external funding.

Institutional Review Board Statement: Not applicable.

Informed Consent Statement: Not applicable.

Data Availability Statement: Not applicable.

Conflicts of Interest: The authors declare no conflict of interest.

References

1. Van Der Meijden, P.E.J.; Heemskerk, J.W.M. Platelet biology and functions: New concepts and clinical perspectives. *Nat. Rev. Cardiol.* **2019**, *16*, 166–179. [CrossRef]
2. Gawaz, M.; Langer, H.; May, A.E. Platelets in inflammation and atherogenesis. *J. Clin. Investig.* **2005**, *115*, 3378–3384. [CrossRef]
3. Mezger, M.; Gobel, K.; Kraft, P.; Meuth, S.G.; Kleinschnitz, C.; Langer, H.F. Platelets and vascular inflammation of the brain. *Hämostaseologie* **2015**, *35*, 244–251. [CrossRef]
4. Engelmann, B.; Massberg, S. Thrombosis as an intravascular effector of innate immunity. *Nat. Rev. Immunol.* **2012**, *13*, 34–45. [CrossRef]
5. Carestia, A.; Mena, H.A.; Olexen, C.M.; Wilczyñski, J.M.O.; Negrotto, S.; Errasti, A.E.; Gómez, R.M.; Jenne, C.N.; Silva, E.A.C.; Schattner, M. Platelets Promote Macrophage Polarization toward Pro-inflammatory Phenotype and Increase Survival of Septic Mice. *Cell Rep.* **2019**, *28*, 896–908.e5. [CrossRef]
6. Garraud, O.; Ecognasse, F. Are Platelets Cells? And if Yes, are They Immune Cells? *Front. Immunol.* **2015**, *6*, 70. [CrossRef]
7. Griffin, B.R.; Bronsert, M.; Reece, T.B.; Pal, J.D.; Cleveland, J.C.; Fullerton, D.A.; Gist, K.M.; Jovanovich, A.; Jalal, D.; Faubel, S.; et al. Thrombocytopenia After Cardiopulmonary Bypass Is Associated With Increased Morbidity and Mortality. *Ann. Thorac. Surg.* **2020**, *110*, 50–57. [CrossRef]
8. Kertai, M.D.; Zhou, S.; Karhausen, J.A.; Cooter, M.; Jooste, E.; Li, Y.-J.; White, W.D.; Aronson, S.; Podgoreanu, M.V.; Gaca, J.G.; et al. Platelet Counts, Acute Kidney Injury, and Mortality after Coronary Artery Bypass Grafting Surgery. *Anesthesiology* **2016**, *124*, 339–352. [CrossRef]
9. Jiritano, F.; Lorusso, R.; Santarpino, G. Causes of Thrombocytopenia in Cardiac Surgery: Looking for the Holy Grail? *Ann. Thorac. Surg.* **2020**, *110*, 751–752. [CrossRef]
10. Squiccimarro, E.; Labriola, C.; Malvindi, P.G.; Margari, V.; Guida, P.; Visicchio, G.; Kounakis, G.; Favale, A.; Dambruoso, P.; Mastrototaro, G.; et al. Prevalence and Clinical Impact of Systemic Inflammatory Reaction After Cardiac Surgery. *J. Cardiothorac. Vasc. Anesthesia* **2019**, *33*, 1682–1690. [CrossRef]
11. Deptula, J.; Glogowski, K.; Merrigan, K.; Hanson, K.; Felix, D.; Hammel, J.; Duncan, K. Evaluation of biocompatible cardiopulmonary bypass circuit use during pediatric open heart surgery. *J. Extra Corporeal Technol.* **2006**, *38*, 22–26.
12. Tabuchi, N.; Shibamiya, A.; Koyama, T.; Fukuda, T.; Van Oeveren, W.; Sunamori, M. Activated Leukocytes Adsorbed on the Surface of an Extracorporeal Circuit. *Artif. Organs* **2003**, *27*, 591–594. [CrossRef]
13. Vardon-Bounes, F.; Ruiz, S.; Gratacap, M.-P.; Garcia, C.; Payrastre, B.; Minville, V. Platelets Are Critical Key Players in Sepsis. *Int. J. Mol. Sci.* **2019**, *20*, 3494. [CrossRef]
14. Mezger, M.; Nording, H.; Sauter, R.; Graf, T.; Heim, C.; Von Bubnoff, N.; Ensminger, S.M.; Langer, H.F. Platelets and Immune Responses During Thromboinflammation. *Front. Immunol.* **2019**, *10*, 1731. [CrossRef]

15. Rossaint, J.; Kühne, K.; Skupski, J.; Van Aken, H.; Looney, M.R.; Hidalgo, A.; Zarbock, A. Directed transport of neutrophil-derived extracellular vesicles enables platelet-mediated innate immune response. *Nat. Commun.* **2016**, *7*, 13464. [CrossRef]
16. Zahler, S.; Massoudy, P.; Hartl, H.; Hähnel, C.; Meisner, H.; Becker, B.F. Acute cardiac inflammatory responses to postischemic reperfusion during cardiopulmonary bypass. *Cardiovasc. Res.* **1999**, *41*, 722–730. [CrossRef]
17. Warltier, D.C.; Laffey, J.G.; Boylan, J.F.; Cheng, D.C.H. The Systemic Inflammatory Response to Cardiac Surgery. *Anesthesiology* **2002**, *97*, 215–252. [CrossRef]
18. Clark, S.R.; Ma, A.C.; A Tavener, S.; McDonald, B.; Goodarzi, Z.; Kelly, M.M.; Patel, K.D.; Chakrabarti, S.; McAvoy, E.; Sinclair, G.D.; et al. Platelet TLR4 activates neutrophil extracellular traps to ensnare bacteria in septic blood. *Nat. Med.* **2007**, *13*, 463–469. [CrossRef]
19. Perdomo, J.; Leung, H.H.L.; Ahmadi, Z.; Yan, F.; Chong, J.J.H.; Passam, F.H.; Chong, B.H. Neutrophil activation and NETosis are the major drivers of thrombosis in heparin-induced thrombocytopenia. *Nat. Commun.* **2019**, *10*, 1322. [CrossRef]
20. Rossaint, J.; Herter, J.M.; Van Aken, H.; Napirei, M.; Döring, Y.; Weber, C.; Soehnlein, O.; Zarbock, A. Synchronized integrin engagement and chemokine activation is crucial in neutrophil extracellular trap–mediated sterile inflammation. *Blood* **2014**, *123*, 2573–2584. [CrossRef]
21. Orlova, V.V.; Choi, E.Y.; Xie, C.; Chavakis, E.; Bierhaus, A.; Ihanus, E.; Ballantyne, C.M.; Gahmberg, C.G.; E Bianchi, M.; Nawroth, P.P.; et al. A novel pathway of HMGB1-mediated inflammatory cell recruitment that requires Mac-1-integrin. *EMBO J.* **2007**, *26*, 1129–1139. [CrossRef]
22. Maugeri, N.; Campana, L.; Gavina, M.; Covino, C.; De Metrio, M.; Panciroli, C.; Maiuri, L.; Maseri, A.; D'Angelo, A.; Bianchi, M.E.; et al. Activated platelets present high mobility group box 1 to neutrophils, inducing autophagy and promoting the extrusion of neutrophil extracellular traps. *J. Thromb. Haemost.* **2014**, *12*, 2074–2088. [CrossRef]
23. Cognasse, F.; Nguyen, K.A.; Damien, P.; McNicol, A.; Pozzetto, B.; Hamzeh-Cognasse, H.; Garraud, O. The inflammatory role of platelets via their TLRs and Siglec receptors. *Front. Immunol.* **2015**, *6*, 83. [CrossRef]
24. Weyrich, A.S.; Elstad, M.R.; McEver, R.P.; McIntyre, T.M.; Moore, K.L.; Morrissey, J.H.; Prescott, S.M.; A Zimmerman, G. Activated platelets signal chemokine synthesis by human monocytes. *J. Clin. Investig.* **1996**, *97*, 1525–1534. [CrossRef] [PubMed]
25. Blair, P.; Flaumenhaft, R. Platelet α-granules: Basic biology and clinical correlates. *Blood Rev.* **2009**, *23*, 177–189. [CrossRef]
26. Rolfes, V.; Ribeiro, L.S.; Hawwari, I.; Böttcher, L.; Rosero, N.; Maasewerd, S.; Santos, M.L.S.; Próchnicki, T.; Silva, C.M.D.S.; Wanderley, C.W.D.S.; et al. Platelets Fuel the Inflammasome Activation of Innate Immune Cells. *Cell Rep.* **2020**, *31*, 107615. [CrossRef]
27. Peerschke, E.I.B.; Yin, W.; Ghebrehiwet, B. Complement activation on platelets: Implications for vascular inflammation and thrombosis. *Mol. Immunol.* **2010**, *47*, 2170–2175. [CrossRef]
28. Del Conde, I.; Crúz, M.A.; Zhang, H.; López, J.A.; Afshar-Kharghan, V. Platelet activation leads to activation and propagation of the complement system. *J. Exp. Med.* **2005**, *201*, 871–879. [CrossRef]
29. Hamad, O.A.; Ekdahl, K.N.; Nilsson, P.H.; Andersson, J.; Magotti, P.; Lambris, J.D.; Nilsson, B. Complement activation triggered by chondroitin sulfate released by thrombin receptor-activated platelets. *J. Thromb. Haemost.* **2008**, *6*, 1413–1421. [CrossRef]
30. Yin, W.; Ghebrehiwet, B.; Peerschke, E.I.B. Expression of complement components and inhibitors on platelet microparticles. *Platelets* **2008**, *19*, 225–233. [CrossRef]
31. Morrell, C.N.; Aggrey, A.A.; Chapman, L.M.; Modjeski, K.L. Emerging roles for platelets as immune and inflammatory cells. *Blood* **2014**, *123*, 2759–2767. [CrossRef]
32. Mause, S.F.; Von Hundelshausen, P.; Zernecke, A.; Koenen, R.R.; Weber, C. Platelet Microparticles. *Arter. Thromb. Vasc. Biol.* **2005**, *25*, 1512–1518. [CrossRef]
33. Rousseau, M.; Duchez, A.-C.; Lee, C.H.C.; Boilard, E.; Laffont, B.; Corduan, A.; Provost, P. Platelet microparticles reprogram macrophage gene expression and function. *Thromb. Haemost.* **2016**, *115*, 311–323. [CrossRef]
34. Gidlöf, O.; Van Der Brug, M.; Öhman, J.; Gilje, P.; Olde, B.; Wahlestedt, C.; Erlinge, D. Platelets activated during myocardial infarction release functional miRNA, which can be taken up by endothelial cells and regulate ICAM1 expression. *Blood* **2013**, *121*, 3908–3917. [CrossRef] [PubMed]
35. Laffont, B.; Corduan, A.; Plé, H.; Duchez, A.-C.; Cloutier, N.; Boilard, E.; Provost, P. Activated platelets can deliver mRNA regulatory Ago2•microRNA complexes to endothelial cells via microparticles. *Blood* **2013**, *122*, 253–261. [CrossRef] [PubMed]
36. Poon, K.-S.; Palanisamy, K.; Chang, S.-S.; Sun, K.-T.; Chen, K.-B.; Li, P.-C.; Lin, T.-C.; Li, C.-Y. Plasma exosomal miR-223 expression regulates inflammatory responses during cardiac surgery with cardiopulmonary bypass. *Sci. Rep.* **2017**, *7*, 1–11. [CrossRef]
37. Müller, I.; Klocke, A.; Alex, M.; Kotzsch, M.; Luther, T.; Morgenstern, E.; Zieseniss, S.; Zahler, S.; Preissner, K.; Engelmann, B. Intravascular tissue factor initiates coagulation via circulating microvesicles and platelets. *FASEB J.* **2003**, *17*, 1–20. [CrossRef] [PubMed]
38. Mukai, N.; Nakayama, Y.; Ishi, S.; Ogawa, S.; Maeda, S.; Anada, N.; Murakami, S.; Mizobe, T.; Sawa, T.; Nakajima, Y. Changes in MicroRNA Expression Level of Circulating Platelets Contribute to Platelet Defect After Cardiopulmonary Bypass. *Crit. Care Med.* **2018**, *46*, e761–e767. [CrossRef]
39. Murase, M.; Nakayama, Y.; Sessler, D.; Mukai, N.; Ogawa, S.; Nakajima, Y. Changes in platelet Bax levels contribute to impaired platelet response to thrombin after cardiopulmonary bypass: Prospective observational clinical and laboratory investigations. *Br. J. Anaesth.* **2017**, *119*, 1118–1126. [CrossRef]

40. De Backer, D.; Dubois, M.-J.; Schmartz, D.; Koch, M.; Ducart, A.; Barvais, L.; Vincent, J.-L. Microcirculatory Alterations in Cardiac Surgery: Effects of Cardiopulmonary Bypass and Anesthesia. *Ann. Thorac. Surg.* **2009**, *88*, 1396–1403. [CrossRef] [PubMed]
41. Koning, N.J.; Atasever, B.; Vonk, A.B.; Boer, C. Changes in Microcirculatory Perfusion and Oxygenation During Cardiac Surgery With or Without Cardiopulmonary Bypass. *J. Cardiothorac. Vasc. Anesthesia* **2014**, *28*, 1331–1340. [CrossRef]
42. Di Dedda, U.; Ranucci, M.; Porta, A.; Bari, V.; Ascari, A.; Fantinato, A.; Baryshnikova, E.; Cotza, M. The combined effects of the microcirculatory status and cardiopulmonary bypass on platelet count and function during cardiac surgery. *Clin. Hemorheol. Microcirc.* **2018**, *70*, 327–337. [CrossRef] [PubMed]
43. Karhausen, J.; Choi, H.W.; Maddipati, K.R.; Mathew, J.P.; Ma, Q.; Boulaftali, Y.; Lee, R.H.; Bergmeier, W.; Abraham, S.N. Platelets trigger perivascular mast cell degranulation to cause inflammatory responses and tissue injury. *Sci. Adv.* **2020**, *6*, eaay6314. [CrossRef]
44. Hill, J.D.; O'Brien, T.G.; Murray, J.J.; Dontigny, L.; Bramson, M.L.; Osborn, J.J.; Gerbode, F. Prolonged Extracorporeal Oxygenation for Acute Post-Traumatic Respiratory Failure (Shock-Lung Syndrome). *N. Engl. J. Med.* **1972**, *286*, 629–634. [CrossRef]
45. Chen, Y.-S.; Lin, J.-W.; Yu, H.-Y.; Ko, W.-J.; Jerng, J.-S.; Chang, W.-T.; Chen, W.-J.; Huang, S.-C.; Chi, N.-H.; Wang, C.-H.; et al. Cardiopulmonary resuscitation with assisted extracorporeal life-support versus conventional cardiopulmonary resuscitation in adults with in-hospital cardiac arrest: An observational study and propensity analysis. *Lancet* **2008**, *372*, 554–561. [CrossRef]
46. Sy, E.; Sklar, M.C.; Lequier, L.; Fan, E.; Kanji, H.D. Anticoagulation practices and the prevalence of major bleeding, thromboembolic events, and mortality in venoarterial extracorporeal membrane oxygenation: A systematic review and meta-analysis. *J. Crit. Care* **2017**, *39*, 87–96. [CrossRef]
47. Yoshimoto, Y.; Hasebe, T.; Takahashi, K.; Amari, M.; Nagashima, S.; Kamijo, A.; Hotta, A.; Takahashi, K.; Suzuki, T. Ultrastructural characterization of surface-induced platelet activation on artificial materials by transmission electron microscopy. *Microsc. Res. Tech.* **2013**, *76*, 342–349. [CrossRef]
48. Chen, Z.; Mondal, N.K.; Zheng, S.; Koenig, S.C.; Slaughter, M.S.; Griffith, B.P.; Wu, Z.J. High shear induces platelet dysfunction leading to enhanced thrombotic propensity and diminished hemostatic capacity. *Platelets* **2017**, *30*, 112–119. [CrossRef]
49. Sun, W.; Wang, S.; Chen, Z.; Zhang, J.; Li, T.; Arias, K.; Griffith, B.P.; Wu, Z.J. Impact of high mechanical shear stress and oxygenator membrane surface on blood damage relevant to thrombosis and bleeding in a pediatric ECMO circuit. *Artif. Organs* **2020**, *44*, 717–726. [CrossRef]
50. Lukito, P.; Wong, A.; Jing, J.; Arthur, J.F.; Marasco, S.F.; Murphy, D.A.; Bergin, P.J.; Shaw, J.A.; Collecutt, M.; Andrews, R.K.; et al. Mechanical circulatory support is associated with loss of platelet receptors glycoprotein Ibα and glycoprotein VI. *J. Thromb. Haemost.* **2016**, *14*, 2253–2260. [CrossRef]
51. Chung, J.H.; Yeo, H.J.; Kim, D.; Lee, S.M.; Han, J.; Kim, M.; Cho, W.H. Changes in the Levels of Beta-thromboglobulin and Inflammatory Mediators during Extracorporeal Membrane Oxygenation Support. *Int. J. Artif. Organs* **2017**, *40*, 575–580. [CrossRef]
52. Kalbhenn, J.; Schlagenhauf, A.; Rosenfelder, S.; Schmutz, A.; Zieger, B. Acquired von Willebrand syndrome and impaired platelet function during venovenous extracorporeal membrane oxygenation: Rapid onset and fast recovery. *J. Hear. Lung Transplant.* **2018**, *37*, 985–991. [CrossRef]
53. Fuchs, G.; Berg, N.; Broman, L.M.; Wittberg, L.P. Flow-induced platelet activation in components of the extracorporeal membrane oxygenation circuit. *Sci. Rep.* **2018**, *8*, 1–9. [CrossRef]
54. Arachchillage, D.J.; Laffan, M.; Khanna, S.; Vandenbriele, C.; Kamani, F.; Passariello, M.; Rosenberg, A.; Aw, T.C.; Banya, W.; Ledot, S.; et al. Frequency of Thrombocytopenia and Heparin-Induced Thrombocytopenia in Patients Receiving Extracorporeal Membrane Oxygenation Compared With Cardiopulmonary Bypass and the Limited Sensitivity of Pretest Probability Score. *Crit. Care Med.* **2020**, *48*, e371–e379. [CrossRef]
55. The Extracorporeal Life Support Organization (ELSO). Extracorporeal Life Support Organization (ELSO) General Guidelines for All ECLS Cases. Available online: https://www.elso.org/Portals/0/Files/elsoanticoagulationguideline8-2014-table-contents.pdf (accessed on 26 July 2020).
56. Jiritano, F.; Serraino, G.F.; Cate, H.T.; Fina, D.; Matteucci, M.; Mastroroberto, P.; Lorusso, R. Platelets and extra-corporeal membrane oxygenation in adult patients: A systematic review and meta-analysis. *Intensiv. Care Med.* **2020**, *46*, 1154–1169. [CrossRef]
57. Abrams, D.; Baldwin, M.R.; Champion, M.; Agerstrand, C.; Eisenberger, A.; Bacchetta, M.; Brodie, D. Thrombocytopenia and extracorporeal membrane oxygenation in adults with acute respiratory failure: A cohort study. *Intensiv. Care Med.* **2016**, *42*, 844–852. [CrossRef]
58. Panigada, M.; Artoni, A.; Passamonti, S.M.; Maino, A.; Mietto, C.; L'Acqua, C.; Cressoni, M.; Boscolo, M.; Tripodi, A.; Bucciarelli, P.; et al. Hemostasis changes during veno-venous extracorporeal membrane oxy-genation for respiratory support in adults. *Minerva Anestesiol.* **2016**, *82*, 170–179.
59. Ang, A.L.; Teo, D.; Lim, C.H.; Leou, K.K.; Tien, S.L.; Koh, M.B.C. Blood transfusion requirements and independent predictors of increased transfusion requirements among adult patients on extracorporeal membrane oxygenation - a single centre experience. *Vox Sang.* **2009**, *96*, 34–43. [CrossRef]
60. Rauova, L.; Poncz, M.; McKenzie, S.E.; Reilly, M.P.; Arepally, G.; Weisel, J.W.; Nagaswami, C.; Cines, D.B.; Sachais, B.S.; Herre, J.; et al. Ultralarge complexes of PF4 and heparin are central to the pathogenesis of heparin-induced thrombocytopenia. *Blood* **2005**, *105*, 131–138. [CrossRef]

61. Ontaneda, A.; Annich, G.M. Novel Surfaces in Extracorporeal Membrane Oxygenation Circuits. *Front. Med.* **2018**, *5*, 321. [CrossRef]
62. Klein, S.; Hesselmann, F.; Djeljadini, S.; Berger, T.; Thiebes, A.L.; Schmitz-Rode, T.; Jockenhoevel, S.; Cornelissen, C.G. EndOxy: Dynamic Long-Term Evaluation of Endothelialized Gas Exchange Membranes for a Biohybrid Lung. *Ann. Biomed. Eng.* **2020**, *48*, 747–756. [CrossRef]
63. Jiritano, F.; Santarpino, G.; Serraino, G.F.; Cate, H.T.; Matteucci, M.; Fina, D.; Mastroroberto, P.; Lorusso, R. Peri-procedural thrombocytopenia after aortic bioprosthesis implant: A systematic review and meta-analysis comparison among conventional, stentless, rapid-deployment, and transcatheter valves. *Int. J. Cardiol.* **2019**, *296*, 43–50. [CrossRef]
64. Steinlechner, B.; Dworschak, M.; Birkenberg, B.; Duris, M.; Zeidler, P.; Fischer, H.; Milosevic, L.; Wieselthaler, G.; Wolner, E.; Quehenberger, P.; et al. Platelet Dysfunction in Outpatients With Left Ventricular Assist Devices. *Ann. Thorac. Surg.* **2009**, *87*, 131–137. [CrossRef]
65. Chen, Z.; Mondal, N.K.; Ding, J.; Koenig, S.C.; Slaughter, M.S.; Wu, Z.J. Paradoxical Effect of Nonphysiological Shear Stress on Platelets and von Willebrand Factor. *Artif. Organs* **2016**, *40*, 659–668. [CrossRef]
66. Vogt, F.; Moscarelli, M.; Pollari, F.; Kalisnik, J.M.; Pfeiffer, S.; Fittkau, M.; Sirch, J.; Pförringer, D.; Jessl, J.; Eckner, D.; et al. Two approaches—one phenomenon—thrombocytopenia after surgical and transcatheter aortic valve replacement. *J. Card. Surg.* **2020**, *35*, 1186–1194. [CrossRef] [PubMed]
67. Le Guyader, A.; Watanabe, R.; Berbé, J.; Boumediene, A.; Cogné, M.; Laskar, M. Platelet activation after aortic prosthetic valve surgery. *Interact. Cardiovasc. Thorac. Surg.* **2005**, *5*, 60–64. [CrossRef]
68. Ravenni, G.; Celiento, M.; Ferrari, G.; Milano, A.; Scioti, G.; Pratali, S.; Bortolotti, U. Reduction in platelet count after aortic valve replacement: Comparison of three bioprostheses. *J. Hear. Valve Dis.* **2012**, *21*, 655–661.
69. Stanger, O.; Grabherr, M.; Gahl, B.; Longnus, S.; Meinitzer, A.; Fiedler, M.; Tevaearai, H.; Carrel, T. Thrombocytopaenia after aortic valve replacement with stented, stentless and sutureless bioprostheses. *Eur. J. Cardio-Thoracic Surg.* **2016**, *51*, 340–346. [CrossRef] [PubMed]
70. Yerebakan, C.; Kaminski, A.; Westphal, B.; Kundt, G.; Ugurlucan, M.; Steinhoff, G.; Liebold, A. Thrombocytopenia after aortic valve replacement with the Freedom Solo stentless bioprosthesis. *Interact. Cardiovasc. Thorac. Surg.* **2008**, *7*, 616–620. [CrossRef]
71. Hilker, L.; Wodny, M.; Ginesta, M.; Wollert, H.-G.; Eckel, L. Differences in the recovery of platelet counts after biological aortic valve replacement. *Interact. Cardiovasc. Thorac. Surg.* **2008**, *8*, 70–73. [CrossRef]
72. Miceli, A.; Gilmanov, D.; Murzi, M.; Parri, M.S.; Cerillo, A.; Bevilacqua, S.; Farneti, P.A.; Glauber, M. Evaluation of platelet count after isolated biological aortic valve replacement with Freedom Solo bioprosthesis. *Eur. J. Cardio-Thoracic Surg.* **2011**, *41*, 69–73. [CrossRef]
73. Piccardo, A.; Rusinaru, D.; Petitprez, B.; Marticho, P.; Vaida, I.; Tribouilloy, C.; Caus, T. Thrombocytopenia After Aortic Valve Replacement With Freedom Solo Bioprosthesis: A Propensity Study. *Ann. Thorac. Surg.* **2010**, *89*, 1425–1430. [CrossRef]
74. Sánchez, E.; Corrales, J.-A.; Fantidis, P.; Tarhini, I.S.; Khan, I.; Pineda, T.; González, J.-R. Thrombocytopenia after Aortic Valve Replacement with Perceval S Sutureless Bioprosthesis. *J. Hear. Valve Dis.* **2016**, *25*, 75–81.
75. Mujtaba, S.S.; Ledingham, S.; Shah, A.R.; Schueler, S.; Clark, S.; Pillay, T. Thrombocytopenia After Aortic Valve Replacement: Comparison Between Sutureless Perceval S Valve and Perimount Magna Ease Bioprosthesis. *Braz. J. Cardiovasc. Surg.* **2018**, *33*, 169–175. [CrossRef]
76. Andreas, M.; Wallner, S.; Habertheuer, A.; Rath, C.; Schauperl, M.; Binder, T.; Beitzke, D.; Rosenhek, R.; Loewe, C.; Wiedemann, D.; et al. Conventional versus rapid-deployment aortic valve replacement: A single-centre comparison between the Edwards Magna valve and its rapid-deployment successor. *Interact. Cardiovasc. Thorac. Surg.* **2016**, *22*, 799–805. [CrossRef]
77. Jiritano, F.; Cristodoro, L.; Malta, E.; Mastroroberto, P. Thrombocytopenia after sutureless aortic valve implantation: Comparison between Intuity and Perceval bioprostheses. *J. Thorac. Cardiovasc. Surg.* **2016**, *152*, 1631–1633. [CrossRef] [PubMed]
78. Gallet, R.; Seemann, A.; Yamamoto, M.; Hayat, D.; Mouillet, G.; Monin, J.-L.; Gueret, P.; Couetil, J.-P.; Dubois-Randé, J.-L.; Teiger, E.; et al. Effect of Transcatheter (via Femoral Artery) Aortic Valve Implantation on the Platelet Count and Its Consequences. *Am. J. Cardiol.* **2013**, *111*, 1619–1624. [CrossRef]
79. Dvir, D.; Généreux, P.; Barbash, I.M.; Kodali, S.; Ben-Dor, I.; Williams, M.; Torguson, R.; Kirtane, A.J.; Minha, S.; Badr, S.; et al. Acquired thrombocytopenia after transcatheter aortic valve replacement: Clinical correlates and association with outcomes. *Eur. Hear. J.* **2014**, *35*, 2663–2671. [CrossRef] [PubMed]
80. McCabe, J.M.; Huang, P.-H.; Riedl, L.A.; Ba, S.R.D.; Rn, J.G.; Rn, A.C.C.; Davidson, M.J.; Eisenhauer, A.C.; Welt, F.G. Incidence and implications of idiopathic thrombocytopenia following transcatheter aortic valve replacement with the Edwards Sapien©valves: A single center experience. *Catheter. Cardiovasc. Interv.* **2013**, *83*, 633–641. [CrossRef]
81. Gul, M.; Uyarel, H.; Akgul, O.; Uslu, N.; Yildirim, A.; Eksik, A.; Aksu, H.U.; Ozal, E.; Pusuroglu, H.; Erol, M.K.; et al. Hematologic and Clinical Parameters After Transcatheter Aortic Valve Implantation (TAVI) in Patients With Severe Aortic Stenosis. *Clin. Appl. Thromb.* **2012**, *20*, 304–310. [CrossRef]
82. Flaherty, M.P.; Mohsen, A.; Moore, J.B.; Bartoli, C.R.; Schneibel, E.; Rawasia, W.; Williams, M.L.; Grubb, K.J.; Hirsch, G.A. Predictors and clinical impact of pre-existing and acquired thrombocytopenia following transcatheter aortic valve replacement. *Catheter. Cardiovasc. Interv.* **2014**, *85*, 118–129. [CrossRef]

83. Sedaghat, A.; Falkenberg, N.; Sinning, J.-M.; Kulka, H.; Hammerstingl, C.; Nickenig, G.; Oldenburg, J.; Pötzsch, B.; Werner, N. TAVI induces an elevation of hemostasis-related biomarkers, which is not causative for post-TAVI thrombocytopenia. *Int. J. Cardiol.* **2016**, *221*, 719–725. [CrossRef] [PubMed]
84. Hernández-Enríquez, M.; Chollet, T.; Bataille, V.; Campelo-Parada, F.; Boudou, N.; Bouisset, F.; Grunenwald, E.; Porterie, J.; Freixa, X.; Regueiro, A.; et al. Comparison of the Frequency of Thrombocytopenia After Transfemoral Transcatheter Aortic Valve Implantation Between Balloon-Expandable and Self-Expanding Valves. *Am. J. Cardiol.* **2019**, *123*, 1120–1126. [CrossRef]
85. Jilaihawi, H.; Doctor, N.; Chakravarty, T.; Kashif, M.; Mirocha, J.; Cheng, W.; Lill, M.; Nakamura, M.; Gheorghiu, M.; Makkar, R. Major thrombocytopenia after balloon-expandable transcatheter aortic valve replacement: Prognostic implications and comparison to surgical aortic valve replacement. *Catheter. Cardiovasc. Interv.* **2015**, *85*, 130–137. [CrossRef]
86. Abu Saleh, W.K.; Tang, G.H.L.; Ahmad, H.; Cohen, M.; Undemir, C.; Lansman, S.L.S.L.; Reyes, M.; Barker, C.M.; Kleiman, N.S.; Reardon, M.J.; et al. Vascular complication can be minimized with a balloon-expandable, re-collapsible sheath in TAVR with a self-expanding bioprosthesis. *Catheter. Cardiovasc. Interv.* **2015**, *88*, 135–143. [CrossRef] [PubMed]
87. Mitrosz, M.; Kazimierczyk, R.; Sobkowicz, B.; Waszkiewicz, E.; Kralisz, P.; Frank, M.; Piszcz, J.; Galar, M.; Dobrzycki, S.; Musial, W.J.; et al. The causes of thrombocytopenia after transcatheter aortic valve implantation. *Thromb. Res.* **2017**, *156*, 39–44. [CrossRef] [PubMed]
88. Mitrosz, M.; Kazimierczyk, R.; Chlabicz, M.; Sobkowicz, B.; Waszkiewicz, E.; Lisowska, A.; Dobrzycki, S.; Musial, W.J.; Hirnle, T.; Kaminski, K.A.; et al. Perioperative thrombocytopenia predicts poor outcome in patients undergoing transcatheter aortic valve implantation. *Adv. Med Sci.* **2018**, *63*, 179–184. [CrossRef]
89. Takagi, H.; Hari, Y.; Nakashima, K.; Ueyama, H.; Kuno, T.; Ando, T. Impact of postprocedural thrombocytopenia on mortality after transcatheter aortic valve implantation. *J. Cardiovasc. Med.* **2020**, *21*, 318–324. [CrossRef]
90. Takahashi, S.; Yokoyama, N.; Watanabe, Y.; Katayama, T.; Hioki, H.; Yamamoto, H.; Kawasugi, K.; Kozuma, K. Predictor and Mid-Term Outcome of Clinically Significant Thrombocytopenia After Transcatheter Aortic Valve Selection. *Circ. J.* **2020**, *84*, 1020–1027. [CrossRef]
91. Mullen, M.P.; Wessel, D.L.; Thomas, K.C.; Gauvreau, K.; Neufeld, E.J.; McGowan, F.X.; Dinardo, J.A. The Incidence and Implications of Anti-Heparin-Platelet Factor 4 Antibody Formation in a Pediatric Cardiac Surgical Population. *Anesthesia Analg.* **2008**, *107*, 371–378. [CrossRef]
92. Dhakal, B.; Kreuziger, L.B.; Rein, L.; Kleman, A.; Fraser, R.; Aster, R.H.; Hari, P.; Padmanabhan, A. Disease burden, complication rates, and health-care costs of heparin-induced thrombocytopenia in the USA: A population-based study. *Lancet Haematol.* **2018**, *5*, e220–e231. [CrossRef]
93. Dhakal, P.; Giri, S.; Pathak, R.; Bhatt, V.R. Heparin Reexposure in Patients With a History of Heparin-Induced Thrombocytopenia. *Clin. Appl. Thromb.* **2013**, *21*, 626–631. [CrossRef] [PubMed]
94. Warkentin, T.E.; Sheppard, J.-A.I.; Sigouin, C.S.; Kohlmann, T.; Eichler, P.; Greinacher, A. Gender imbalance and risk factor interactions in heparin-induced thrombocytopenia. *Blood* **2006**, *108*, 2937–2941. [CrossRef]
95. Stein, P.D.; Hull, R.D.; Matta, F.; Yaekoub, A.Y.; Liang, J. Incidence of Thrombocytopenia in Hospitalized Patients with Venous Thromboembolism. *Am. J. Med.* **2009**, *122*, 919–930. [CrossRef] [PubMed]
96. Karnes, J.H.; Cronin, R.M.; Rollin, J.; Teumer, A.; Pouplard, C.; Shaffer, C.M.; Blanquicett, C.; Bowton, E.A.; Cowan, J.D.; Mosley, J.D.; et al. A genome-wide association study of heparin-induced thrombocyto-penia using an electronic medical record. *Thromb. Haemost.* **2015**, *113*, 772–781. [CrossRef]
97. Karnes, J.H.; Shaffer, C.M.; Cronin, R.; Bastarache, L.; Gaudieri, S.; James, I.; Pavlos, R.; Steiner, H.E.; Mosley, J.D.; Mallal, S.; et al. Influence of Human Leukocyte Antigen (HLA) Alleles and Killer Cell Immunoglobulin-Like Receptors (KIR) Types on Heparin-Induced Thrombocytopenia (HIT). *Pharmacother. J. Hum. Pharmacol. Drug Ther.* **2017**, *37*, 1164–1171. [CrossRef]
98. Witten, A.; Bolbrinker, J.; Barysenka, A.; Huber, M.; Rühle, F.; Nowak-Göttl, U.; Garbe, E.; Kreutz, R.; Stoll, M. Targeted resequencing of a locus for heparin-induced thrombocytopenia on chromosome 5 identified in a genome-wide association study. *J. Mol. Med.* **2018**, *96*, 765–775. [CrossRef]
99. Smythe, M.A.; Koerber, J.M.; Mattson, J.C. The Incidence of Recognized Heparin-Induced Thrombocytopenia in a Large, Tertiary Care Teaching Hospital. *Chest* **2007**, *131*, 1644–1649. [CrossRef] [PubMed]
100. Amiral, J.; Peynaud-Debayle, E.; Wolf, M.; Bridey, F.; Vissac, A.M.; Meyer, D. Generation of antibodies to heparin-PF4 com-plexes without thrombocytopenia in patients treated with unfractionated or low-molecular-weight heparin. *Am. J. Hematol.* **1996**, *52*, 90–95. [CrossRef]
101. Warkentin, T.E.; Sheppard, J.A.; Horsewood, P.; Simpson, P.J.; Moore, J.C.; Kelton, J.G. Impact of the patient population on the risk for heparin-induced thrombocytopenia. *Blood* **2000**, *96*, 1703–1708. [CrossRef] [PubMed]
102. Cuker, A.; Cines, U.B. How I treat heparin-induced thrombocytopenia. *Blood* **2012**, *119*, 2209–2218. [CrossRef]
103. McGowan, K.E.; Makari, J.; Diamantouros, A.; Bucci, C.; Rempel, P.; Selby, R.; Geerts, W. Reducing the hospital burden of heparin-induced thrombocytopenia: Impact of an avoid-heparin program. *Blood* **2016**, *127*, 1954–1959. [CrossRef]
104. Suvarna, S.; Espinasse, B.; Qi, R.; Lubica, R.; Poncz, M.; Cines, U.B.; Wiesner, M.R.; Arepally, G.M. Determinants of PF4/heparin immunogenicity. *Blood* **2007**, *110*, 4253–4260. [CrossRef]
105. Arepally, G.M.; Cines, D.B. Pathogenesis of heparin-induced thrombocytopenia. *Transl. Res.* **2020**, *225*, 131–140. [CrossRef]
106. Francis, J.L.; Palmer, G.J.; Moroose, R.; Drexler, A. Comparison of bovine and porcine heparin in heparin antibody formation after cardiac surgery. *Ann. Thorac. Surg.* **2003**, *75*, 17–22. [CrossRef]

107. Ahmad, S. Heparin-induced thrombocytopenia: Impact of bovine versus porcine heparin in HIT pathogenesis. *Front. Biosci.* **2007**, *12*, 3312–3320. [CrossRef] [PubMed]
108. Greinacher, A.; Warkentin, T.E.; Chong, B.H. Heparin-induced thrombocytopenia. In *Platelets*, 4th ed.; Michelson, A.D., Ed.; Academic Press: New York, NY, USA, 2019; pp. 741–767.
109. Hayes, V.; Johnston, I.; Arepally, G.M.; McKenzie, S.E.; Cines, D.B.; Rauova, L.; Poncz, M. Endothelial antigen assembly leads to thrombotic complications in heparin-induced thrombocytopenia. *J. Clin. Investig.* **2017**, *127*, 1090–1098. [CrossRef] [PubMed]
110. Gollomp, K.; Kim, M.; Johnston, I.; Hayes, V.; Welsh, J.; Arepally, G.M.; Kahn, M.; Lambert, M.P.; Cuker, A.; Cines, D.B.; et al. Neutrophil accumulation and NET release contribute to thrombosis in HIT. *JCI Insight* **2018**, *3*, 99445. [CrossRef] [PubMed]
111. Bauer, T.L.; Arepally, G.; Konkle, B.A.; Mestichelli, B.; Shapiro, S.S.; Cines, D.B.; Poncz, M.; McNulty, S.; Amiral, J.; Hauck, W.W.; et al. Prevalence of Heparin-Associated Antibodies Without Thrombosis in Patients Undergoing Cardiopulmonary Bypass Surgery. *Circ.* **1997**, *95*, 1242–1246. [CrossRef]
112. Pouplard, C.; May, M.-A.; Iochmann, S.; Amiral, J.; Vissac, A.-M.; Marchand, M.; Gruel, Y. Antibodies to Platelet Factor 4–Heparin After Cardiopulmonary Bypass in Patients Anticoagulated With Unfractionated Heparin or a Low-Molecular-Weight Heparin. *Circ.* **1999**, *99*, 2530–2536. [CrossRef]
113. Koster, A.; Sänger, S.; Hansen, R.; Sodian, R.; Mertzlufft, F.; Harke, C.; Kuppe, H.; Hetzer, R.; Loebe, M. Prevalence and Persistence of Heparin/Platelet Factor 4 Antibodies in Patients with Heparin Coated and Noncoated Ventricular Assist Devices. *ASAIO J.* **2000**, *46*, 319–322. [CrossRef]
114. Schenk, S.; El-Banayosy, A.; Prohaska, W.; Arusoglu, L.; Morshuis, M.; Koester-Eiserfunke, W.; Kizner, L.; Murray, E.; Eichler, P.; Koerfer, R.; et al. Heparin-induced thrombocytopenia in patients receiving mechanical circulatory support. *J. Thorac. Cardiovasc. Surg.* **2006**, *131*, 1373–1381.e4. [CrossRef]
115. Warkentin, T.E.; Sheppard, J.I.; Sun, J.C.J.; Jung, H.; Eikelboom, J.W. Anti-PF4/heparin antibodies and venous graft occlusion in postcoronary artery bypass surgery patients randomized to postoperative unfractionated heparin or fondaparinux thromboprophylaxis. *J. Thromb. Haemost.* **2013**, *11*, 253–260. [CrossRef]
116. Demma, L.J.; Winkler, A.M.; Levy, J.H. A Diagnosis of Heparin-Induced Thrombocytopenia with Combined Clinical and Laboratory Methods in Cardiothoracic Surgical Intensive Care Unit Patients. *Anesthesia Analg.* **2011**, *113*, 697–702. [CrossRef]
117. Warkentin, T.E.; Arsenault, K.A.; Whitlock, R.; Eikelboom, J.; Yusuf, A.M. Prognostic importance of preoperative anti-PF4/heparin antibodies in patients undergoing cardiac surgery. *Thromb. Haemost.* **2012**, *107*, 8–14. [CrossRef] [PubMed]
118. Bennett-Guerrero, E.; Slaughter, T.F.; White, W.D.; Welsby, I.J.; Greenberg, C.S.; El-Moalem, H.; Ortel, T.L. Preoperative anti-PF4/heparin antibody level predicts adverse outcome after cardiac surgery. *J. Thorac. Cardiovasc. Surg.* **2005**, *130*, 1567–1572. [CrossRef] [PubMed]
119. Everett, B.M.; Yeh, R.; Foo, S.Y.; Criss, D.; Van Cott, E.M.; Laposata, M.; Avery, E.G.; Hoffman, W.D.; Walker, J.; Torchiana, D.; et al. Prevalence of Heparin/Platelet Factor 4 Antibodies Before and After Cardiac Surgery. *Ann. Thorac. Surg.* **2007**, *83*, 592–597. [CrossRef] [PubMed]
120. Selleng, S.; Malowsky, B.; Itterman, T.; Bagemühl, J.; Wessel, A.; Wollert, H.-G.; Warkentin, T.E.; Greinacher, A. Incidence and clinical relevance of anti–platelet factor 4/heparin antibodies before cardiac surgery. *Am. Hear. J.* **2010**, *160*, 362–369. [CrossRef] [PubMed]
121. Mattioli, A.V.; Bonetti, L.; Zennaro, M.; Ambrosio, G.; Mattioli, G. Heparin/PF4 antibodies formation after heparin treatment: Temporal aspects and long-term follow-up. *Am. Hear. J.* **2009**, *157*, 589–595. [CrossRef]
122. Dyke, C.M.; Smedira, N.G.; Koster, A.; Aronson, S.; McCarthy, H.L.; Kirshner, R.; Lincoff, A.M.; Spiess, B.D. A comparison of bivalirudin to heparin with protamine reversal in patients undergoing cardiac surgery with cardiopulmonary bypass: The EVOLUTION-ON study. *J. Thorac. Cardiovasc. Surg.* **2006**, *131*, 533–539. [CrossRef] [PubMed]
123. Koster, A.; Dyke, C.M.; Aldea, G.; Smedira, N.G.; Ii, H.L.M.; Aronson, S.; Hetzer, R.; Avery, E.; Spiess, B.; Lincoff, A.M. Bivalirudin During Cardiopulmonary Bypass in Patients With Previous or Acute Heparin-Induced Thrombocytopenia and Heparin Antibodies: Results of the CHOOSE-ON Trial. *Ann. Thorac. Surg.* **2007**, *83*, 572–577. [CrossRef] [PubMed]
124. Follis, F.; Filippone, G.; Montalbano, G.; Floriano, M.; Lobianco, E.; D'Ancona, G.; Follis, M. Argatroban as a substitute of heparin during cardiopulmonary bypass: A safe alternative? *Interact. Cardiovasc. Thorac. Surg.* **2010**, *10*, 592–596. [CrossRef] [PubMed]
125. Agarwal, S.; Ullom, B.; Al-Baghdadi, Y.; Okumura, M. Challenges encountered with argatroban anticoagulation during cardiopulmonary bypass. *Journal of Anaesthesiology, Clinical Pharmacology* **2012**, *28*, 106–110. [CrossRef] [PubMed]
126. Antoniou, T.; Kapetanakis, E.I.; Theodoraki, K.; Rellia, P.; Thanopoulos, A.; Kotiou, M.; Zarkalis, D.; Alivizatos, P. Cardiac surgery in patients with heparin-induced thrombocytopenia using preoperatively determined dosages of iloprost. *Hear. Surg. Forum* **2002**, *5*, 354–357.
127. Voeller, R.K.; Melby, S.J.; Grizzell, B.E.; Moazami, N. Novel use of plasmapheresis in a patient with heparin-induced thrombocytopenia requiring urgent insertion of a left ventricular assist device under cardiopulmonary bypass. *J. Thorac. Cardiovasc. Surg.* **2010**, *140*, e56–e58. [CrossRef]
128. Jaben, E.A.; Torloni, A.S.; Pruthi, R.K.; Winters, J.L. Use of plasma exchange in patients with heparin-induced thrombocytopenia: A report of two cases and a review of the literature. *J. Clin. Apher.* **2011**, *26*, 219–224. [CrossRef]

129. A Cannon, M.; Butterworth, J.; Riley, R.D.; Hyland, J.M. Failure of argatroban anticoagulation during off-pump coronary artery bypass surgery. *Ann. Thorac. Surg.* **2004**, *77*, 711–713. [CrossRef] [PubMed]
130. Dyke, C.M.; Aldea, G.; Koster, A.; Smedira, N.; Avery, E.; Aronson, S.; Spiess, B.D.; Lincoff, A.M. Off-Pump Coronary Artery Bypass with Bivalirudin for Patients with Heparin-Induced Thrombocytopenia or Antiplatelet Factor Four/Heparin Antibodies. *Ann. Thorac. Surg.* **2007**, *84*, 836–839. [CrossRef] [PubMed]

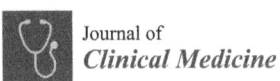

Review

Heparin-Induced Thrombocytopenia: A Review of New Concepts in Pathogenesis, Diagnosis, and Management

Matteo Marchetti [1,2,†], Maxime G. Zermatten [1,†], Debora Bertaggia Calderara [1], Alessandro Aliotta [1] and Lorenzo Alberio [1,*]

[1] Division of Hematology and Central Hematology Laboratory, Lausanne University Hospital (CHUV) and University of Lausanne (UNIL), CH-1011 Lausanne, Switzerland; matteo.marchetti@ghol.ch (M.M.); Maxime.Zermatten@chuv.ch (M.G.Z.); Debora.Bertaggia-Calderara@chuv.ch (D.B.C.); Alessandro.Aliotta@chuv.ch (A.A.)

[2] Service de Médecine Interne, Hôpital de Nyon, CH-1260 Nyon, Switzerland

* Correspondence: lorenzo.alberio@chuv.ch

† These authors contributed equally to this work.

Abstract: Knowledge on heparin-induced thrombocytopenia keeps increasing. Recent progress on diagnosis and management as well as several discoveries concerning its pathogenesis have been made. However, many aspects of heparin-induced thrombocytopenia remain partly unknown, and exact application of these new insights still need to be addressed. This article reviews the main new concepts in pathogenesis, diagnosis, and management of heparin-induced thrombocytopenia.

Keywords: heparin-induced thrombocytopenia (HIT); new concepts; pathogenesis; diagnosis; management; immune PF4/heparin/antibody complexes; Bayesian diagnostic thinking; therapeutic plasma exchange; intravenous immunoglobulins (IVIG)

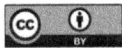

1. Introduction

Heparin-induced thrombocytopenia (HIT) is a fascinating, complex, and still partially obscure immunological syndrome. It is associated with a very high prothrombotic risk and may cause limb and life-threatening complications. Thus, a rapid accurate clinical and laboratory recognition as well as a prompt and effective management are required. Since its discovery, knowledge on HIT has been impressively growing, and all fields have been evolving: from pathogenesis to diagnostic approaches and management. In this review, we will particularly focus on the most relevant clinical new insights and advances on HIT.

2. Pathophysiology

The pathophysiology of heparin-induced thrombocytopenia (HIT) is complex and far exceeds simple platelet activation. Its spectrum is broad. Here, we will describe each step of HIT pathophysiology, beginning with antigen formation, followed by immune reaction and antibody synthesis, development of a severe prothrombotic state, and ending with thromboembolism, which has the potential to be life threatening.

2.1. Antigen Formation: Platelet Factor 4-Heparin (PF4/H) Complexes

The HIT antigen is situated on the platelet factor 4 (PF4), a chemokine that is contained in platelet α-granules. PF4 is not immunogenic in its primary form. Conformational PF4 changes are needed to expose a neo-epitope, which is the HIT antigen. These changes occur by the formation of complexes between PF4 and negatively charged molecules, especially heparin and other glycosaminoglycans (GAGs) [1]. The size and the charge of the complexes play a central role in pathogenicity. These two parameters depend on the relative amounts of PF4 and heparin. The PF4/heparin complexes are electrostatically formed by at least 16 PF4 molecules (positively charged) assembled with heparin chains (negatively charged) in multimolecular ultralarge complexes (ULCs), which will participate to platelet activation (see below) [2]. Quantitatively, the maximal amount of these ULCs is formed at equimolar PF4/heparin ratio [2,3]. Of note, when performing these analyses in presence of platelets, the ratio has been reported to be 20:1, indicating that, in vivo, a proportion of the heparin chains could be replaced by endogenous glycosaminoglycans in the glycocalyx of the cell surface [4]. Importantly and compared to unfractionated heparin (UFH), far fewer ULCs are formed with low molecular weight heparins (LMWH), and none with fondaparinux [2], because heparin chains with at least 12 saccharides are necessary to form ULCs [2,5]. This explains the lower risk to develop HIT with LMWH. Qualitatively, the immunogenicity of the complexes depends on their net charge and not their size. A positive net charge facilitates the interaction with immune cells [3]. Therefore, the highest immunogenicity is reached when PF4—in absence of platelets (see above)—is in excess and at a molar PF4/heparin ratio of 20/1 [3]. Of note, these mechanisms explain why fondaparinux is immunogenic but only rarely has been reported as a cause HIT [6]. Similarly, the immunogenicity of a high PF4/heparin ratio also explains the high incidence of HIT in patients with high amounts of circulating PF4 (e.g., orthopedic and vascular surgery) and prophylactic doses of UFH.

2.2. Anti-PF4/H Antibodies Synthesis

Innate and adaptive humoral and cellular reactions lead to anti-PF4/H antibodies synthesis. Briefly, once formed, ULCs activate complement, leading to the deposition of C3/C4 on the complexes. This allows their binding to cluster of differentiation 21 (CD21, the complement receptor 2) on B cells, which facilitates their activation, antigen transport to secondary lymphoid follicles, and antigen transfer. This culminates in an adaptive humoral immune response and anti-PF4/H antibodies production [7].

2.3. Antigen Formation on the Platelet Surface and Platelet Activation

The antigenic complex formation occurs on the platelet surface in a dynamic and potentially reversible manner. In presence of PF4, increasing heparin initially leads to an increasing antigen-complex size. HIT antibodies will then bind to these ULCs [8]. With further increase, heparin would then displace PF4 from the platelet surface and diminish the size of the antigen-complexes, thus decreasing their capacity to activate platelets [8]. The antigen–antibody binding on the platelet surface induces platelet activation via FcγRIIa (CD32, the low affinity IgG receptor) and leads to platelet degranulation and aggregation. Degranulation increases the available PF4 concentration for further antigen-complex formation [9,10]. Besides these "classical" platelet activation endpoints, platelet activation also induces the production of procoagulant platelets and platelet-derived procoagulant microparticles [11], dramatically enhancing thrombin generation. Moreover, in presence of an excess of PF4, further cells, including monocytes, endothelial cells, and neutrophils, can be recruited. The interactions and roles of these cells are summed up below and graphically presented in Figure 1.

2.4. Other Cells Beyond Platelets Involved in HIT Prothrombotic State
2.4.1. Monocytes

Monocytes participate in HIT hypercoagulability. Indeed, PF4 binds monocytes with a higher affinity than platelets. This is due to the different GAGs proportion in their glycocalyx and to a variable PF4 affinity for the different GAGs. Indeed, PF4 binds with decreasing intensity to heparin, heparan sulfate, dermatan sulfate, chondroitin-6-sulfate, and chondroitin-4-sulfate [12]. This facilitates the binding of HIT antibodies [13–16], which appears to be optimal in absence of heparin [13]. This could be due to the higher availability of PF4, which is not bound by heparin. The formation of antibody/antigen complexes on the monocyte surface leads to their activation [15], inducing (i) secretion of IL-8 [13] and surface expression of tissue factor (TF) [13,16] and (ii production of tissue-factor expressing microparticles (TF-MPs) [13]. TF expression seems to depend on FcγRIIa [16], while the de novo synthesis and production of TF-MPs appears to depend on FcγRI [13]. Moreover, monocyte activation leads to their glycocalyx sulfation, which induces a higher affinity for PF4 binding, thus sustaining an amplification loop [14]. These changes provoke a procoagulant activity of the monocytes [17], culminating in thrombin generation. The generated thrombin will in turn activate platelets in other amplification loops leading to procoagulant platelets due to platelet co-activation via FcγRIIa [18], whose downstream signaling is similar to that observed upon glycoprotein (GP) VI engagement [19]. Of note, monocyte activation can also occur via P-selectin expressed on platelets [20]. To summarize, monocytes are activated by antigen/antibody HIT complexes, which lead to thrombin generation via TF expression and TF-MPs production.

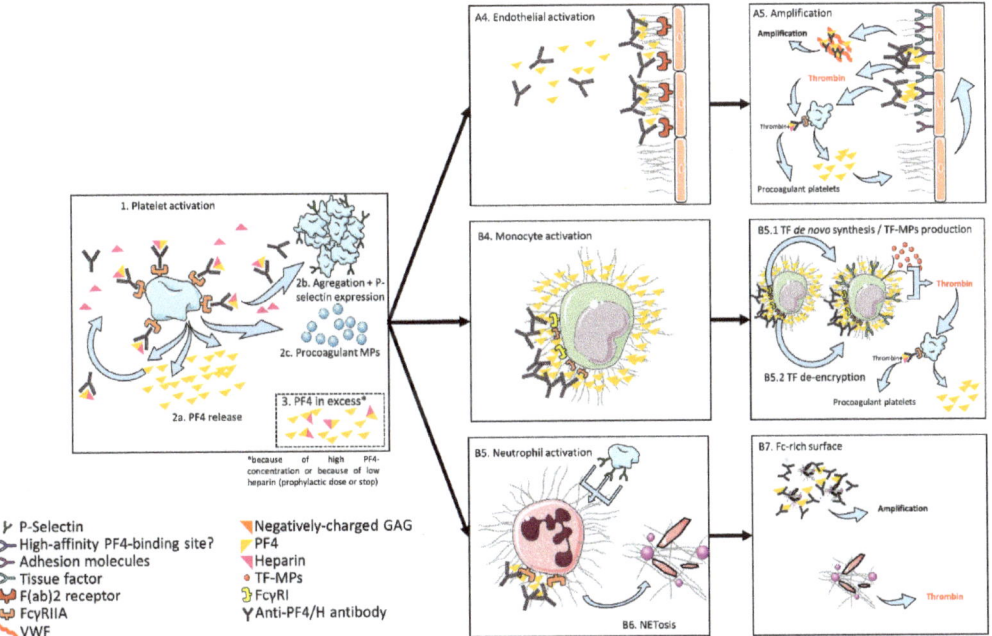

Figure 1. Pathophysiology of HIT. Platelets are activated by ultralarge complexes (ULCs) of PF4 and heparin via FcγRIIa. The activation leads to PF4 release, aggregation, P-selectin expression, and to production of procoagulant microparticles. After platelet activation, PF4 is in excess compared to heparin and can bind to endogenous glycosaminoglycans (GAG) on endothelial cells, monocytes, and neutrophils. Complexes of PF4 and GAG are recognized by HIT antibodies with consecutive activation of the cells. The activation of monocytes and endothelial cells leads to thrombin generation via expression of tissue factor (TF) and microparticles with TF (TF-MP), with further activation of platelets, creating a positive feedback loop. Moreover, the activation of endothelial cells leads to von Willebrand factor (VWF) secretion, on which PF4 binds, creating a Fc-rich surface, which leads to further activation of platelets. Activation of neutrophils leads to NETosis offering a Fc-rich surface with further activation of platelets and supporting thrombin generation (see text).

2.4.2. Endothelial Cells

HIT antibodies bind to PF4 on endothelial cells as well [21,22], possibly via the F(ab) region of the antibodies [22]. This binding, which seems to be preferentially directed towards microvascular endothelial cells, requires an endothelial preactivation, possibly caused by TNFα released during platelet activation [22]. Because PF4 is required, the primary step remains platelet activation and degranulation. This leads to the required high PF4 concentrations that exceed the PF4-neutralization capacity of heparin. In presence of vascular lesions, PF4 could mainly bind to endothelial cells [23], and these lesions could be the preferred sites for thrombosis development in HIT [24]. The formation of antigen–antibody complexes on the cell surface induces additional endothelial injuries and activation [21,22,25], which leads to the expression of TF [21] and adhesion molecules [22] and to changes in the glycocalyx of the endothelial cells. Indeed, injured endothelial cells seem to release thrombomodulin [22,25], which could lead to locally decreased anticoagulant potential. Of note, the binding of PF4 could be more intense on injured endothelial cells [23], despite loss of negative charges. This could indicate the existence of a high-affinity PF4-binding site being unveiled and inducing a positive feedback loop with increased formation of immune complexes and sensitization of neighbor endothelial cells [23].

Moreover, PF4 could bind to extended strings of von Willebrand factor, which have been released from activated or injured endothelial cells, consecutively exposing the HIT antigen on bound PF molecules [26]. This is recognized by HIT antibodies leading to the formation of a IgG Fc-rich network with complement activation and activation of additional cells.

2.4.3. Neutrophils

Neutrophils are thought to play an essential role in HIT hypercoagulability and in thrombosis development. They are activated by P-selectin on platelets and via FcγRIIa [27] by anti-PF4/H antibodies and heparin immune complexes formed on their surface, which are bound to chondroitin sulfate [28]. This induces neutrophil extracellular traps (NET) formation and release (NETosis). NETs participate in the hypercoagulability in HIT. First, they can bind to PF4, developing a surface rich in fragment crystallizable regions (Fc-domain) and an amplification loop [29]. Second, they are thought to be essential for thrombosis development [27], via their procoagulant activities, in particular direct activation of the contact phase of thrombin generation.

2.5. HIT, A Side Effect of an Immune Mechanism?

PF4 and anti-PF4/polyanion antibodies could play a physiologic role in the host immune defense, particularly against Gram-negative bacterial infections. Indeed, bacteria can activate platelets, leading to degranulation and release of PF4 and polyphosphates. PF4 and polyphosphates can successively bind on lipid A on Gram-negative bacteria [30–32], leading to opsonization of bacteria by anti-PF4/polyanion antibodies, enabling better host defense against infection. The formation of anti-PF4/heparin antibodies would therefore be a pathological molecular-mimicry activation of a physiologic mechanism.

2.6. Importance of Specific Gene Polymorphisms

As widely known, not all patients developing HIT antibodies develop HIT, and not all patients with HIT develop thromboembolic complications. The mechanisms underlying these variable responses are not completely understood. However, specific gene polymorphisms could be involved, especially in the risk to develop thromboembolic complications in HIT. Indeed, an association between the polymorphism of FcγRIIIA 158VV [30] and occurrence of HIT and between the polymorphism of FcγRIIA 131R and thromboembolic complications in HIT [31–33] has been observed in different studies. Further genetic polymorphisms could be identified in the future, explaining the different responses to HIT antibodies.

2.7. HIT without Heparin

Heparin is the most frequent negatively charged molecule that induces HIT. However, some patients develop symptoms and signs of HIT without exposition to heparin, especially after orthopedic surgery, which is known as spontaneous or autoimmune HIT (aHIT) [34–38]. This could be due to the presence of others polyanions that can induce "HIT". This is the case for chondroitin sulfate [39,40], polyphosphates [41], nucleic acid [42], or bacterial components [43]. A brief comparison between classical HIT and aHIT is presented in Table 1. For further details on aHIT, we refer the reader to the excellent review of Greinacher, Selleng, and Warkentin [44].

Table 1. Comparison of classical and autoimmune HIT.

	Classical HIT	Autoimmune HIT
Antigen	Neoepitope on PF4, revealed by a conformational change due to binding to a negatively-charged surface	
Negatively-charged molecule	Heparin	Other polyanions: chondroitin sulfate, polyphosphates, nucleic acid, bacterial components
Pathogenesis	Similar (see text: part 1a–d)	
Therapy	Heparin avoidance, alternative non-heparin anticoagulation	Intravenous immunoglobulins (IVIG), plasmapheresis

To summarize, HIT is a complex immune-mediated pathology. Its mechanisms depend on the concentrations of PF4 and heparin, particularly their ratio to each other and involve platelets, monocytes, endothelial cells, and neutrophils as well. The activation of these cells induces, besides thrombocytopenia, a coagulation cascade activation leading to a severe hypercoagulant state.

3. Diagnostic Approach

Making a correct and rapid diagnosis of HIT is challenging and of utmost importance [45]. It requires the association of clinical parameters to estimate the pre-test probability and laboratory assays to confirm or infirm the diagnosis [46].

3.1. Clinical Pre-Test Probability

At the bedside, the cornerstones are thinking of HIT when appropriate (e.g., fall in platelet count, thrombosis despite heparin anticoagulation) and subsequently assess the clinical pre-test probability of HIT with validated clinical scores. To do so, the 4T score (thrombocytopenia, timing, thrombosis, other causes of thrombocytopenia; 0–8 points) has been developed [47], and its use is currently recommended by the American Society of Hematology (ASH) [48]. The HEP score is a more recent clinical score [49]. Compared to the 4T score, it showed a higher specificity among ICU patients [50]. However, it still needs broader implementation studies and is not yet recommended [48,50]. The clinical probability can rule out HIT or establish the indication for laboratory testing. Currently, it is considered that a low (0–3 points) 4T score can rule out HIT, while an intermediate (4–5) or high (6–8) score requires laboratory testing [48]. However, different studies observed HIT cases despite low 4T scores, which raised concern about ruling out HIT among patients with a 4T score of 3 [51–54].

3.2. Laboratory Work-Up

Different types of laboratory assays exist. In this review, we will focus on two platelet-activation assays (i.e., the serotonin-release assay (SRA) and the heparin-induced platelet aggregation test (HIPA)), on some broadly available immunoassays (IA) for HIT, and on emerging diagnostic strategies.

3.2.1. Platelet-Activation Assays: The Gold Standard for HIT

Two platelet-activation assays using donor washed platelets are considered as diagnostic gold standards for HIT [55]. These assays are considered to be functional because they detect heparin-dependent platelet activation by either aggregation (HIPA) or degranulation and release of serotonin (SRA) when the patient's plasma, possibly containing anti-PF4/heparin platelet-activating antibodies, is added in presence of pharmacological concentrations of heparin. However, these assays are technically demanding, time consuming, and unavailable for many hospitals, which delays definitive diagnostic work-up and optimal management [52]. As a consequence, their use is currently only recommended after a first clinical-biological work-up, namely among patients with intermediate and/or high clinical suspicion (i.e., 4T score > 3 points) and a positive IA [48]. Moreover, recent studies described the possibility of false-negative functional assays [52,56,57]. Ticagrelor can induce false negative HIPA among HIT patients, and other anti-platelet drugs might also cause false negative HIT functional assays [56]. Another mechanism is the novel concept of seroconversion preceding functional positivity in vitro [58]. To address this lack of sensitivity, several methods to avoid false-negative functional assays have been reported, but not validated by a dedicated study: (i) removing/inhibiting antiplatelet agents in the first case and (ii) performing a PF4-enhanced assay (PF4-SRA) [59,60] when suspecting the second case, although this approach could lead to false positive results [56–58,61]. Although such methods increase the performances of the gold standards functional assays, HIPA and SRA, false negative-negative results are still possible. Therefore, when the 4T score is high and the IA are strongly positive, HIT should still be considered despite a negative functional assay [45,48]. Apart from the SRA and the HIPA assays, many other platelet-activating assays have been developed, and for a more detailed review on this topic, we refer to the recent review of Tardy et al. [62].

3.2.2. Immunoassays (IA): Rapid and Broadly Available Alternatives

Many laboratory techniques detecting anti-PF4/heparin antibodies exist.

The Classical IA

Enzyme-linked immunosorbent assays (ELISA) were the first wide available techniques [46]. They are nowadays still broadly used, and the ASH guidelines recommend their use as first-line laboratory test [48]. They are recognized to be highly sensitive (i.e., allow to accurately rule out HIT), but unspecific (i.e., leading to false-positive results and unnecessary non-heparin anticoagulation while awaiting the definitive result of a functional assay or for long course) [46,58]. Recently, Warkentin et al. highlighted that ELISA are not considered as rapid immunoassays anymore [58]. In addition, they underscored the original observation of Lindhoff-Last [58], that IgG-specific ELISA are more specific without being less sensitive for HIT, echoing a communication of the scientific and standardization committee of the International Society on Thrombosis and Haemostasis (ISTH) [63] in favor of use of IgG-specific immunoassays [58]. In a review published in 2017, Arepally also underscored that anti-PF4/H IgG antibodies are the most relevant isotype for HIT pathogenesis, IgA and IgM contribution to HIT being subordinate [46].

Other "Rapid" IA

Many other techniques detecting anti-PF4/H antibodies have been developed and studied. In 2016, two very relevant meta-analyses about rapid IA for HIT were published. Nagler et al. identified five tests as highly sensitive and specific for HIT, namely the polyspecific ELISA with an intermediate threshold (Genetic Testing Institute, Asserachrom), particle-gel immunoassay (PaGIA), lateral flow immunoassay (LFIA), polyspecific chemiluminescent immunoassay (CLIA) with a high threshold, and IgG-specific CLIA with a low threshold [64]. Sun et al. reached the conclusion that PaGIA, IgG-specific CLIA, and LFIA showed excellent sensitivity and specificity [65].

Emerging Diagnostic Strategies

Moreover, both meta-analyses highlighted that combining results of some of the different aforementioned rapid IA might improve diagnostic performance for HIT and thus further improve care in patients with suspected HIT. Additionally, Sun et al. highlighted that combining clinical assessment (i.e., pre-test probability) with rapid immunoassays in a Bayesian approach was likely to be the most powerful way to estimate an overall likelihood of HIT in real-world clinical practice [64,65]. In 2018, the ASH guidelines identified "integration of emerging rapid immuno-assays into diagnostic algorithms" as a pressing research priority [48].

Regarding the Bayesian diagnostic approach, Nellen et al. showed in 2012 for the first time ever that the combination of clinical pre-test probability (assessed by the 4T score) with the quantitative result of a rapid immunoassay detecting anti-PF4/heparin antibodies was valuable not only for excluding [66], but also for predicting a positive heparin-induced platelet aggregation test, i.e., for diagnosing HIT rapidly [51]. Other groups confirmed that a Bayesian diagnostic approach for HIT that combines clinical probability assessed with validated scores with rapid immunoassay results was a promising approach towards improvement of HIT diagnostic work-up, especially when semi-quantitative immunoassay results were used [53,54,67,68].

Recently, two groups described diagnostic approaches that combine two rapid immunoassays. Our group developed and prospectively validated a Bayesian diagnostic algorithm (the "Lausanne algorithm") based on the 4T score and the combination of IgG-specific CLIA and PaGIA that correctly classifies >95% of patients within a 60 min laboratory work-up time [52]. This algorithm was recognized by Cuker and Cines to perform better than the ASH algorithm, correctly classifying "all patients with HIT and 95.4% of patients without HIT, whereas the ASH algorithm correctly classified only 91.1% of the patients with HIT and 93.2% of patients without HIT" [45]. Warkentin et al. described a diagnostic laboratory scoring system (0–6 points) based on the combination of IgG-specific CLIA and latex immunoturbidimetric assay (LIA) that reached a 99% sensitivity when both assays (CLIA and LIA negative threshold <1.0 U/mL) were negative and a positive predictive value for platelet-activating antibodies (i.e., positive SRA or PF4-SRA) of 97.1% for scores ≥5 points [69]. Of particular relevant note, these diagnostic approaches use the PaGIA and the IgG-specific CLIA or the LIA as rapid IAs. Thus, integrating other IAs in such Bayesian approaches that combine two rapid IAs still needs to be studied.

4. Management of Acute HIT

As described previously, HIT is a complex and severe prothrombotic state. Briefly, current cornerstones of HIT management are (i) immediate cessation of any heparin administration and (ii) introduction of non-heparin therapeutic anticoagulation, such as argatroban or bivalirudin (direct parenteral thrombin inhibitors), or danaparoid or fondaparinux (indirect parenteral factor Xa inhibitors) [48]. Recently, direct oral anticoagulants (DOACs) are emerging as an alternative in acute HIT or HIT with thrombosis, but the data on their use remain very limited [70]. For a detailed review and updated recommendation on the use and monitoring of these different non-heparin anticoagulants, we refer the interested readers to Table 2 and a recent comprehensive article [70]. In the present review, we will focus on other emerging and second-line management strategies in HIT that either directly target platelet-activating anti-PF4/heparin antibodies or inhibit antibody-mediated platelet activation (Table 3).

Table 2. Key information on alternative parenteral non-heparin anticoagulants (adapted from [70]).

	Argatroban	Bivalirudin	Danaparoid	Fondaparinux
Mechanism of action	Direct thrombin inhibitor	Direct thrombin inhibitor	Indirect factor Xa inhibitor (mediated by antithrombin)	Indirect factor Xa inhibitor (mediated by antithrombin)
Half-life	45 min	25 min	19–25 h	17–21 h
Route of administration	IV	IV	IV/SC	SC
Main elimination pathway	Hepatobiliary	Proteolytic (80%) and renal (20%)	Renal	Renal
Monitoring	Calibrated diluted anti-factor IIa assay	Calibrated diluted anti-factor IIa assay	Calibrated anti-factor Xa assay	Calibrated anti-factor Xa assay

Legend: IV, intravenous, SC, subcutaneous.

Table 3. Key information on second-line treatments of HIT.

	Therapeutic Plasmapheresis (TPE)	Intravenous Immunoglobulins (IVIG)	Cangrelor	IdeS (Imlifidase)
Rationale	Removal of pathological antibodies	Binding of pathological antibodies	Rapid-acting, reversible platelet inhibitor	Endopeptidase specifically cleaving IgG antibodies
Dose and mode/frequency of administration	A single TPE removes about 2/3 of the HIT-antibodies [71]. Exact number of TPE and duration of action unknown [72,73]	1 g/kg/day IV for 2 consecutive days. NB: use calculated dosing-weight among obese patients [74]	30 µg/kg IV bolus, followed by 4 µg/kg IV infusion [75,76]	0.24–0.5 mg/kg [77,78]. NB: Appropriate dosage has to be established in HIT
Indications	1. Acute HIT or positive functional assay + immediate cardiovascular surgery with heparin [48] 2. Alternative anticoagulation contraindicated [73,79] 3. Clinical course worsening despite non-heparin anticoagulation [72]	1. Clinical course worsening despite non-heparin anticoagulation [74,80] 2. aHIT [74,80] 3. Alternative anticoagulation contraindicated	Cardiovascular surgery when anti-PF4/heparin are present and intraoperative heparin use is mandatory [76,81,82]	To date, no clear indication
Pros	Effective for managing HIT in many conditions, regional anticoagulation possible	Favorable experience, especially in patients with refractory HIT and aHIT [74,80]	Favorable experience with this treatment	Promising results in mice HIT model [77] and kidney transplant patients [78]
Cons	Cost; infectious, metabolic complications; difficulty in predicting how often and how long to perform [72,73]	Adjunctive to anticoagulation, high cost, standard dose insufficient in severe cases	Cost; efficacy to be assessed for each patient with a functional assay before its use [82]	Not yet studied in HIT patients

Legend: aHIT, autoimmune HIT; IV, intravenous. For more details, please refer to the text and to the cited references.

4.1. Therapeutic Plasmapheresis (TPE)

Experience with TPE in patients with HIT remains limited, as underscored in 2018 by Cho et al. who performed a national survey (USA) of academic apheresis services regarding practices in managing patients with HIT and found only 15.4% of respondents reporting having performed TPE on patients with HIT during the past year [83].

To date, case reports are the major source of evidence. Additionally, although a single TPE removes about two-thirds of the HIT antibodies [71], the exact number of required plasma exchanges in order to effectively lower the plasmatic HIT antibodies concentration and the duration of action of TPE due to mobilization of the extravascular antibody compartment remain unknown and difficult to predict. Thus, TPE is probably best guided by biological monitoring [72,73].

TPE has been described as an effective option for managing HIT in three particular situations [72]. First, pre/perioperative plasmapheresis along with intraoperative heparin anticoagulation is one of the three management options for patients with acute HIT or persisting positive functional assay and anti-PF4/H antibodies who require immediate cardiovascular surgery [48]. When doing so, sensitive functional platelet aggregation assays are best suited to determine readiness for heparin re-exposure [84]. The second situation is when non-heparin anticoagulation is contraindicated because of a major bleeding event, such as intracerebral hemorrhage (ICH) [79]. The third situation is when HIT clinical and biological course worsens/does not improve under well-conducted non-heparin anticoagulation (i.e., refractory HIT). For further details, we refer the reader to the recent excellent review of Onuoha et al. [72].

4.2. Intravenous Immunoglobulin (IVIG)

In the latest guidelines on HIT management, elucidation of the role of IVIG treatment in acute HIT has been defined as a key research priority for the management of HIT [48].

Regarding safety of IVIG use, a consensus of 15 Canadian hematologists stated in 2007 that IVIG were contraindicated for treatment of HIT because of a potential increased thrombotic risk [85]. However, in their recent study, Dhakal et al. found no increased risk for arterial or venous thrombosis incidence among patients with HIT treated with IVIG [86].

In clinical practice, many groups have reported favorable experience with this treatment, especially in patients with refractory HIT [72,87]. Recently, Warkentin underscored IVIG use as an adjunctive treatment, especially when thrombocytopenia persists in the setting of auto-immune HIT (aHIT) [74]. Briefly, aHIT is a subgroup of HIT including different disorders and is characterized by in vivo and in vitro heparin-dependent and heparin-independent platelet-activating antibodies. Because of high-titer, heparin-independent, platelet-activating antibodies, clinical course of aHIT is often severe and characterized by worsening or persisting HIT, even after beginning an alternative anticoagulation [74]. For a detailed clinical and biological description of aHIT, we refer to the excellent review of Greinacher, Selleng, and Warkentin [44].

Interestingly and in relationship with elements discussed above, in vitro IVIG have been shown to preferentially inhibit heparin-independent platelet-activating antibodies, explaining thus the rationale of their use in aHIT and/or refractory HIT [74]. Even if their exact mechanism of action remains unknown, they are believed to inhibit platelet (and other cells, see above) activation through FcγRIIa receptors [88].

4.3. New Insights of the Translational Research: The Quest for Inhibiting FcγRIIa-Mediated Platelet Activation

A chimeric anti-PF4/H antibody composed of a mouse IgG1 and a human Fc fragment was developed, namely the 5B9. It was obtained after immunization of transgenic mice with heparin and purified human PF4. 5B9 was proven to (i) induce platelet degranulation and release of serotonin when added in whole blood of healthy donors containing UFH (i.e., result in a positive SRA) and (ii) induce thrombocytopenia and thrombin generation when administered with UFH to another species of transgenic mice expressing human FcγRIIa and PF4 (i.e., cause HIT). Thus, 5B9 was described to fully mimic the effects of human HIT antibodies [89].

One emerging and appealing option that still needs further study is the IgG-degrading enzyme of *Streptococcus pyogenes* (IdeS), which cleaves a region that is critical in the interaction of IgG with FcγRIIa and thus disables platelet activation via this pathway [77]. Kizlik-Masson showed in vitro that IdeS selectively prevented platelet activation in the presence of heparin and 5B9 or human anti-PF4/heparin platelet-activating IgG antibodies without altering platelet aggregation induced by ADP and/or collagen. Moreover, the same group showed in vivo that IdeS prevented thrombocytopenia and thrombin activation (i.e., HIT) when 5B9 and UFH were administered to transgenic mice expressing human FcγRIIa and PF4 [77]. Summarizing, IdeS has already been studied in different mice models (immune thrombocytopenia, IgG-dependent glomerulonephritis, IgG-dependent arthritis, IgG-HIT models) showing promising effects [77]. Thus, in the field of HIT, IdeS is a promising emerging novel tool that might expand the available therapeutic arsenal.

5. Management of Patients Requiring Cardiovascular Surgery

On the one hand, according to Selleng et al. [90] and Warkentin et al. [91], anticoagulation with unfractionated heparin (UFH) for patients undergoing cardiac surgery in patients with a history of HIT is safe and effective, if circulating anti-PF4/heparin antibodies are no longer detectable [90–92]. On the other hand, management of patients requiring cardiovascular surgery and who have either (i) acute HIT, (ii) persisting positive functional assay and anti-PF4/heparin antibodies, or iii) negative functional assay, but persisting anti-PF4/heparin antibodies, is very challenging because the perioperative balance between both thrombotic and bleeding risk is fragile and can lead to fatal complications.

5.1. Patients with Acute HIT or Persisting Positive Functional Assay and Anti-PF4/Heparin Antibodies

To date, the ASH recommends delaying cardiovascular surgery among these patients. Because of a low level of evidence, there are only suggestions for management strategies in patients requiring immediate cardiovascular surgery [48].

The three main management options in these patients are (i) alternative intraoperative anticoagulation with bivalirudin, (ii) intraoperative anticoagulation with heparin and simultaneous antiaggregation with a potent platelet inhibitor (iloprost or tirofiban), or (iii) intraoperative anticoagulation with heparin and peri-operative plasma exchanges (see above) [48].

Bivalirudin is considered a safe alternative option for intraoperative anticoagulation in patients who undergo cardiovascular surgery when the interdisciplinary team is experienced and familiar with this technique, in particular avoiding blood stasis in the extracorporeal circuit and monitoring bivalirudin [93].

Alternatively, anticoagulation with intraoperative heparin and simultaneous short-acting and reversible anti-aggregation seems to be a valid strategy. In this context, apart from tirofiban (GP IIb/IIIa receptor blocker, half-life of 1.4 to 2.2 h, dependent on renal function) [94] and iloprost (synthetic analogue of epoprostenol PGI2 inhibiting platelet aggregation, adhesion and release reaction, half-life of 30 min) [95], cangrelor is a recent, potent, rapid-acting and reversible ADP receptor P2Y12 inhibitor with a very short half-life of 3–6 min [75]. Its use has been reported to be successful by different groups [81,96]. However, Scala et al. observed that cangrelor unreliably inhibits heparin-induced platelet aggregation in vitro when anti-PF4/heparin platelet-activating antibodies are present, concluding that cangrelor should not be used for HIT patients undergoing cardiac surgery unless its efficacy was confirmed in a particular patient with a presurgery negative aggregation test [82]. Cangrelor has a theoretical optimal profile (potent P2Y12 antagonist, rapid and very short-acting, reversible), but it needs to be further studied before being recommended or advised against.

A novel approach with limited published experience thus far is the use of IVIG to prevent HIT antibodies activating platelets and other cells as well (see above), possibly combined with additional cangrelor, in order to perform cardiovascular surgery with heparin [93].

5.2. Patients with Negative Functional Assay and Persisting Anti-PF4/Heparin Antibodies

To date, the ASH recommends with low level of evidence to favor intraoperative heparin for these patients on the basis of a few cases series [48,90,91]. However, SRA may not be sensitive enough to rule out the presence of pathogenic antibodies before cardiac surgery. Indeed, PF4-enhanced SRA has been described to be more sensitive than SRA, and since cardiac surgery induces a burst in PF4 plasma concentration, elevated intraoperative PF4 plasma concentrations might result in a positive SRA, mimicking thus in vivo a PF4-enhanced SRA [97]. HIT recurrence among patients with persisting anti-PF4/heparin antibodies who receive a single heparin dose is possible, especially if antibodies levels are high [98] and close medical and platelet follow-up is essential. Scala et al. reported the successful use of intraoperative heparin and simultaneous cangrelor in a patient with initial negative functional assay and persisting anti-PF4/heparin antibodies. They observed subsequent anti-PF4/heparin antibodies rise and positive functional assay seroconversion, concluding that even a short heparin administration (<90 min) induced boosting of clinically relevant anti-PF4/heparin antibodies. For similar patients, Scala et al. [76] and

Warkentin et al. [91] underscored that (i) postoperative monitoring of platelet counts [76,91] and anti-PF4/heparin antibodies [76] is mandatory, even after single intraoperative heparin exposition [76,91], (ii) performing a functional assay is necessary when anti-PF4/heparin antibodies rise and/or platelet count decreases [76,91], and (iii) a platelet fall [76,91] or increase in D-dimers [76] must be considered as presumptive recurrent HIT and requires, thus, beginning of non-heparin anticoagulation [76,91]. It remains to be verified whether the administration of IVIG in this context may modulate HIT antibodies boosting [93].

6. Conclusions

In this review, we described novel insights in the pathophysiology of HIT, recent improvements for the accuracy and speed of its diagnostic work-up, as well as new concepts for its management.

The current model of HIT is that of a multi-step immune pathology in response to the simultaneous exposition to an endogenous (i.e., PF4) and an exogenous molecule (i.e., heparin), at specific molar ratios. Moreover, the importance of platelets has been well known for years, but the central roles of other cells (monocytes, endothelial cells, and neutrophils) and specific receptors have only been recognized a few years ago. The comprehension of the pathophysiology of HIT is key to improve the therapeutic arsenal and the management of patients. This is well shown by the opportunity offered by IVIG and IdeS and their inhibitory effects in the interaction of IgG and FcγRIIa. A further and more precise comprehension of the pathophysiology could allow to develop more specific therapy for HIT.

Clinically, the work-up of HIT has improved in the past few years with the emergence of rapid and accurate diagnostic algorithms combining clinical parameters (4T score) and rapid quantitative laboratory assays. It is now possible to rapidly and accurately rule in or out HIT. This drastically improves the management of patients with HIT suspicion.

In conclusion, our knowledge about HIT is rapidly improving, which leads to a better management of this pathology and a better prognosis for patients.

Author Contributions: Conceptualization: M.M., M.G.Z. and L.A. Writing—original draft preparation: M.M., M.G.Z. and L.A. Writing—review and editing: M.M., M.G.Z., D.B.C., A.A. and L.A. Supervision: L.A. All authors have read and agreed to the published version of the manuscript.

Funding: This research received no external funding.

Conflicts of Interest: The authors declare no conflict of interest.

References

1. Mikhailov, D.; Young, H.C.; Linhardt, R.J.; Mayo, K.H. Heparin Dodecasaccharide Binding to Platelet Factor-4 and Growth-related Protein-α. *J. Biol. Chem.* **1999**, *274*, 25317–25329. [CrossRef] [PubMed]
2. Rauova, L.; Poncz, M.; McKenzie, S.E.; Reilly, M.P.; Arepally, G.; Weisel, J.W.; Nagaswami, C.; Cines, D.B.; Sachais, B.S.; Herre, J.; et al. Ultralarge complexes of PF4 and heparin are central to the pathogenesis of heparin-induced thrombocytopenia. *Blood* **2005**, *105*, 131–138. [CrossRef]
3. Suvarna, S.; Espinasse, B.; Qi, R.; Lubica, R.; Poncz, M.; Cines, U.B.; Wiesner, M.R.; Arepally, G.M. Determinants of PF4/heparin immunogenicity. *Blood* **2007**, *110*, 4253–4260. [CrossRef]
4. Krauel, K.; Fürll, B.; Warkentin, T.E.; Weitschies, W.; Kohlmann, T.; Sheppard, J.I.; Greinacher, A. Heparin-induced thrombocytopenia—Therapeutic concentrations of danaparoid, unlike fondaparinux and direct thrombin inhibitors, inhibit formation of platelet factor 4-heparin complexes. *J. Thromb. Haemost.* **2008**, *6*, 2160–2167. [CrossRef]
5. Visentin, G.P.; Moghaddam, M.; Beery, S.E.; McFarland, J.G.; Aster, R.H. Heparin is not required for detection of antibodies associated with heparin-induced thrombocytopenia/thrombosis. *J. Lab. Clin. Med.* **2001**, *138*, 22–31. [CrossRef]
6. Warkentin, T.E.; Maurer, B.T.; Aster, R.H. Heparin-Induced Thrombocytopenia Associated with Fondaparinux. *N. Engl. J. Med.* **2007**, *356*, 2653–2655. [CrossRef]
7. Khandelwal, S.; Lee, G.M.; Hester, C.G.; Poncz, M.; McKenzie, S.E.; Sachais, B.S.; Rauova, L.; Kelsoe, G.; Cines, D.B.; Frank, M.; et al. The antigenic complex in HIT binds to B cells via complement and complement receptor 2 (CD21). *Blood* **2016**, *128*, 1789–1799. [CrossRef]
8. Cines, D.B.; Rauova, L.; Arepally, G.; Reilly, M.P.; McKenzie, S.E.; Sachais, B.S.; Poncz, M. Heparin-induced thrombocytopenia: An autoimmune disorder regulated through dynamic autoantigen assembly/disassembly. *J. Clin. Apher.* **2007**, *22*, 31–36. [CrossRef]

9. Newman, P.M.; Chong, B.H. Heparin-induced thrombocytopenia: New evidence for the dynamic binding of purified anti-PF4-heparin antibodies to platelets and the resultant platelet activation. *Blood* **2000**, *96*, 182–187. [CrossRef]
10. Greinacher, A.; Pötzsch, B.; Amiral, J.; Dummel, V.; Eichner, A.; Mueller-Eckhardt, C. Heparin-associated thrombocytopenia: Isolation of the antibody and characterization of a multimolecular PF4-heparin complex as the major antigen. *Thromb. Haemost.* **1994**, *71*, 247–251.
11. Warkentin, T.; Hayward, C.; Boshkov, L.; Santos, A.; Sheppard, J.; Bode, A.; Kelton, J. Sera from patients with heparin-induced thrombocytopenia generate platelet-derived microparticles with procoagulant activity: An explanation for the thrombotic complications of heparin-induced thrombocytopenia. *Blood* **1994**, *84*, 3691–3699. [CrossRef] [PubMed]
12. Zucker, M.B.; Katz, I.R. Platelet Factor 4: Production, Structure, and Physiologic and Immunologic Action. *Exp. Biol. Med.* **1991**, *198*, 693–702. [CrossRef]
13. Arepally, G.M.; Mayer, I.M. Antibodies from patients with heparin-induced thrombocytopenia stimulate monocytic cells to express tissue factor and secrete interleukin-8. *Blood* **2001**, *98*, 1252–1254. [CrossRef] [PubMed]
14. Rauova, L.; Hirsch, J.D.; Greene, T.K.; Zhai, L.; Hayes, V.M.; Kowalska, M.A.; Cines, U.B.; Poncz, M. Monocyte-bound PF4 in the pathogenesis of heparin-induced thrombocytopenia. *Blood* **2010**, *116*, 5021–5031. [CrossRef] [PubMed]
15. Kasthuri, R.S.; Glover, S.L.; Jonas, W.; Mceachron, T.; Pawlinski, R.; Arepally, G.M.; Key, N.S.; Mackman, N. PF4/heparin-antibody complex induces monocyte tissue factor expression and release of tissue factor positive microparticles by activation of FcγRI. *Blood* **2012**, *119*, 5285–5293. [CrossRef]
16. Tutwiler, V.; Madeeva, D.; Ahn, H.S.; Andrianova, I.; Hayes, V.; Zheng, X.L.; Cines, D.B.; McKenzie, S.E.; Poncz, M.; Rauova, L. Platelet transactivation by monocytes promotes thrombosis in heparin-induced thrombocytopenia. *Blood* **2016**, *127*, 464–472. [CrossRef]
17. Pouplard, C.; Iochmann, S.; Renard, B.; Herault, O.; Colombat, P.; Amiral, J.; Gruel, Y. Induction of monocyte tissue factor expression by antibodies to heparin–platelet factor 4 complexes developed in heparin-induced thrombocytopenia. *Blood* **2001**, *97*, 3300–3302. [CrossRef] [PubMed]
18. Batár, P.; Dale, G.L. Simultaneous engagement of thrombin and FcγRIIA receptors results in platelets expressing high levels of procoagulant proteins. *J. Lab. Clin. Med.* **2001**, *138*, 393–402. [CrossRef]
19. Alberio, L.; Dale, G.L. Platelet-collagen interactions: Membrane receptors and intracellular signalling pathways. *Eur. J. Clin. Investig.* **1999**, *29*, 1066–1076. [CrossRef]
20. Celi, A.; Pellegrini, G.; Lorenzet, R.; De Blasi, A.; Ready, N.; Furie, B.C. P-selectin induces the expression of tissue factor on monocytes. *Proc. Natl. Acad. Sci. USA* **1994**, *91*, 8767–8771. [CrossRef]
21. Visentin, G.P.; Ford, S.E.; Scott, J.P.; Aster, R.H. Antibodies from patients with heparin-induced thrombocytopenia/thrombosis are specific for platelet factor 4 complexed with heparin or bound to endothelial cells. *J. Clin. Investig.* **1994**, *93*, 81–88. [CrossRef]
22. Blank, M.; Shoenfeld, Y.; Tavor, S.; Praprotnik, S.; Boffa, M.C.; Weksler, B.; Walenga, M.J.; Amiral, J.; Eldor, A. Anti-platelet factor 4/heparin antibodies from patients with heparin-induced thrombocytopenia provoke direct activation of microvascular endothelial cells. *Int. Immunol.* **2002**, *14*, 121–129. [CrossRef]
23. Hayes, V.; Johnston, I.; Arepally, G.M.; McKenzie, S.E.; Cines, D.B.; Rauova, L.; Poncz, M. Endothelial antigen assembly leads to thrombotic complications in heparin-induced thrombocytopenia. *J. Clin. Investig.* **2017**, *127*, 1090–1098. [CrossRef]
24. Hong, A.P.; Cook, D.J.; Sigouin, C.S.; Warkentin, T.E. Central venous catheters and upper-extremity deep-vein thrombosis complicating immune heparin-induced thrombocytopenia. *Blood* **2003**, *101*, 3049–3051. [CrossRef] [PubMed]
25. Davidson, S.J.; Wadham, P.; Rogers, L.; Burman, J.F. Endothelial cell damage in heparin-induced thrombocytopenia. *Blood Coagul. Fibrinolysis* **2007**, *18*, 317–320. [CrossRef]
26. Johnston, I.H.; Sarkar, A.; Hayes, V.M.; Koma, G.T.; Arepally, G.M.; Chen, J.; Chung, D.W.; López, J.A.; Cines, D.B.; Rauova, L.; et al. Recognition of PF4-VWF complexes by heparin-induced thrombocytopenia antibodies contributes to thrombus propagation. *Blood* **2020**, *135*, 1270–1280. [CrossRef] [PubMed]
27. Perdomo, J.; Leung, H.H.L.; Ahmadi, Z.; Yan, F.; Chong, J.J.H.; Passam, F.H.; Chong, B.H. Neutrophil activation and NETosis are the major drivers of thrombosis in heparin-induced thrombocytopenia. *Nat. Commun.* **2019**, *10*, 1322. [CrossRef] [PubMed]
28. Xiao, Z.; Visentin, G.P.; Dayananda, K.M.; Neelamegham, S. Immune complexes formed following the binding of anti–platelet factor 4 (CXCL4) antibodies to CXCL4 stimulate human neutrophil activation and cell adhesion. *Blood* **2008**, *112*, 1091–1100. [CrossRef] [PubMed]
29. Gollomp, K.; Kim, M.; Johnston, I.; Hayes, V.; Welsh, J.; Arepally, G.M.; Kahn, M.; Lambert, M.P.; Cuker, A.; Cines, D.B.; et al. Neutrophil accumulation and NET release contribute to thrombosis in HIT. *JCI Insight* **2018**, *3*. [CrossRef]
30. Gruel, Y.; Pouplard, C.; Lasne, D.; Magdelaine-Beuzelin, C.; Charroing, C.; Watier, H. The homozygous FcγRIIIa-158V genotype is a risk factor for heparin-induced thrombocytopenia in patients with antibodies to heparin-platelet factor 4 complexes. *Blood* **2004**, *104*, 2791–2793. [CrossRef]
31. Gruel, Y.; Vayne, C.; Rollin, J.; Weber, P.; Faille, D.; Bauters, A.; Macchi, L.; Alhenc-Gelas, M.; Lebreton, A.; De Maistre, E.; et al. Comparative Analysis of a French Prospective Series of 144 Patients with Heparin-Induced Thrombocytopenia (FRIGTIH) and the Literature. *Thromb. Haemost.* **2020**, *120*, 1096–1107. [CrossRef] [PubMed]
32. Rollin, J.; Pouplard, C.; Sung, H.C.; Leroux, D.; Saada, A.; Gouilleux-Gruart, V.; Thibault, G.; Gruel, Y. Increased risk of thrombosis in FcγRIIA 131RR patients with HIT due to defective control of platelet activation by plasma IgG2. *Blood* **2015**, *125*, 2397–2404. [CrossRef] [PubMed]

33. Pouplard, C.; May, M.-A.; Iochmann, S.; Amiral, J.; Vissac, A.-M.; Marchand, M.; Gruel, Y. Antibodies to Platelet Factor 4–Heparin After Cardiopulmonary Bypass in Patients Anticoagulated With Unfractionated Heparin or a Low-Molecular-Weight Heparin. *Circulation* **1999**, *99*, 2530–2536. [CrossRef]
34. Warkentin, T.E.; Basciano, P.A.; Knopman, J.; Bernstein, R.A. Spontaneous heparin-induced thrombocytopenia syndrome: 2 new cases and a proposal for defining this disorder. *Blood* **2014**, *123*, 3651–3654. [CrossRef] [PubMed]
35. Poudel, D.R.; Ghimire, S.; Dhital, R.; Forman, D.A.; Warkentin, T.E. Spontaneous HIT syndrome post-knee replacement surgery with delayed recovery of thrombocytopenia: A case report and literature review. *Platelets* **2017**, *28*, 614–620. [CrossRef] [PubMed]
36. Jay, R.M.; Warkentin, T.E. Fatal heparin-induced thrombocytopenia (HIT) during warfarin thromboprophylaxis following orthopedic surgery: Another example of 'spontaneous' HIT? *J. Thromb. Haemost.* **2008**, *6*, 1598–1600. [CrossRef] [PubMed]
37. Warkentin, T.E.; Makris, M.; Jay, R.M.; Kelton, J.G. A Spontaneous Prothrombotic Disorder Resembling Heparin-induced Thrombocytopenia. *Am. J. Med.* **2008**, *121*, 632–636. [CrossRef]
38. Pruthi, R.K.; Daniels, P.; Nambudiri, G.; Warkentin, T.E. Heparin-induced thrombocytopenia (HIT) during postoperative warfarin thromboprophylaxis: A second example of postorthopedic surgery 'spontaneous' HIT. *J. Thromb. Haemost.* **2009**, *7*, 499–501. [CrossRef]
39. Padmanabhan, A.; Jones, C.G.; Bougie, D.W.; Curtis, B.R.; McFarland, J.G.; Wang, D.; Aster, R.H. Heparin-independent, PF4-dependent binding of HIT antibodies to platelets: Implications for HIT pathogenesis. *Blood* **2015**, *125*, 155–161. [CrossRef]
40. Greinacher, A.; Warkentin, T.E. Contaminated Heparin. *N. Engl. J. Med.* **2008**, *359*, 1291–1293. [CrossRef]
41. Brandt, S.; Krauel, K.; Jaax, M.; Renné, T.; Helm, C.A.; Hammerschmidt, S.; Delcea, M.; Greinacher, A. Polyphosphates form antigenic complexes with platelet factor 4 (PF4) and enhance PF4-binding to bacteria. *Thromb. Haemost.* **2015**, *114*, 1189–1198. [CrossRef]
42. Jaax, M.E.; Krauel, K.; Marschall, T.; Brandt, S.; Gansler, J.; Fürll, B.; Appel, B.; Fischer, S.; Block, S.; Helm, C.A.; et al. Complex formation with nucleic acids and aptamers alters the antigenic properties of platelet factor 4. *Blood* **2013**, *122*, 272–281. [CrossRef] [PubMed]
43. Krauel, K.; Pötschke, C.; Weber, C.; Kessler, W.; Fürll, B.; Ittermann, T.; Maier, S.; Hammerschmidt, S.; Bröker, B.M.; Greinacher, A. Platelet factor 4 binds to bacteria, inducing antibodies cross-reacting with the major antigen in heparin-induced thrombocytopenia. *Blood* **2011**, *117*, 1370–1378. [CrossRef] [PubMed]
44. Greinacher, A.; Selleng, K.; Warkentin, T.E. Autoimmune heparin-induced thrombocytopenia. *J. Thromb. Haemost.* **2017**, *15*, 2099–2114. [CrossRef]
45. Cuker, A.; Cines, D.B. Diagnosing HIT: The need for speed. *Blood* **2020**, *135*, 1082–1083. [CrossRef]
46. Arepally, G.M. Heparin-induced thrombocytopenia. *Blood* **2017**, *129*, 2864–2872. [CrossRef] [PubMed]
47. Lo, G.K.; Juhl, D.; Warkentin, T.E.; Sigouin, C.S.; Eichler, P.; Greinacher, A. Evaluation of pretest clinical score (4 T's) for the diagnosis of heparin-induced thrombocytopenia in two clinical settings. *J. Thromb. Haemost.* **2006**, *4*, 759–765. [CrossRef]
48. Cuker, A.; Arepally, G.M.; Chong, B.H.; Cines, D.B.; Greinacher, A.; Gruel, Y.; Linkins, L.-A.; Rodner, S.B.; Selleng, S.; Warkentin, T.E.; et al. American Society of Hematology 2018 guidelines for management of venous thromboembolism: Heparin-induced thrombocytopenia. *Blood Adv.* **2018**, *2*, 3360–3392. [CrossRef]
49. Cuker, A.; Arepally, G.; Crowther, M.A.; Rice, L.; Datko, F.; Hook, K.; Propert, K.J.; Kuter, D.J.; Ortel, T.L.; Konkle, B.A.; et al. The HIT Expert Probability (HEP) Score: A novel pre-test probability model for heparin-induced thrombocytopenia based on broad expert opinion. *J. Thromb. Haemost.* **2010**, *8*, 2642–2650. [CrossRef]
50. Pishko, A.M.; Fardin, S.; Lefler, D.S.; Paydary, K.; Vega, R.; Arepally, G.M.; Crowther, M.A.; Rice, L.; Cines, D.B.; Cuker, A. Prospective comparison of the HEP score and 4Ts score for the diagnosis of heparin-induced thrombocytopenia. *Blood Adv.* **2018**, *2*, 3155–3162. [CrossRef]
51. Nellen, V.; Sulzer, I.; Barizzi, G.; Lämmle, B.; Alberio, L. Rapid exclusion or confirmation of heparin-induced thrombocytopenia: A single-center experience with 1,291 patients. *Haematologia* **2012**, *97*, 89–97. [CrossRef]
52. Marchetti, M.; Barelli, S.; Zermatten, M.G.; Monnin-Respen, F.; Matthey-Guirao, E.; Nicolas, N.; Gomez, F.; Goodyer, M.; Gerschheimer, C.; Alberio, L. Rapid and Accurate Bayesian Diagnosis of Heparin-induced thrombocytopenia. *Blood* **2020**, *135*, 1171–1184. [CrossRef]
53. Warkentin, T.E.; Sheppard, J.-A.I.; Linkins, L.-A.; Arnold, D.M.; Nazy, I. High sensitivity and specificity of an automated IgG-specific chemiluminescence immunoassay for diagnosis of HIT. *Blood* **2018**, *132*, 1345–1349. [CrossRef]
54. Linkins, L.-A.; Bates, S.M.; Lee, A.Y.Y.; Heddle, N.M.; Wang, G.; Warkentin, T.E. Combination of 4Ts score and PF4/H-PaGIA for diagnosis and management of heparin-induced thrombocytopenia: Prospective cohort study. *Blood* **2015**, *126*, 597–603. [CrossRef]
55. Greinacher, A. Heparin-Induced Thrombocytopenia. *N. Engl. J. Med.* **2015**, *373*, 252–261. [CrossRef]
56. Eekels, J.J.M.; Pachler, C.; Krause, N.; Muhr, T.; Waltl, G.; Greinacher, A. Ticagrelor causes false-negative functional tests for heparin-induced thrombocytopenia. *Blood* **2020**, *135*, 875–878. [CrossRef]
57. Warkentin, T.E.; Nazy, I.; Sheppard, J.I.; Smith, J.W.; Kelton, J.G.; Arnold, D.M. Serotonin-release assay-negative heparin-induced thrombocytopenia. *Am. J. Hematol.* **2020**, *95*, 38–47. [CrossRef]
58. Warkentin, T.E. Challenges in Detecting Clinically Relevant Heparin-Induced Thrombocytopenia Antibodies. *Hämostaseologie* **2020**, *40*, 472–484. [CrossRef]
59. Rubino, J.G.; Arnold, D.M.; Warkentin, T.E.; Smith, J.W.; Kelton, J.G.; Nazy, I. A Comparative Study of Platelet Factor 4-Enhanced Platelet Activation Assays for the Diagnosis of Heparin-Induced Thrombocytopenia. *J. Thromb. Haemost.* **2021**. [CrossRef]

60. Vayne, C.; Guery, E.-A.; Kizlik-Masson, C.; Rollin, J.; Bauters, A.; Gruel, Y.; Pouplard, C. Beneficial effect of exogenous platelet factor 4 for detecting pathogenic heparin-induced thrombocytopenia antibodies. *Br. J. Haematol.* **2017**, *179*, 811–819. [CrossRef]
61. Padmanabhan, A.; Jones, C.G.; Curtis, B.R.; Bougie, D.W.; Sullivan, M.J.; Peswani, N.; McFarland, J.G.; Eastwood, D.; Wang, D.; Aster, R.H. A Novel PF4-Dependent Platelet Activation Assay Identifies Patients Likely to Have Heparin-Induced Thrombocytopenia/Thrombosis. *Chest* **2016**, *150*, 506–515. [CrossRef]
62. Tardy-Poncet, B.; Lecompte, T.; Mullier, F.; Vayne, C.; Pouplard, C. Detection of Platelet-Activating Antibodies Associated with Heparin-Induced Thrombocytopenia. *J. Clin. Med.* **2020**, *9*, 1226. [CrossRef]
63. Warkentin, T.E.; Greinacher, A.; Gruel, Y.; Aster, R.H.; Chong, B.H. On behalf of the scientific and standardization committee of the international society on thrombosis and haemostasis Laboratory testing for heparin-induced thrombocytopenia: A conceptual framework and implications for diagnosis. *J. Thromb. Haemost.* **2011**, *9*, 2498–2500. [CrossRef]
64. Nagler, M.; Bachmann, L.M.; Cate, H.T.; Cate-Hoek, A.T. Diagnostic value of immunoassays for heparin-induced thrombocytopenia: A systematic review and meta-analysis. *Blood* **2016**, *127*, 546–557. [CrossRef]
65. Sun, L.; Gimotty, P.A.; Lakshmanan, S.; Cuker, A. Diagnostic accuracy of rapid immunoassays for heparin-induced thrombocytopenia. *Thromb. Haemost.* **2016**, *115*, 1044–1055. [CrossRef]
66. Pouplard, C.; Gueret, P.; Fouassier, M.; Ternisien, C.; Trossaert, M.; Régina, S.; Gruel, Y. Prospective evaluation of the ?4Ts? score and particle gel immunoassay specific to heparin/PF4 for the diagnosis of heparin-induced thrombocytopenia. *J. Thromb. Haemost.* **2007**, *5*, 1373–1379. [CrossRef]
67. Warkentin, T.E. Scoring systems for heparin-induced thrombocytopenia (HIT): Whither now? *Thromb. Haemost.* **2015**, *113*, 437–438. [CrossRef]
68. Raschke, R.A.; Gallo, T.; Curry, S.C.; Whiting, T.; Padilla-Jones, A.; Warkentin, T.E.; Puri, A. Clinical effectiveness of a Bayesian algorithm for the diagnosis and management of heparin-induced thrombocytopenia. *J. Thromb. Haemost.* **2017**, *15*, 1640–1645. [CrossRef]
69. Warkentin, T.E.; Sheppard, J.-A.I.; Smith, J.W.; Li, N.; Moore, J.C.; Arnold, D.M.; Nazy, I.; Na, L. Combination of two complementary automated rapid assays for diagnosis of heparin-induced thrombocytopenia (HIT). *J. Thromb. Haemost.* **2020**, *18*, 1435–1446. [CrossRef]
70. Alberio, L.; Angelillo-Scherrer, A.; Asmis, L.; Casini, A.; Fontana, P.; Graf, L.; Hegemann, I.; Hovinga, J.A.K.; Korte, W.; Lecompte, T.; et al. Recommendations on the use of anticoagulants for the treatment of patients with heparin-induced thrombocytopenia in Switzerland. *Swiss Med. Wkly.* **2020**, *150*, w20210. [CrossRef]
71. Welsby, I.J.; Um, J.; Milano, C.A.; Ortel, T.L.; Arepally, G. Plasmapheresis and Heparin Reexposure as a Management Strategy for Cardiac Surgical Patients with Heparin-Induced Thrombocytopenia. *Anesthesia Analg.* **2010**, *110*, 30–35. [CrossRef] [PubMed]
72. Onuoha, C.; Barton, K.D.; Wong, E.C.; Raval, J.S.; Rollins-Raval, M.A.; Ipe, T.S.; Kiss, J.E.; Boral, L.I.; Adamksi, J.; Zantek, N.D.; et al. Therapeutic plasma exchange and intravenous immune globulin in the treatment of heparin-induced thrombocytopenia: A systematic review. *Transfusion* **2020**, *60*, 2714–2736. [CrossRef]
73. Iluonakhamhe, E.; Ibekwe, O.; Samuel, S.; Zakaria, A. Plasmapheresis May Be an Option in Urgent Management of Heparin-Induced Thrombocytopenia in the Setting of Acute Intracerebral Hemorrhage. *Neurocrit. Care* **2015**, *22*, 140–145. [CrossRef]
74. Warkentin, T.E. High-dose intravenous immunoglobulin for the treatment and prevention of heparin-induced thrombocytopenia: A review. *Expert Rev. Hematol.* **2019**, *12*, 685–698. [CrossRef] [PubMed]
75. Cada, D.J.; Baker, D.E.; Ingram, K.T. Cangrelor. *Hosp. Pharm.* **2015**, *50*, 922–929. [CrossRef]
76. Scala, E.; Pitta-Gros, B.; Pantet, O.; Iafrate, M.; Kirsch, M.; Marcucci, C.; Alberio, L. Cardiac Surgery Successfully Managed With Cangrelor in a Patient With Persistent Anti-PF4/Heparin Antibodies 8 Years After Heparin-Induced Thrombocytopenia. *J. Cardiothorac. Vasc. Anesth.* **2019**, *33*, 3073–3077. [CrossRef] [PubMed]
77. Kizlik-Masson, C.; Deveuve, Q.; Zhou, Y.; Vayne, C.; Thibault, G.; McKenzie, S.E.; Pouplard, C.; Loyau, S.; Gruel, Y.; Rollin, J. Cleavage of anti-PF4/heparin IgG by a bacterial protease and potential benefit in heparin-induced thrombocytopenia. *Blood* **2019**, *133*, 2427–2435. [CrossRef]
78. Jordan, S.C.; Lorant, T.; Choi, J.; Kjellman, C.; Winstedt, L.; Bengtsson, M.; Zhang, X.; Eich, T.; Toyoda, M.; Eriksson, B.-M.; et al. IgG Endopeptidase in Highly Sensitized Patients Undergoing Transplantation. *N. Engl. J. Med.* **2017**, *377*, 442–453. [CrossRef]
79. Tun, N.M.; Bo, Z.M.; Ahluwalia, M.; Guevara, E.; Villani, G.M. A rare case of intracerebral hemorrhage complicating heparin-induced thrombocytopenia with thrombosis: A clinical dilemma ameliorated by novel use of plasmapheresis. *Int. J. Hematol.* **2012**, *96*, 513–515. [CrossRef]
80. Aryal, M.R.; Gosain, R.; Donato, A.; Katel, A.; Chakradhar, R.; Dhital, R.; Kouides, P.A. Effectiveness of intravenous immunoglobulin use in heparin-induced thrombocytopenia. *Blood Coagul. Fibrinolysis* **2020**, *31*, 287–292. [CrossRef]
81. Mazzeffi, M.A.; Patel, P.A.; Bolliger, D.; Erdoes, G.; Tanaka, K. The Year in Coagulation: Selected Highlights from 2019. *J. Cardiothorac. Vasc. Anesth.* **2020**, *34*, 1745–1754. [CrossRef] [PubMed]
82. Scala, E.; Gerschheimer, C.; Gomez, F.J.; Alberio, L.; Marcucci, C. Potential and Limitations of the New P2Y12 Inhibitor, Cangrelor, in Preventing Heparin-Induced Platelet Aggregation During Cardiac Surgery: An In Vitro Study. *Anesth. Analg.* **2020**, *131*, 622–630. [CrossRef] [PubMed]
83. Miller, J.L.; Parilla, M.; Treml, A.; Wool, G. Plasma exchange for heparin-induced thrombocytopenia in patients on extracorporeal circuits: A challenging case and a survey of the field. *J. Clin. Apher.* **2019**, *34*, 64–72. [CrossRef]

84. Warkentin, T.E.; Sheppard, J.-A.I.; Chu, F.V.; Kapoor, A.; Crowther, M.A.; Gangji, A. Plasma exchange to remove HIT antibodies: Dissociation between enzyme-immunoassay and platelet activation test reactivities. *Blood* **2015**, *125*, 195–198. [CrossRef]
85. Anderson, D.R.; Ali, K.; Blanchette, V.; Brouwers, M.; Couban, S.; Radmoor, P.; Huebsch, L.; Hume, H.; McLeod, A.; Meyer, R.; et al. Guidelines on the Use of Intravenous Immune Globulin for Hematologic Conditions. *Transfus. Med. Rev.* **2007**, *21*, S9–S56. [CrossRef] [PubMed]
86. Dhakal, B.; Rein, L.; Szabo, A.; Padmanabhan, A. Use of IV Immunoglobulin G in Heparin-Induced Thrombocytopenia Patients Is Not Associated With Increased Rates of Thrombosis. *Chest* **2020**, *158*, 1172–1175. [CrossRef] [PubMed]
87. Padmanabhan, A.; Jones, C.G.; Pechauer, S.M.; Curtis, B.R.; Bougie, D.W.; Irani, M.S.; Bryant, B.J.; Alperin, J.B.; Deloughery, T.G.; Mulvey, K.P.; et al. IVIg for Treatment of Severe Refractory Heparin-Induced Thrombocytopenia. *Chest* **2017**, *152*, 478–485. [CrossRef]
88. Warkentin, T.E.; Climans, T.H.; Morin, P.-A. Intravenous Immune Globulin to Prevent Heparin-Induced Thrombocytopenia. *N. Engl. J. Med.* **2018**, *378*, 1845–1848. [CrossRef]
89. Kizlik-Masson, C.; Vayne, C.; McKenzie, S.E.; Poupon, A.; Zhou, Y.; Champier, G.; Pouplard, C.; Gruel, Y.; Rollin, J. 5B9, a monoclonal antiplatelet factor 4/heparin IgG with a human Fc fragment that mimics heparin-induced thrombocytopenia antibodies. *J. Thromb. Haemost.* **2017**, *15*, 2065–2075. [CrossRef]
90. Selleng, S.; Haneya, A.; Hirt, S.; Selleng, K.; Schmid, C.; Greinacher, A. Management of anticoagulation in patients with subacute heparin-induced thrombocytopenia scheduled for heart transplantation. *Blood* **2008**, *112*, 4024–4027. [CrossRef] [PubMed]
91. Warkentin, T.E.; Anderson, J.A.M. How I treat patients with a history of heparin-induced thrombocytopenia. *Blood* **2016**, *128*, 348–359. [CrossRef]
92. Pötzsch, B.; Klövekorn, W.-P.; Madlener, K. Use of Heparin during Cardiopulmonary Bypass in Patients with a History of Heparin-Induced Thrombocytopenia. *N. Engl. J. Med.* **2000**, *343*, 515. [CrossRef]
93. Koster, A.; Erdoes, G.; Nagler, M.; Birschmann, I.; Alberio, L. How Would Our Own Heparin-Induced Thrombocytopenia Be Treated During Cardiac Surgery? *J. Cardiothorac. Vasc. Anesth.* **2020**. [CrossRef] [PubMed]
94. Koster, A.; Meyer, O.; Fischer, T.; Kukucka, M.; Krabatsch, T.; Bauer, M.; Kuppe, H.; Hetzer, R. One-year experience with the platelet glycoprotein IIb/IIIa antagonist tirofiban and heparin during cardiopulmonary bypass in patients with heparin-induced thrombocytopenia type II. *J. Thorac. Cardiovasc. Surg.* **2001**, *122*, 1254–1255. [CrossRef] [PubMed]
95. Palatianos, G.; Michalis, A.; Alivizatos, P.; Lacoumenda, S.; Geroulanos, S.; Karabinis, A.; Iliopoulou, E.; Soufla, G.; Kanthou, C.; Khoury, M.; et al. Perioperative use of iloprost in cardiac surgery patients diagnosed with heparin-induced thrombocytopenia-reactive antibodies or with true HIT (HIT-reactive antibodies plus thrombocytopenia): An 11-year experience. *Am. J. Hematol.* **2015**, *90*, 608–617. [CrossRef]
96. Gernhofer, Y.K.; Ross, M.; Khoche, S.; Pretorius, V. The use of cangrelor with heparin for left ventricular assist device implantation in a patient with acute heparin-induced thrombocytopenia. *J. Cardiothorac. Surg.* **2018**, *13*, 30. [CrossRef] [PubMed]
97. Gruel, Y.; De Maistre, E.; Pouplard, C.; Mullier, F.; Susen, S.; Roullet, S.; Blais, N.; Le Gal, G.; Vincentelli, A.; Lasne, D.; et al. Diagnosis and management of heparin-induced thrombocytopenia. *Anaesth. Crit. Care Pain Med.* **2020**, *39*, 291–310. [CrossRef]
98. Warkentin, T.E.; Sheppard, J.-A.I. Serological investigation of patients with a previous history of heparin-induced thrombocytopenia who are reexposed to heparin. *Blood* **2014**, *123*, 2485–2493. [CrossRef]

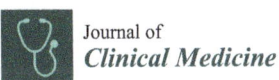

Review

Primary Immune Thrombocytopenia: Novel Insights into Pathophysiology and Disease Management

Anurag Singh [1,†], Günalp Uzun [2,†] and Tamam Bakchoul [1,2,*]

1. Institute for Clinical and Experimental Transfusion Medicine (IKET), University Hospital of Tuebingen, 72076 Tuebingen, Germany; anurag.singh@med.uni-tuebingen.de
2. Centre for Clinical Transfusion Medicine, University Hospital of Tuebingen, 72076 Tuebingen, Germany; guenalp.uzun@med.uni-tuebingen.de
* Correspondence: tamam.bakchoul@med.uni-tuebingen.de; Tel.: +49-7071-29-81601
† These authors contributed equally to this work.

Abstract: Immune thrombocytopenia (ITP) is an autoimmune disorder defined by a significantly reduced number of platelets in blood circulation. Due to low levels of platelets, ITP is associated with frequent bruising and bleeding. Current evidence suggests that low platelet counts in ITP are the result of multiple factors, including impaired thrombopoiesis and variations in immune response leading to platelet destruction during pathological conditions. Patient outcomes as well as clinic presentation of the disease have largely been shown to be case-specific, hinting towards ITP rather being a group of clinical conditions sharing common symptoms. The most frequent characteristics include dysfunction in primary haemostasis and loss of immune tolerance towards platelet as well as megakaryocyte antigens. This heterogeneity in patient population and characteristics make it challenging for the clinicians to choose appropriate therapeutic regimen. Therefore, it is vital to understand the pathomechanisms behind the disease and to consider various factors including patient age, platelet count levels, co-morbidities and patient preferences before initiating therapy. This review summarizes recent developments in the pathophysiology of ITP and provides a comprehensive overview of current therapeutic strategies as well as potential future drugs for the management of ITP.

Keywords: immune thrombocytopenia; bleeding; platelets; platelet destruction; immune tolerance; megakaryocytes; ITP treatment

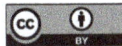

1. Introduction

Primary immune thrombocytopenia (ITP) is a haematological autoimmune disorder characterised by bleeding and a low platelet count of less than 100×10^9/L [1–4]. There are several factors contributing to the onset of ITP, and the exact mechanisms behind how host immune response turns against own system (autoimmunity) and leads to ITP are still incompletely understood. There is growing evidence suggesting that the main event during ITP is a misbalanced interaction between effectors and regulatory immune cells [5]. This lack of an equitable response leads to a distorted immune tolerance, resulting in increased platelet clearance by immune cells, as well as an impairment in thrombopoiesis. Earlier studies suggested that a low platelet count is largely a consequence of anti-platelet antibodies opsonizing the cells and hence an increased clearance from the circulation [6–8]. However, lately, it has been demonstrated by many researchers that cytotoxic T cells also play a vital role in ITP pathomechanism by impairing megakaryopoiesis.

During ITP, it has been observed that although brief, spontaneous remissions can occur frequently in children. On the other hand, adult patients rather display a more chronic form of ITP that correlates with significant clinical presentations including bleeding disorders, haemorrhages in skin or mucous membranes, namely purpura, petechiae and rarely intracranial manifestations of the disease [9,10]. Treatment strategies for ITP are mostly prescribed on the basis of clinical symptoms of the patients with a focus on reducing the risk of severe bleeding, and they do not essentially include the boosting of platelet numbers. As per the guidelines of International Working Group [2,11], patients with acute ITP and without a history suggesting severe bleeding risk are advised to be managed with observation strategy (wait and see). On the other hand, ITP patients require urgent treatment if they are prone to a higher risk of bleeding or carry a severe case of chronic thrombocytopenia.

In this review, we discuss the pathomechanisms that lead to platelet destruction in ITP with a particular focus on recent findings regarding various diversifications during thrombopoiesis. Furthermore, we will provide a broad overview regarding various management strategies of ITP patients. We also outline different treatment options including efficacy and safety of therapeutic medicaments, management of bleeding emergencies as well as a summary of different approved drugs as well as drugs under clinical trials for ITP treatment.

2. Pathophysiology of ITP

One of the crucial steps during pathophysiology of ITP is described as the loss of immunological tolerance to autoantigens on patient's own platelets [12]. Many studies demonstrate that during ITP, a dysregulated T-cell response leads to a distorted balance of helper T cells (Th1/Th2) ratio [13,14], and imbalance further leads to an enhanced number as well as hyperactivity of cytotoxic T cells. Subsequently, this enhanced activity of cytotoxic T cells results in an increase in platelet destruction, combined with improved survival of B cells. An enhanced survival rate of B cells hence facilitates a larger production of autoantibodies, leading to an accelerated rate of platelet clearance. Autoantibodies opsonize platelets leading to enhanced phagocytosis, apoptosis, complement activation and impaired thrombopoiesis [15–17] (Figure 1).

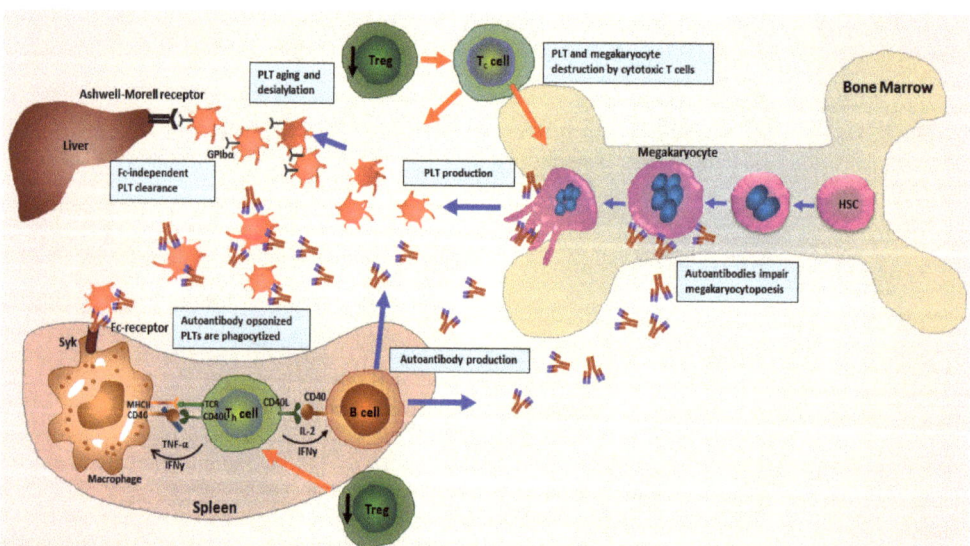

Figure 1. Graphical representation of the pathophysiology of immune thrombocytopenia (ITP) illustrating involvement of multiple immune cells. Impairment of regulatory T cells leads to a disruption in regulation of helper T cell-mediated activation of B cells. B cells in turn produce autoantibodies in abundance leading to opsonisation, phagocytosis and complement activation, desialylation and finally destruction of platelets. Autoantibodies further hinder megakaryocyte maturation (megakaryocytopoiesis), and autoreactive cytotoxic T cells destroy megakaryocytes and platelets. (Adapted from Kashiwagi et al. 2013 [18]).

Although platelet destruction in the spleen primarily involves constant fragment (Fc)-dependent mechanisms, various researchers have also described novel mechanisms independent of Fc-mediation [19–21]. In a study, it was shown that ITP-autoantibodies can induce glycan modifications on platelet surface glycoproteins (GPs). Upon further recognition by Ashwell–Morell receptors which are expressed on hepatocytes, this GPs modification leads to accelerated platelet clearance in the liver [22]. CD8+ T cells from ITP patients also induce platelet desialylation and platelet phagocytosis by hepatocytes [23]. This might explain a potential mechanism how splenectomy remains ineffective in some ITP patients. In an intriguing retrospective study with a cohort of 61 ITP patients, it was shown that platelet desialylation and subsequent reduction in response to first line of treatments was independent of any Fc-mediated mechanism [24].

A recent study by Quach and colleagues demonstrated that ITP patients who did not respond to therapy were more likely to produce autoantibodies against the ligand binding domain (LBD) of GPIb/IX [25]. This specific binding leads to activation of GPIb/IX via crosslinking of platelet receptors and unfolding of a mechanosensory domain and platelet destruction, providing further a pivotal evidence of Fc-independent mechanism [25]. Recently, we demonstrated that novel effector functions of autoantibodies in ITP modulate the disease and might interfere with the clinical outcome for patients. We showed that a subgroup of autoantibodies induces cleavage of sialic acid residues from the surface of human platelets and megakaryocytes during ITP. Furthermore, autoantibody-mediated desialylation was found to interfere with the cell–extracellular matrix protein interaction and hence leading to impaired platelet adhesion and megakaryocyte differentiation [26]. This hints towards a potential use of sialidase inhibitors as a treatment approach in combination with other therapies to boost platelet numbers in some patients who have failed to respond to previous therapies.

It is well established that intrinsic apoptotic pathway plays a significant role in platelet life cycle. Many research groups have demonstrated the role of ITP-autoantibodies in regulating platelet apoptosis and pathways involved. There is ample evidence showing that various apoptosis markers including phosphatidylserine (PS) exposure, depolarisation of the mitochondrial transmembrane potential, Bcl-2 family protein expression, activation of caspase-3 as well as of caspase-9 are significantly involved in platelet apoptosis in ITP [27,28]. Immunoglobin infusion was shown to successfully mitigate platelet apoptosis in adult as well as paediatric patients [29,30]. Interestingly, it was shown that apoptotic platelets were not found in ITP patients harbouring anti-GPIa/IIa autoantibodies but only in those who carried anti-GPIIb/IIIa and anti-GPIb autoantibodies [31], indicating a potential role of autoantibody specificity.

Autoantibodies produced during ITP not only affect platelet survival but also platelet formation by megakaryocytes [32]. It has been shown that autoantibodies bind and hinder the megakaryocyte maturation, resulting in reduced platelet formation [33,34]. It was demonstrated in vitro, that autoantibodies inhibit platelet production by impairing megakaryopoiesis and maturation [35–37]. However, the role of megakaryocyte apoptosis still needs to be investigated in terms of involvement in the pathophysiology of ITP. There have been some hints and contradicting claims through results generated via earlier and recent investigations. A study in fact demonstrated that treatment with ITP plasma rather leads to a reduced apoptosis of megakaryocytes [38]. Haematopoietic stem cells (HSCs) isolated from healthy umbilical cord blood were co-cultured with plasma of ITP patients, resulting into a decrease in apoptosis, reduced expression of tumour necrosis factor-related apoptosis inducing ligand (TRAIL) and increased expression of the anti-apoptotic protein Bcl-xL in differentiated megakaryocytes [39]. On the other hand, in contrast to these findings, an earlier in vivo study suggested that megakaryocytes in fact undergo enhanced apoptosis in the presence of autoantibodies [40]. It was observed in biopsies of ITP patients that increased apoptosis involves nuclear fragmentation, chromatin condensation and activation of caspase 3. This further leads to phagocytosis of the polyploid cells by resident macrophages in the bone marrow [40]. Another recent study showed that an increased megakaryocyte apoptosis occurs in the bone marrow samples obtained from ITP patients [41].

3. Clinical Manifestations

The overall annual incidence rate of ITP is 1.6–5.3 per 100,000 persons, and it is more frequent in women than men [42–44]. ITP can be classified according to disease duration as acute (<3 months), persistent (3 to 12 months) or chronic (>12 months). Compared to children, adults are more likely to develop chronic ITP disease. While up to 60% of adults develop chronic diseases [45,46], only 20–30% of children have persistent thrombocytopenia at 12 months [47,48].

Most patients are presented with bleeding symptoms such as petechiae, purpura, haemorrhages of the mucous membranes of the mouth and nose, urogenital bleeding or increased menstrual bleeding [49]. Some patients can be asymptomatic at presentation and 30–40% of patients with chronic ITP do not have any bleeding symptom [50]. Bleeding risk is calculated as 8% per year in ITP patients [51].

Major bleedings are associated with a high rate of mortality [52,53]. Reported rates of severe bleeding vary depending on the population studied. In a recent literature review including 108 studies reporting on 10,908 patients, the weighted proportion for intracerebral haemorrhage (ICH) was 1.0% (95% CI, 0.7–1.3) and for non-ICH severe bleeding was 15.0% (95% CI, 9.3–21.8) [54]. Forsthye and colleagues reported a severe bleeding episode that required rescue medication (intravenous immunoglobulin, corticosteroid injections or platelet transfusions) in 10,2% of adult ITP patients within 6 months after starting therapy with thrombopoietin receptor agonists (TRO-RA) [55]. In a retrospective evaluation of the McMaster ITP registry, Arnold et al. found that 56% of ITP patients experience clinically significant bleeding at some point during their disease course and 2.2% had ICH [56].

Compared to ITP patients with normal platelet counts, those with a platelet count between 25 to 49 $\times 10^9$ /L and <25 $\times 10^9$ /L had 2.4 fold and 4.5 fold increased bleeding rates, respectively [51]. Furthermore, bleeding requiring a hospital contact within 1 year prior to ITP diagnosis was associated with a 3-fold increased rate of subsequent bleeding [51]. The use of non-steroidal anti-inflammatory drugs (NSAIDs) was found to be associated with any bleeding (OR 4.8, 95% CI 1.1–20.7) and anticoagulant drugs were associated with severe bleeding (OR 4.3, 95% CI 1.3–14.1) [57]. In a large patient cohort, Hato et. al. found that age (>60 years), platelet count (<10 $\times 10^9$ /L), and the presence of haematuria are associated with increased risk for ICH [58].

Fatigue is common in patients with ITP, and its impact on health-related quality of life in ITP patients has been until recently underappreciated [59]. Treatments that increase platelet count also reduce fatigue [60,61]. However, it is also recommended to use treatment strategies that directly target fatigue to improve the health-related quality of life in ITP patients [62].

Paradoxically, an increased frequency of thromboembolic events has been reported in ITP patients [63,64]. Therefore, it is crucial that ITP patients should be aware of the risk of thromboembolic events. Patients should be educated that ITP can increase not only the risk of bleeding but also the risk of venous and arterial thromboembolism [50]. Furthermore, patients at risk of embolic events should be followed more closely. Presence of lupus anticoagulants is related to thrombotic events [65]. The increased levels of prothrombotic, platelet-derived microparticles and complement activation on antibody-coated platelets also contribute to the development of thrombosis in ITP [66]. In addition to disease and patient related factors, ITP treatments such as TPO-RA and splenectomy could also increase the individual risk of thromboembolic events [64,67,68]. Clinical management of thrombocytopenic patients who require anticoagulant or antiplatelet therapy due to cardiovascular comorbidities is a serious challenge. An aggressive treatment of ITP may be required in these patients to achieve a safe platelet count over 50 $\times 10^9$L [50].

The overall mortality rate is slightly higher than general population in ITP patients, predominantly due to increased cardiovascular disease, infection, bleeding and haematological cancer related mortalities [69].

4. Diagnosis

ITP is usually diagnosed after precluding other potential causes of thrombocytopenia. A diagnosis is performed in patients with a low platelet count (<100 10^9/L) with no evidence or history of an underlying condition, which can lead to thrombocytopenia, including a physical examination, evaluation of blood counts and visual examination of blood smears. However, since thrombocytopenia may be a multifactorial condition, it is indeed complicated to identity substitute causes, and examining physician needs to have a broad knowledge in platelet disorders. A confirmation of ITP is achieved via detection of characteristic platelet-specific autoantibodies, free in patient serum or bound to own platelets [70]. As per recommendations of various regulatory guidelines, GP-specific assays, for example direct monoclonal antibody immobilisation of platelet antigens (MAIPA test) or direct immunobead assays prove the diagnosis of ITP, and further laboratory tests are deemed unnecessary [71]. However, current ASH-guidelines of 2019 do not give any clear recommendations for antibody evaluation in ITP patients, as there is still lack of strong evidence supporting clinical advantage of the assays [4]. We strongly recommended that as a part of initial assessment, presence of platelet autoantibodies should be evaluated. A positive test result at this stage establishes a sound basis for further diagnostic procedures and paves ways for initiating the treatment. It is notable to mention that although GP-specific tests have shown an excellent specificity, the lack of sensitivity is an important issue to consider. The low sensitivity of the test can often produce negative results, and care needs to be taken while interpretation and subsequent recommendation. Other potential hurdles in implementing antibody testing as a part of mandatory diagnostic regime for ITP also include unavailability of experienced staff, equipment and set up, as well as cost effectiveness.

Therefore, it is recommended to establish an appropriate diagnostic set up to analyse ITP during early phase of patient examination.

5. Treatment of ITP

The main goals of ITP treatment are to intervene in the case of an acute severe bleeding and to prevent future bleeding events (Figure 2).

5.1. First-Line Treatments and Treatment of Bleeding Emergencies

The decision to start a treatment in newly diagnosed ITP depends on several factors. Current guidelines recommend a platelet count of 20 to 30 × 10^3/μL as a cut-off value to start intervention in adult ITP patients [4]. Other than thrombocyte count, patient related factors can help to determine the risk of bleeding such as age (e.g., >65 years), previous bleeding events, comorbidities associated with high bleeding risk (i.e., hypertension, cerebrovascular disease), renal or hepatic impairment, medication with anticoagulants and platelet inhibitors, surgical interventions and risky life style (i.e., combat sports) [51,57,73]. A higher platelet count (>50,000 μL) should be considered for these patient populations.

As emphasized in the current guidelines, the decision regarding ITP treatment should be made in agreement between physician and patient. The patient should be informed about the benefits and possible side effects of treatment options. It should be considered that some side effects of treatments might pose a greater risk for the patient than ITP itself [74]. Advantages and disadvantages of ITP treatments are summarized in Table 1.

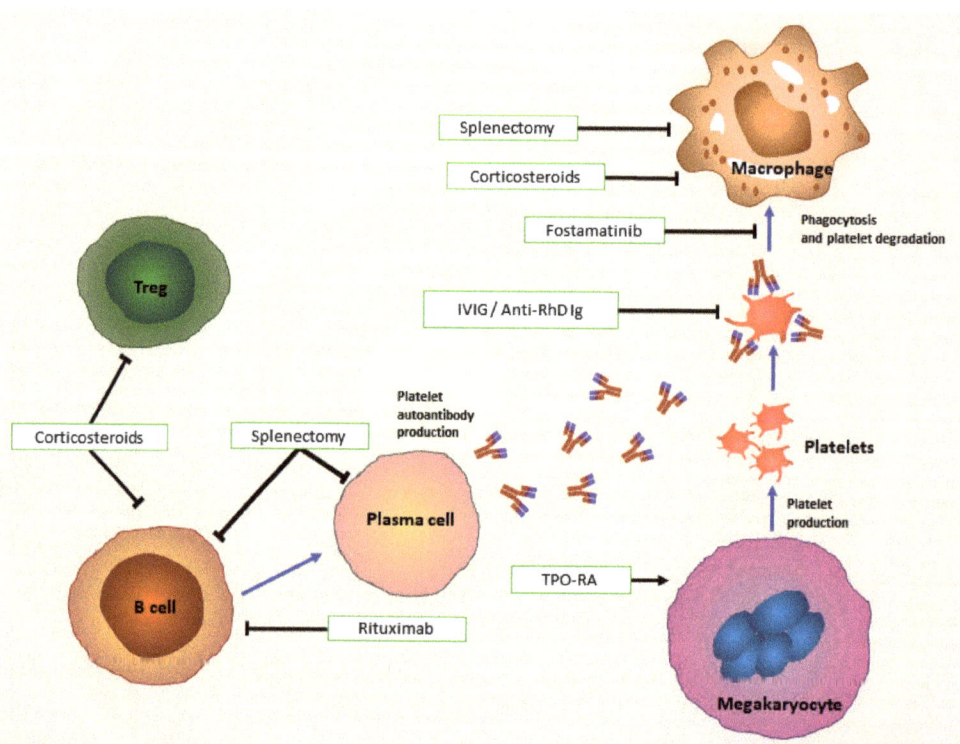

Figure 2. Treatments for immune thrombocytopenia: Corticosteroids used as first line of treatment modulate Treg, B-cell and FcR function. In combination with or without IVIg and anti-D, they impair antigen presentation and recognition of autoantibody-coated platelets by macrophages. Second-line treatments such as surgical splenectomy remove spleen as a site of platelet destruction, and drugs as rituximab target antibody-producing B cells. TPO-RAs, such as romiplostim and eltrombopag work by stimulating platelet production by megakaryocytes. Fostamatinib impairs Syk-mediated phagocytosis of platelets. FcR: Fc receptors; IVIg: Intravenous immunoglobulin; TPO-RA: Thrombopoietin receptor agonist; Syk: spleen tyrosine kinase. (Adapted from Newland et al. 2018 [72]).

Table 1. Treatment options for ITP.

Agent	Application Route and Dosage	Advantages	Disadvantages and Complications
First-line Therapies			
Glucocorticoids			
Predniso(lo)ne	Oral 1 mg/kg of body weight for 2–3 weeks (maximum 80 mg/d), gradual tapering	Response within 1–2 weeks Early response rate 60–80%	Low durable response rate after discontinuation (30–50%) Complications: hypertension, hyperglycaemia, sleep and mood disturbances, gastric ulceration, myopathy, glaucoma and osteoporosis
Dexamethasone	Oral 40 mg for 4 days Maximum 3 cycles		
Immunoglobulin	Intravenous 0.4–1 gr/kg of body weight, total maximal dose of 2 gr/kg of body weight	Response within 1–4 days Early response rate 70–80%	Only a transient rise of platelet count Complications: headache, pyrexia, vomiting, acute kidney injury, aseptic meningitis and thrombotic events
Anti-Rhesus D Ig	Intravenous 50 to 75 µg/kg	Early response rate 65%	Only effective in Rh-positive patients Not approved for ITP in Europe Complications: headache, nausea, chills, fever and mild to moderate haemolysis Severe intravascular haemolysis and disseminated intravascular coagulation

Table 1. Cont.

Agent	Application Route and Dosage	Advantages	Disadvantages and Complications
Second-line Therapies			
Thrombopoietin-receptor Agonists			
Romiplostim	Subcutaneous 1–10 microg/kg/week	Response rate 70–80% Remission rate 10–30%	Cost Headache, arthralgia, myalgia, dizziness and insomnia Thromboembolism and bone marrow fibrosis
Eltrombobag	Oral 25–75 mg/day	Response rate 70–80% Remission rate 10–30%	Cost Dietary restrictions Gastrointestinal symptoms (nausea, vomiting, diarrhoea), mild transaminase elevations and headache Thromboembolism and bone marrow fibrosis
Avatrombopag	Oral 20–40 mg/day	Response rate 60% No dietary restrictions	Cost Headache, arthralgia, fatigue and diarrhoea
Immunomodulators			
Rituximab	Intravenous 375 mg/m^2 per week for 4 weeks 100 mg/m^2 per week for 4 weeks	Response rate 60% at 6 months No need for chronic treatment	High relapse rate Contraindicated by patients with evidence of an active or previous HBV infection Increased tendency to minor infections; progressive multifocal leukoencephalopathy
Fostamatinib	Oral 100–150 mg twice daily	Response rate 43% within 12 weeks after treatment	Diarrhoea, hypertension and nausea Monthly follow up for hypertension, hepatotoxicity and neutropenia.
Splenectomy	Open or laparoscopic surgery	Durable remission rate 60 to 70% No need for chronic treatment	Surgical complications, thromboembolic events, infection with encapsulated bacteria, Sepsis

5.1.1. Glucocorticoids

Glucocorticoid treatment is the most-commonly used first-line therapy in patients with ITP [43,75]. The beneficial effects of glucocorticoids include reduction of platelet clearance by reticuloendothelial system [76,77]. Platelet count usually increases within a couple of days after therapy initiation [49]. Two most-commonly used glucocorticoids are prednisone (1 mg/kg orally per day for 2–3 weeks, with a gradual withdraw and discontinuation by 6 to 8 weeks) and high-dose dexamethasone (one or more cycles of 40 mg orally, once daily for 4 days, usually 4 weeks apart) [78]. Current ASH guideline recommends against the use of glucocorticoids longer than 6 weeks [4]. On the other hand, some others suggested that a longer low-dose steroid therapy could be considered to keep the platelet counts over 30×10^3/ml if a response with initial steroid therapy has been achieved [11]. Several studies demonstrated more rapid response with dexamethasone as compared to prednisone, but overall response rates are not significantly different in the long term after 6 and 12 months [79]. Similarly, Wang et al. reported a rapid response with high-dose dexamethasone compared to prednisolone, but sustained response rates were similar at 12 months and later [78]. Of note, dexamethasone seems to have a better safety profile (fewer Cushing's disease, weight gain and infection rates) in comparison to prednisolone [80].

Despite the high early-response rate, most of the patients do not have a sustained response after the cessation of glucocorticoids. In fact, approximately 80% of patients respond initially to corticosteroids, but only 20 to 40% of these patients achieve sustained response when steroids are discontinued [81,82]. As a predictive factor, Wang et al. measured anti-platelet antibody levels in ITP patients under glucocorticoid treatment [78]. They found that presence of anti-GPIb-IX antibodies predicts a poor initial response to corticosteroids [78]. Further studies are needed to determine the role of antiplatelet antibodies in predicting the corticosteroid response.

It is crucial to closely monitor the patients for possible side-effects of glucocorticoids such as hypertension, hyperglycaemia, sleep and mood disturbances, gastric ulceration, myopathy, glaucoma and osteoporosis [4]. To prevent severe toxicities, corticosteroids should be tapered appropriately and discontinued in non-responding patients. Non-responders and patients with contraindication to steroid therapy such as (pregnancy, diabetes mellitus, active infection and psychiatric disorders) can be treated with other first-line treatments-IVIG and IV anti-D [4].

To increase the rate of sustained response, combination of dexamethasone with second line treatments such as rituximab have been investigated. A recent meta-analysis compared the effectiveness of the combination of high-dose dexamethasone and rituximab with dexamethasone alone in ITP [83]. Overall response rate at month 3 (RR = 5.07, 95% CI: 2.91–8.86, and $p < 0.00001$) and sustained response rate at 12 months (RR = 1.73, 95% CI: 1.36–2.91, and $p < 0.00001$) was significantly higher in combination arm than that in monotherapy. Furthermore, the rate of adverse events has not significantly increased with combination therapy [83].

5.1.2. Intravenous Immunoglobulin (IVIG)

IVIG has been introduced into the treatment of ITP in 1980s [84]. IVIG is prepared by purification from the pooled plasma of healthy donors [84]. It contains polyvalent IgG (80 to >95%) and irrelevant amount of IgA and IgM. IVIG is thought to inhibit Fc-mediated phagocytosis of antibody coated platelets by reticuloendothelial system [85]. Platelet count usually increases within 48 hours after IVIG application [86]. The preferred treatment regime is 1 g/kg per day, which should be repeated for two consecutive days [2]. A lower dose of 0.2–0.4 g/kg/day can also be used for 4–5 days [87]. In a meta-analysis of 13 randomized studies, low dose IVIG regimes were found to be as effective as high dose IVIG, and low-dose-IVIG was associated with a significantly reduced risk of side-effects (OR = 0.39 (95% CI = 0.18–0.83) [88].

Limited number of randomized controlled studies compared the effectiveness of IVIG and corticosteroids as a first line therapy in ITP in adults [89,90]. Godeau et al. demonstrated that IVIG increases platelet count more effectively than high-dose methyl-prednisolone in adults with newly diagnosed ITP (79% vs. 60% response rate) [90]. In a smaller study, adult ITP patients were treated with oral prednisone (1 mg/kg/day; $n = 17$), high-dose IVIG (400 mg/kg on days 1 through 5; $n = 13$) or a combination of both agents ($n = 13$). A platelet response (>50 × 10^9/L) was achieved in 82%, 54% and 92% of patients, respectively [89].

There may be a relationship between the presence of anti-platelet antibody and the response to IVIG. Peng et al. found that the response rate was significantly higher in patients without anti-GPIb-IX autoantibodies compared to those with anti-GPIb-IX autoantibodies (80.0% vs. 36.4%), while the presence of the anti-GPIIb/IIIa autoantibodies had no effect on response to treatment [91]. However, others failed to show a significant relationship between an autoantibody and nonresponse to IVIG [92].

Most frequent adverse effects of IVIG include headache, pyrexia and vomiting [93]. Severe side effects such as acute kidney injury, aseptic meningitis and thrombotic events are rare [94].

5.1.3. Anti-RhD Immunoglobulin (Ig)

Anti-RhD consists of IgG selectively taken from the plasma of donors immunized to the Rhesus D antigen [85]. Anti-RhD Ig binds to Rh-positive erythrocytes and these antibody-coated erythrocytes competitively inhibit the destruction of antibody-coated platelets by binding and occupying Fc receptors on phagocytes in the spleen [95]. Anti-RhD is therefore only effective in Rh-positive patients with an intact spleen. A single intravenous dose of 50 to 75 µg/kg is recommended [96]. A safe subcutaneous administration in small children or patients is also described in the literature [97]. Side effects include mild infusion reactions such as headache, nausea, chills, fever and mild to moderate haemolysis [98]. However, life-threatening episodes of severe intravascular haemolysis and disseminated intravascular coagulation after Anti-RhD Ig administration have also been reported [99,100]. These reports led to the withdrawal of an Anti-RhD product (WinRho® SDF, Cangene Europe Ltd, London, UK) from European markets in 2009 [50].

5.2. Treatment of Active Bleeding

In case of clinically relevant bleeding, glucocorticoids, IVIG and platelet transfusion are used alone or in combination to increase the platelet count rapidly [11]. Besides, other interventions such as endoscopy or surgery may be necessary depending on the severity and the site of the bleeding [52]. Furthermore, anticoagulant and antiplatelet medications should be ceased immediately, if possible. Since the effect of platelet transfusion is limited due to rapid clearance of platelets by the circulating autoantibodies, combining platelet transfusion with IVIG or corticosteroids might be useful [11]. Although IVIG increases platelet count in most of the cases within 48 hours, its effect is temporary, and platelet count decreases after 1 to 2 weeks. Therefore, concomitant use of glucocorticoids with IVIG can be considered to achieve a more sustained response than that with IVIG alone [90]. Of note, the recommendations for the treatment of active bleeding in ITP are based on small observational studies, and randomized controlled studies are urgently needed.

The Updated International Consensus Report recommends the use of TPO-RA in the case of a life-threatening bleeding if initial treatments with corticosteroids, IVIG and thrombocyte transfusion fails to increase the platelet count [11]. Roumier et al. used high dose romiplostim (10 µg/kg body weight) together with vinca alkaloids in 30 patients with severe bleeding and compared the results with a historical patient group treated with vinca alkaloids only [101]. Both groups constituted of patients who failed to achieve a response after initial therapy with IVIG, corticosteroids and/or platelet transfusion [101]. At day 7, complete response (60% vs. 29%, $p < 0.05$), and at day 14, both partial response (80% vs. 43%, $p < 0.05$) and complete response (70 vs. 17%, $p < 0.0001$) were significantly higher in the romiplostim plus vinca alkaloid group compared to the vinca alkaloid group alone [101]. Although this study shows the effective use of high dose romiplostim in life-threatening bleeding in ITP patients, two patients (6.6%) treated with high dose romiplostim developed major thromboembolic events. Therefore, the risk over benefit ratio should be carefully assessed for each patient.

Antifibrinolytics (tranexamic acid and aminocaproic acid) are successfully used to control significant bleeding in patients with ITP [102–104]. Oral contraceptives can be used in female patients with menorrhagia. In life threatening bleeding emergencies, recombinant activated factor VII may be a useful supportive treatment [105–107].

5.3. Second-line treatments
5.3.1. Thrombopoietin-Receptor Agonists (TPO-RA)

Romiplostim is an Fc-peptide fusion protein and administered as a once-weekly subcutaneous injection. The recommended initial dose is 1 µg/kg per week, which can be adjusted by weekly increments of 1 µg/kg according to platelet response to achieve a platelet count of $>50 \times 10^9$ platelets/L. The maximum dose is 10 µg/kg/week. Romiplostim is indicated in adult ITP patients who have had an insufficient response to corticosteroids, immunoglobulins or splenectomy. Self-administration of romiplostim by patients can help in reducing healthcare costs and increase patient comfort by eliminating the need to visit the hospital every week for applications [108].

Owing to the effectiveness and safety-profile of TPO-RAs recent studies explored the use of these drugs in other patient groups also. Kuter et al. investigated the effectiveness of romiplostim in patients with ITP for less than 12 months by analysing the data from 9 studies [109]. They found that the number of patients with a platelet response at $\geq$75% of measurements were higher for romiplostim (74% (204/277)) than for placebo/standard of care (18% (6/34)) in patients with ITP $\leq$1 year. More importantly the rate of treatment free remission (platelet counts $\geq$50 $\times$ 10^9 /l for $\geq$6 months) was higher in patients with ITP $\leq$ 1 year compared to those with ITP >1 year [109]. Clinically relevant bleeding-related episodes are significantly lower in patients on romiplostim therapy [110,111]. Kuter et al. followed 292 adult ITP patients receiving romiplostim as weekly treatment and observed that the platelet response is maintained with stable dosing for up to 5 years of continuous treatment [67].

Most frequently observed side effects are headache, arthralgia, myalgia, dizziness and insomnia [112]. Thromboembolism and bone marrow fibrosis are the most feared complications of TPO-RA in ITP patients. Gernsheimer reported that romiplostim does not present an increased risk of thromboembolic events compared to placebo [111]. However, close monitoring of patients for thromboembolic events is recommended. Bone marrow changes were observed in a small proportion of patients receiving romiplostim [113]. But the bone marrow fibrosis is reversed after the end of treatment [114,115].

Eltrombopag, which is a synthetic non-peptide molecule, binds selectively with thrombopoietin receptors on megakaryocytes and induces thrombopoiesis [116]. Eltrombopag is recommended for adult ITP patients who have had an insufficient response to corticosteroids, immunoglobulins or splenectomy. Eltrombopag is administered orally as a daily tablet. Daily dose is 25–75 mg according to the age and hepatic function status of the patient. To ensure an adequate absorption of eltrombopag, it should be taken at least 2 hours before or 4 hours after any medications or products containing polyvalent cations (such as antacids, calcium-rich foods and mineral supplements). Many patients have difficulty meeting these dietary requirements and an alternative intermittent dosing 1–5 times weekly have been recommended [117]. Due to the risk of hepatotoxicity, a dose reduction is necessary in patients with hepatic impairment and a close monitoring of liver enzymes and bilirubin every two weeks throughout the treatment is indicated [118].

Randomized controlled studies showed that eltrombopag achieved early platelet response in 70–80% of the patients and a remission rate of 20–30% [119–122]. In an open-label extension study, 85% of the patients achieved a platelet response, and 52% of them had a continuous response of 25 weeks or longer [123]. Furthermore, the incidence of bleeding episodes in patients receiving eltrombopag decreased from 57% to 16% at 1 year [123]. Although some patients seem to have a prolonged/complete remission after pausing TPO-RA, no prognostic marker is currently available to identify such patients [124]. However, recently, an inverse relation between TPO level and response to eltrombopag or romiplostim has been shown [125]. Patients with a normal baseline TPO level are more likely to benefit from a therapy with these drugs [125].

Forsthye et al. compared the bleeding related adverse events in patients receiving romiplostim or eltrombopag in a retrospective cross-sectional study. Patients on eltrombopag (n = 1617) had significantly fewer bleeding episodes compared to those on romiplostim (n = 1140) (7% vs. 14%) [55].

In terms of adverse effects, liver functions, thromboembolism and bone marrow fibrosis have been the areas of concern in the long-term use of eltrombopag [126]. Gastrointestinal symptoms (nausea, vomiting and diarrhoea), mild transaminase elevations and headache are the most commonly observed adverse events in clinical studies [122]. In a prospective safety and efficacy study, thromboembolic events were observed in 6% of patients and hepatobiliary side effects in 15% of patients with a median eltrombopag treatment duration of >2 years [123]. Regular follow-up of patients for these side effects is justified.

Avatrombopag is an orally administered TRO-RA and recently received FDA approval for treatment of resistant ITP in adults. Unlike eltrombopag, avatrombopag can be administered without dietary restrictions. Furthermore, avatrombopag does not require monitoring of liver functions [127]. The phase 3 clinical trial showed a longer median number of weeks with platelet count of 50×10^9/L or higher during the first 26 weeks in patients who received avatrombopag than in those who received placebo [128]. A platelet response (a platelet count $\geq 30 \times 10^9$/L, with at least a two-fold increase in platelet count from baseline and an absence of bleeding) has been observed in 56.3% of the avatrombopag treated patients [128]. The recommended initial dose is 20 mg/day. The doses or dosing frequency should be adjusted individually to maintain platelet count greater than 50×10^9/L. The maximum daily dose is 40 mg [127]. The treatment should be discontinued if a platelet response is not achieved in 4 weeks of avatrombopag therapy at a dose of 40 mg/day. Most common side effects are headache, arthralgia, fatigue and diarrhoea. Further studies are needed to ensure the long-term safety of avatrombopag.

5.3.2. Immunomodulators

Rituximab is an anti-CD20 monoclonal antibody that depletes CD20+ B cells and reduces antiplatelet antibody production directly [129]. Rituximab achieves a significantly higher incidence of complete response at 6 months compared to glucocorticoids or placebo in non-splenectomised ITP patients (46.8% vs. 32.5%) [130]. More than one-half of the responders had their response last for at least 1 year, resulting in a 1-year response rate of 38%. Patel et al. reported a 2-year response rate of 31% and a 5-year response rate of 21% in adults treated with rituximab [131]. Sustained platelet response lasts more than 2 years in 50% of patients who have an initial response to rituximab [131,132]. Low dose rituximab therapy has been recommended to avoid treatment related adverse events. A recent systematic review found an overall response rate of 63% and complete response rate of 44% in ITP patients treated with low-dose (100 mg or 100 mg/m^2 per week for 4 weeks) rituximab instead of the standard dose of 375 mg/m^2 per week for 4 weeks [133]. Low dose rituximab has a satisfactory efficacy and safety profile [133]. In a long-term follow-up study (median follow-up of 6 years), median duration of response was longer (17 months vs. 11 months), and splenectomy rate was lower (17.2% vs. 26.4) in rituximab-treated patients. However, 70% of the rituximab-treated patients relapsed within two years after response [134]. Hammond et al. showed that response rate at 2 years was 70% in ITP patients treated with rituximab after unsuccessful splenectomy [135]. Wang et al. have recently demonstrated that a positive ANA test is associated with a better initial response but with an unfavourable long-term outcome in ITP patients treated with rituximab [136].

Rituximab should not be prescribed to patients with evidence of an active or previous HBV infection due to the risk of fulminant hepatitis, and other treatment options should be considered [129]. An increased tendency to minor infections after rituximab therapy has been reported. On the other hand, progressive multifocal leukoencephalopathy seem to be rare [137]. Taken together, due to the lower efficacy and higher complications compared with TPO-RAs [138], rituximab should be avoided as first line therapy and used only if there is high evidence for remission [4].

Fostamatinib is an orally available spleen tyrosine kinase (Syk) inhibitor. Syk-dependent phagocytosis of FcγR-bound platelets plays a role in the pathophysiology of ITP, and fostamatinib inhibits antibody-mediated destruction of platelets [139]. Pooled analyses of two randomized controlled trials demonstrated a response within 12 weeks in 43% of the patients compared to 14% of those receiving placebo [140]. In addition, a sustained platelet count $\geq 50 \times 10^9$/L for up to 24 weeks was observed in 18% of refractory ITP patients compared to 2% of those receiving placebo [140]. In the open label extension study with the patients who had a stable response, 21 (78%) patients had maintained the response for 1 year and 15 (56%) for 2 years [141]. In a post-hoc analysis of the phase 3 and open-label extension study, Boccia et al. observed a higher platelet response rate ($\geq 50 \times 10^9$/L) (78% vs. 48%) and lower bleeding events (28% vs. 45%) when fostamatinib was used as a second line therapy as compared to its use as a third-or-later-line of therapy [142]. The recommended initial dose is 100 mg twice daily, and the dose can be increased to 150 mg twice daily, if platelet count has not increased to at least 50×10^9 /L after 4 weeks of therapy. Most common adverse reactions are diarrhoea, hypertension and nausea. A monthly monitoring for hepatotoxicity and neutropenia is recommended [143]. Long-term studies are needed to better understand the efficacy and safety profile of fostamatinib in patients with chronic ITP.

5.3.3. Splenectomy

Spleen is the main site of the autoantibody production and platelet destruction. Splenectomy is long regarded as the gold standard therapy for ITP patients who are unresponsive to corticosteroids [144]. Compared to other treatment options, splenectomy has a higher sustainable response rate [4]. However, with the introduction of new medicaments, splenectomy has lost its place in the treatment of ITP [75,145].

Splenectomy achieves a high rate of durable remissions in 60 to 70% of the patients [146]. The need for the third-line treatment is significantly lower in patients who have undergone splenectomy (20%) compared to patients treated with second-line therapy (39–44%) [147]. Vianelli et al. reported a relapse free survival in 67% of the patients for up to 20 years after splenectomy [148]. However, due to the surgical risks and potential long-term complications, splenectomy is usually reserved to chronic ITP patients who failed to respond to standard medical therapies or when therapies are contraindicated [50,144].

Furthermore, the lack of reliable predictors of response to splenectomy hinders the selection of the patients who will benefit from splenectomy [146]. Revealing the main site of platelet sequestration can help to predict the success of splenectomy. Autologous platelet scanning can be used to detect the site of platelet sequestration, but it is technically challenging and not widely available [149]. Knowledge of desialylation capacity of the anti-platelet autoantibodies might also be helpful to detect Fc-independent clearance of platelets in the liver [22].

Complications associated with splenectomy are post-operative bleeding, infection with encapsulated bacteria, sepsis as well as thromboembolic events in venous and arterial circulation (i.e., coronary artery disease, stroke and chronic thromboembolic pulmonary hypertension) [144]. In a retrospective analysis of medical records, among second line treatments, splenectomy had the highest frequency of deep vein thrombosis and pulmonary embolism [147]. Compared to open surgery, laparoscopic splenectomy has a lower rate of postoperative mortality and morbidity and a shorter hospitalization [146,150]. Moreover, the immediate as well as the persistent risks of venous thromboembolism have been shown to be higher among patients with ITP who have undergone splenectomy as compared those who have not [151,152].

Patient's age must also be taken into consideration during the selection process for splenectomy. Maria et al. showed that patients age at the time of the surgery predicted the response in children [153]. Older children show a better outcome after splenectomy. Recently, Kwiatkowska et al. showed that age (<41 years) together with (BMI < 24.3 kg/m^2) and preoperative platelet count ($\geq$97 × 103 mm^3) are independent prognostic factors for ITP remission after splenectomy [154]. Geriatric patients are prone to surgical complications and an increased relapse has been reported in ITP patients over 60 years [155,156]. Therefore, splenectomy should be implemented as a last resort in elderly patients. Last but not the least; splenectomy should not be performed in the first 12 to 24 months after ITP diagnosis because of the chances of spontaneous remission or disease stabilization [11].

5.4. New Drugs under Investigation

Rozanolixizumab is anti-neonatal Fc receptor (FcRn) antibody that reduces plasma IgG levels. In a recent phase 2 study, >50% patients with persistent/chronic primary ITP achieved clinically relevant platelet responses ($\geq 50 \times 10^9$/L) by day 8 after a single injection of rozanolixizumab at a dose of 15 and 20 mg/kg [157]. Treatment related mild-to-moderate adverse events have been seen in 15 of 66 (21%) patients, and no serious infections have been reported. A phase 3 study is currently recruiting participants (NCT04224688).

Bortezomib, a proteosom inhibitor, induces apoptosis of long-lived autoreactive plasmocytes and reduces secretion of anti-platelet antibodies. In murine models of ITP, bortezomib eliminated long-lived plasmocytes and alleviated thrombocytopenia [158]. Beckman et al. used bortezomib to treat a 63-year-old female patient who had severe thrombocytopenia and bleeding episodes despite the utilization of several treatments including splenectomy [159]. The patient received bortezomib injections in addition to other treatments, and platelet count increased rapidly after the initiation of bortezomib. The results of the ongoing clinical trials (NCT03443570, NCT04083014) will help us to better define, if any, the role of bortezomib in ITP.

Efgartigimod is an Fc fragment that blocks FcRn. In a recent study, patients with a platelet count <30 × 10^9/L despite treatment received four weekly intravenous injections of either placebo or efgartigimod, at a dose of 5 mg/kg or 10 mg/kg [160]. Antiplatelet antibody levels reduced 40% or more in 8/12 (66.7%) patients treated with efgartigimod at 5 mg/kg and in 7/10 (70.0%) patients treated with efgartigimod at 10 mg/kg. A platelet response >50 × 10^9/L on 2 occasions has been achieved in 46.2% of the patients on efgartigimod as compared to 25% on placebo [160]. A Phase 3 Study investigating the safety and efficacy of efgartigimod at a dose of 10 mg/kg is ongoing (NCT04225156).

Decitabine is an inhibitor of DNA methylation and used in the treatment of myelodysplastic syndrome. Considering the possible role of DNA-methylation in the aetiology of ITP [161], decitabine seems to be a potential treatment option. Low dose decitabine promotes megakaryocyte maturation and platelet production in patients with myelodysplastic syndrome and ITP [162,163]. In a prospective open label study, Zhou et. al. showed that an overall response rate of 51% with a median initial response time of 28 days in ITP patients [164]. The sustained response rates at 6, 12 and 18 months were 44.44% (20/45), 31.11% (14/45) and 20.0% (9/45), respectively [164].

6. Conclusions

In recent years, ITP guidelines have been updated in the context of improved understanding of the pathophysiology of ITP and evidence supporting newly introduced treatments. Despite recent developments, the expected increase in the success rate of treatments has not been achieved yet. A substantial number of patients either do not respond at all or respond only transiently to many treatment interventions. The use of different treatment regimens targeting different key points in the pathophysiology of the disease may increase the success rate. In addition, the development of patient-specific testing methods, which can predict treatment success, may assist in avoiding complications, wasted time and associated costs from unnecessary treatments.

The management of ITP during ongoing 2019 coronavirus disease (COVID-19) pandemic has emerged as an additional challenge for clinicians. COVID-19, caused by severe acute respiratory syndrome coronavirus 2 (SARS-CoV-2), is known to be associated with increased coagulopathy and thrombotic complications [165]. Current data are insufficient to make evidence-based recommendations related to the ITP management. Pavord et al. published a series of recommendations based on expert opinion on the management of ITP during the COVID-19 pandemic [166]. They drew attention to a possible further increased risk of thrombosis in patients with COVID-19 from ITP or its treatment (particularly with TPO-RA). Mahevas et al. reported in a case series that COVID-19-associated ITP can lead to profound thrombocytopenia and severe bleeding manifestations but has a favourable outcome in most cases [167]. More studies are needed to make evidence-based decisions on managing ITP during the pandemic.

Current guidelines state that patient preferences should be prioritized when choosing a treatment regimen. Important factors that determine patient preferences include treatment efficacy and the potential for complications. Efficacy and safety data from post-marketing studies of new treatments will be helpful in this regard. In addition, randomized controlled trials comparing existing treatments not only in terms of treatment response or safety but also in terms of their impact on the health-related quality of life of patients with ITP are needed.

Author Contributions: A.S. conducted the literature search, created the figures and wrote the sections on pathophysiology and diagnosis of ITP. G.U. conducted the literature search and wrote the sections on clinical manifestations and treatment of ITP. T.B. designed the original layout and edited the manuscript. All authors have read and agreed to the published version of the manuscript.

Funding: This work was supported by grants from the German Research Foundation, the Herzstiftung (BA5158/4), Günther Landbeck Foundation and German Red Cross to T.B.

Institutional Review Board Statement: Not applicable.

Informed Consent Statement: Not applicable.

Data Availability Statement: Not applicable.

Acknowledgments: We thank Karina Althaus for insightful suggestions.

Conflicts of Interest: The authors declare no conflict of interest.

References

1. Provan, D.; Stasi, R.; Newland, A.C.; Blanchette, V.S.; Bolton-Maggs, P.; Bussel, J.B.; Chong, B.H.; Cines, D.B.; Gernsheimer, T.B.; Godeau, B.; et al. International consensus report on the investigation and management of primary immune thrombocytopenia. *Blood* **2010**, *115*, 168–186. [CrossRef]
2. Neunert, C.; Lim, W.; Crowther, M.; Cohen, A.; Solberg, L.; Crowther, M.A. The American Society of Hematology 2011 evidence-based practice guideline for immune thrombocytopenia. *Blood* **2011**, *117*, 4190–4207. [CrossRef]
3. Moulis, G.; Palmaro, A.; Montastruc, J.-L.; Godeau, B.; Lapeyre-Mestre, M.; Sailler, L. Epidemiology of incident immune thrombocytopenia: a nationwide population-based study in France. *Blood* **2014**, *124*, 3308–3315. [CrossRef] [PubMed]
4. Neunert, C.; Terrell, D.R.; Arnold, D.M.; Buchanan, G.; Cines, D.B.; Cooper, N.; Cuker, A.; Despotovic, J.M.; George, J.N.; Grace, R.F.; et al. American Society of Hematology 2019 guidelines for immune thrombocytopenia. *Blood Adv.* **2019**, *3*, 3829–3866. [CrossRef]
5. McKenzie, C.G.J.; Guo, L.; Freedman, J.; Semple, J.W. Cellular immune dysfunction in immune thrombocytopenia (ITP). *Br. J. Haematol.* **2013**, *163*, 10–23. [CrossRef] [PubMed]
6. Shulman, N.R.; Marder, V.J.; Weinrach, R.S. Similarities between known antiplatelet antibodies and the factor responsible for thrombocytopenia in idiopathic purpura. Physiologic, serologic and isotopic studies. *Ann. NY Acad. Sci.* **1965**, *124*, 499–542. [CrossRef]
7. Ku, F.-C.; Tsai, C.-R.; Der Wang, J.; Wang, C.H.; Chang, T.-K.; Hwang, W.-L. Stromal-derived factor-1 gene variations in pediatric patients with primary immune thrombocytopenia. *Eur. J. Haematol.* **2013**, *90*, 25–30. [CrossRef] [PubMed]
8. Rank, A.; Weigert, O.; Ostermann, H. Management of chronic immune thrombocytopenic purpura: targeting insufficient megakaryopoiesis as a novel therapeutic principle. *Biologics* **2010**, *4*, 139–145. [CrossRef] [PubMed]
9. Cines, D.B.; Liebman, H.A. The Immune Thrombocytopenia Syndrome: A Disorder of Diverse Pathogenesis and Clinical Presentation. *Hematol. Oncol. Clin. North Am.* **2009**, *23*, 1155–1161. [CrossRef] [PubMed]
10. D'Orazio, J.A.; Neely, J.; Farhoudi, N. ITP in Children. *J. Pediatric Hematol. Oncol.* **2013**, *35*, 1–13. [CrossRef] [PubMed]
11. Provan, D.; Arnold, D.M.; Bussel, J.B.; Chong, B.H.; Cooper, N.; Gernsheimer, T.; Ghanima, W.; Godeau, B.; González-López, T.J.; Grainger, J.; et al. Updated international consensus report on the investigation and management of primary immune thrombocytopenia. *Blood Adv.* **2019**, *3*, 3780–3817. [CrossRef] [PubMed]
12. Bakchoul, T.; Sachs, U.J. Platelet destruction in immune thrombocytopenia. Understanding the mechanisms. *Hamostaseologie* **2016**, *36*, 187–194. [CrossRef]
13. Zhao, Z.; Yang, L.; Yang, G.; Zhuang, Y.; Qian, X.; Zhou, X.; Xiao, D.; Shen, Y. Contributions of T Lymphocyte Abnormalities to Therapeutic Outcomes in Newly Diagnosed Patients with Immune Thrombocytopenia. *PLoS ONE* **2015**, *10*, e0126601. [CrossRef] [PubMed]
14. Ji, X.; Zhang, L.; Peng, J.; Hou, M. T cell immune abnormalities in immune thrombocytopenia. *J. Hematol. Oncol.* **2014**, *7*. [CrossRef] [PubMed]
15. Zhang, F.; Chu, X.; Wang, L.; Zhu, Y.; Li, L.; Ma, D.; Peng, J.; Hou, M. Cell-mediated lysis of autologous platelets in chronic idiopathic thrombocytopenic purpura. *Eur. J. Haematol.* **2006**, *76*, 427–431. [CrossRef] [PubMed]
16. Zhao, C.; Li, X.; Zhang, F.; Wang, L.; Peng, J.; Hou, M. Increased cytotoxic T-lymphocyte-mediated cytotoxicity predominant in patients with idiopathic thrombocytopenic purpura without platelet autoantibodies. *Haematologica* **2008**, *93*, 1428–1430. [CrossRef]
17. Bakchoul, T.; Walek, K.; Krautwurst, A.; Rummel, M.; Bein, G.; Santoso, S.; Sachs, U.J. Glycosylation of autoantibodies: insights into the mechanisms of immune thrombocytopenia. *Thromb. Haemost.* **2013**, *110*, 1259–1266. [CrossRef]

18. Kashiwagi, H.; Tomiyama, Y. Pathophysiology and management of primary immune thrombocytopenia. *Int. J. Hematol.* **2013**, *98*, 24–33. [CrossRef]
19. Nieswandt, B.; Bergmeier, W.; Rackebrandt, K.; Gessner, J.E.; Zirngibl, H. Identification of critical antigen-specific mechanisms in the development of immune thrombocytopenic purpura in mice. *Blood* **2000**, *96*, 2520–2527. [CrossRef]
20. Nieswandt, B.; Bergmeier, W.; Schulte, V.; Rackebrandt, K.; Gessner, J.E.; Zirngibl, H. Expression and function of the mouse collagen receptor glycoprotein VI is strictly dependent on its association with the FcRgamma chain. *J. Biol. Chem.* **2000**, *275*, 23998–24002. [CrossRef] [PubMed]
21. Webster, M.L.; Sayeh, E.; Crow, M.; Chen, P.; Nieswandt, B.; Freedman, J.; Ni, H. Relative efficacy of intravenous immunoglobulin G in ameliorating thrombocytopenia induced by antiplatelet GPIIbIIIa versus GPIbalpha antibodies. *Blood* **2006**, *108*, 943–946. [CrossRef] [PubMed]
22. Li, J.; van der Wal, D.E.; Zhu, G.; Xu, M.; Yougbare, I.; Ma, L.; Vadasz, B.; Carrim, N.; Grozovsky, R.; Ruan, M.; et al. Desialylation is a mechanism of Fc-independent platelet clearance and a therapeutic target in immune thrombocytopenia. *Nat. Commun.* **2015**, *6*. [CrossRef] [PubMed]
23. Qiu, J.; Liu, X.; Li, X.; Zhang, X.; Han, P.; Zhou, H.; Shao, L.; Hou, Y.; Min, Y.; Kong, Z.; et al. CD8(+) T cells induce platelet clearance in the liver via platelet desialylation in immune thrombocytopenia. *Sci. Rep.* **2016**, *6*, 27445. [CrossRef] [PubMed]
24. Tao, L.; Zeng, Q.; Li, J.; Xu, M.; Wang, J.; Pan, Y.; Wang, H.; Tao, Q.; Chen, Y.; Peng, J.; et al. Platelet desialylation correlates with efficacy of first-line therapies for immune thrombocytopenia. *J. Hematol. Oncol.* **2017**, *10*. [CrossRef] [PubMed]
25. Quach, M.E.; Dragovich, M.A.; Chen, W.; Syed, A.K.; Cao, W.; Liang, X.; Deng, W.; de Meyer, S.F.; Zhu, G.; Peng, J.; et al. Fc-independent immune thrombocytopenia via mechanomolecular signaling in platelets. *Blood* **2018**, *131*, 787–796. [CrossRef]
26. Marini, I.; Zlamal, J.; Faul, C.; Holzer, U.; Hammer, S.; Pelzl, L.; Bethge, W.; Althaus, K.; Bakchoul, T. Autoantibody-mediated desialylation impairs human thrombopoiesis and platelet lifespan. *Haematologica* **2020**, *106*, 196–207. [CrossRef]
27. Mason, K.D.; Carpinelli, M.R.; Fletcher, J.I.; Collinge, J.E.; Hilton, A.A.; Ellis, S.; Kelly, P.N.; Ekert, P.G.; Metcalf, D.; Roberts, A.W.; et al. Programmed Anuclear Cell Death Delimits Platelet Life Span. *Cell* **2007**, *128*, 1173–1186. [CrossRef]
28. Van der Wal, D.E.; Gitz, E.; Du, V.X.; Lo, K.S.L.; Koekman, C.A.; Versteeg, S.; Akkerman, J.W.N. Arachidonic acid depletion extends survival of cold-stored platelets by interfering with the glycoprotein Ibα–14-3-3ζ association. *Haematologica* **2012**, *97*, 1514–1522. [CrossRef]
29. Álvarez Román, M.; Bello, I.; Arias-Salgado, E.G.; Pollmar, M.I.; Yuste, V.; Salces, M.; Butta, N.V. Effects of thrombopoietin receptor agonists on procoagulant state in patients with immune thrombocytopenia. *Thromb. Haemost.* **2014**, *112*, 65–72. [CrossRef]
30. Winkler, J.; Kroiss, S.; Rand, M.L.; Azzouzi, I.; Annie Bang, K.W.; Speer, O.; Schmugge, M. Platelet apoptosis in paediatric immune thrombocytopenia is ameliorated by intravenous immunoglobulin. *Br. J. Haematol.* **2012**, *156*, 508–515. [CrossRef]
31. Goette, N.P.; Glembotsky, A.C.; Lev, P.R.; Grodzielski, M.; Contrufo, G.; Pierdominici, M.S.; Espasandin, Y.R.; Riveros, D.; García, A.J.; Molinas, F.C.; et al. Platelet Apoptosis in Adult Immune Thrombocytopenia: Insights into the Mechanism of Damage Triggered by Auto-Antibodies. *PLoS ONE* **2016**, *11*, e0160563. [CrossRef]
32. Marini, I.; Bakchoul, T. Pathophysiology of Autoimmune Thrombocytopenia: Current Insight with a Focus on Thrombopoiesis. *Hamostaseologie* **2019**, *39*, 227–237. [CrossRef]
33. McMillan, R.; Luiken, G.A.; Levy, R.; Yelenosky, R.; Longmire, R.L. Antibody against megakaryocytes in idiopathic thrombocytopenic purpura. *JAMA* **1978**, *239*, 2460–2462. [CrossRef]
34. Takahashi, R.; Sekine, N.; Nakatake, T. Influence of monoclonal antiplatelet glycoprotein antibodies on in vitro human megakaryocyte colony formation and proplatelet formation. *Blood* **1999**, *93*, 1951–1958. [CrossRef]
35. Chang, M.; Nakagawa, P.A.; Williams, S.A.; Schwartz, M.R.; Imfeld, K.L.; Buzby, J.S.; Nugent, D.J. Immune thrombocytopenic purpura (ITP) plasma and purified ITP monoclonal autoantibodies inhibit megakaryocytopoiesis in vitro. *Blood* **2003**, *102*, 887–895. [CrossRef]
36. McMillan, R.; Wang, L.; Tomer, A.; Nichol, J.; Pistillo, J. Suppression of in vitro megakaryocyte production by antiplatelet autoantibodies from adult patients with chronic ITP. *Blood* **2004**, *103*, 1364–1369. [CrossRef]
37. Iraqi, M.; Perdomo, J.; Yan, F.; Choi, P.Y.-I.; Chong, B.H. Immune thrombocytopenia: antiplatelet autoantibodies inhibit proplatelet formation by megakaryocytes and impair platelet production in vitro. *Haematologica* **2015**, *100*, 623–632. [CrossRef]
38. Yang, L.; Wang, L.; Zhao, C.; Zhu, X.; Hou, Y.; Jun, P.; Hou, M. Contributions of TRAIL-mediated megakaryocyte apoptosis to impaired megakaryocyte and platelet production in immune thrombocytopenia. *Blood* **2010**, *116*, 4307–4316. [CrossRef] [PubMed]
39. Radley, J.M.; Haller, C.J. Fate of senescent megakaryocytes in the bone marrow. *Br. J. Haematol.* **1983**, *53*, 277–287. [CrossRef] [PubMed]
40. Houwerzijl, E.J.; Blom, N.R.; van der Want, J.J.L.; Esselink, M.T.; Koornstra, J.J.; Smit, J.W.; Louwes, H.; Vellenga, E.; de Wolf, J.T.M. Ultrastructural study shows morphologic features of apoptosis and para-apoptosis in megakaryocytes from patients with idiopathic thrombocytopenic purpura. *Blood* **2004**, *103*, 500–506. [CrossRef] [PubMed]
41. Vrbensky, J.R.; Nazy, I.; Toltl, L.J.; Ross, C.; Ivetic, N.; Smith, J.W.; Kelton, J.G.; Arnold, D.M. Megakaryocyte apoptosis in immune thrombocytopenia. *Platelets* **2018**, *29*, 729–732. [CrossRef] [PubMed]
42. Neylon, A.J.; Saunders, P.W.G.; Howard, M.R.; Proctor, S.J.; Taylor, P.R.A. Clinically significant newly presenting autoimmune thrombocytopenic purpura in adults: A prospective study of a population-based cohort of 245 patients. *Br. J. Haematol.* **2003**, *122*, 966–974. [CrossRef]

43. Lee, J.Y.; Lee, J.-H.; Lee, H.; Kang, B.; Kim, J.-W.; Kim, S.H.; Lee, J.-O.; Kim, J.W.; Kim, Y.J.; Lee, K.-W.; et al. Epidemiology and management of primary immune thrombocytopenia: A nationwide population-based study in Korea. *Thromb. Res.* **2017**, *155*, 86–91. [CrossRef]
44. Schoonen, W.M.; Kucera, G.; Coalson, J.; Li, L.; Rutstein, M.; Mowat, F.; Fryzek, J.; Kaye, J.A. Epidemiology of immune thrombocytopenic purpura in the General Practice Research Database. *Br. J. Haematol.* **2009**, *145*, 235–244. [CrossRef]
45. Grimaldi-Bensouda, L.; Nordon, C.; Michel, M.; Viallard, J.-F.; Adoue, D.; Magy-Bertrand, N.; Durand, J.-M.; Quittet, P.; Fain, O.; Bonnotte, B.; et al. Immune thrombocytopenia in adults: A prospective cohort study of clinical features and predictors of outcome. *Haematologica* **2016**, *101*, 1039–1045. [CrossRef]
46. Sailer, T.; Lechner, K.; Panzer, S.; Kyrle, P.A.; Pabinger, I. The course of severe autoimmune thrombocytopenia in patients not undergoing splenectomy. *Haematologica* **2006**, *91*, 1041–1045. [CrossRef]
47. Kühne, T.; Buchanan, G.R.; Zimmerman, S.; Michaels, L.A.; Kohan, R.; Berchtold, W.; Imbach, P. A prospective comparative study of 2540 infants and children with newly diagnosed idiopathic thrombocytopenic purpura (ITP) from the Intercontinental Childhood ITP Study Group. *J. Pediatrics* **2003**, *143*, 605–608. [CrossRef]
48. Imbach, P.; Kühne, T.; Müller, D.; Berchtold, W.; Zimmerman, S.; Elalfy, M.; Buchanan, G.R. Childhood ITP: 12 months follow-up data from the prospective registry I of the Intercontinental Childhood ITP Study Group (ICIS). *Pediatr. Blood Cancer* **2006**, *46*, 351–356. [CrossRef]
49. Jaime-Pérez, J.C.; Aguilar-Calderón, P.; Jiménez-Castillo, R.A.; Ramos-Dávila, E.M.; Salazar-Cavazos, L.; Gómez-Almaguer, D. Treatment outcomes and chronicity predictors for primary immune thrombocytopenia: 10-year data from an academic center. *Ann. Hematol.* **2020**, *99*, 2513–2520. [CrossRef] [PubMed]
50. Matzdorff, A.; Meyer, O.; Ostermann, H.; Kiefel, V.; Eberl, W.; Kühne, T.; Pabinger, I.; Rummel, M. Immune Thrombocytopenia—Current Diagnostics and Therapy: Recommendations of a Joint Working Group of DGHO, ÖGHO, SGH, GPOH, and DGTI. *Oncol. Res. Treat.* **2018**, *41* (Suppl. 5), 1–30. [CrossRef] [PubMed]
51. Adelborg, K.; Kristensen, N.R.; Nørgaard, M.; Bahmanyar, S.; Ghanima, W.; Kilpatrick, K.; Frederiksen, H.; Ekstrand, C.; Sørensen, H.T.; Fynbo Christiansen, C. Cardiovascular and bleeding outcomes in a population-based cohort of patients with chronic immune thrombocytopenia. *J. Thromb. Haemost.* **2019**, *17*, 912–924. [CrossRef] [PubMed]
52. Mithoowani, S.; Cervi, A.; Shah, N.; Ejaz, R.; Sirotich, E.; Barty, R.; Li, N.; Nazy, I.; Arnold, D.M. Management of major bleeds in patients with immune thrombocytopenia. *J. Thromb. Haemost.* **2020**, *18*, 1783–1790. [CrossRef]
53. Cohen, Y.C.; Djulbegovic, B.; Shamai-Lubovitz, O.; Mozes, B. The bleeding risk and natural history of idiopathic thrombocytopenic purpura in patients with persistent low platelet counts. *Arch. Intern. Med.* **2000**, *160*, 1630–1638. [CrossRef] [PubMed]
54. Neunert, C.; Noroozi, N.; Norman, G.; Buchanan, G.R.; Goy, J.; Nazi, I.; Kelton, J.G.; Arnold, D.M. Severe bleeding events in adults and children with primary immune thrombocytopenia: a systematic review. *J. Thromb. Haemost.* **2015**, *13*, 457–464. [CrossRef]
55. Forsythe, A.; Schneider, J.; Pham, T.; Bhor, M.; Said, Q.; Allepuz, A.; Socorro O Portella, M.D.; Kwon, C.S.; Roy, A.N. Real-world evidence on clinical outcomes in immune thrombocytopenia treated with thrombopoietin receptor agonists. *J. Comp. Eff. Res.* **2020**, *9*, 447–457. [CrossRef]
56. Arnold, D.M.; Nazy, I.; Clare, R.; Jaffer, A.M.; Aubie, B.; Li, N.; Kelton, J.G. Misdiagnosis of primary immune thrombocytopenia and frequency of bleeding: Lessons from the McMaster ITP Registry. *Blood Adv.* **2017**, *1*, 2414–2420. [CrossRef]
57. Piel-Julian, M.-L.; Mahévas, M.; Germain, J.; Languille, L.; Comont, T.; Lapeyre-Mestre, M.; Payrastre, B.; Beyne-Rauzy, O.; Michel, M.; Godeau, B.; et al. Risk factors for bleeding, including platelet count threshold, in newly diagnosed immune thrombocytopenia adults. *J. Thromb. Haemost.* **2018**, *16*, 1830–1842. [CrossRef]
58. Hato, T.; Shimada, N.; Kurata, Y.; Kuwana, M.; Fujimura, K.; Kashiwagi, H.; Takafuta, T.; Murata, M.; Tomiyama, Y. Risk factors for skin, mucosal, and organ bleeding in adults with primary ITP: A nationwide study in Japan. *Blood Adv.* **2020**, *4*, 1648–1655. [CrossRef] [PubMed]
59. Newton, J.L.; Reese, J.A.; Watson, S.I.; Vesely, S.K.; Bolton-Maggs, P.H.B.; George, J.N.; Terrell, D.R. Fatigue in adult patients with primary immune thrombocytopenia. *Eur. J. Haematol.* **2011**, *86*, 420–429. [CrossRef]
60. Kuter, D.J.; Mathias, S.D.; Rummel, M.; Mandanas, R.; Giagounidis, A.A.; Wang, X.; Deuson, R.R. Health-related quality of life in nonsplenectomized immune thrombocytopenia patients receiving romiplostim or medical standard of care. *Am. J. Hematol.* **2012**, *87*, 558–561. [CrossRef]
61. Blatt, J.; Weston, B.; Gold, S. Fatigue as marker of thrombocytopenia in childhood idiopathic thrombocytopenic purpura. *Pediatr. Hematol. Oncol.* **2010**, *27*, 65–67. [CrossRef]
62. Hill, Q.A.; Newland, A.C. Fatigue in immune thrombocytopenia. *Br. J. Haematol.* **2015**, *170*, 141–149. [CrossRef] [PubMed]
63. Severinsen, M.T.; Engebjerg, M.C.; Farkas, D.K.; Jensen, A.Ø.; Nørgaard, M.; Zhao, S.; Sørensen, H.T. Risk of venous thromboembolism in patients with primary chronic immune thrombocytopenia: A Danish population-based cohort study. *Br. J. Haematol.* **2011**, *152*, 360–362. [CrossRef] [PubMed]
64. Doobaree, I.U.; Nandigam, R.; Bennett, D.; Newland, A.; Provan, D. Thromboembolism in adults with primary immune thrombocytopenia: A systematic literature review and meta-analysis. *Eur. J. Haematol.* **2016**, *97*, 321–330. [CrossRef]
65. Hollenhorst, M.A.; Al-Samkari, H.; Kuter, D.J. Markers of autoimmunity in immune thrombocytopenia: Prevalence and prognostic significance. *Blood Adv.* **2019**, *3*, 3515–3521. [CrossRef] [PubMed]
66. Peerschke, E.I.; Yin, W.; Ghebrehiwet, B. Complement activation on platelets: Implications for vascular inflammation and thrombosis. *Mol. Immunol.* **2010**, *47*, 2170–2175. [CrossRef] [PubMed]

67. Kuter, D.J.; Bussel, J.B.; Newland, A.; Baker, R.I.; Lyons, R.M.; Wasser, J.; Viallard, J.-F.; Macik, G.; Rummel, M.; Nie, K.; et al. Long-term treatment with romiplostim in patients with chronic immune thrombocytopenia: Safety and efficacy. *Br. J. Haematol.* **2013**, *161*, 411–423. [CrossRef]
68. Rodeghiero, F.; Stasi, R.; Giagounidis, A.; Viallard, J.-F.; Godeau, B.; Pabinger, I.; Cines, D.; Liebman, H.; Wang, X.; Woodard, P. Long-term safety and tolerability of romiplostim in patients with primary immune thrombocytopenia: A pooled analysis of 13 clinical trials. *Eur. J. Haematol.* **2013**, *91*, 423–436. [CrossRef]
69. Frederiksen, H.; Maegbaek, M.L.; Nørgaard, M. Twenty-year mortality of adult patients with primary immune thrombocytopenia: A Danish population-based cohort study. *Br. J. Haematol.* **2014**, *166*, 260–267. [CrossRef]
70. Vollenberg, R.; Jouni, R.; Norris, P.A.A.; Burg-Roderfeld, M.; Cooper, N.; Rummel, M.J.; Bein, G.; Marini, I.; Bayat, B.; Burack, R.; et al. Glycoprotein V is a relevant immune target in patients with immune thrombocytopenia. *Haematologica* **2019**, *104*, 1237–1243. [CrossRef] [PubMed]
71. Kiefel, V.; Freitag, E.; Kroll, H.; Santoso, S.; Mueller-Eckhardt, C. Platelet autoantibodies (IgG, IgM, IgA) against glycoproteins IIb/IIIa and Ib/IX in patients with thrombocytopenia. *Ann. Hematol.* **1996**, *72*, 280–285. [CrossRef] [PubMed]
72. Newland, A.; Lee, E.-J.; McDonald, V.; Bussel, J.B. Fostamatinib for persistent/chronic adult immune thrombocytopenia. *Immunotherapy* **2018**, *10*, 9–25. [CrossRef]
73. Page, L.K.; Psaila, B.; Provan, D.; Michael Hamilton, J.; Jenkins, J.M.; Elish, A.S.; Lesser, M.L.; Bussel, J.B. The immune thrombocytopenic purpura (ITP) bleeding score: Assessment of bleeding in patients with ITP. *Br. J. Haematol.* **2007**, *138*, 245–248. [CrossRef]
74. Palau, J.; Jarque, I.; Sanz, M.A. Long-term management of chronic immune thrombocytopenic purpura in adults. *Int. J. Gen. Med.* **2010**, *3*, 305–311. [CrossRef]
75. McGrath, L.J.; Kilpatrick, K.; Overman, R.A.; Reams, D.; Sharma, A.; Altomare, I.; Wasser, J.; Brookhart, M.A. Treatment Patterns Among Adults with Primary Immune Thrombocytopenia Diagnosed in Hematology Clinics in the United States. *Clin. Epidemiol.* **2020**, *12*, 435–445. [CrossRef]
76. Branehög, I.; Weinfeld, A. Platelet survival and platelet production in idiopathic thrombocytopenic purpura (ITP) before and during treatment with corticosteroids. *Scand. J. Haematol.* **1974**, *12*, 69–79. [CrossRef] [PubMed]
77. Gernsheimer, T.; Stratton, J.; Ballem, P.J.; Slichter, S.J. Mechanisms of response to treatment in autoimmune thrombocytopenic purpura. *N. Engl. J. Med.* **1989**, *320*, 974–980. [CrossRef]
78. Wang, L.; Xu, L.; Hao, H.; Jansen, A.J.G.; Liu, G.; Li, H.; Liu, X.; Zhao, Y.; Peng, J.; Hou, M. First line treatment of adult patients with primary immune thrombocytopenia: A real-world study. *Platelets* **2020**, *31*, 55–61. [CrossRef]
79. Mithoowani, S.; Gregory-Miller, K.; Goy, J.; Miller, M.C.; Wang, G.; Noroozi, N.; Kelton, J.G.; Arnold, D.M. High-dose dexamethasone compared with prednisone for previously untreated primary immune thrombocytopenia: A systematic review and meta-analysis. *Lancet Haematol.* **2016**, *3*, e489–e496. [CrossRef]
80. Ma, J.; Fu, L.; Chen, Z.; Gu, H.; Ma, J.; Wu, R. High-dose dexamethasone as a replacement for traditional prednisone as the first-line treatment in children with previously untreated primary immune thrombocytopenia: A prospective, randomized single-center study. *Int. J. Hematol.* **2020**, *112*, 773–779. [CrossRef] [PubMed]
81. Frederiksen, H.; Ghanima, W. Response of first line treatment with corticosteroids in a population-based cohort of adults with primary immune thrombocytopenia. *Eur. J. Intern. Med.* **2017**, *37*, e23–e25. [CrossRef] [PubMed]
82. Cheng, Y.; Wong, R.S.; Soo, Y.O.; Chui, C.H.; Lau, F.Y.; Chan, N.P.; Wong, W.S.; Cheng, G. Initial Treatment of Immune Thrombocytopenic Purpura with High-Dose Dexamethasone. *N. Engl. J. Med.* **2003**, *349*, 831–836. [CrossRef]
83. Wang, J.; Li, Y.; Wang, C.; Zhang, Y.; Gao, C.; Lang, H.; Chen, X. Efficacy and Safety of the Combination Treatment of Rituximab and Dexamethasone for Adults with Primary Immune Thrombocytopenia (ITP): A Meta-Analysis. *Biomed Res. Int.* **2018**, *2018*, 1316096. [CrossRef] [PubMed]
84. Imbach, P. Treatment of immune thrombocytopenia with intravenous immunoglobulin and insights for other diseases. A historical review. *Swiss Med. Wkly.* **2012**, *142*, w13591. [CrossRef]
85. Lazarus, A.H.; Crow, A.R. Mechanism of action of IVIG and anti-D in ITP. *Transfus. Apher. Sci.* **2003**, *28*, 249–255. [CrossRef]
86. Beck, C.E.; Nathan, P.C.; Parkin, P.C.; Blanchette, V.S.; Macarthur, C. Corticosteroids Versus Intravenous Immune Globulin for the Treatment of Acute Immune Thrombocytopenic Purpura in Children: A Systematic Review and Meta-Analysis of Randomized Controlled Trials. *J. Pediatrics* **2005**, *147*, 521–527. [CrossRef]
87. Zhou, Z.; Qiao, Z.; Li, H.; Luo, N.; Zhang, X.; Xue, F.; Yang, R. Different dosages of intravenous immunoglobulin (IVIg) in treating immune thrombocytopenia with long-term follow-up of three years: Results of a prospective study including 167 cases. *Autoimmunity* **2016**, *49*, 50–57. [CrossRef] [PubMed]
88. Qin, Y.-H.; Zhou, T.-B.; Su, L.-N.; Lei, F.-Y.; Zhao, Y.-J.; Huang, W.-F. The efficacy of different dose intravenous immunoglobulin in treating acute idiopathic thrombocytopenic purpura: a meta-analysis of 13 randomized controlled trials. *Blood Coagul. Fibrinolysis* **2010**, *21*, 713–721. [CrossRef]
89. Jacobs, P.; Wood, L.; Novitzky, N. Intravenous gammaglobulin has no advantages over oral corticosteroids as primary therapy for adults with immune thrombocytopenia: A prospective randomized clinical trial. *Am. J. Med.* **1994**, *97*, 55–59. [CrossRef]
90. Godeau, B.; Chevret, S.; Varet, B.; Lefrère, F.; Zini, J.-M.; Bassompierre, F.; Chèze, S.; Legouffe, E.; Hulin, C.; Grange, M.-J.; et al. Intravenous immunoglobulin or high-dose methylprednisolone, with or without oral prednisone, for adults with untreated severe autoimmune thrombocytopenic purpura: A randomised, multicentre trial. *Lancet* **2002**, *359*, 23–29. [CrossRef]

91. Peng, J.; Ma, S.-H.; Liu, J.; Hou, Y.; Liu, X.-M.; Niu, T.; Xu, R.-R.; Guo, C.-S.; Wang, X.-M.; Cheng, Y.-F.; et al. Association of autoantibody specificity and response to intravenous immunoglobulin G therapy in immune thrombocytopenia: A multicenter cohort study. *J. Thromb. Haemost.* **2014**, *12*, 497–504. [CrossRef]
92. Al-Samkari, H.; Rosovsky, R.P.; Karp Leaf, R.S.; Smith, D.B.; Goodarzi, K.; Fogerty, A.E.; Sykes, D.B.; Kuter, D.J. A modern reassessment of glycoprotein-specific direct platelet autoantibody testing in immune thrombocytopenia. *Blood Adv.* **2020**, *4*, 9–18. [CrossRef]
93. Dash, C.H.; Gillanders, K.R.; Stratford Bobbitt, M.E.; Gascoigne, E.W.; Leach, S.J. Safety and efficacy of Gammaplex® in idiopathic thrombocytopenic purpura (ClinicalTrials.gov–NCT00504075). *PLoS ONE* **2014**, *9*, e96600. [CrossRef] [PubMed]
94. Bonilla, F.A. Intravenous immunoglobulin: Adverse reactions and management. *J. Allergy Clin. Immunol.* **2008**, *122*, 1238–1239. [CrossRef] [PubMed]
95. Bussel, J.B.; Graziano, J.N.; Kimberly, R.P.; Pahwa, S.; Aledort, L.M. Intravenous anti-D treatment of immune thrombocytopenic purpura: Analysis of efficacy, toxicity, and mechanism of effect. *Blood* **1991**, *77*, 1884–1893. [CrossRef]
96. Cheung, E.; Liebman, H.A. Anti-RhD immunoglobulin in the treatment of immune thrombocytopenia. *Biologics* **2009**, *3*, 57–62. [PubMed]
97. Meyer, O.; Kiesewetter, H.; Hermsen, M.; Petriedes, P.; Rose, M.; Seibt, H.; Salama, A. Replacement of intravenous administration of anti-D by subcutaneous administration in patients with autoimmune thrombocytopenia. *Pediatr. Blood Cancer* **2006**, *47*, 721–722. [CrossRef] [PubMed]
98. Scaradavou, A.; Woo, B.; Woloski, B.M.; Cunningham-Rundles, S.; Ettinger, L.J.; Aledort, L.M.; Bussel, J.B. Intravenous anti-D treatment of immune thrombocytopenic purpura: Experience in 272 patients. *Blood* **1997**, *89*, 2689–2700. [CrossRef]
99. Gaines, A.R. Disseminated intravascular coagulation associated with acute hemoglobinemia or hemoglobinuria following Rh(0)(D) immune globulin intravenous administration for immune thrombocytopenic purpura. *Blood* **2005**, *106*, 1532–1537. [CrossRef]
100. Tarantino, M.D.; Bussel, J.B.; Cines, D.B.; McCrae, K.R.; Gernsheimer, T.; Liebman, H.A.; Wong, W.-Y.; Kulkarni, R.; Grabowski, E.; McMillan, R. A closer look at intravascular hemolysis (IVH) following intravenous anti-D for immune thrombocytopenic purpura (ITP). *Blood* **2007**, *109*, 5527. [CrossRef]
101. Roumier, M.; Le Burel, S.; Audia, S.; Chauchet, A.; Gousseff, M.; Hamidou, M.; Liferman, F.; Moulis, G.; Lioger, B.; Galicier, L.; et al. High dose romiplostim as a rescue therapy for adults with severe bleeding and refractory immune thrombocytopenia. *Am. J. Hematol.* **2020**. [CrossRef]
102. Mayer, B.; Salama, A. Successful treatment of bleeding with tranexamic acid in a series of 12 patients with immune thrombocytopenia. *Vox Sang.* **2017**, *112*, 767–772. [CrossRef] [PubMed]
103. Bartholomew, J.R.; Salgia, R.; Bell, W.R. Control of bleeding in patients with immune and nonimmune thrombocytopenia with aminocaproic acid. *Arch. Intern. Med.* **1989**, *149*, 1959–1961. [CrossRef] [PubMed]
104. Randall, M.M.; Nurse, J.; Singh, K.P. Tranexamic Acid in a Case Report of Life-threatening Nontraumatic Hemorrhage in Immune Thrombocytopenic Purpura. *Clin. Pract. Cases Emerg. Med.* **2020**, *4*, 421–423. [CrossRef]
105. Gurion, R.; Siu, A.; Weiss, A.R.; Masterson, M. Use of Recombinant Factor VIIa in a Pediatric Patient with Initial Presentation of Refractory Acute Immune Thrombocytopenic Purpura and Severe Bleeding. *J. Pediatr. Pharmacol. Ther.* **2012**, *17*, 274–280. [CrossRef]
106. Gerotziafas, G.T.; Zervas, C.; Gavrielidis, G.; Tokmaktsis, A.; Hatjiharissi, E.; Papaioannou, M.; Lazaridou, A.; Constantinou, N.; Samama, M.M.; Christakis, J. Effective hemostasis with rFVIIa treatment in two patients with severe thrombocytopenia and life-threatening hemorrhage. *Am. J. Hematol.* **2002**, *69*, 219–222. [CrossRef]
107. Waddington, D.P.; McAuley, F.T.; Hanley, J.P.; Summerfield, G.P. The use of recombinant factor viia in a jehovah's witness with auto-immune thrombocytopenia and post-splenectomy haemorrhage. *Br. J. Haematol.* **2002**, *119*, 286–288. [CrossRef]
108. Kuter, D.J.; Arnold, D.M.; Rodeghiero, F.; Janssens, A.; Selleslag, D.; Bird, R.; Newland, A.; Mayer, J.; Wang, K.; Olie, R. Safety and efficacy of self-administered romiplostim in patients with immune thrombocytopenia: Results of an integrated database of five clinical trials. *Am. J. Hematol.* **2020**, *95*, 643–651. [CrossRef]
109. Kuter, D.J.; Newland, A.; Chong, B.H.; Rodeghiero, F.; Romero, M.T.; Pabinger, I.; Chen, Y.; Wang, K.; Mehta, B.; Eisen, M. Romiplostim in adult patients with newly diagnosed or persistent immune thrombocytopenia (ITP) for up to 1 year and in those with chronic ITP for more than 1 year: A subgroup analysis of integrated data from completed romiplostim studies. *Br. J. Haematol.* **2019**, *185*, 503–513. [CrossRef] [PubMed]
110. Stasi, R.; Murali, M.; Michel, M.; Viallard, J.-F.; Giagounidis, A.; Janssens, A.; Legg, J.; Deuson, R.; Danese, M.D. Evaluation of bleeding-related episodes in patients with immune thrombocytopenia (ITP) receiving romiplostim or medical standard of care. *Int. J. Hematol.* **2012**, *96*, 26–33. [CrossRef]
111. Gernsheimer, T.B.; George, J.N.; Aledort, L.M.; Tarantino, M.D.; Sunkara, U.; Matthew Guo, D.; Nichol, J.L. Evaluation of bleeding and thrombotic events during long-term use of romiplostim in patients with chronic immune thrombocytopenia (ITP). *J. Thromb. Haemost.* **2010**, *8*, 1372–1382. [CrossRef]
112. Kuter, D.J.; Rummel, M.; Boccia, R.; Macik, B.G.; Pabinger, I.; Selleslag, D.; Rodeghiero, F.; Chong, B.H.; Wang, X.; Berger, D.P. Romiplostim or standard of care in patients with immune thrombocytopenia. *N. Engl. J. Med.* **2010**, *363*, 1889–1899. [CrossRef]

113. Janssens, A.; Rodeghiero, F.; Anderson, D.; Chong, B.H.; Boda, Z.; Pabinger, I.; Červinek, L.; Terrell, D.R.; Wang, X.; Franklin, J. Changes in bone marrow morphology in adults receiving romiplostim for the treatment of thrombocytopenia associated with primary immune thrombocytopenia. *Ann. Hematol.* **2016**, *95*, 1077–1087. [CrossRef] [PubMed]
114. Lambert, M.P. TPO-mimetics and myelofibrosis? A reticulin question! *Blood* **2009**, *114*, 3722–3723. [CrossRef] [PubMed]
115. Kuter, D.J.; Mufti, G.J.; Bain, B.J.; Hasserjian, R.P.; Davis, W.; Rutstein, M. Evaluation of bone marrow reticulin formation in chronic immune thrombocytopenia patients treated with romiplostim. *Blood* **2009**, *114*, 3748–3756. [CrossRef] [PubMed]
116. Garnock-Jones, K.P. Spotlight on eltrombopag in treatment-refractory chronic primary immune thrombocytopenia. *BioDrugs* **2011**, *25*, 401–404. [CrossRef]
117. Al-Samkari, H.; Kuter, D.J. An alternative intermittent eltrombopag dosing protocol for the treatment of chronic immune thrombocytopenia. *Br. J. Clin. Pharmacol.* **2018**, *84*, 2673–2677. [CrossRef]
118. Promacta®Prescription Information. Available online: www.accessdata.fda.gov/drugsatfda_docs/label/2015/207027s000lbl.pdf (accessed on 2 January 2021).
119. Bussel, J.B.; Provan, D.; Shamsi, T.; Cheng, G.; Psaila, B.; Kovaleva, L.; Salama, A.; Jenkins, J.M.; Roychowdhury, D.; Mayer, B.; et al. Effect of eltrombopag on platelet counts and bleeding during treatment of chronic idiopathic thrombocytopenic purpura: A randomised, double-blind, placebo-controlled trial. *Lancet* **2009**, *373*, 641–648. [CrossRef]
120. Tomiyama, Y.; Miyakawa, Y.; Okamoto, S.; Katsutani, S.; Kimura, A.; Okoshi, Y.; Ninomiya, H.; Kosugi, H.; Nomura, S.; Ozaki, K.; et al. A lower starting dose of eltrombopag is efficacious in Japanese patients with previously treated chronic immune thrombocytopenia. *J. Thromb. Haemost.* **2012**, *10*, 799–806. [CrossRef]
121. Yang, R.; Hou, M.; Li, J. Effect of eltrombopag on platelet response and safety results in Chinese adults with chronic ITP-primary result of a phase III study (abstract). *Blood* **2014**, *124*, 1464. [CrossRef]
122. Cheng, G.; Saleh, M.N.; Marcher, C.; Vasey, S.; Mayer, B.; Aivado, M.; Arning, M.; Stone, N.L.; Bussel, J.B. Eltrombopag for management of chronic immune thrombocytopenia (RAISE): A 6-month, randomised, phase 3 study. *Lancet* **2011**, *377*, 393–402. [CrossRef]
123. Wong, R.S.M.; Saleh, M.N.; Khelif, A.; Salama, A.; Portella, M.S.O.; Burgess, P.; Bussel, J.B. Safety and efficacy of long-term treatment of chronic/persistent ITP with eltrombopag: Final results of the EXTEND study. *Blood* **2017**, *130*, 2527–2536. [CrossRef] [PubMed]
124. González-López, T.J.; Pascual, C.; Álvarez-Román, M.T.; Fernández-Fuertes, F.; Sánchez-González, B.; Caparrós, I.; Jarque, I.; Mingot-Castellano, M.E.; Hernández-Rivas, J.A.; Martín-Salces, M.; et al. Successful discontinuation of eltrombopag after complete remission in patients with primary immune thrombocytopenia. *Am. J. Hematol.* **2015**, *90*, E40–E43. [CrossRef]
125. Al-Samkari, H.; Kuter, D.J. Thrombopoietin level predicts response to treatment with eltrombopag and romiplostim in immune thrombocytopenia. *Am. J. Hematol.* **2018**, *93*, 1501–1508. [CrossRef]
126. Mishra, K.; Pramanik, S.; Jandial, A.; Sahu, K.K.; Sandal, R.; Ahuja, A.; Yanamandra, U.; Kumar, R.; Kapoor, R.; Verma, T.; et al. Real-world experience of eltrombopag in immune thrombocytopenia. *Am. J. Blood Res.* **2020**, *10*, 240–251. [PubMed]
127. Doptelet®Prescribtion Information. Available online: www.accessdata.fda.gov/drugsatfda_docs/label/2018/210238s000lbl.pdf (accessed on 8 January 2021).
128. Jurczak, W.; Chojnowski, K.; Mayer, J.; Krawczyk, K.; Jamieson, B.D.; Tian, W.; Allen, L.F. Phase 3 randomised study of avatrombopag, a novel thrombopoietin receptor agonist for the treatment of chronic immune thrombocytopenia. *Br. J. Haematol.* **2018**, *183*, 479–490. [CrossRef] [PubMed]
129. Godeau, B. B-cell depletion in immune thrombocytopenia. *Semin. Hematol.* **2013**, *50* (Suppl. 1), S75–S82. [CrossRef] [PubMed]
130. Chugh, S.; Darvish-Kazem, S.; Lim, W.; Crowther, M.A.; Ghanima, W.; Wang, G.; Heddle, N.M.; Kelton, J.G.; Arnold, D.M. Rituximab plus standard of care for treatment of primary immune thrombocytopenia: A systematic review and meta-analysis. *Lancet Haematol.* **2015**, *2*, e75–e81. [CrossRef]
131. Patel, V.L.; Mahévas, M.; Lee, S.Y.; Stasi, R.; Cunningham-Rundles, S.; Godeau, B.; Kanter, J.; Neufeld, E.; Taube, T.; Ramenghi, U.; et al. Outcomes 5 years after response to rituximab therapy in children and adults with immune thrombocytopenia. *Blood* **2012**, *119*, 5989–5995. [CrossRef]
132. Ghanima, W.; Khelif, A.; Waage, A.; Michel, M.; Tjønnfjord, G.E.; Romdhan, N.B.; Kahrs, J.; Darne, B.; Holme, P.A. Rituximab as second-line treatment for adult immune thrombocytopenia (the RITP trial): a multicentre, randomised, double-blind, placebo-controlled trial. *Lancet* **2015**, *385*, 1653–1661. [CrossRef]
133. Li, Y.; Shi, Y.; He, Z.; Chen, Q.; Liu, Z.; Yu, L.; Wang, C. The efficacy and safety of low-dose rituximab in immune thrombocytopenia: a systematic review and meta-analysis. *Platelets* **2019**, *30*, 690–697. [CrossRef]
134. Tjønnfjord, E.; Holme, P.A.; Darne, B.; Khelif, A.; Waage, A.; Michel, M.; Ben Romdhan, N.; Ghanima, W. Long-term outcomes of patients treated with rituximab as second-line treatment for adult immune thrombocytopenia - Follow-up of the RITP study. *Br. J. Haematol.* **2020**, *191*, 460–465. [CrossRef]
135. Hammond, W.A.; Vishnu, P.; Rodriguez, E.M.; Li, Z.; Dholaria, B.; Shreders, A.J.; Rivera, C.E. Sequence of Splenectomy and Rituximab for the Treatment of Steroid-Refractory Immune Thrombocytopenia: Does It Matter? *Mayo Clin. Proc.* **2019**, *94*, 2199–2208. [CrossRef]
136. Wang, Y.-M.; Yu, Y.-F.; Liu, Y.; Liu, S.; Hou, M.; Liu, X.-G. The association between antinuclear antibody and response to rituximab treatment in adult patients with primary immune thrombocytopenia. *Hematology* **2020**, *25*, 139–144. [CrossRef] [PubMed]

137. Khellaf, M.; Charles-Nelson, A.; Fain, O.; Terriou, L.; Viallard, J.-F.; Cheze, S.; Graveleau, J.; Slama, B.; Audia, S.; Ebbo, M.; et al. Safety and efficacy of rituximab in adult immune thrombocytopenia: Results from a prospective registry including 248 patients. *Blood* **2014**, *124*, 3228–3236. [CrossRef] [PubMed]
138. Puavilai, T.; Thadanipon, K.; Rattanasiri, S.; Ingsathit, A.; McEvoy, M.; Attia, J.; Thakkinstian, A. Treatment efficacy for adult persistent immune thrombocytopenia: A systematic review and network meta-analysis. *Br. J. Haematol.* **2020**, *188*, 450–459. [CrossRef] [PubMed]
139. Podolanczuk, A.; Lazarus, A.H.; Crow, A.R.; Grossbard, E.; Bussel, J.B. Of mice and men: an open-label pilot study for treatment of immune thrombocytopenic purpura by an inhibitor of Syk. *Blood* **2009**, *113*, 3154–3160. [CrossRef] [PubMed]
140. Bussel, J.; Arnold, D.M.; Grossbard, E.; Mayer, J.; Treliński, J.; Homenda, W.; Hellmann, A.; Windyga, J.; Sivcheva, L.; Khalafallah, A.A.; et al. Fostamatinib for the treatment of adult persistent and chronic immune thrombocytopenia: Results of two phase 3, randomized, placebo-controlled trials. *Am. J. Hematol.* **2018**, *93*, 921–930. [CrossRef]
141. Bussel, J.B.; Arnold, D.M.; Boxer, M.A.; Cooper, N.; Mayer, J.; Zayed, H.; Tong, S.; Duliege, A.-M. Long-term fostamatinib treatment of adults with immune thrombocytopenia during the phase 3 clinical trial program. *Am. J. Hematol.* **2019**, *94*, 546–553. [CrossRef]
142. Boccia, R.; Cooper, N.; Ghanima, W.; Boxer, M.A.; Hill, Q.A.; Sholzberg, M.; Tarantino, M.D.; Todd, L.K.; Tong, S.; Bussel, J.B. Fostamatinib is an effective second-line therapy in patients with immune thrombocytopenia. *Br. J. Haematol.* **2020**, *190*, 933–938. [CrossRef]
143. Tavalisse®Prescription Information. Available online: https://www.accessdata.fda.gov/drugsatfda_docs/label/2018/209299lbl.pdf (accessed on 2 January 2021).
144. Chaturvedi, S.; Arnold, D.M.; McCrae, K.R. Splenectomy for immune thrombocytopenia: Down but not out. *Blood* **2018**, *131*, 1172–1182. [CrossRef]
145. Palandri, F.; Polverelli, N.; Sollazzo, D.; Romano, M.; Catani, L.; Cavo, M.; Vianelli, N. Have splenectomy rate and main outcomes of ITP changed after the introduction of new treatments? A monocentric study in the outpatient setting during 35 years. *Am. J. Hematol.* **2016**, *91*, E267–E272. [CrossRef]
146. Kojouri, K.; Vesely, S.K.; Terrell, D.R.; George, J.N. Splenectomy for adult patients with idiopathic thrombocytopenic purpura: a systematic review to assess long-term platelet count responses, prediction of response, and surgical complications. *Blood* **2004**, *104*, 2623–2634. [CrossRef]
147. Lal, L.S.; Said, Q.; Andrade, K.; Cuker, A. Second-line treatments and outcomes for immune thrombocytopenia: A retrospective study with electronic health records. *Res. Pract. Thromb. Haemost.* **2020**, *4*, 1131–1140. [CrossRef] [PubMed]
148. Vianelli, N.; Palandri, F.; Polverelli, N.; Stasi, R.; Joelsson, J.; Johansson, E.; Ruggeri, M.; Zaja, F.; Cantoni, S.; Catucci, A.E.; et al. Splenectomy as a curative treatment for immune thrombocytopenia: A retrospective analysis of 233 patients with a minimum follow up of 10 years. *Haematologica* **2013**, *98*, 875–880. [CrossRef] [PubMed]
149. Amini, S.N.; Nelson, V.S.; Sobels, A.; Schoones, J.W.; Zwaginga, J.J.; Schipperus, M.R. Autologous platelet scintigraphy and clinical outcome of splenectomy in immune thrombocytopenia: A systematic review and meta-analysis. *Crit. Rev. Oncol. Hematol.* **2020**, *153*, 103040. [CrossRef] [PubMed]
150. Qu, Y.; Xu, J.; Jiao, C.; Cheng, Z.; Ren, S. Long-Term Outcomes of Laparoscopic Splenectomy Versus Open Splenectomy for Idiopathic Thrombocytopenic Purpura. *Int. Surg.* **2014**, *99*, 286–290. [CrossRef] [PubMed]
151. Nørgaard, M.; Cetin, K.; Maegbaek, M.L.; Kristensen, N.R.; Ghanima, W.; Bahmanyar, S.; Stryker, S.; Christiansen, C.F. Risk of arterial thrombotic and venous thromboembolic events in patients with primary chronic immune thrombocytopenia: A Scandinavian population-based cohort study. *Br. J. Haematol.* **2016**, *174*, 639–642. [CrossRef]
152. Boyle, S.; White, R.H.; Brunson, A.; Wun, T. Splenectomy and the incidence of venous thromboembolism and sepsis in patients with immune thrombocytopenia. *Blood* **2013**, *121*, 4782–4790. [CrossRef]
153. Maria, L.A.; Nour, A.; Eleanor, P.; Victor, B.; Paul, I.; Thomas, K.; Intercontinental, C.I.S.G. Long-term outcomes after splenectomy in children with immune thrombocytopenia: An update on the registry data from the Intercontinental Cooperative ITP Study Group. *Haematologica* **2019**, *105*, 2682–2685. [CrossRef]
154. Kwiatkowska, A.; Radkowiak, D.; Wysocki, M.; Torbicz, G.; Gajewska, N.; Lasek, A.; Kulawik, J.; Budzyński, A.; Pędziwiatr, M. Prognostic Factors for Immune Thrombocytopenic Purpura Remission after Laparoscopic Splenectomy: A Cohort Study. *Medicina (Kaunas)* **2019**, *55*. [CrossRef]
155. Gonzalez-Porras, J.R.; Escalante, F.; Pardal, E.; Sierra, M.; Garcia-Frade, L.J.; Redondo, S.; Arefi, M.; Aguilar, C.; Ortega, F.; de Cabo, E.; et al. Safety and efficacy of splenectomy in over 65-yrs-old patients with immune thrombocytopenia. *Eur. J. Haematol.* **2013**, *91*, 236–241. [CrossRef] [PubMed]
156. Park, Y.H.; Yi, H.G.; Kim, C.S.; Hong, J.; Park, J.; Lee, J.H.; Kim, H.Y.; Kim, H.J.; Zang, D.Y.; Kim, S.H.; et al. Clinical Outcome and Predictive Factors in the Response to Splenectomy in Elderly Patients with Primary Immune Thrombocytopenia: A Multicenter Retrospective Study. *Acta Haematol.* **2016**, *135*, 162–171. [CrossRef]
157. Robak, T.; Kaźmierczak, M.; Jarque, I.; Musteata, V.; Treliński, J.; Cooper, N.; Kiessling, P.; Massow, U.; Woltering, F.; Snipes, R.; et al. Phase 2 multiple-dose study of an FcRn inhibitor, rozanolixizumab, in patients with primary immune thrombocytopenia. *Blood Adv.* **2020**, *4*, 4136–4146. [CrossRef]

158. Li, G.; Wang, S.; Li, N.; Liu, Y.; Feng, Q.; Zuo, X.; Li, X.; Hou, Y.; Shao, L.; Ma, C.; et al. Proteasome Inhibition with Bortezomib Induces Apoptosis of Long-Lived Plasma Cells in Steroid-Resistant or Relapsed Immune Thrombocytopaenia. *Thromb. Haemost.* **2018**, *118*, 1752–1764. [CrossRef] [PubMed]
159. Beckman, J.D.; Rollins-Raval, M.A.; Raval, J.S.; Park, Y.A.; Mazepa, M.; Ma, A. Bortezomib for Refractory Immune-Mediated Thrombocytopenia Purpura. *Am. J. Ther.* **2018**, *25*, e270–e272. [CrossRef]
160. Newland, A.C.; Sánchez-González, B.; Rejtő, L.; Egyed, M.; Romanyuk, N.; Godar, M.; Verschueren, K.; Gandini, D.; Ulrichts, P.; Beauchamp, J.; et al. Phase 2 study of efgartigimod, a novel FcRn antagonist, in adult patients with primary immune thrombocytopenia. *Am. J. Hematol.* **2020**, *95*, 178–187. [CrossRef]
161. Chen, Z.; Guo, Z.; Ma, J.; Ma, J.; Liu, F.; Wu, R. Foxp3 methylation status in children with primary immune thrombocytopenia. *Hum. Immunol.* **2014**, *75*, 1115–1119. [CrossRef]
162. Ding, K.; Fu, R.; Liu, H.; Nachnani, D.A.; Shao, Z.-H. Effects of decitabine on megakaryocyte maturation in patients with myelodysplastic syndromes. *Oncol. Lett.* **2016**, *11*, 2347–2352. [CrossRef]
163. Zhou, H.; Hou, Y.; Liu, X.; Qiu, J.; Feng, Q.; Wang, Y.; Zhang, X.; Min, Y.; Shao, L.; Liu, X.; et al. Low-dose decitabine promotes megakaryocyte maturation and platelet production in healthy controls and immune thrombocytopenia. *Thromb. Haemost.* **2015**, *113*, 1021–1034. [CrossRef] [PubMed]
164. Zhou, H.; Qin, P.; Liu, Q.; Yuan, C.; Hao, Y.; Zhang, H.; Wang, Z.; Ran, X.; Chu, X.; Yu, W.; et al. A prospective, multicenter study of low dose decitabine in adult patients with refractory immune thrombocytopenia. *Am. J. Hematol.* **2019**, *94*, 1374–1381. [CrossRef] [PubMed]
165. Levi, M.; Thachil, J. Coronavirus Disease 2019 Coagulopathy: Disseminated Intravascular Coagulation and Thrombotic Microangiopathy-Either, Neither, or Both. *Semin. Thromb. Hemost.* **2020**, *46*, 781–784. [CrossRef] [PubMed]
166. Pavord, S.; Thachil, J.; Hunt, B.J.; Murphy, M.; Lowe, G.; Laffan, M.; Makris, M.; Newland, A.C.; Provan, D.; Grainger, J.D.; et al. Practical guidance for the management of adults with immune thrombocytopenia during the COVID-19 pandemic. *Br. J. Haematol.* **2020**, *189*, 1038–1043. [CrossRef] [PubMed]
167. Mahévas, M.; Moulis, G.; Andres, E.; Riviere, E.; Garzaro, M.; Crickx, E.; Guillotin, V.; Malphettes, M.; Galicier, L.; Noel, N.; et al. Clinical characteristics, management and outcome of COVID-19-associated immune thrombocytopenia: a French multicentre series. *Br. J. Haematol.* **2020**, *190*, e224–e229. [CrossRef] [PubMed]

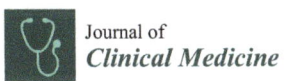

Review

Thrombocytopenia in Virus Infections

Matthijs Raadsen [1], Justin Du Toit [2], Thomas Langerak [1], Bas van Bussel [3,4], Eric van Gorp [1,5] and Marco Goeijenbier [1,5,*]

1. Department of Viroscience, Erasmus MC Rotterdam, Doctor molewaterplein 40, 3015 GD Rotterdam, The Netherlands; m.p.raadsen@erasmusmc.nl (M.R.); thomas.langerak@erasmusmc.nl (T.L.); e.vangorp@erasmusmc.nl (E.v.G.)
2. Department of Haematology, Wits University Donald Gordon Medical Centre Johannesburg, Johannesburg 2041, South Africa; justinr_dutoit@yahoo.com
3. Department of Intensive Care Medicine, Maastricht University Medical Center Plus, 6229 HX Maastricht, The Netherlands; bas.van.bussel@mumc.nl
4. Care and Public Health Research Institute (CAPHRI), Maastricht University, 6229 GT Maastricht, The Netherlands
5. Department of Internal Medicine, Erasmus MC Rotterdam, 3000 CA Rotterdam, The Netherlands
* Correspondence: m.goeijenbier@erasmusmc.nl

Abstract: Thrombocytopenia, which signifies a low platelet count usually below 150×10^9/L, is a common finding following or during many viral infections. In clinical medicine, mild thrombocytopenia, combined with lymphopenia in a patient with signs and symptoms of an infectious disease, raises the suspicion of a viral infection. This phenomenon is classically attributed to platelet consumption due to inflammation-induced coagulation, sequestration from the circulation by phagocytosis and hypersplenism, and impaired platelet production due to defective megakaryopoiesis or cytokine-induced myelosuppression. All these mechanisms, while plausible and supported by substantial evidence, regard platelets as passive bystanders during viral infection. However, platelets are increasingly recognized as active players in the (antiviral) immune response and have been shown to interact with cells of the innate and adaptive immune system as well as directly with viruses. These findings can be of interest both for understanding the pathogenesis of viral infectious diseases and predicting outcome. In this review, we will summarize and discuss the literature currently available on various mechanisms within the relationship between thrombocytopenia and virus infections.

Keywords: virus infection; thrombocytopenia; thrombocytopathy; aggregation; HIV; SARS-CoV-2; hantavirus; coronavirus; influenza

1. Introduction

In patients presenting to care with signs or symptoms of infectious disease, a full blood count is part of a routine diagnostic evaluation. Mild thrombocytopenia, often combined with lymphocytopenia is typical of most acute viral infections, but neither are sufficiently sensitive nor specific to reliably distinguish viral from bacterial or parasitic pathogens. Except for viral hemorrhagic fevers and rare cases of severe disseminated viral infections, virus-induced thrombocytopenia does not lead to significant bleeding, rarely requires platelet transfusions, and is therefore easily dismissed as clinically irrelevant. However, when the relationship between platelets and viral infection is studied more closely and in larger study populations, important findings emerge which shed light on previously unrecognized aspects of viral diseases. The incidence of thromboembolic complications is elevated in individuals during and after influenza virus infection, for example, a relation which may not be apparent to physicians diagnosing and treating influenza-like illness [1]. Platelet counts during peak symptomatic disease have also been found to be a marker of disease severity in certain viral infections, [2–19] or can serve as a first clue towards diagnosing chronic viral infections [20–23]. These phenomena are typically not explained by changes in platelet quantity, but rather by the effects of viral infections on platelet function.

Platelets are small, anucleate cells that circulate in the blood for approximately 7 to 10 days after being formed. Their main physiological role is hemostasis, forming blood clots (thrombi) to safeguard vascular integrity. Platelets originate from megakaryocytes, which are giant polyploid cells residing in the bone marrow that have themselves formed from hematopoietic stem cells. Megakaryocytes develop proplatelets that bud off numerous platelets into the blood stream, after endoplasmic maturation [24]. In individuals with normal bone marrow function, platelets circulate at levels between 150 to 450 $\times$ 10^9/L [25]. Megakaryopoiesis is stimulated by a number of cytokines, with Stromal Derived Factor 1 (SDF-1), Granulocyte-Monocyte Colony Stimulating Factor (GM-CSF) Interleukins (IL-3, IL-6, and IL-11) Fibroblast Growth factor 4 (FGF-4) and thrombopoietin (TPO) being the most important [26]. Whereas TPO plays a crucial role in maintenance of hematopoietic stem cells [27], most of these cytokines are proinflammatory and induce rapid maturation and activation of leukocytes, as well as stimulating megakaryopoiesis, which illustrates how platelet production is affected by inflammatory processes.

Conversely, platelets also affect the inflammatory response to viral infection and can even internalize several viruses directly. In response to infection, platelets interact with leukocytes and vascular endothelial cells before activating and secreting soluble prothrombotic and inflammatory mediators stored within granules [28]. Despite not having a nucleus, platelets do contain some RNA and maintain a limited ability for protein translation, enabling some regulation of this response [29], but also potentially supporting replication of some RNA viruses [30].

In this review, all of the literature on the relationship between platelets and viral infectious diseases published between 2010 and late 2020 has been systematically assessed and summarized in a narrative format, classified per virus category.

2. Search Strategy

The online database from the national Center of biotechnology information, Pubmed, was queried on August 3rd 2020 using the search term available in the supplemental information section included with this paper. This search was repeated on December 21st 2020, in order to include the latest publications on the currently pandemic Severe Acute Respiratory Syndrome Coronavirus 2 (SARS-CoV-2).

Additional filters were applied to restrict results to original research papers published during the previous 10 years, related to humans and with full text available. Individual papers were assessed by the first author, based on title and abstract for relevance, originality and quality and sorted based on virus species or virus family. The findings of the papers that are relevant for the subject matter of this review were presented in a narrative format within the following subgroups: "General Topics", "Arboviruses", "Blood Borne Viruses", "Rodent Borne Viruses", "Gastrointestinal Viruses", "Herpesviruses" and "Respiratory tract Viruses". Additional references were added to provide more context when necessary.

3. Results

The search yielded 413 papers. The results of the author classification process are summarized in Figure 1.

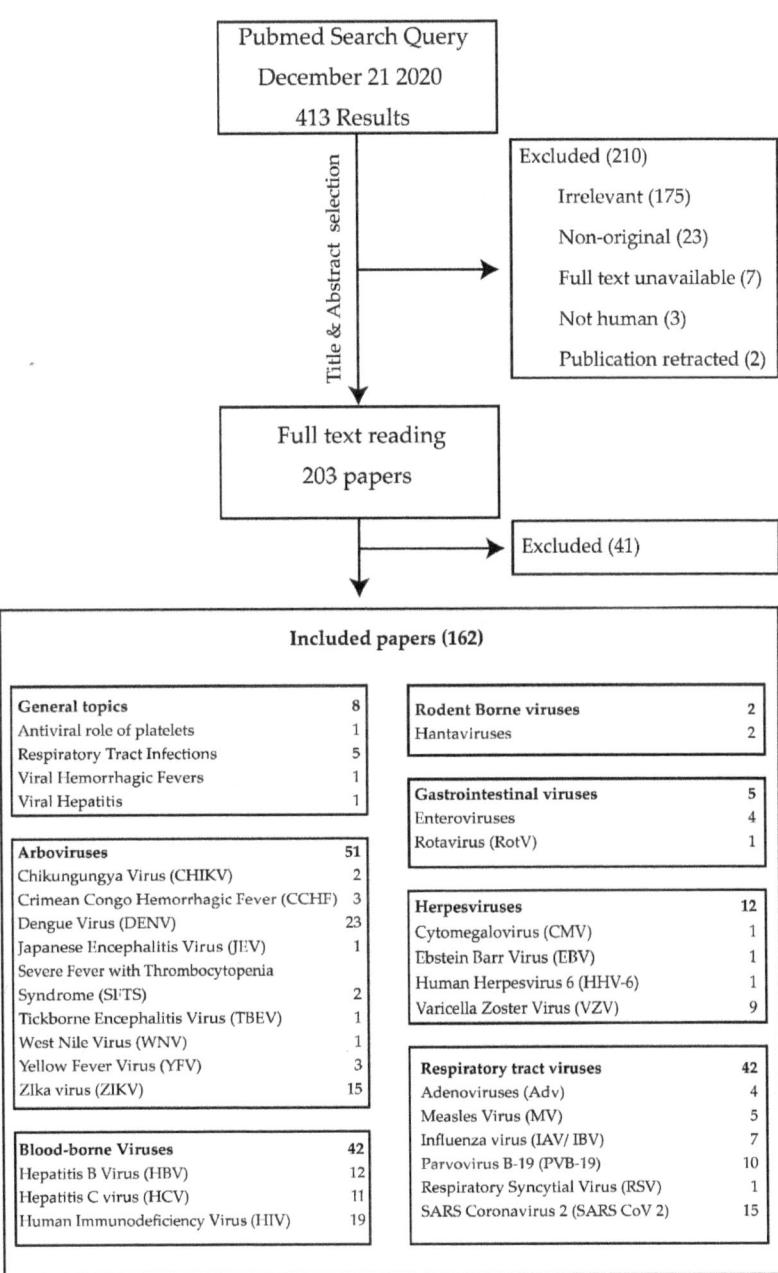

Figure 1. Flow diagram of PubMed search results.

3.1. Platelets and Viral Infections: General Principles

An overview of the mechanisms that contribute to thrombocytopenia in the main viral infections discussed in this review, including references, can be found in Table 1.

3.1.1. Aggregation

Platelet agglutination or adhesion to leukocytes is often found in patients with systemic inflammatory diseases, including viral infections. Standard automated hematology analyzers are often unable to accurately detect leukocyte-bound platelets or platelet aggregates, leading to a false finding of a reduced platelet count (pseudo-thrombocytopenia). This can also be caused by drawing blood into tubes containing EDTA, the most common anticoagulant used for complete blood counts. If pseudo-thrombocytopenia is suspected, performing a manual peripheral blood smear or repeating the platelet count in using different anticoagulants, can help avoid unnecessary diagnostic procedures or transfusions [31]. Isolated thrombocytopenia should prompt investigation into chronic viral infections, such as hepatitis B, C and HIV, whereas leukocyte abnormalities and rise in other infection biomarkers, raises suspicions of an acute viral illness [32].

3.1.2. Impaired Hematopoiesis

One of the most common accepted etiologies underlying virus-induced thrombocytopenia is the one where viruses can directly infect bone marrow stromal cells and hematopoietic stem cells leading to defective hematopoiesis and thrombocytopenia [33]. Furthermore, decreased platelet production can be the result of changed cytokine profiles, during infection, leading to lower TPO production in the liver, reducing megakaryopoiesis [34,35]. Finally, viruses can infect and replicate in megakaryocytes while other viruses modulate megakaryocyte function or decrease the expression of Myeloproliferative Leukemia Protein (c-MPL), the receptor for TPO, leading megakaryocyte destruction and subsequent lowered platelet production [36–38].

3.1.3. Sequestration and Intravascular Destruction

Platelet destruction can occur via direct interaction of platelets with viruses. This interaction occurs via a range of receptors including Toll-Like Receptors (TLRs), integrins (GPIIb/IIIa) and c-type lectins (CLEC), that interact with the different viruses leading to platelet activation, degranulation and clearance in liver and spleen [39–41]. Upon viral infection the host defense generally induces a systemic inflammatory response, which leads to platelet activation and subsequent clearance [42]. Furthermore, platelets can bind to neutrophils, forming platelet-neutrophil aggregates, which in turn triggers the phagocytosis of platelets [43,44]. Additionally, many viruses can activate the coagulation system by induction of tissue factor leading to thrombin generation and platelet activation with subsequent platelet clearance via protease activating receptor (PAR) signaling. PARs are present on platelets, leucocytes and endothelial cells which modulate the innate immune responses [45]. Platelets can bind immunoglobulins (attached to viruses) via Fc-gamma-RII receptors leading to platelet activation, aggregation and clearance [46,47], while immunoglobulins produced by B-lymphocytes that target viruses can cross-react with platelet surface integrins (GPIIb/IIIa or GPIb-IX-V) leading to immune thrombocytopenia (ITP) [48]. In depth, more virus specific mechanisms will be discussed in the specific virus groups.

3.1.4. Platelet Expression of Pattern Recognition Receptors (PRR)

PRRs such as TLRs and CLECs, [49] or messenger ribonucleic acids (mRNAs) can identify pathogen associated molecular patterns (PAMPs) from viruses and many are expressed by platelets [44]. This direct interaction of a virus or its genome with PRR can lead to platelet activation and subsequent release of chemokines. This enhances endothelial cell signaling, leucocyte migration and direct interaction and activation of leucocytes [50]. These complex interactions may have both an immune protective mechanism, [44] or be injurious to the host.

3.1.5. Platelets Can Induce Inflammation and Secrete Anti-Microbial Proteins

Activated platelets undergo degranulation and release numerous inflammatory mediators, cytokines and chemokines stored in granules. Three types of granules exist: α granules, dense granules and lysosomal granules. These granules contain different molecules that can exert pro-thrombotic and immune effects leading to direct and indirect interactions with different pro-inflammatory immune cells, causing a local or systemic inflammatory milieu [51]. In addition, the α-granules can secrete platelet microbicidal peptides (PMPs) that have direct anti-viral effects, for example, it has previously been shown that synthetic PMPs have strong viricidal effects against vaccinia virus [52].

3.1.6. Platelets Act as Antigen Presenting Cells (APCs)

APCs require MHC-I molecules to present antigen to CD8+ T cells. There is evidence now that platelets and megakaryocytes contain all the MHC-I and co-stimulatory molecules necessary for antigen presentation including the entire proteome [53,54]. In addition, it has been shown that platelets can successfully present ovalbumin and malarial antigens to activate CD8+ T cells [55].

3.2. Arboviruses

Arthropod borne viruses (arboviruses) are viruses that are transmitted to humans through arthropods, mainly mosquitoes and ticks. Some of these arboviruses, especially flaviviruses, potentially cause hemorrhagic fever. In this section, we will discuss the most prevalent arboviruses as well as potentially emerging arboviruses.

3.2.1. Dengue Virus

With an estimated 390 million annual infections, dengue virus (DENV) is the most prevalent arbovirus worldwide [56]. Thrombocytopenia is a hallmark of severe DENV infection and platelet levels are lower in DENV infected patients compared to other febrile illnesses [57]. Severe thrombocytopenia $<20 \times 10^9$/L occurs frequently in hospitalized dengue patients, and is associated with prolonged admission, plasma leakage and the presence of clinical warning signs [58,59]. Severe DENV infections with severe thrombocytopenia, hemorrhage and plasma leakage, occur more often in secondary DENV infection compared to primary DENV infection, due to antibody-dependent enhancement [60–62]. Below, the many mechanisms for thrombocytopenia in DENV disease that have been identified will be discussed.

Platelets can directly be activated by circulating DENV particles and by immune factors released during the acute phase of DENV infection. This activation induces upregulation of platelet adhesion molecules on the surface of vascular endothelial cells, causing more indirect platelet activation [63,64]. Activated platelets undergo degranulation, attach themselves to the vascular wall and form thrombi, effectively removing them from the circulation, which results in thrombocytopenia. Despite this activation, platelets from dengue patients are hyporesponsive to procoagulant stimuli in aggregometry assays, which is likely the result of exhaustion [65]. This illustrates thrombocytopenia and platelet dysfunction go hand in hand during DENV infection. The DENV NS1 protein interacts with both TLR 4 and TLR 2, expressed by platelets, leading to platelet activation, aggregation, adherence to endothelial cells and phagocytosis by macrophages [66]. DENV can also activate platelets via CLEC2, that in turn stimulate macrophages and neutrophils via CLEC5A and TLR 2. Activated neutrophils subsequently form Neutrophil Extracellular Traps (NETs), providing a scaffold for prothrombotic factors, such as platelets, red blood cells and molecules involved in both the intrinsic and extrinsic coagulation pathways. NETs also activate platelets via TLR-4, creating a positive feedback loop between NETosis and platelet activation. These mechanisms contribute to thrombocytopenia, bleeding, vascular leakage and lethality in mouse models of dengue hemorrhagic shock syndrome [66,67]. The formation of platelet-monocyte aggregates in DENV infection has also been demonstrated and correlates with thrombocytopenia and clinical signs of vascular leakage [68,69]. These platelets alter the monocyte's innate immune response, by inducing production of IL-10 [68] and inhibiting the production of interferon α [70]. Serotonin enhances DENV-mediated platelet activation and is released by perivascular mast cells in a mouse model of DENV infection, leading to thrombocytopenia, suggesting serotonin-blocking drugs might be beneficial [71]. Platelet activating factor (PAF) is another inducer of platelet aggregation and vascular leakage elevated in plasma of acute dengue patients. A recent small phase II randomized placebo-controlled clinical trial showed that Rupatadine, a licensed antihistamine with PAF receptor blocking activity, is safe in acute dengue patients, but not clinically beneficial, with no effect on nadir platelet counts [72].

In response to DENV infection, the immune system also depletes platelets through direct cytotoxic effects. This occurs through complement factor C3 binding to the platelet surface and opsonization of platelets by DENV NS1 specific IgG, leading to subsequent phagocytosis by macrophages [73,74]. The observation that patients with severe DENV infection have increased afucosylated IgG1 antibodies and that these antibodies can cross-react with platelet antigens, further supports the notion that platelet-NS1 cross-reactive antibodies contribute to the depletion of platelets during severe DENV infection [75]. Infusion of anti-NS1 IgG cannot elicit thrombocytopenia in mouse models. However, it does enhance thrombocytopenia when administered during DENV infection. This could indicate that platelet binding and destruction is mediated by IgG bound NS1 dimers, rather than a direct interaction between cross-reactive IgG and platelets. This could have implications for vaccine design [76,77]. Platelets upregulate their expression of Human Leukocyte Antigen (HLA) class I molecules in the presence of DENV, suggesting a possible role in viral antigen presentation and T cell mediated cytotoxicity as a mechanism for thrombocytopenia [64].

A third mechanism is direct infection of platelets and megakaryocytes by DENV, leading to viral replication, cell lysis and impaired production of platelets. DENV infects platelets by binding DC-SIGN (CD209) and heparan sulfate proteoglycan (HSP) on the platelet surface and indirectly via Fc receptor FcγR2A (CD32), after binding of antibodies to the virus particle [30]. The presence of DENV specific antibodies is not required for platelet infection [78]. Especially during the viremic stage and in those patients with more severe dengue, less DC-SIGN and FcγR2A expression is detected on platelets when compared to patients suffering from other febrile illnesses. The relation between this phenomenon with thrombocytopenia has not been explored however and it is unclear whether the presence of DENV particles in the blood could interfere with the binding of the detection antibodies. There could also be a survival advantage of platelets with low DC-SIGN and FcγR2A expression [79]. DENV productively infects a megakaryoblast-like cell line, using Glycoprotein Ib (GPIb) and was found circulating megakaryocyte-like cells in Rhesus Macaques [80]. This suggests that DENV can infect mature megakaryocytes and impair platelet production and survival through replication, although this has not been confirmed in vivo [81].

3.2.2. Chikungunya virus (CHIKV)

Despite sharing many clinical characteristics with DENV, thrombocytopenia has only been occasionally described in CHIKV infected patients [82]. In a cross-sectional study of arbovirus infections in Pakistan, thrombocytopenia was observed in 18% of CHIKV infections, compared to 74% in DENV. Furthermore, thrombocytosis was significantly associated with CHIKV infection (OR 2.2) [83].

3.2.3. Crimean Congo Hemorrhagic Fever (CCHF)

CCHF is a tick-borne virus from the Bunyaviridae family that is associated with pronounced thrombocytopenia, accompanied by bleeding complications [84]. CCHF cases with bleeding have lower platelet counts and slightly raised platelet distribution width compared to those who do not bleed [85]. A lower platelet lymphocyte ratio (PLR) upon presentation to hospital care is predictive of adverse clinical outcomes in CCHF patients [6].

3.2.4. Japanese Encephalitis Virus (JEV)

This vaccine preventable flavivirus has a wide distribution in eastern Asia. Although central nervous system infection has a substantial mortality rate of 20–30%, most cases are either asymptomatic or mild, without clinically overt signs of encephalitis [86]. A recent prospective study performed in hospitalized patients with dengue-negative febrile illness in Indonesia found that 6% had serological evidence of recent JEV infection. Thrombocytopenia was common during the acute phase of illness in these non-encephalitic cases (69%) but did not occur as frequently as dengue cases from the same study (92%) [87].

3.2.5. Severe Fever with Thrombocytopenia Syndrome (SFTS)

SFTS is an emerging infectious disease caused by a recently discovered Bunyavirus that, as the name suggests, is associated with profound thrombocytopenia [88]. DC-SIGN, which is expressed by human platelets, was identified as a receptor for Bunya viruses, but no studies have shown virus entry or replication of SFTS in platelets [89]. A recent detailed study in Chinese SFTS patients revealed a severity-dependent depletion of the essential amino acid arginine due to arginase released by granulocytic Myeloid-derived suppressor cells (gMDSC's), which are recruited during the acute stage of the disease. The resulting lack of both arginine and its metabolite, nitric oxide, are believed to disinhibit platelet activation, leading to platelet aggregation, destruction and thrombocytopenia. A randomized, non-controlled clinical trial was performed were arginine supplementation with best supportive care was compared with supportive care alone. Whilst not demonstrating a statistically significant survival benefit, platelet counts returned to normal more rapidly in the treatment arm [90].

3.2.6. Tick-Borne Encephalitis Virus (TBEV)

TBEV is a flavivirus that is transmitted through bites of ticks and is prevalent in Europe and northeastern Asia [91]. After initial viremia, the central nervous system may become infected, which can result in severe neurological damage and occasionally death. Like most other viruses that can enter the bloodstream, TBEV causes thrombocytopenia, albeit generally mild and not typically associated with bleeding. A case–control study in patients with suspected and confirmed central nervous system infections, reported a decreased mean platelet count in TBE cases versus neuroborreliosis cases. However, the mean platelet count (173.8×10^9/L) remained above the lower limit of normal in the TBE group. In addition, platelet counts correlated positively with concentrations in serum of IL-23, a cytokine secreted by dendritic cells, which is believed to stimulate essential host-defense mechanisms against viruses [92]. This could indicate a role for IL-23 in stimulating megakaryopoiesis during TBEV infection.

3.2.7. Viral Hemorrhagic Fevers (VHF)

The extreme containment precautions required to study the most highly pathogenic VHF's, such as Ebolavirus, Marburgvirus and Lassavirus, makes studying the interactions of live virus with human platelets an expensive and labor intensive endeavor. Only a small number of laboratories worldwide are equipped with biosafety level 4 facilities and only two are located on the African continent, where most VHF infections occur [93]. Lymphocytic Choriomeningitis Virus (LCMV) is an arenavirus, which has sporadically caused severe Lassavirus-like illness in humans. Its reservoir host is mice, who only develop very mild disease. Experimental infections of mice with LCMV, after platelet depletion treatment, however, result in a more severe VHF with uncontrolled viral replication and dissemination, similar to that observed in humans. The platelet-depleted mice had impaired LCMV specific CD8+ T Cell responses. Severe disease and mortality only occurred in mice whose platelet reduction treatment was initiated shortly before LCMV infection. This may suggest that the innate antiviral response against LCMV requires platelets. However, Interferon α and β production appeared to be unaffected by platelet depletion treatment, indicating this part of the innate immune response had remained intact. Further examination of the spleen in LCMV infected mice who underwent platelet depletion demonstrated extensive disruption of the splenic architecture and cellular necrosis, which could be the common mechanism of both the defective innate and T cell responses. These experiments provided novel insights in the role of platelets in controlling VHF through protection of splenic vascular integrity and the importance of this organ in mounting sufficient cellular and innate immune responses to eliminate the virus [94].

3.2.8. West Nile Virus (WNV)

West Nile Virus (WNV) is a neurotropic flavivirus that mainly causes asymptomatic infections, while severe complications such as meningitis or encephalitis can occur, but are rare. WNV infections with hemorrhagic complications have sporadically been reported but severe thrombocytopenia and hemorrhage typically do not occur during WNV infection [95]. A case of WNV transmission through a platelet transfusion unit from a donor that tested negative on whole blood on the day of transfusion has been described, raising the possibility that the virus may concentrate in platelets, although the platelet unit itself was never tested [96].

3.2.9. Yellow Fever Virus (YFV)

Yellow fever virus (YFV) is a flavivirus that can be transmitted through Aedes mosquitoes and other vectors and is endemic in Africa and the Americas but not in Asia [97]. Even though there is an effective vaccine against YFV, annually several tens of thousands of persons die of YFV infection in Africa [98]. Disseminated yellow fever is characterized by hepatitis and hepatic failure, with resulting thrombocytopenia, deficiencies in plasma coagulation factors, prolonged activated Partial Thromboplastin Time (aPTT) and an elevated International Normalized Ratio (INR) [99,100]. A Brazilian retrospective cohort study of patients suffering severe YFV infections, showed severe hemorrhagic complications, mostly from the gastrointestinal tract. Despite this, only mild thrombocytopenia was present, with a median platelet count of 74×10^9/L, indicating platelet consumption as a result of hemorrhage, rather than thrombocytopenia-induced bleeding [100]. This is supported by the presence of ischemic and hemorrhagic microvascular pathology upon fundoscopic examination of hospitalized yellow fever patients, which correlate with the degree of thrombocytopenia present, disease severity and markers for renal and hepatic disease [101].

3.2.10. Zika Virus (ZIKV)

Like DENV, ZIKV is a flavivirus that is mainly transmitted through Aedes mosquitoes. In 2015/2016, there was a large outbreak of ZIKV in the Americas, which led to an increase in the incidence of Guillain-Barré syndrome in adults and congenital abnormalities in newborns [102]. Seroprevalence studies indicate that, depending on the country and location, up to 60% of inhabitants got infected with ZIKV during this outbreak [103–105]. A large prospective cohort study of ZIKV infected patients in Puerto Rico identified thrombocytopenia (defined in this study as a platelet count below 100×10^9/L) in 1.2% of confirmed cases. Only 25% of those had platelet counts below 20×10^9/L and 16% had etiologies other than ZIKV infection [106]. Platelet counts below 150×10^9/L are present in a small minority of ZIKV infections, although profound thrombocytopenia has been described in fulminant cases, associated with bleeding, liver failure and other coagulation disorders [107,108]. Most ZIKV patients have platelet counts between 150 and 300×10^9/L [109–111]. Thrombocytopenia on first diagnosis was significantly associated with higher odds of hospitalization in a case series study of U.S. veterans with laboratory-confirmed or presumptive ZIKV infection (OR 6.4, 95% CI 4.0–10.1) [3]. Suspected diagnosis of de novo Immune Thrombocytopenic Purpura (ITP) has been reported in patients presenting with severe thrombocytopenia during ZIKV convalescence, who responded to treatment with corticosteroids, intravenous immunoglobulin (IVIG), or both [112–114]. Exacerbation of pre-existing ITP during the acute phase of ZIKV disease has also been described [115]. ZIKV infects monocytes, macrophages and dendritic cells, but is unable to propagate in megakaryocyte-differentiated human hematopoietic stem cells and platelets [116]. Thrombocytopenia presents more often in DENV infections compared to ZIKV and can be used to distinguish the two otherwise similar diseases to a limited extent [117–119].

3.3. Blood-Borne Viruses

3.3.1. Hepatitis B and C (HBV and HBC)

Chronic hepatitis B and C virus infections are associated with hepatic cirrhosis, portal hypertension, liver failure and hepatocellular carcinoma (HCC). Thrombocytopenia is a predictor of such adverse outcomes, especially when combined in clinical scoring systems with other parameters such as age, gamma-glutamyl transpeptidase, Alanine and Aspartate aminotransferase [7–10,13–15,17,19,120–122] However, in individuals that have already developed HCC, thrombocytosis carries a negative prognosis rather than thrombocytopenia. Elevated platelet counts, when combined in a ratio with lymphocyte counts (PLR), is a biomarker of malignant inflammation and elevation is predictive of a poor prognosis in patients with HCC [123,124]. However, this marker does not appear to have much added value when tumor size and histological parameters are known or in patients with either no cirrhosis of very severe cirrhosis [11,125].

A likely explanation for the lower platelet counts observed in patients with hepatic cirrhosis, including those with a non-viral etiology, is portal hypertension leading to increased sequestration of platelets and red blood cells in the liver and spleen [126].

Another factor more specific to HBV and HCV infection could be increased platelet activation and consumption due to chronic inflammatory processes caused by these viruses. Mean platelet volume (MPV), a biomarker of platelet activation, was found to be increased in patients with chronic hepatitis B infection, compared to controls with no documented HBV infection [127]. Chronic HBV infection is also associated with a low platelet response to clopidogrel, which could be due to platelet activation by the virus or changes in drug metabolism caused by liver disease [128].

HBV and hepatitis Delta (HDV) co-infection also appears to lower platelet counts compared to HBV mono-infection, independently of the severity of liver disease, though the mechanism is unknown [129].

In hepatitis C infection, intravascular destruction of platelets is likely also mediated by anti-platelet antibodies and ITP related to HCV has been reported in the literature [130]. In HCV infected patients, platelet auto-antibodies were more commonly identified as a cause in mild (platelet count 126–149 $\times 10^9$/L) thrombocytopenia, whereas decreased megakaryopoiesis was a more prominent contributing factor in more severely (platelet count < 100 $\times 10^9$/L) thrombocytopenic patients [131].

Since both hepatitis B and C are blood-borne pathogens, a direct interaction between these viruses and platelets is possible. Hepatitis C virus RNA appears more stable when incubated with platelets than with platelet-free plasma, although there is no evidence of replication [132]. Instead, platelets may shield the virus from complement, interferons, cytokines, antibodies or other antiviral factors present in serum, perhaps through internalization. There have been reported cases of HCV infected patients with much higher viral loads in the platelet compartment compared to plasma [130]. One study found that, while HCV viral load was higher in plasma compared to platelets in patients before interferon/Ribavirin treatment, some patients had detectable RNA in platelets after treatment, but not in serum, resulting in relapse [133]. This could indicate that platelets and their megakaryocyte precursors can provide a site for therapeutic drug and immune evasion, either perhaps due to diminished response to interferons or a relative impermeability for nucleoside analogues or both, while extrahepatic replication is of minor importance during untreated HCV infection. The therapeutic relevance of this finding today is questionable however, given the high curation rate that can be achieved using the novel direct antiviral agents that have become available. The effect of direct interactions between HCV and platelets on platelet lifespan remains to be established.

3.3.2. Human Immunodeficiency Virus (HIV)

Thrombocytopenia is a common finding in HIV infection and HIV testing is part of a routine evaluation for unexplained thrombocytopenia. Screening individuals with thrombocytopenia and other so-called indicator conditions, has been shown to be a cost-effective and more efficient compared to universal screening [20–22]. HIV as the underlying cause for otherwise unexplained thrombocytopenia is frequently missed [23]. Decline of platelet count over time in HIV patients has been associated with development of dementia and reduced gray matter volume on MRI scans, although univariate and multivariate analyses were not entirely consistent [134]. Several mechanisms for thrombocytopenia in HIV infected individuals have been proposed and these will be discussed in more detail below.

Chronically infected HIV patients, even when adequately suppressed with combination Anti-Retroviral Therapy (c-ART), have a substantially increased risk of developing cardiovascular disease and deep venous thrombosis compared to HIV negative individuals. Platelet activation is believed to be a major driving factor behind this phenomenon. Untreated HIV positive individuals have elevated platelet activation markers in plasma compared to matched healthy controls, which positively correlate with viral load and negatively with CD4+ T cell counts. In addition, platelets from HIV patients express more oxidative stress-related proteins [135]. Studies investigating platelet morphology (MPV, PDW) in HIV patients, report contradictory results [136,137]. Platelets can bind HIV-1 virus through DC-SIGN and serve as a carrier, protecting virions in the circulation from antiviral factors through formation of RBC-platelet aggregates [138]. Platelets may also become activated after binding to HIV and release platelet factor 4 (PF4/CXCL4), from their α granules, which has been shown to inhibit cell attachment and entry of several HIV-1 strains through binding of its main envelope glycoprotein, GP-120 [139]. PF4 and other α-granule cytokines such as CCL5 likely also contribute to a chronic proinflammatory state in HIV patients. Interestingly, HIV patients on c-ART who become infected with DENV, were found to have milder disease and their platelets released less proinflammatory PF4 and CCL5 from α granules, likely resulting from previous HIV-associated depletion [140].

Very recently, platelets from long-term virologically suppressed HIV-infected individuals were shown to contain infectious HIV-1, demonstrating its ability to infect platelets and remain viable. Both viral RNA and proviral DNA of HIV was detected in bone marrow megakaryocytes from these same individuals, indicating platelets may already be infected upon formation. Platelets phagocytosis by macrophages was shown to lead to productive infection in this cell type [141]. The effects of HIV-1 infection on the activation status or lifespan of platelets were not investigated, meaning the role this mechanism plays in thrombocytopenia in people living with HIV remains unclear.

Another factor contributing to the prothrombotic state of HIV patients is the induction of platelet-monocyte aggregates (PMA) by the virus, which causes mutual activation of these two cell types [142,143]. Monocytes expressing CD16 (nonclassical and intermediate monocytes) appear to be primarily involved in the formation of PMA [144]. Electron microscopy (EM) studies of PMA in HIV infected individuals show a maximum of 4 simultaneously attached platelets per monocyte [145]. However, a single monocyte is likely capable of transiently interacting with many more platelets during its lifetime, leading to platelet activation and cumulative loss over time. The formation of PMA is mediated by binding of P-selectin on the platelet surface with P-Selectin Glycoprotein Ligand-1 (PSGL-1) on the monocyte surface. This leads to monocyte activation, including secretion of proinflammatory cytokines and Tissue Factor (TF), which initiates the extrinsic coagulation pathway. Monocytes may be able to downregulate PSGL-1 expression in response to platelet binding, but this has not been definitively established [143]. HIV transactivating factor (Tat) interacts with platelet integrin β3 and CCL3, resulting in the secretion of soluble

CD40 ligand (sCD40L), a platelet activator [146]. Subsequently, activated platelets initiate the formation of PMA [144,145]. The CD40L released, also increases B cell activation and secretion of immunoglobulins in vitro and in vivo in mouse models, which has been associated with ITP in non-HIV infected individuals and could play a similar role in HIV positives [147]. Platelets isolated from HIV patients secrete significantly more sCD40L in response to stimulation compared to healthy controls. The same effect was seen for other proinflammatory molecules, such as CCL5 and P-selectin expression. Patients who are not on c-ART can also have diminished responses however, which is attributed to exhaustion [148]. Overall, this evidence suggests that HIV infection sensitizes platelets to procoagulant and proinflammatory stimuli, which in response release more procoagulant and proinflammatory factors and induce monocytes to do the same. This creates a positive feedback loop underlying chronic inflammation and risk of thromboembolic complication. Although initiation of c-ART normalizes both platelet and monocyte activation markers in plasma within 12 weeks [149], these studies using isolated platelets and monocytes demonstrate that virological suppression seems unable to completely disrupt this inflammation-coagulation cycle present in people living with HIV.

3.4. Rodent-Borne Viruses

Hantavirus

Hemorrhagic Fever and Renal Syndrome *(HFRS)* caused by Eurasian hantaviruses is associated with severity-dependent thrombocytopenia. The clinical characteristics of the disease include both hemorrhagic and thrombotic complications. This suggests that platelet consumption plays a significant role in the pathogenesis of thrombocytopenia. A longitudinal study of 35 hospitalized HFRS patients with Puumala virus (PUUV) infection revealed a biphasic pattern in platelet counts over time. This started with marked thrombocytopenia upon first presentation to the clinic, followed by a rise to just below the upper limit of normal approximately 2 weeks after symptom onset, and subsequent normalization of platelet counts. Elevated plasma TPO levels, reticulated platelet counts and MPV (each peaking at the platelet count nadir) suggest a compensatory myeloproliferative response to an acute loss of platelets within the circulation during early infection. Ex vivo expression of platelet surface activation markers was higher during the acute disease stage compared to follow-up, although the opposite was found for in vitro stimulation assays, indicating platelet exhaustion. Finally, patients who had signs of Disseminated Intravascular Coagulation (DIC) or thrombosis during the disease had higher plasma platelet activation markers, such as soluble P-selectin and soluble Glycoprotein IV (GP IV) compared to those who had not [150]. Another longitudinal study measured Von Willebrand Factor, Fibrinogen, fibronectin and A Disintegrin Additionally, Metalloproteinase with a ThromboSpondin type 1 domain (ADAMTS13) concentrations in plasma of PUUV infected patients during the acute and recovery phase. These factors where indeed elevated during acute disease when compared to recovery. Thrombocytopenia was present in 15 out of the 19 patients studied, but the exact numbers and how they correlate with the markers measured in plasma is not described [151]. Furthermore, during the acute phase of PUUV infection platelet aggregation appears impaired, especially when induced with thrombin, when tested on impedance aggregometry. Platelet adhesive mechanisms on collagen are intact, despite thrombocytopenia, while thrombopoiesis is active [152]. Potential mechanisms explaining the decrease in platelet count based on In vitro data include decreased production due to bone marrow invasion and megakaryocyte infection [153] and binding of platelets to infected endothelial cells [154].

3.5. Gastrointestinal Tract Viruses

3.5.1. Enteroviruses

Since the near-eradication of poliomyelitis, severe enterovirus infections have become rare, typically causing mild cold-like illness in children and hand-foot and mouth disease. Coxsackievirus infections occasionally cause myocarditis in adults, and Enterovirus 68 has recently been implicated in episodes of acute flaccid myelitis in children. Thrombocytopenia has been described in neonatal cases of coxsackievirus B3 (CoxV B3) infections, both in Japan, with one case being related to secondary Hemophagocytic Lymphohistiocytosis (HLH) triggered by CoxV B13 [155,156]. A cross-al study of neonatal cases with severe enteroviral infection in Japan demonstrated significantly decreased platelet and WBC counts in Human Parechovirus 3 infections compared to RSV infected controls. In addition, the Human Parachovirus 3 infected patients showed elevated plasma ferritin and lactate dehydrogenase (LDH) levels, both compared to the RSV controls and infants with other enterovirus infections. This may suggest an HLH-like illness secondary to this viral infection [157]. Human platelets express the Coxsackie-Adeno Receptor (CAR), aCoxVB3 cell entry receptor. Whether this mechanism plays a role remains unclear, in particular as the virus appears to be unable to replicate in platelets in vitro. However, platelets become activated after incubation with CoxVB3, increasing their expression of P-selectin and showing signs of apoptosis (i.e., increased phospatidylserine (PS) expression) [158].

3.5.2. Rotavirus (RotV)

Viral gastroenteritis is a major cause of child mortality in the developing world and a significant burden on the healthcare system in developed countries [159]. Outbreaks of norovirus and rotavirus frequently occur in childcare institutions and nursing homes, where those most vulnerable to dehydration are affected. These infections are typically limited to the gastrointestinal epithelium and rarely cause severe systemic disease with involvement of multiple organs or severe inflammation. It is therefore not surprising that thrombocytopenia is not a dominant clinical feature of viral gastroenteritis. Mean platelet counts in children with rotavirus gastroenteritis are reported within the normal range and not diverging from children with other viral causes of gastroenteritis [160]. It is important to recognize both concentration and dilution effects of intravascular fluid shifts when assessing platelet counts or other blood cell counts in patients with conditions such as severe gastroenteritis or other critical illnesses.

3.6. Herpesviruses

3.6.1. Cytomegalovirus (CMV)

CMV is present in nearly all humans and remains latent for life after primary infection, which is usually asymptomatic in immunocompetent hosts. In contrast, severe immune suppression can lead to reactivation in later life leading most notably to CMV-mediated enterocolitis, hepatitis, retitinis or encephalitis [161]. However, very little is known about platelet counts during primary infection in immunocompetent hosts, because CMV infection comes to the attention of clinicians only when these rare complications develop. In vitro, CMV has been shown to interact with platelets through TLR-2. However, rather than directly resulting in platelet aggregation, these activated platelets produce a proinflammatory response, form aggregates with leukocytes and increase their adhesion to human vascular endothelial cells (HUVEC). Thus, in this model of CMV infection, platelets act as an intermediary between the virus and circulating immune cells [39].

3.6.2. Epstein Barr Virus (EBV)

Like all other human herpesviruses, infection with EBV occurs in the majority of the population at an early age. This leads frequently to a mild but sometimes protracted viral symptomatic episode called infectious mononucleosis, which is followed by lifelong latency. Occasionally reactivation occurs in immunocompromised hosts, most commonly in organ transplant recipients. Recently, primary EBV infection has been associated with a variety of auto-immune diseases, whereas latent EBV infection and reactivation plays a role in the pathogenesis of Hodgkin's lymphoma and B and T cell lymphoma's, through poorly understood mechanisms. EBV infection is also a well described trigger for secondary Hemophagocytic Lymphohistiocytosis (HLH) [162].

In the case of EBV reactivation, the relation with lymphoproliferative disorders is important to keep in mind when evaluating a patient with thrombocytopenia, especially when other cell-lineages are involved.

In cases of primary EBV infection, thrombocytopenia and hemolytic anemia are occasionally also found and have been associated with the presence of platelet and erythrocyte auto-antibodies. Typical of primary EBV infection is the production of heterophile antibodies by naïve B cells that have become infected with latent-phase EBV [162]. Some of these antibodies may be autoreactive and bind to platelets, leading to their destruction. Due to EBV's restriction to human hosts, well established animal models to study viral-platelet interactions in vivo do not exist. However, experimental infections with the related murine gammaherpesvirus 68 (γHV68) produce a mononucleosis-like illness in mice. This shows a significantly reduced platelet count during the early latent replication phase (nadir 17 days post infection). In this model, thrombocytopenia was found to be the result of antibodies induced by the infection and depended on viral latency, supporting the notion that polyclonal antibodies produced by latently infected B cells include autoantibodies against platelets [163]. This mechanism appears to be unique to EBV infection and is separate from auto-antibodies induced by other viral infection, which is believed to be the result of molecular mimicry between viral and self-antigens.

3.6.3. Human Herpesvirus 6 (HHV-6)

HHV-6 causes a near universal childhood illness, exanthema subitum, before entering its latent stage. Reactivation is rare, and generally only occurs during profound immunosuppression, such as during allogenic hematopoietic stem cell transplantation. In this population, HHV-6 reactivation (defined as a positive PCR on blood samples) was significantly associated with delayed platelet engraftment and the development of graft versus host disease (GVHD) [164].

3.6.4. Varicella Zostervirus (VZV)

Primary VZV infection almost universally presents itself as a self-limiting childhood illness, with more significant sequalae emerging later in life, ranging from common herpes zoster to rare cases of severe disseminated disease. The latter is typically only found in immunocompromised hosts, although not exclusively [165]. Typical Herpes Zoster manifests itself as a vesicular cutaneous eruption restricted to one dermatome and is most frequently seen in the elderly and patients who received chemotherapy for solid or hematological malignancies. Herpes Zoster can have long-term sequalae, such as post-herpetic neuralgia, but does not cause systemic disease and patients usually have normal platelet counts [166]. Profound thrombocytopenia has been described in reports of disseminated VZV infection, combined with DIC, hemorrhaging, ischemic strokes, ileus, abdominal pain, hepatitis, meningoencephalitis and vasculitis [167–170]. The vasculitis is believed to be caused by VZV infection of the arterial walls themselves and can be found in arteries in various organs, including smaller cerebral arteries, where it is associated with stroke [171]. Case series describing VZV related strokes report elevated platelet activation markers, such as PF-4 and β-thromboglobulin levels in some patients [172]. Splenomegaly with associated hypersplenism is a common feature of systemic herpesvirus infections, which contributes to thrombocytopenia and sometimes leads to splenic rupture [173]. The differential diagnosis of thrombocytopenia during a VZV infection is broad, because of comorbidity-related immune suppression, and includes immune thrombocytopenia, drug induced thrombocytopenia [174] and bone marrow dysfunction, particularly if other lineages are affected. First presentation or relapse of ITP has been reported during primary VZV infection in adulthood [175,176]. A platelet count <200 × 10^9/L was found to be predictive of a poor outcome in patients suffering from Ramsey Hunt Syndrome [2]. A large prospective cohort study identified thrombocytopenia as an independent risk factor for ICU admission in hospitalized children with VZV infection, although the rate of underlying hematological comorbidities and bacterial coinfections was high, suggesting VZV was not the sole cause of this phenomenon [177].

3.7. Respiratory Tract Infections

A platelet count close to the lower reference limit is a common finding in more severe viral respiratory tract infections [178]. Data on platelet counts in mild respiratory infections are scarce, possibly due to the fact that these cases typically do not present to care and blood counts are rarely performed. Interestingly, the literature reports thrombocytosis in infants hospitalized with respiratory tract infections, especially RSV and rhinoviruses, with platelet counts decreasing with age [179–181]. Platelet counts in patients with acute exacerbations of heart failure who tested positive for respiratory viruses by PCR, did not differ significantly from those who tested negative [182]. The lungs have recently been found to host resident megakaryocytes, which contribute to platelet production [183]. Investigating the interactions between respiratory viruses and platelets could be key to understanding the high rate of thromboembolic complications that arise during viral acute respiratory distress syndrome (ARDS).

3.7.1. Adenoviruses (Adv)

Among viruses causing mild upper respiratory tract infection, adenoviruses appear to be most studied in relation to platelets. Coxsackie and Adenovirus receptor (CAR) is the receptor adenoviruses use for cellular attachment. Expression of this receptor has been reported in healthy human platelets, albeit at a very low frequency (3.5%) [184]. In vitro studies where platelet rich plasma was incubated with very high concentrations of human adenovirus 3 and 5, showed a moderate increase in platelet aggregation and platelet activation marker expression, with uptake of adenovirus 5 by platelets demonstrated using EM [185,186]. Since natural infection in humans is unlikely to expose platelets to the high viral titers used in these incubation experiments, the clinical relevance for this finding is mostly related to the potential future use of adenoviruses for gene therapy purposes. Indeed, cancer patients experimentally treated intravenously with oncolytic adenovirus where serially sampled to determine relative abundance of viral DNA in various blood cell populations. Although very little platelet-associated virus was found in vivo, in vitro experiments where whole blood was incubated with the studied adenoviruses revealed a large proportion of virus bound to platelets. Given the thrombocytopenia observed during adenovirus-based treatments, this discrepancy could be the result of a survival disadvantage of adenovirus bound platelets in the circulation [187].

3.7.2. Influenza Virus (IAV/IBV)

Influenza virus infection is associated with a severity-dependent thrombocytopenia. Pediatric outpatients with confirmed IAV or IBV infection showed slightly, though significantly, lower mean platelet counts compared to asymptomatic controls. Children with influenza-like illness who were IAV and IBV PCR negative had platelet counts in between the confirmed positive and healthy groups, and platelet counts could not reliably distinguish between influenza positive and negative children [188]. In adults, severe influenza infection is accompanied by an increased risk of pulmonary thromboembolisms and cardiovascular events (Sellers, 2017 #1) suggesting platelet activation occurs during infection. Whole-blood transcriptome studies have found gene expression signatures in patients during H1N1 infection that are associated with a poor response to antiplatelet agents. Conversely, patients undergoing coronary catheterization that had a gene expression signature associated with viral infection, where more likely to have a confirmed myocardial infarction compared to those that did not express this signature [189]. Pathogenic H3N2 and H1N1 strains are capable of infecting pulmonary vascular endothelial cells, which increases platelet adhesion to both infected and nearby uninfected cells through interaction between endothelial fibronectin and platelet integrins [190]. Various influenza A strains cause thrombocytopenia in experimentally infected ferrets, with highly pathogenic strains

(H5N1) showing a stronger decrease compared to moderate (H1N1) or mildly pathogenic (H3N2) strains. In addition, these viruses are capable of directly infecting platelets in vivo through binding of sialic acids on glycans on their cell surface. EM imaging has demonstrated the ability of platelets to phagocytose influenza virus particles. This infection of platelets results in their activation, aggregation and subsequent clearance from the circulation. Interestingly, desialylation of platelet glycans by viral neuraminidase is hypothesized to reduce the lifespan of affected platelets through increased hepatic clearance [191]. Influenza virus can also interact with platelets through TLR7, which leads to the formation of platelet-neutrophil aggregates and neutrophil NETosis, through complement (C3) secreted by the platelets [192]. Immune-complexes of antibodies against influenza virus are also capable of activating platelets through an interaction with the Fc-YIIA receptor present on the platelet surface, leading to thrombocytopenia in a humanized mouse model. These findings, combined with reported influenza vaccine induced ITP, point to a link between influenza virus-specific adaptive immunity and thrombocytopenia [193–195].

3.7.3. Measles Virus (MV)

Likely the most contagious virus known to affect humans, this virus first infects the respiratory tract and subsequently spreads to lymphoid organs, infecting lymphocytes, including memory B and T cells [196]. A highly effective vaccine has been available for several decades, yet immunization programs have not been able to reach sufficient coverage to eradicate the disease, leading to sporadic outbreaks [197]. Studies published in the past 10 years describing natural infection in adults report mild leukocytopenia and thrombocytopenia as a frequent finding, occasionally with minor bleeding complications, but no thromboembolisms [198–200]. A link between Subacute Sclerosing Panencephalitis (SSPE), a late complication of Measles caused by persistence of MV in the brain, and ITP has been proposed, based on the co-occurrence of both extremely rare diseases in 3 pediatric cases [201]. This is further supported by an increased incidence of ITP after MV vaccination, where platelet binding anti-MV (and anti-rubella) IgG and IgM was demonstrated [202].

3.7.4. Parvovirus B19 (PVB-19)

While best known as a mild, self-limiting childhood illness (fifth disease), PVB-19 can occasionally cause more severe disease, especially during pregnancy, resulting in hydrops fetalis. Due to its tropism for erythroid progenitor cells and megakaryocytes, fetal PVB-19 infection causes severe anemia and thrombocytopenia, requiring Intrauterine Transfusion (IUT) of platelets and erythrocytes in some cases [203,204]. While most severe and best described in fetal infections, PVB-19 can also cause thrombocytopenia, anemia, leukopenia or pancytopenia in children and adults [205–208]. A retrospective cohort study reports PVB19 infection in children undergoing chemo- and radiation therapy for non-hematological malignancies increases the risk of thrombocytopenia and transfusion of blood products [209]. A similar study comparing malignant and nonmalignant hematological disease in a pediatric population found that PVB-19 DNA positivity was not associated with a higher risk of transfusion, but the number of platelet transfusion units administered per patient was over 3-fold higher in PVB-19 DNA positive patients [210]. PVB-19 is also able to infect myocardial tissue, leading to clinical myocarditis and dilated cardiomyopathy. This raises the question whether PVB-19 is also capable of infecting vascular endothelium and cause vasculitis and platelet adhesion to infected vessel walls. A case–control study exploring differences in microparticle (MP) profiles in the peripheral circulation of patients with myocarditis caused by PVB-19 versus other causes, found significant increases in apoptotic endothelial, platelet and leukocyte-derived MPs in PVB-19 mediated disease. This suggests that, in addition to impaired hematopoiesis, PVB also causes platelet destruction and vascular damage [211]. In vitro studies suggest PVB-19 nonstructural protein 1 (NS1) causes endothelial activation, upregulation of adhesion molecules and an increase in platelet and monocyte binding [212].

3.7.5. Respiratory Syncytial Virus

Severe respiratory infections with RSV occur mainly in children, the immunocompromised and those with underlying pulmonary disease [213]. In contrast to other respiratory infections, thrombocytosis rather than thrombocytopenia appears to be a common phenomenon found during acute RSV disease [181]. In vitro experiments demonstrate a reduction of monocyte RSV infection when platelets are added to the culture, possibly by binding and internalization of RSV. Platelets increase surface P selectin expression in the process, but why this would lead to thrombocytosis rather than thrombocytopenia is unclear [214].

3.7.6. SARS Coronavirus 2 (SARS-CoV-2, COVID-19)

The literature cited in this part of the review was updated shortly before submission to include the high volume of scientific work that has been published on this virus, which has caused a pandemic of severe pneumonia of historical proportions. Besides bilateral pneumonia, critical COVID-19 cases are characterized by multi-organ disease [215], and a remarkably high incidence of pulmonary embolisms [216,217]. Several mechanisms involving hypercoagulability and inflammation interact resulting in thrombotic phenomena both in the microvasculature and in the larger, mostly pulmonary blood vessels [218].

In fact, upon autopsy these embolisms were found to be mainly composed of platelets, fibrinogen and neutrophils [219–221]. Another typical finding during autopsy of deceased COVID-19 patients is the presence of widespread microvascular thrombosis in both pulmonary and extrapulmonary vessels, including in patients without true thromboembolisms, indicating a systemic prothrombotic state [220].

A low to low-normal platelet count is present during peak symptomatic illness, with increased MPV and PDW, and expression of surface activation markers [222,223]. However, one study identified subpopulations of platelets with a downregulated phenotype, which were highly enriched in severe, but not in intermediate COVID-19 cases, suggesting exhaustion of circulating platelets [220]. The total platelet population from these patients still showed hyperresponsiveness to procoagulant stimuli in vitro, likely driven by a hyperactive minority that was also present. This hyperresponsiveness was also found in other studies [224]. Some clinical studies report that thrombocytopenia is associated with increased mortality [4,5], whereas other do not [215,225]. This discrepancy might depend on disease severity, comorbidities or the type of care provided. For example, a well-defined cohort of mechanically ventilated critically ill patients showed that daily platelet concentrations were not associated with intensive care unit survival [215]. However, this observation does not exclude a role for platelet (dys)function in immunothrombosis. Other coagulation-related markers during acute illness show strongly elevated levels of D-dimers and fibrinogen degradation product (FDP), normal to slightly prolonged PT, APTT, elevated plasma viscosity and coagulability and normal to mildly increased INR [5,12,222,223]. Whether these markers have diagnostic or prognostic value requires investigation and might differ along the course of infection depending on disease severity, comorbidities and type of care provided. Platelet counts appear to rise slowly over the course of the disease, which coincides with a sharp peak in IL-6, suggesting this cytokine may play a role in the thrombopoietic response [220]. Plasma TPO levels are elevated in severe COVID-19 patients, but gene expression of its receptor, c-MPL is decreased, suggesting desensitization of the bone marrow as an additional mechanism for thrombocytopenia in COVID-19. When thrombocytopenia is present, it is often accompanied by relative deficiencies in other myeloid and lymphoid cell lineages [226,227], which could indicate bone marrow displacement caused by a proliferative response to hyperinflammation, either as a toxic effect of cytokines to progenitor cells in the bone marrow or a result of homing to inflamed tissues and extravasation.

Considerable work within a relatively short timespan has been done unraveling the mechanisms through which SARS-CoV-2 infection causes platelet activation. One study shows that platelet activation in severe COVID-19 is associated with detectable viral RNA in blood. Furthermore, the viral Spike protein enhanced platelet activation, aggregation, thrombus formation and degranulation in vitro and in a mouse model. This effect was only seen when the full Spike protein or its ACE-2 binding S1 subdomain were used, not the S2 domain. This suggests that ACE-2 signaling mediates this platelet activation. Further analysis of intracellular messaging points towards involvement of the MAPK signaling pathway. The same study confirmed expression of ACE-2 in human platelets using immunofluorescence [223]. However, another study did not detect any ACE-2 mRNA or protein expression in COVID-19 patients by RNA-seq, qPCR or Western blot [224]. To date, no study has demonstrated SARS-CoV-2 internalization by platelets.

It is also clear that platelets influence the host immune response to SARS-CoV-2. Platelet gene expression profiles in severe and critically ill COVID-19 patients showed shared pathways with sepsis and Influenza H1N1 infection. These show related antigen presentation and immune regulation, including differential expression of interferon-induced transmembrane protein 3, which has antiviral properties [224]. The formation of platelet-leukocyte aggregates was also found, with neutrophil-platelet aggregates correlating with the severity of lung injury and leading to the formation of NETs [220,221,224,228,229]. Similar to observations in HIV and DENV, platelet-monocyte complexes are formed in severe COVID-19 patients via platelet P-selectin, which results in overexpression of Tissue Factor on the monocyte surface, the key initiator of the extrinsic coagulation pathway [230].

As with many other viral infections, reports have been published of cases of ITP associated with COVID-19 infection, including one case of Evans syndrome [231]. Another case report illustrates the importance of performing a peripheral blood smear in COVID-19 patients with severe thrombocytopenia to exclude EDTA dependent pseudo-thrombocytopenia [232].

4. Conclusions

The topic of thrombocytopenia in viral infectious diseases has been actively studied for many decades, with the last 10 years yielding many new insights. A scientific field combining the disciplines of virology, hematology and increasingly immunology is revealing a complex system of interactions between various viruses, the coagulation cascade and the innate and adaptive immune system. Increasingly, platelets are regarded as part of the immune system, in addition to being capable of forming blood clots. The rapidly changing world of viruses ensures that this field is constantly forced to adapt to new outbreaks and is therefore equally dynamic. The current COVID-19 pandemic has brought platelet-virus interactions to the forefront, with many publications addressing this topic being available within a year after the SARS-CoV-2 virus first emerged.

The absence of research on the "classical" hemorrhagic fevers, such as Ebola, Lassa and Marburgvirus, has been notable however, despite two large outbreaks of Ebola occurring in the last decade. The high level of biological containment required to safely study these viruses, combined with the extremely resource-limited settings in which these outbreaks occurred make doing research into these viral diseases extremely challenging. Nonetheless, significant progress has been made in preventive and therapeutic interventions for Ebolavirus, with the successful trials of several vaccines, [233] antiviral drugs and monoclonal antibodies [234].

Table 1. Overview of mechanisms contributing to thrombocytopenia in a selection of major viral infections. U = unknown.

Virus	Platelet Binding (Receptors)	Platelet Activation (Receptors, Markers)	Platelet Infection (Receptors)	Platelet Replication	Vascular Endothelial Disruption	Impairs Platelet Production	Associated with Hemorrhage	Associated with Thromboembolism	Platelet Sequestration	PLA Formation	Autoimmunity
DENV	DC-SIGN, HSP, FcγR2A, GPIb, CLEC2, CLEC5A [66,67,81]	Receptors: CLEC2, CLEC5A, TLR 2/4, 5HT2 [66,67,71] Markers: P-Selectin, Integrin α2b, PF4, CCL5, PS, CD40L, CD63, GPIb, GPIIb/IIIa, microparticle release, aggregation [63–67,70,73]	DC-SIGN, HSP, FcγR2A (Ig bound virus) [30]	Yes [30]	Plasma leakage [59,67]	Infects megakaryocyte like cells [80,81]	With endothelial and platelet dysfunction [56–58]	Rare [235]	Phagocytosis [73,76]	PMA, PNA, inducing NETosis [68,69]	Immune complexes [75]
ZIKV	U	U	No [116]	No [116]	Infects vascular endothelial cells in vitro [236]	U	In severe cases [107,108]	Rare [237]	U	U	ITP [112–114]
YFV	U	U	U	U	Fundoscopic abnormalities [101]	U		Microvascular thrombosis [101]	U	U	U
HBV	U	Markers: Morphological changes [127] resistance to antiplatelet agents [128]	U	U	Polyarteritis nodosa (rare) [238]	Impaired hepatic TPO production [131,234]	Hepatic failure and deficiency of plasma coagulation factors. [99,100] Cirrhosis associated varices (HBV/HCV)	Increased risk of VTE [240] Portal vein thrombosis in cirrhosis [241]. Risk of ischemic cardiovascular disease elevated for HCV only [242,243]	Portal hypertension and hypersplenism [239]	U	U
HCV	Likely, Mechanisms unknown. [130,132,133]	U	Greater stability of HCV in platelets, [130,132] persistence in platelets during treatment [133]	No [132]	Endothelial activation [244], capillarization of liver sinusoidal endothelial cells [245], (non)cryoglobulinemic vasculitis [246]					U	ITP [130]

Table 1. Cont.

Virus	Platelet Binding (Receptors)	Platelet Activation (Receptors, Markers)	Platelet Infection (Receptors)	Platelet Replication	Vascular Endothelial Disruption	Impairs Platelet Production	Associated with Hemorrhage	Associated with Thromboembolism	Platelet Sequestration	PLA Formation	Autoimmunity
HIV	DC-SIGN, [138] GPIIIa, CCL-3 [146]	Receptors: CXCL4, CCR3, GPIIIa. Markers: PF-4, CCL5, P-selectin, sCD40L, CCL5, Conflicting reports on morphological changes, oxidative stress. (135–137, 139)	Yes, via megakaryocyte precursors [141]	No	HIV-associated vasculopathy [247], Infects arterial smooth muscle cells [248]	Infection and impairment of hematopoietic progenitor cells [249]	No	Increased risk of VTE [250], myocardial infarction [251] and cerebrovascular disease [247]	Hypersplenism [252]	PMA, increasing monocyte TF expression [144,145].	ITP [253], HLH [254]
IAV/IBV	Likely NA binding of glycans [191]	Receptors: Glycans, TLR7, [44] Immune complexes via Fc-γIIA receptor [193] Markers: P-selectin, [191] CD40L, C3, CD63[192] Resistance to antiplatelet agents.[189]	Phagocytosis [191]	U	Infection of pulmonary vascular endothelial cells [190]	U	No	VTE, myocardial infarction, ischemic cerebrovascular accidents. [1]	U	PNA, inducing NETosis [192]	ITP [194,195]
SARS CoV 2	ACE2, conflicting evidence on platelet expression [223,224]	Receptors: ACE2, TLR4, CLEC2, CXCR-4. Markers: P-selectin, GPIb, GP IIa GPIIIb, GPIIb/IIIa, CD40L, CD63, morphological changes, aggregation, degranulation [220,222–224]	U	U	U	Decreased cGMP expression [224]	No	Microvascular thrombosis and VTE. [216–219]	U	PMA increasing monocyte TF expression, PNA inducing NETosis [221,230]	ITP, Evans Syndrome [231]

DENV, another viral infection disproportionately affecting people in resource limited settings, was the virus we found most publications about in relation to platelets in the past decade. This is not surprising, given the considerable role platelets play in the pathophysiology of severe disease and the enormous public health burden associated with the virus. Despite the considerable knowledge gained, this has so far not been translated into clinically effective interventions. However, we did find several studies investigating therapeutics aimed at modifying platelet function in DENV infection, which will hopefully bear fruit in the coming decade.

Looking in detail at the interactions between viral infections and platelets revealed several common pathways connecting inflammation and platelet activation, which has been termed "Immunothrombosis". This is a term which has not yet been clearly defined as a clinical or pathological entity and has some overlapping features with DIC, with the main clinical difference being the absence of significant bleeding. COVID-19 may provide us the opportunity to increase our overall understanding of thrombocytopenia in viral infections and perhaps to study a new dimension of immunothrombosis which could be translated to other viral infections. It is especially important to gain more understanding about which interventions could aid in reducing the morbidity and mortality related to immunothrombosis. As platelet dysfunction is often accompanied by an increased risk of both bleeding and thrombosis, approaching this issue with conventional anticoagulants often involves having to choose the lesser of two evils. Immunomodulation therapy is a rapidly evolving field, with many newly available therapeutics, most of which have not yet been trialed in viral infectious diseases. This approach warrants further study, but here caution is also advisable, given the possibility that some mechanisms involved in immunothrombosis are required in the antiviral response in the host.

Author Contributions: Conceptualization: M.R., M.G., E.v.G. Writing: M.R., J.D.T., M.G., T.L. Search strategy & literature review: MPR. Editing & expert contribution: B.v.B., J.D.T., E.v.G., M.G. All authors have read and agreed to the published version of the manuscript.

Funding: This research received no external funding.

Data Availability Statement: Data available in a publicly accessible repository. The data presented in this study are available via the national Center of biotechnology information.

Conflicts of Interest: The authors declare no conflict of interest.

Abbreviations

Abbreviation	Meaning
ACE	Angiotensin Converting Enzyme
ADAMTS13	A Disintegrin And Metalloproteinase with a ThromboSpondin type 1 domain
AdV	Adenovirus
APC	Antigen Presenting Cell
aPTT	activated Partial Thromboplastin Time
ARDS	Acute Respiratory Distress Syndrome
CAR	Coxsackie-Adeno Receptor
c-ART	combination Anti-Retroviral Therapy
CCHF	Crimean Congo Hemorrhagic Fever
CCL	Chemokine Ligand
CD	Cluster of Differentiation
CHIKV	Chikungungya Virus
CLEC	C-type Lectin
c-MPL	Myeloproliferative Leukemia Protein
CMV	Cytomegalovirus
COVID-19	Coronavirus Disease 2019
CoxV	Coxsackie virus
DC-SIGN	Dendritic Cell-Specific Intercellular adhesion molecule-3-Grabbing Non-integrin

DENV	Dengue Virus
DIC	Disseminated Intravascular Coagulation
DNA	Desoxyribonucleic Acid
EBV	Ebstein Barr Virus
EDTA	Ethylenediaminetetraacetic acid
EM	Electron Microscopy
FcYR2A	Fc Gamma Receptor 2a
FDP	Fibrinogen Degradation Product
FGF-4	Fibroblast Growth Factor
GM-CSF	Granulocyte-Monocyte Colony Stimulating Factor
gMDSC	Granulocytic Myeloid-derived suppressor cell
GP	Glycoprotein
GVHD	graft versus host disease
HBV	Hepatitis B Virus
HCC	Hepatocellular Carcinoma
HCV	Hepatitis C Virus
HDV	Hepatitis Delta Virus
HFRS	Hemorrhagic Fever and Renal Syndrome
HHV-6	Human Herpesvirus 6
HIV	Human Immunodeficiency Virus
HLA	Human Leukocyte Antigen
HLH	Hemophagocytic Lymphohistiocytosis
HSP	Heparan Sulfate Proteoglycan
HUVEC	human vascular endothelial cells
IAV/IBV	Influenza A/B Virus
ICU	Intensive Care Unit
Ig	Immunoglobulin
IL	Interleukin
INR	International Normalized Ratio
ITP	Immune Thrombocytopenia
IUT	Intrauterine Transfusion
IVIG	Intravenous Immunoglobulin
JEV	Japanese Encephalitis Virus
LCMV	Lymphocytic Choriomeningitis Virus
LDH	Lactate Dehydrogenase
MHC	Major Histocompatibility Complex
MPV	Mean Platelet Volume
MRI	Magnetic Resonance Imaging
MV	Measles Virus
NET	Neutrophil Extracellular Trap
NS1	Nonstructural Protein 1
OR	Odds Ratio
PAF	Platelet Activating Factor
PAMP	Pattern Associated Molecular Pattern
PAR	Protease Activating Receptor
PCR	Polymerase Chain Reaction
PDW	Platelet Distribution Width
PF4	Platelet Factor 4
PLR	Platelet Lymphocyte Ratio
PMA	Platelet-Monocyte Aggregate
PMP	Platelet Microbicidal Peptides
PRR	Pattern Recognition Receptor
PS	phospatidylserine
PSGL-1	P-Selectin Glycoprotein Ligand-1
PT	Prothrombin Time
PUUV	Puumala virus
PVB-19	Parvovirus B19

RBC	Red Blood Cell
RNA	Ribonucleic Acid
RotV	Rotavirus
RSV	Respiratory Syncytial Virus
SARS-CoV-2	SARS Coronavirus 2
sCD40L	soluble CD40 ligand
SDF-1	Stromal Derived Factor 1
SFTS	Severe Fever with Thrombocytopenia Syndrome
Tat	Transactivating factor
TBEV	Tickborne Encephalitis Virus
TF	Tissue Factor
TLR	Toll-Like Receptor
TPO	Thrombopoietin
VHF	Viral Hemorrhagic Fever
VZV	Varicella Zoster Virus
WBC	White Blood Cell
WNV	West Nile Virus
YFV	Yellow Fever Virus
ZIKV	Zika Virus
γHV68	murine gammaherpesvirus 68

References

1. Sellers, S.A.; Hagan, R.S.; Hayden, F.G.; Fischer, W.A., 2nd. The hidden burden of influenza: A review of the extra-pulmonary complications of influenza infection. *Influenza Other Respir. Viruses.* **2017**, *11*, 372–393. [CrossRef]
2. Wasano, K.; Ishikawa, T.; Kawasaki, T.; Yamamoto, S.; Tomisato, S.; Shinden, S.; Minami, S.; Wakabayashi, T.; Ogawa, K. Novel pre-therapeutic scoring system using patient and haematological data to predict facial palsy prognosis. *Clin. Otolaryngol.* **2017**, *42*, 1224–1228. [CrossRef] [PubMed]
3. Schirmer, P.L.; Wendelboe, A.; Lucero-Obusan, C.A.; Ryono, R.A.; Winters, M.A.; Oda, G.; Martinez, M.; Saavedra, S.; Holodniy, M. Zika virus infection in the Veterans Health Administration (VHA), 2015–2016. *PLoS Negl. Trop. Dis.* **2018**, *12*, e0006416. [CrossRef] [PubMed]
4. Pakos, I.S.; Lo, K.B.; Salacup, G.; Pelayo, J.; Bhargav, R.; Peterson, E.; Gul, F.; DeJoy, R., 3rd; Albano, J.; Patarroyo-Aponte, G.; et al. Characteristics of peripheral blood differential counts in hospitalized patients with COVID-19. *Eur. J. Haematol.* **2020**, *105*, 773–778. [CrossRef] [PubMed]
5. Martín-Rojas, R.M.; Pérez-Rus, G.; Delgado-Pinos, V.E.; Domingo-González, A.; Regalado-Artamendi, I.; Alba-Urdiales, N.; Demelo-Rodríguez, P.; Monsalvo, S.; Rodríguez-Macías, G.; Ballesteros, M.; et al. COVID-19 coagulopathy: An in-depth analysis of the coagulation system. *Eur. J. Haematol.* **2020**, *105*, 741–750. [CrossRef]
6. Eren, S.H.; Zengin, S.; Büyüktuna, S.A.; Gözel, M.G. Clinical severity in forecasting platelet to lymphocyte ratio in Crimean-Congo hemorrhagic fever patients. *J. Med Microbiol.* **2016**, *65*, 1100–1104. [CrossRef]
7. Kuo, Y.H.; Kee, K.M.; Hsu, N.T.; Wang, J.H.; Hsiao, C.C.; Chen, Y.; Lu, S.N. Using AST-platelet ratio index and fibrosis 4 index for detecting chronic hepatitis C in a large-scale community screening. *PLoS ONE* **2019**, *14*, e0222196. [CrossRef]
8. Zhu, Y.F.; Tan, Y.F.; Xu, X.; Zheng, J.L.; Zhang, B.H.; Tang, H.R.; Yang, J.Y. Gamma-glutamyl transpeptidase-to-platelet ratio and the fibrosis-4 index in predicting hepatitis B virus-related hepatocellular carcinoma development in elderly chronic hepatitis B patients in China: A single-center retrospective study. *Medicine* **2019**, *98*, e18319. [CrossRef] [PubMed]
9. Liu, L.; Lan, Q.; Lin, L.; Lu, J.; Ye, C.; Tao, Q.; Cui, M.; Zheng, S.; Zhang, X.; Xue, Y. Gamma-glutamyl transpeptidase-to-platelet ratio predicts the prognosis in HBV-associated acute-on-chronic liver failure. *Clin. Chim. Acta* **2018**, *476*, 92–97. [CrossRef]
10. Zhao, Z.; Liu, J.; Wang, J.; Xie, T.; Zhang, Q.; Feng, S.; Deng, H.; Zhong, B. Platelet-to-lymphocyte ratio (PLR) and neutrophil-to-lymphocyte ratio (NLR) are associated with chronic hepatitis B virus (HBV) infection. *Int. Immunopharmacol.* **2017**, *51*, 1–8. [CrossRef]
11. Wang, Q.; Blank, S.; Fiel, M.I.; Kadri, H.; Luan, W.; Warren, L.; Zhu, A.; Deaderick, P.A.; Sarpel, U.; Labow, D.M.; et al. The Severity of Liver Fibrosis Influences the Prognostic Value of Inflammation-Based Scores in Hepatitis B-Associated Hepatocellular Carcinoma. *Ann. Surg. Oncol.* **2015**, *22* (Suppl. 3), S1125–S1132. [CrossRef]
12. Wang, X.; Li, X.; Shang, Y.; Wang, J.; Zhang, X.; Su, D.; Zhao, S.; Wang, Q.; Liu, L.; Li, Y.; et al. Ratios of neutrophil-to-lymphocyte and platelet-to-lymphocyte predict all-cause mortality in inpatients with coronavirus disease 2019 (COVID-19): A retrospective cohort study in a single medical centre. *Epidemiol. Infect.* **2020**, *148*, e211. [CrossRef]
13. Thandassery, R.B.; Al Kaabi, S.; Soofi, M.E.; Mohiuddin, S.A.; John, A.K.; Al Mohannadi, M.; Al Ejji, K.; Yakoob, R.; Derbala, M.F.; Wani, H.; et al. Mean Platelet Volume, Red Cell Distribution Width to Platelet Count Ratio, Globulin Platelet Index, and 16 Other Indirect Noninvasive Fibrosis Scores: How Much Do Routine Blood Tests Tell About Liver Fibrosis in Chronic Hepatitis C? *J. Clin. Gastroenterol.* **2016**, *50*, 518–523. [CrossRef]

14. Ng, K.J.; Tseng, C.W.; Chang, T.T.; Tzeng, S.J.; Hsieh, Y.H.; Hung, T.H.; Huang, H.T.; Wu, S.F.; Tseng, K.C. Aspartate aminotransferase to platelet ratio index and sustained virologic response are associated with progression from hepatitis C associated liver cirrhosis to hepatocellular carcinoma after treatment with pegylated interferon plus ribavirin. *Clin. Interv. Aging* **2016**, *11*, 1035–1041. [PubMed]
15. Tseng, P.L.; Wang, J.H.; Hung, C.H.; Tung, H.D.; Chen, T.M.; Huang, W.S.; Liu, S.L.; Hu, T.H.; Lee, C.M.; Lu, S.N. Comparisons of noninvasive indices based on daily practice parameters for predicting liver cirrhosis in chronic hepatitis B and hepatitis C patients in hospital and community populations. *Kaohsiung J. Med Sci.* **2013**, *29*, 385–395. [CrossRef] [PubMed]
16. Zhang, C.; Wu, J.; Xu, J.; Xu, J.; Xian, J.; Xue, S.; Ye, J. Association between Aspartate Aminotransferase-to-Platelet Ratio Index and Hepatocellular Carcinoma Risk in Patients with Chronic Hepatitis: A Meta-Analysis of Cohort Study. *Dis. Markers* **2019**, *2019*, 2046825. [CrossRef]
17. Jun, B.G.; Park, E.J.; Lee, W.C.; Jang, J.Y.; Jeong, S.W.; Kim, Y.D.; Cheon, G.J.; Cho, Y.S.; Lee, S.H.; Kim, H.S.; et al. Platelet count is associated with sustained virological response rates in treatments for chronic hepatitis C. *Korean J. Intern. Med.* **2019**, *34*, 989–997. [CrossRef]
18. Lee, J.; Kim, M.Y.; Kang, S.H.; Kim, J.; Uh, Y.; Yoon, K.J.; Kim, H.S. The gamma-glutamyl transferase to platelet ratio and the FIB-4 score are noninvasive markers to determine the severity of liver fibrosis in chronic hepatitis B infection. *Br. J. Biomed. Sci.* **2018**, *75*, 128–132. [CrossRef]
19. Nishikawa, H.; Iguchi, E.; Koshikawa, Y.; Ako, S.; Inuzuka, T.; Takeda, H.; Nakajima, J.; Matsuda, F.; Sakamoto, A.; Henmi, S.; et al. The effect of pegylated interferon-alpha2b and ribavirin combination therapy for chronic hepatitis C infection in elderly patients. *BMC Res. Notes* **2012**, *5*, 135. [CrossRef]
20. Menacho, I.; Sequeira, E.; Muns, M.; Barba, O.; Leal, L.; Clusa, T.; Fernandez, E.; Moreno, L.; Raben, D.; Lundgren, J.; et al. Comparison of two HIV testing strategies in primary care centres: Indicator-condition-guided testing vs. testing of those with non-indicator conditions. *HIV Med.* **2013**, *14* (Suppl. 3), 33–37. [CrossRef] [PubMed]
21. Sullivan, A.K.; Raben, D.; Reekie, J.; Rayment, M.; Mocroft, A.; Esser, S.; Leon, A.; Begovac, J.; Brinkman, K.; Zangerle, R.; et al. Feasibility and effectiveness of indicator condition-guided testing for HIV: Results from HIDES I (HIV indicator diseases across Europe study). *PLoS ONE* **2013**, *8*, e52845. [CrossRef]
22. Søgaard, O.S.; Lohse, N.; Østergaard, L.; Kronborg, G.; Røge, B.; Gerstoft, J.; Sørensen, H.T.; Obel, N. Morbidity and risk of subsequent diagnosis of HIV: A population based case control study identifying indicator diseases for HIV infection. *PLoS ONE* **2012**, *7*, e32538.
23. Tominski, D.; Katchanov, J.; Driesch, D.; Daley, M.B.; Liedtke, A.; Schneider, A.; Slevogt, H.; Arastéh, K.; Stocker, H. The late-presenting HIV-infected patient 30 years after the introduction of HIV testing: Spectrum of opportunistic diseases and missed opportunities for early diagnosis. *HIV Med.* **2017**, *18*, 125–132. [CrossRef] [PubMed]
24. Kuter, D.J. Milestones in understanding platelet production: A historical overview. *Br. J. Haematol.* **2014**, *165*, 248–258. [CrossRef] [PubMed]
25. Vinholt, P.J. The role of platelets in bleeding in patients with thrombocytopenia and hematological disease. *Clin. Chem. Lab. Med.* **2019**, *57*, 1808–1817. [CrossRef] [PubMed]
26. Behrens, K.; Alexander, W.S. Cytokine control of megakaryopoiesis. *Growth Factors (Chur, Switzerland)* **2018**, *36*, 89–103. [CrossRef]
27. de Graaf, C.A.; Metcalf, D. Thrombopoietin and hematopoietic stem cells. *Cell Cycle (Georgetown, Tex)* **2011**, *10*, 1582–1589. [CrossRef] [PubMed]
28. Assinger, A. Platelets and infection—An emerging role of platelets in viral infection. *Front. Immunol.* **2014**, *5*, 649. [CrossRef] [PubMed]
29. Rowley, J.W.; Schwertz, H.; Weyrich, A.S. Platelet mRNA: The meaning behind the message. *Curr. Opin. Hematol.* **2012**, *19*, 385–391. [CrossRef]
30. Sutherland, M.R.; Simon, A.Y.; Serrano, K.; Schubert, P.; Acker, J.P.; Pryzdial, E.L. Dengue virus persists and replicates during storage of platelet and red blood cell units. *Transfusion* **2016**, *56*, 1129–1137. [CrossRef]
31. Zhang, L.; Xu, J.; Gao, L.; Pan, S. Spurious Thrombocytopenia in Automated Platelet Count. *Lab. Med.* **2018**, *49*, 130–133. [CrossRef]
32. Stasi, R. How to approach thrombocytopenia. *Hematol. Amer. Society Hematol. Educ. Prog.* **2012**, *2012*, 191–197. [CrossRef]
33. Kolb-Mäurer, A.; Goebel, W. Susceptibility of hematopoietic stem cells to pathogens: Role in virus/bacteria tropism and path-ogenesis. *FEMS Microbiol. Lett.* **2003**, *226*, 203–207. [CrossRef]
34. Metcalf Pate, K.A.; Lyons, C.E.; Dorsey, J.L.; Queen, S.E.; Adams, R.J.; Morrell, C.N.; Mankowski, J.L. TGFβ-Mediated Downregulation of Throm-bopoietin Is Associated with Platelet Decline in Asymptomatic SIV Infection. *J. Acquir. Immune Defic. Syndr.* **2014**, *65*, 510–516. [CrossRef] [PubMed]
35. Isomura, H.; Yoshida, M.; Namba, H.; Fujiwara, N.; Ohuchi, R.; Uno, F.; Oda, M.; Seino, Y.; Yamada, M. Suppressive effects of human herpesvirus-6 on thrombopoietin-inducible megakaryocytic colony formation in vitro. *J. Gen. Virol.* **2000**, *81* Pt 3, 663–673. [CrossRef]
36. Chelucci, C.; Federico, M.; Guerriero, R.; Mattia, G.; Casella, I.; Pelosi, E.; Testa, U.; Mariani, G.; Hassan, H.J.; Peschle, C. Productive Human Immunodeficiency Virus-1 Infection of Purified Megakaryocytic Progenitors/Precursors and Maturing Megakaryocytes. *Blood* **1998**, *91*, 1225–1234. [CrossRef] [PubMed]

37. Crapnell, K.; Zanjani, E.D.; Chaudhuri, A.; Ascensao, J.L.; St Jeor, S.; Maciejewski, J.P. In vitro infection of megakaryocytes and their precursors by human cytomegalovirus. *Blood* **2000**, *95*, 487–493. [CrossRef] [PubMed]
38. Li, X.; Jeffers, L.J.; Garon, C.; Fischer, E.R.; Scheffel, J.; Moore, B.; Reddy, K.R.; Demedina, M.; Schiff, E.R. Persistence of hepatitis C virus in a human megakaryoblastic leukaemia cell line. *J. Viral Hepat.* **1999**, *6*, 107–114. [CrossRef] [PubMed]
39. Assinger, A.; Kral, J.B.; Yaiw, K.C.; Schrottmaier, W.C.; Kurzejamska, E.; Wang, Y.; Mohammad, A.A.; Religa, P.; Rahbar, A.; Schabbauer, G.; et al. Human Cytomegalovirus–Platelet Interaction Triggers Toll-Like Receptor 2–Dependent Proinflammatory and Proangiogenic Responses. *Arter. Thromb. Vasc. Biol.* **2014**, *34*, 801–809. [CrossRef]
40. Flaujac, C.; Boukour, S.; Cramer-Bordé, E. Platelets and viruses: An ambivalent relationship. *Cell. Mol. Life Sci.* **2009**, *67*, 545–556. [CrossRef] [PubMed]
41. Speth, C.; Löffler, J.; Krappmann, S.; Lass-Flörl, C.; Rambach, G. Platelets as immune cells in infectious diseases. *Future Microbiol.* **2013**, *8*, 1431–1451. [CrossRef] [PubMed]
42. Seyoum, M.; Enawgaw, B.; Melku, M. Human blood platelets and viruses: Defense mechanism and role in the removal of viral pathogens. *Thromb. J.* **2018**, *16*, 16. [CrossRef]
43. Maugeri, N.; Cattaneo, M.; Rovere-Querini, P.; Manfredi, A.A. Platelet clearance by circulating leukocytes: A rare event or a determinant of the "immune continuum"? *Platelets* **2014**, *25*, 224–225. [CrossRef] [PubMed]
44. Koupenova, M.; Vitseva, O.; MacKay, C.R.; Beaulieu, L.M.; Benjamin, E.J.; Mick, E.; Kurt-Jones, E.A.; Ravid, K.; Freedman, J.E. Platelet-TLR7 mediates host survival and platelet count during viral infection in the absence of platelet-dependent thrombosis. *Blood* **2014**, *124*, 791–802. [CrossRef]
45. Antoniak, S.; Mackman, N. Multiple roles of the coagulation protease cascade during virus infection. *Blood* **2014**, *123*, 2605–2613. [CrossRef] [PubMed]
46. Anderson, C.L.; Chacko, G.W.; Osborne, J.M.; Brandt, J.T. The Fc receptor for immunoglobulin G (Fc gamma RII) on human platelets. *Semin. Thromb. Hemost.* **1995**, *21*, 1–9. [CrossRef]
47. Cox, D.; Kerrigan, S.W.; Watson, S.P. Platelets and the innate immune system: Mechanisms of bacterial-induced platelet activation. *J. Thromb. Haemost.* **2011**, *9*, 1097–1107. [CrossRef]
48. Goeijenbier, M.; van Wissen, M.; van de Weg, C.; Jong, E.; Gerdes, V.E.; Meijers, J.C.; Brandjes, D.P.; van Gorp, E.C. Review: Viral infections and mechanisms of thrombosis and bleeding. *J. Med Virol.* **2012**, *84*, 1680–1696. [CrossRef]
49. Brubaker, S.W.; Bonham, K.S.; Zanoni, I.; Kagan, J.C. Innate Immune Pattern Recognition: A Cell Biological Perspective. *Annu. Rev. Immunol.* **2015**, *33*, 257–290. [CrossRef]
50. Hottz, E.D.; Bozza, F.A.; Bozza, P.T. Platelets in Immune Response to Virus and Immunopathology of Viral Infections. *Front. Med.* **2018**, *5*, 121. [CrossRef]
51. Morrell, C.N.; Aggrey, A.A.; Chapman, L.M.; Modjeski, K.L. Emerging roles for platelets as immune and inflammatory cells. *Blood* **2014**, *123*, 2759–2767. [CrossRef]
52. Mohan, K.V.; Rao, S.S.; Atreya, C.D. Antiviral activity of selected antimicrobial peptides against vaccinia virus. *Antivir. Res.* **2010**, *86*, 306–311. [CrossRef]
53. Zufferey, A.; Schvartz, D.; Nolli, S.; Reny, J.-L.; Sanchez, J.-C.; Fontana, P. Characterization of the platelet granule proteome: Evidence of the presence of MHC1 in alpha-granules. *J. Proteom.* **2014**, *101*, 130–140. [CrossRef]
54. Colberg, L.; Cammann, C.; Greinacher, A.; Seifert, U. Structure and function of the ubiquitin-proteasome system in platelets. *J. Thromb. Haemost.* **2020**, *18*, 771–780. [CrossRef]
55. Chapman, L.M.; Aggrey, A.A.; Field, D.J.; Srivastava, K.; Ture, S.; Yui, K.; Topham, D.J.; Baldwin, W.M., 3rd; Morrell, C.N. Platelets Present Antigen in the Context of MHC Class I. *J. Immunol.* **2012**, *189*, 916–923. [CrossRef] [PubMed]
56. Bhatt, S.; Gething, P.W.; Brady, O.J.; Messina, J.P.; Farlow, A.W.; Moyes, C.L.; Drake, J.M.; Brownstein, J.S.; Hoen, A.G.; Sankoh, O.; et al. The global distribution and burden of dengue. *Nature* **2013**, *496*, 504–507. [CrossRef]
57. Tomashek, K.M.; Lorenzi, O.D.; Andújar-Pérez, D.A.; Torres-Velásquez, B.C.; Hunsperger, E.A.; Munoz-Jordan, J.L.; Perez-Padilla, J.; Rivera, A.; Gonzalez-Zeno, G.E.; Sharp, T.M.; et al. Clinical and epidemiologic characteristics of dengue and other etiologic agents among patients with acute febrile illness, Puerto Rico, 2012–2015. *PLoS Negl. Trop. Dis.* **2017**, *11*, e0005859. [CrossRef] [PubMed]
58. Dhanoa, A.; Rajasekaram, G.; Hassan, S.S.; Ramadas, A.; Azreen Adnan, N.A.; Lau, C.F.; Chan, T.S.; Ngim, C.F. Risk factors and clinical outcome of profound thrombocytopenia in adult patients with DENV infections. *Platelets* **2017**, *28*, 724–727. [CrossRef]
59. Tramontini Gomes de Sousa Cardozo, F.; Baimukanova, G.; Lanteri, M.C.; Keating, S.M.; Moraes Ferreira, F.; Heitman, J.; Pannuti, C.S.; Pati, S.; Romano, C.M.; Cerdeira Sabino, E. Serum from dengue virus-infected patients with and without plasma leakage differentially affects endothelial cells barrier function in vitro. *PLoS ONE* **2017**, *12*, e0178820. [CrossRef]
60. Katzelnick, L.C.; Gresh, L.; Halloran, M.E.; Mercado, J.C.; Kuan, G.; Gordon, A.; Balmaseda, A.; Harris, E. Antibody-dependent enhancement of severe dengue disease in humans. *Science* **2017**, *358*, 929–932. [CrossRef] [PubMed]
61. Arya, S.C.; Agarwal, N.; Parikh, S.C. Detection of dengue NS1 antigen, alongside IgM plus IgG and concurrent platelet enumeration during an outbreak. *Asian Pac. J. Trop. Med.* **2011**, *4*, 672. [CrossRef]
62. Arya, S.C.; Agarwal, N. Thrombocytopenia progression in dengue cases during the 2010 outbreak in Indian capital metropolis. *Platelets* **2011**, *22*, 476–477. [CrossRef] [PubMed]

63. Núñez-Avellaneda, D.; Mosso-Pani, M.A.; Sánchez-Torres, L.E.; Castro-Mussot, M.E.; Corona-de la Peña, N.A.; Salazar, M.I. Dengue Virus Induces the Release of sCD40L and Changes in Levels of Membranal CD42b and CD40L Molecules in Human Platelets. *Viruses* **2018**, *10*, 357. [CrossRef] [PubMed]
64. Trugilho, M.R.O.; Hottz, E.D.; Brunoro, G.V.F.; Teixeira-Ferreira, A.; Carvalho, P.C.; Salazar, G.A.; Zimmerman, G.A.; Bozza, F.A.; Bozza, P.T.; Perales, J. Platelet proteome reveals novel pathways of platelet activation and platelet-mediated immunoregulation in dengue. *PLoS Pathog.* **2017**, *13*, e1006385. [CrossRef]
65. de Jong, W.; Asmarawati, T.P.; Verbeek, I.; Rusli, M.; Hadi, U.; van Gorp, E.; Goeijenbier, M. Point-of-care thrombocyte function testing using multiple-electrode aggregometry in dengue patients: An explorative study. *BMC Infect. Dis.* **2020**, *20*, 580. [CrossRef]
66. Chao, C.H.; Wu, W.C.; Lai, Y.C.; Tsai, P.J.; Perng, G.C.; Lin, Y.S.; Yeh, T.M. Dengue virus nonstructural protein 1 activates platelets via Toll-like receptor 4, leading to thrombocytopenia and hemorrhage. *PLoS Pathog.* **2019**, *15*, e1007625. [CrossRef]
67. Sung, P.S.; Huang, T.F.; Hsieh, S.L. Extracellular vesicles from CLEC2-activated platelets enhance dengue virus-induced lethality via CLEC5A/TLR2. *Nat. Commun.* **2019**, *10*, 2402. [CrossRef]
68. Hottz, E.D.; Medeiros-de-Moraes, I.M.; Vieira-de-Abreu, A.; de Assis, E.F.; Vals-de-Souza, R.; Castro-Faria-Neto, H.C.; Weyrich, A.S.; Zimmerman, G.A.; Bozza, F.A.; Bozza, P.T. Platelet Activation and Apoptosis Modulate Monocyte Inflammatory Responses in Dengue. *J. Immunol.* **2014**, *193*, 1864–1872. [CrossRef]
69. Tsai, J.J.; Jen, Y.H.; Chang, J.S.; Hsiao, H.M.; Noisakran, S.; Perng, G.C. Frequency Alterations in Key Innate Immune Cell Components in the Peripheral Blood of Dengue Patients Detected by FACS Analysis. *J. Innate Immun.* **2011**, *3*, 530–540. [CrossRef]
70. Ojha, A.; Bhasym, A.; Mukherjee, S.; Annarapu, G.K.; Bhakuni, T.; Akbar, I.; Seth, T.; Vikram, N.K.; Vrati, S.; Basu, A.; et al. Platelet Factor 4 Promotes Rapid Replication and Propagation of Dengue and Japanese Encephalitis Viruses. *EBioMedicine* **2019**, *39*, 332–347. [CrossRef]
71. Masri, M.F.B.; Mantri, C.K.; Rathore, A.P.S.; John, A.L.S. Peripheral serotonin causes dengue virus–induced thrombocytopenia through 5HT2 receptors. *Blood* **2019**, *133*, 2325–2337. [CrossRef] [PubMed]
72. Malavige, G.N.; Wijewickrama, A.; Fernando, S.; Jeewandara, C.; Ginneliya, A.; Samarasekara, S.; Madushanka, P.; Punchihewa, C.; Paranavitane, S.; Idampitiya, D.; et al. A preliminary study on efficacy of rupatadine for the treatment of acute dengue infection. *Sci. Rep.* **2018**, *8*, 3857. [CrossRef]
73. Ojha, A.; Nandi, D.; Batra, H.; Singhal, R.; Annarapu, G.K.; Bhattacharyya, S.; Seth, T.; Dar, L.; Medigeshi, G.R.; Vrati, S.; et al. Platelet activation determines the severity of thrombocytopenia in dengue infection. *Sci. Rep.* **2017**, *7*, 41697. [CrossRef] [PubMed]
74. Wan, S.W.; Yang, Y.W.; Chu, Y.T.; Lin, C.F.; Chang, C.P.; Yeh, T.M.; Anderson, R.; Lin, Y.S. Anti-dengue virus nonstructural protein 1 antibodies contribute to platelet phagocytosis by macrophages. *Thromb. Haemost.* **2016**, *115*, 646–656.
75. Wang, T.T.; Sewatanon, J.; Memoli, M.J.; Wrammert, J.; Bournazos, S.; Bhaumik, S.K.; Pinsky, B.A.; Chokephaibulkit, K.; Onlamoon, N.; Pattanapanyasat, K.; et al. IgG antibodies to dengue enhanced for FcγRIIIA binding determine disease severity. *Science* **2017**, *355*, 395–398. [CrossRef]
76. Wan, S.W.; Lu, Y.T.; Huang, C.H.; Lin, C.F.; Anderson, R.; Liu, H.S.; Yeh, T.M.; Yen, Y.T.; Wu-Hsieh, B.A.; Lin, Y.S. Protection against dengue virus infection in mice by ad-ministration of antibodies against modified nonstructural protein 1. *PLoS ONE* **2014**, *9*, e92495. [CrossRef]
77. Wan, S.W.; Chen, P.W.; Chen, C.Y.; Lai, Y.C.; Chu, Y.T.; Hung, C.Y.; Lee, H.; Wu, H.F.; Chuang, Y.C.; Lin, J.; et al. Therapeutic Effects of Monoclonal Antibody against Dengue Virus NS1 in a STAT1 Knockout Mouse Model of Dengue Infection. *J. Immunol.* **2017**, *199*, 2834–2844. [CrossRef] [PubMed]
78. Simon, A.Y.; Sutherland, M.R.; Pryzdial, E.L. Dengue virus binding and replication by platelets. *Blood* **2015**, *126*, 378–385. [CrossRef]
79. Tomo, S.; Mohan, S.; Ramachandrappa, V.S.; Samadanam, D.M.; Suresh, S.; Pillai, A.B.; Tamilarasu, K.; Ramachandran, R.; Rajendiran, S. Dynamic modulation of DC-SIGN and FcγR2A receptors expression on platelets in dengue. *PLoS ONE* **2018**, *13*, e0206346. [CrossRef]
80. Noisakran, S.; Onlamoon, N.; Pattanapanyasat, K.; Hsiao, H.M.; Songprakhon, P.; Angkasekwinai, N.; Chokephaibulkit, K.; Villinger, F.; Ansari, A.A.; Perng, G.C. Role of CD61+ cells in thrombocytopenia of dengue patients. *Int. J. Hematol.* **2012**, *96*, 600–610. [CrossRef]
81. Attatippaholkun, N.; Kosaisawe, N.; Yaowalak, U.P.; Supraditaporn, P.; Lorthongpanich, C.; Pattanapanyasat, K.; Issaragrisil, S. Selective Tropism of Dengue Virus for Human Glycoprotein Ib. *Sci. Rep.* **2018**, *8*, 2688. [CrossRef]
82. Torres, J.R.; Falleiros-Arlant, L.H.; Dueñas, L.; Pleitez-Navarrete, J.; Salgado, D.M.; Castillo, J.B. Congenital and perinatal complications of chikungunya fever: A Latin American experience. *Int. J. Infect. Dis.* **2016**, *51*, 85–88. [CrossRef] [PubMed]
83. Shahid, U.; Farooqi, J.Q.; Barr, K.L.; Mahmood, S.F.; Jamil, B.; Imitaz, K.; Azizullah, Z.; Malik, F.R.; Prakoso, D.; Long, M.T.; et al. Comparison of clinical presentation and out-comes of Chikungunya and Dengue virus infections in patients with acute undifferentiated febrile illness from the Sindh region of Pa-kistan. *PLoS Negl. Trop. Dis.* **2020**, *14*, e0008086. [CrossRef] [PubMed]
84. Doğan, H.O.; Büyüktuna, S.A.; Kapancik, S.; Bakir, S. Evaluation of the associations between endothelial dysfunction, inflammation and coagulation in Crimean-Congo hemorrhagic fever patients. *Arch. Virol.* **2018**, *163*, 609–616. [CrossRef]
85. Yilmaz, H.; Yilmaz, G.; Menteşe, A.; Kostakoğlu, U.; Karahan, S.C.; Köksal, İ. Prognostic impact of platelet distribution width in patients with Crimean-Congo hemorrhagic fever. *J. Med Virol.* **2016**, *88*, 1862–1866. [CrossRef]
86. Solomon, T.; Dung, N.M.; Kneen, R.; Gainsborough, M.; Vaughn, D.W.; Khanh, V.T. Japanese encephalitis. *J. Neurol. Neurosurg. Psychiatry* **2000**, *68*, 405. [CrossRef]

87. Ma'roef, C.N.; Dhenni, R.; Megawati, D.; Fadhilah, A.; Lucanus, A.; Artika, I.M.; Masyeni, S.; Lestarini, A.; Sari, K.; Suryana, K.; et al. Japanese encephalitis virus infection in non-encephalitic acute febrile illness patients. *PLoS Negl. Trop. Dis.* **2020**, *14*, e0008454. [CrossRef]
88. Liu, S.; Chai, C.; Wang, C.; Amer, S.; Lv, H.; He, H.; Sun, J.; Lin, J. Systematic review of severe fever with thrombocytopenia syndrome:virology, epidemiology, and clinical characteristics. *Rev. Med Virol.* **2013**, *24*, 90–102. [CrossRef]
89. Hofmann, H.; Li, X.; Zhang, X.; Liu, W.; Kühl, A.; Kaup, F.; Soldan, S.S.; González-Scarano, F.; Weber, F.; He, Y.; et al. Severe fever with thrombocytopenia virus glycoproteins are targeted by neutralizing antibodies and can use DC-SIGN as a receptor for pH-dependent entry into human and animal cell lines. *J. Virol.* **2013**, *87*, 4384–4394. [CrossRef]
90. Li, X.K.; Lu, Q.B.; Chen, W.W.; Xu, W.; Liu, R.; Zhang, S.F.; Du, J.; Li, H.; Yao, K.; Zhai, D.; et al. Arginine deficiency is involved in thrombocytopenia and immuno-suppression in severe fever with thrombocytopenia syndrome. *Sci. Transl. Med.* **2018**, *10*, eaat4162. [CrossRef] [PubMed]
91. Ruzek, D.; Avšič Županc, T.; Borde, J.; Chrdle, A.; Eyer, L.; Karganova, G.; Kholodilov, I.; Knap, N.; Kozlovskaya, L.; Matveev, A.; et al. Tick-borne encephalitis in Europe and Russia: Review of pathogenesis, clinical features, therapy, and vaccines. *Antivir. Res.* **2019**, *164*, 23–51. [CrossRef]
92. Moniuszko, A.; Pancewicz, S.; Czupryna, P.; Grygorczuk, S.; Świerzbińska, R.; Kondrusik, M.; Penza, P.; Zajkowska, J. ssICAM-1, IL-21 and IL-23 in patients with tick borne encephalitis and neuroborreliosis. *Cytokine* **2012**, *60*, 468–472. [CrossRef]
93. Ahmad, A.; Ashraf, S.; Komai, S. Are developing countries prepared to face Ebola-like outbreaks? *Virol. Sin.* **2015**, *30*, 234–237. [CrossRef]
94. Loria, G.D.; Romagnoli, P.A.; Moseley, N.B.; Rucavado, A.; Altman, J.D. Platelets support a protective immune response to LCMV by preventing splenic necrosis. *Blood* **2013**, *121*, 940–950. [CrossRef]
95. Paddock, C.D.; Nicholson, W.L.; Bhatnagar, J.; Goldsmith, C.S.; Greer, P.W.; Hayes, E.B.; Risko, J.A.; Henderson, C.; Blackmore, C.G.; Lanciotti, R.S.; et al. Fatal Hemorrhagic Fever Caused by West Nile Virus in the United States. *Clin. Infect. Dis.* **2006**, *42*, 1527–1535. [CrossRef]
96. Hayes, C.; Stephens, L.; Fridey, J.L.; Snyder, R.E.; Groves, J.A.; Stramer, S.L.; Klapper, E. Probable transfusion transmission of West Nile virus from an apheresis platelet that screened non-reactive by individual donor-nucleic acid testing. *Transfusion* **2019**, *60*, 424–429. [CrossRef]
97. Lataillade, L.G.; Vazeille, M.; Obadia, T.; Madec, Y.; Mousson, L.; Kamgang, B.; Chen, C.H.; Failloux, A.B.; Yen, P.S. Risk of yellow fever virus transmission in the Asia-Pacific region. *Nat. Commun.* **2020**, *11*, 5801. [CrossRef] [PubMed]
98. Garske, T.; Van Kerkhove, M.D.; Yactayo, S.; Ronveaux, O.; Lewis, R.F.; Staples, J.E.; Perea, W.; Ferguson, N.M. Yellow Fever in Africa: Estimating the Burden of Disease and Impact of Mass Vaccination from Outbreak and Serological Data. *PLoS Med.* **2014**, *11*, e1001638. [CrossRef] [PubMed]
99. Oliosi, E.; Serero Corcos, C.; Barroso, P.F.; Bleibtreu, A.; Grard, G.; De Filippis, B.A.M.; Caumes, E. Yellow fever in two unvaccinated French tourists to Brazil, January and March, 2018. *Eurosurveillance* **2018**, *23*, 1800240. [CrossRef] [PubMed]
100. Ho, Y.L.; Joelsons, D.; Leite, G.F.C.; Malbouisson, L.M.S.; Song, A.T.W.; Perondi, B.; Andrade, L.C.; Pinto, L.F.; D'Albuquerque, L.A.C.; Segurado, A.A.C. Severe yellow fever in Brazil: Clinical charac-teristics and management. *J. Travel Med.* **2019**, *26*, taz040. [CrossRef] [PubMed]
101. Brandão-de-Resende, C.; Cunha, L.H.M.; Oliveira, S.L.; Pereira, L.S.; Oliveira, J.G.F.; Santos, T.A.; Vasconcelos-Santos, D.V. Characterization of Retinopathy Among Patients with Yellow Fever During 2 Outbreaks in Southeastern Brazil. *JAMA Ophthalmol.* **2019**, *137*, 996–1002. [CrossRef] [PubMed]
102. Musso, D.; Ko, A.I.; Baud, D. Zika Virus Infection—After the Pandemic. *N. Engl. J. Med.* **2019**, *381*, 1444–1457. [CrossRef]
103. Langerak, T.; Brinkman, T.; Mumtaz, N.; Arron, G.; Hermelijn, S.; Baldewsingh, G.; Wongsokarijo, M.; Resida, L.; Rockx, B.; Koopmans, M.P.G.; et al. Zika virus seroprevalence in urban and rural areas of Suriname in 2017. *J. Infect. Dis.* **2019**, *220*, 28–31. [CrossRef]
104. Saba Villarroel, P.M.; Nurtop, E.; Pastorino, B.; Roca, Y.; Drexler, J.F.; Gallian, P.; Jaenisch, T.; Leparc-Goffart, I.; Priet, S.; Ninove, L.; et al. Zika virus epidemiology in Bolivia: A sero-prevalence study in volunteer blood donors. *PLoS Negl. Trop. Dis.* **2018**, *12*, e0006239. [CrossRef]
105. Netto, E.M.; Moreira-Soto, A.; Pedroso, C.; Höser, C.; Funk, S.; Kucharski, A.J.; Rockstroh, A.; Kümmerer, B.M.; Sampaio, G.S.; Luz, E.; et al. High Zika Virus Seroprevalence in Salvador, Northeastern Brazil Limits the Potential for Further Outbreaks. *mBio* **2017**, *8*. [CrossRef]
106. Van Dyne, E.A.; Neaterour, P.; Rivera, A.; Bello-Pagan, M.; Adams, L.; Munoz-Jordan, J.; Baez, P.; Garcia, M.; Waterman, S.H.; Reyes, N.; et al. Incidence and Outcome of Severe and Nonsevere Thrombocytopenia Associated with Zika Virus Infection-Puerto Rico, 2016. *Open Forum Infect. Dis.* **2019**, *6*, ofy325. [CrossRef] [PubMed]
107. Wu, Y.; Cui, X.; Wu, N.; Song, R.; Yang, W.; Zhang, W.; Fan, D.; Chen, Z.; An, J. A unique case of human Zika virus infection in association with severe liver injury and coagulation disorders. *Sci. Rep.* **2017**, *7*, 11393. [CrossRef] [PubMed]
108. Azevedo, R.S.; Araujo, M.T.; Martins Filho, A.J.; Oliveira, C.S.; Nunes, B.T.; Cruz, A.C.; Nascimento, A.G.; Medeiros, R.C.; Caldas, C.A.; Araujo, F.C.; et al. Zika virus epidemic in Brazil. I. Fatal disease in adults: Clinical and laboratorial aspects. *J. Clin. Virol.* **2016**, *85*, 56–64. [CrossRef] [PubMed]
109. Sokal, A.; D'Ortenzio, E.; Houhou-Fidouh, N.; Brichler, S.; Dorchies, J.; Cabras, O.; Leparc-Goffart, I.; Yazdanpanah, Y.; Matheron, S. Zika virus infection: Report of the first imported cases in a Paris travel centre. *J. Travel Med.* **2016**, *24*. [CrossRef]

110. Bandeira, A.C.; Gois, L.L.; Campos, G.S.; Sardi, S.; Yssel, H.; Vieillard, V.; Autran, B.; Grassi, M.F.R. Clinical and laboratory findings of acute Zika virus infection in patients from Salvador during the first Brazilian epidemic. *Braz. J. Infect. Dis.* **2020**, *24*, 405–411. [CrossRef] [PubMed]
111. Ng, D.H.L.; Ho, H.J.; Chow, A.; Wong, J.; Kyaw, W.M.; Tan, A.; Chia, P.Y.; Choy, C.Y.; Tan, G.; Yeo, T.W.; et al. Correlation of clinical illness with viremia in Zika virus disease during an outbreak in Singapore. *BMC Infect. Dis.* **2018**, *18*, 301. [CrossRef] [PubMed]
112. Sharp, T.M.; Muñoz-Jordán, J.; Perez-Padilla, J.; Bello-Pagán, M.I.; Rivera, A.; Pastula, D.M.; Salinas, J.L.; Martínez Mendez, J.H.; Méndez, M.; Powers, A.M.; et al. Zika Virus Infection Associated With Severe Thrombocytopenia. *Clin. Infect. Dis.* **2016**, *63*, 1198–1201. [CrossRef] [PubMed]
113. Chraïbi, S.; Najioullah, F.; Bourdin, C.; Pegliasco, J.; Deligny, C.; Résière, D.; Meniane, J.C. Two cases of thrombocytopenic purpura at onset of Zika virus infection. *J. Clin. Virol.* **2016**, *83*, 61–62. [CrossRef] [PubMed]
114. Boyer Chammard, T.; Schepers, K.; Breurec, S.; Messiaen, T.; Destrem, A.L.; Mahevas, M.; Soulillou, A.; Janaud, L.; Curlier, E.; Herrmann-Storck, C.; et al. Severe Thrombocytopenia after Zika Virus Infection, Guadeloupe, 2016. *Emerg. Infect. Dis.* **2017**, *23*, 696–698. [CrossRef] [PubMed]
115. Zea-Vera, A.F.; Parra, B. Zika virus (ZIKV) infection related with immune thrombocytopenic purpura (ITP) exacerbation and antinuclear antibody positivity. *Lupus* **2016**, *26*, 890–892. [CrossRef] [PubMed]
116. Roth, H.; Schneider, L.; Eberle, R.; Lausen, J.; Modlich, U.; Blümel, J.; Baylis, S.A. Zika virus infection studies with CD34 + hematopoietic and megakaryocyte-erythroid progenitors, red blood cells and platelets. *Transfusion* **2020**, *60*, 561–574. [CrossRef] [PubMed]
117. Hunsberger, S.; Ortega-Villa, A.M.; Powers, J.H., 3rd; León, H.A.R.; Sosa, S.C.; Hernández, E.R.; Nájera Cancino, J.G.; Nason, M.; Lumbard, K.; Sepulveda, J.; et al. Patterns of signs, symptoms and laboratory values associated with Zika, dengue and undefined acute illnesses in a dengue endemic region: Secondary analysis of a prospective cohort study in southern México. *Int. J. Infect. Dis.* **2020**, *98*, 241–248. [CrossRef]
118. Musso, D.; Nhan, T.X.; de Pina, J.J.; Marchi, J.; Texier, G. The Use of Simple Laboratory Parameters in the Differential Diagnosis of Acute-Phase Zika and Dengue Viruses. *Intervirology* **2019**, *62*, 51–56. [CrossRef]
119. Yan, G.; Pang, L.; Cook, A.R.; Ho, H.J.; Win, M.S.; Khoo, A.L.; Wong, J.G.X.; Lee, C.K.; Yan, B.; Jureen, R.; et al. Distinguishing Zika and Dengue Viruses through Simple Clinical Assessment, Singapore. *Emerg. Infect. Dis.* **2018**, *24*, 1565–1568. [CrossRef]
120. Wang, R.Q.; Zhang, Q.S.; Zhao, S.X.; Niu, X.M.; Du, J.H.; Du, H.J.; Nan, Y.M. Gamma-glutamyl transpeptidase to platelet ratio index is a good noninvasive biomarker for predicting liver fibrosis in Chinese chronic hepatitis B patients. *J. Int. Med Res.* **2016**, *44*, 1302–1313. [CrossRef]
121. Zhang, W.; Sun, M.; Chen, G.; An, Y.; Lv, C.; Wang, Y.; Shang, Q. Reassessment of gamma-glutamyl transpeptidase to platelet ratio (GPR): A large-sample, dynamic study based on liver biopsy in a Chinese population with chronic hepatitis B virus (HBV) infection. *Gut* **2017**, *67*, 989–991. [CrossRef]
122. Lee, H.S.; Kweon, Y.O.; Tak, W.Y.; Park, S.Y.; Kang, E.J.; Lee, Y.L.; Yang, H.M.; Park, H.W. Advanced fibrosis is not a negative pretreatment predictive factor for genotype 2 or 3 chronic hepatitis C patients. *Clin. Mol. Hepatol.* **2013**, *19*, 148–155. [CrossRef] [PubMed]
123. Ismael, M.N.; Forde, J.; Milla, E.; Khan, W.; Cabrera, R. Utility of Inflammatory Markers in Predicting Hepatocellular Carcinoma Survival after Liver Transplantation. *BioMed Res. Int.* **2019**, *2019*, 7284040. [CrossRef] [PubMed]
124. Tian, X.C.; Liu, X.L.; Zeng, F.R.; Chen, Z.; Wu, D.H. Platelet-to-lymphocyte ratio acts as an independent risk factor for patients with hepatitis B virus-related hepatocellular carcinoma who received transarterial chemoembolization. *Eur. Rev. Med Pharmacol. Sci.* **2016**, *20*, 2302–2309. [PubMed]
125. Shen, S.L.; Fu, S.J.; Chen, B.; Kuang, M.; Li, S.Q.; Hua, Y.P.; Liang, L.J.; Guo, P.; Hao, Y.; Peng, B.G. Preoperative aspartate aminotransferase to platelet ratio is an inde-pendent prognostic factor for hepatitis B-induced hepatocellular carcinoma after hepatic resection. *Ann. Surg. Oncol.* **2014**, *21*, 3802–3809. [CrossRef]
126. Dou, J.; Lou, Y.; Wu, Z.; Lu, Y.; Jin, Y. Thrombocytopenia in patients with hepatitis B virus-related chronic hepatitis: Evaluation of the immature platelet fraction. *Platelets* **2014**, *25*, 399–404. [CrossRef]
127. Cho, S.Y.; Lee, A.; Lee, H.J.; Suh, J.T.; Park, T.S. Mean platelet volume in Korean patients with hepatic diseases. *Platelets* **2012**, *23*, 648–649. [CrossRef] [PubMed]
128. Ying, L.; Wang, F.; Zhang, J.; Yang, L.; Gong, X.; Fan, Y.; Xu, K.; Li, J.; Lu, Y.; Mei, L.; et al. Impact of hepatitis B virus (HBV) infection on platelet response to clopidogrel in patients undergoing coronary stent implantation. *Thromb. Res.* **2018**, *167*, 119–124. [CrossRef]
129. Lima, D.S.; Murad Júnior, A.J.; Barreira, M.A.; Fernandes, G.C.; Coelho, G.R.; Garcia, J.H.P. Liver Transplantation in Hepatitis Delta: South America Experience. *Arquivos de Gastroenterologia* **2018**, *55*, 14–17. [CrossRef]
130. Onan, E.; Uskudar, O.; Coşkun, Y.; Akkız, H. Higher hepatitis C [correction of hepatis C] virus concentration in platelets than in plasma in a patient with ITP. *Platelets* **2012**, *23*, 413–414. [CrossRef]
131. Olariu, M.; Olariu, C.; Olteanu, D. Thrombocytopenia in chronic hepatitis C. *J. Gastrointest. Liver Dis.* **2010**, *19*, 381–385.
132. Ariede, J.R.; Pardini, M.I.; Silva, G.F.; Grotto, R.M. Platelets can be a biological compartment for the Hepatitis C Virus. *Braz. J. Microbiol.* **2015**, *46*, 627–629. [CrossRef]

133. Espírito-Santo, M.P.; Brandão-Mello, C.E.; Marques, V.A.; Lampe, E.; Almeida, A.J. Analysis of hepatitis C virus (HCV) RNA load in platelets of HCV-monoinfected patients receiving antiviral therapy. *Ann. Hepatol.* **2013**, *12*, 373–379. [CrossRef]
134. Ragin, A.B.; D'Souza, G.; Reynolds, S.; Miller, E.; Sacktor, N.; Selnes, O.A.; Martin, E.; Visscher, B.R.; Becker, J.T. Platelet decline as a predictor of brain injury in HIV infection. *J. NeuroVirology* **2011**, *17*, 487–495. [CrossRef] [PubMed]
135. Pastori, D.; Esposito, A.; Carnevale, R.; Bartimoccia, S.; Novo, M.; Fantauzzi, A.; Di Campli, F.; Pignatelli, P.; Violi, F.; Mezzaroma, I. HIV-1 induces in vivo platelet activation by enhancing platelet NOX2 activity. *J. Infect.* **2015**, *70*, 651–658. [CrossRef] [PubMed]
136. Nkambule, B.B.; Davison, G.M.; Ipp, H. The evaluation of platelet indices and markers of inflammation, coagulation and disease progression in treatment-naïve, asymptomatic HIV-infected individuals. *Int. J. Lab. Hematol.* **2015**, *37*, 450–458. [CrossRef]
137. Mena, Á.; Meijide, H.; Vázquez, P.; Castro, Á.; López, S.; Bello, L.; Serrano, J.; Baliñas, J.; Pedreira, J.D. HIV Increases Mean Platelet Volume During Asymptomatic HIV Infection in Treatment-Naive Patients. *J. Acquir. Immune Defic. Syndr.* **2011**, *57*, e112–e113. [CrossRef]
138. Beck, Z.; Jagodzinski, L.L.; Eller, M.A.; Thelian, D.; Matyas, G.R.; Kunz, A.N.; Alving, C.R. Platelets and erythrocyte-bound platelets bind in-fectious HIV-1 in plasma of chronically infected patients. *PLoS ONE* **2013**, *8*, e81002. [CrossRef]
139. Auerbach, D.J.; Lin, Y.; Miao, H.; Cimbro, R.; Difiore, M.J.; Gianolini, M.E.; Furci, L.; Biswas, P.; Fauci, A.S.; Lusso, P. Identification of the platelet-derived chemokine CXCL4/PF-4 as a broad-spectrum HIV-1 inhibitor. *Proc. Natl. Acad. Sci. USA* **2012**, *109*, 9569–9574. [CrossRef] [PubMed]
140. Hottz, E.D.; Quirino-Teixeira, A.C.; Valls-de-Souza, R.; Zimmerman, G.A.; Bozza, F.A.; Bozza, P.T. Platelet function in HIV plus dengue coinfection associates with reduced inflammation and milder dengue illness. *Sci. Rep.* **2019**, *9*, 7096. [CrossRef]
141. Real, F.; Capron, C.; Sennepin, A.; Arrigucci, R.; Zhu, A.; Sannier, G.; Zheng, J.; Xu, L.; Massé, J.M.; Greffe, S.; et al. Platelets from HIV-infected individuals on antiretroviral drug therapy with poor CD4+ T cell recovery can harbor replication-competent HIV despite viral suppression. *Sci. Transl. Med.* **2020**, *12*, eaat6263. [CrossRef]
142. Nkambule, B.B.; Davison, G.; Ipp, H. Platelet leukocyte aggregates and markers of platelet aggregation, immune activation and disease progression in HIV infected treatment naive asymptomatic individuals. *J. Thromb. Thrombolysis* **2015**, *40*, 458–467. [CrossRef]
143. Liang, H.; Duan, Z.; Li, D.; Li, D.; Wang, Z.; Ren, L.; Shen, T.; Shao, Y. Higher levels of circulating monocyte–platelet aggregates are correlated with viremia and increased sCD163 levels in HIV-1 infection. *Cell. Mol. Immunol.* **2015**, *12*, 435–443. [CrossRef] [PubMed]
144. Singh, M.V.; Davidson, D.C.; Kiebala, M.; Maggirwar, S.B. Detection of circulating platelet–monocyte complexes in persons infected with human immunodeficiency virus type-1. *J. Virol. Methods* **2012**, *181*, 170–176. [CrossRef]
145. Singh, M.V.; Davidson, D.C.; Jackson, J.W.; Singh, V.B.; Silva, J.; Ramirez, S.H.; Maggirwar, S.B. Characterization of Platelet–Monocyte Complexes in HIV-1–Infected Individuals: Possible Role in HIV-Associated Neuroinflammation. *J. Immunol.* **2014**, *192*, 4674–4684. [CrossRef]
146. Davidson, D.C.; Hirschman, M.P.; Spinelli, S.L.; Morrell, C.N.; Schifitto, G.; Phipps, R.P.; Maggirwar, S.B. Antiplatelet Activity of Valproic Acid Contributes to Decreased Soluble CD40 Ligand Production in HIV Type 1-Infected Individuals. *J. Immunol.* **2011**, *186*, 584–591. [CrossRef]
147. Wang, J.; Zhang, W.; Nardi, M.A.; Li, Z. HIV-1 Tat-induced platelet activation and release of CD154 contribute to HIV-1-associated autoimmune thrombocytopenia. *J. Thromb. Haemost.* **2011**, *9*, 562–573. [CrossRef]
148. Damien, P.; Cognasse, F.; Lucht, F.; Suy, F.; Pozzetto, B.; Garraud, O.; Hamzeh-Cognasse, H. Highly Active Antiretroviral Therapy Alters Inflammation Linked to Platelet Cytokines in HIV-1-Infected Patients. *J. Infect. Dis.* **2013**, *208*, 868–870. [CrossRef] [PubMed]
149. O'Halloran, J.A.; Dunne, E.; Gurwith, M.; Lambert, J.S.; Sheehan, G.J.; Feeney, E.R.; Pozniak, A.; Reiss, P.; Kenny, D.; Mallon, P. The effect of initiation of antiretroviral therapy on monocyte, endothelial and platelet function in HIV-1 infection. *HIV Med.* **2015**, *16*, 608–619. [CrossRef]
150. Connolly-Andersen, A.M.; Sundberg, E.; Ahlm, C.; Hultdin, J.; Baudin, M.; Larsson, J.; Dunne, E.; Kenny, D.; Lindahl, T.L.; Ramström, S.; et al. Increased Thrombopoiesis and Platelet Activation in Hantavirus-Infected Patients. *J. Infect. Dis.* **2015**, *212*, 1061–1069. [CrossRef] [PubMed]
151. Laine, O.; Mäkelä, S.; Mustonen, J.; Helminen, M.; Vaheri, A.; Lassila, R.; Joutsi-Korhonen, L. Platelet ligands and ADAMTS13 during Puumala hantavirus infection and associated thrombocytopenia. *Blood Coagul. Fibrinolysis* **2011**, *22*, 468–472. [CrossRef] [PubMed]
152. Laine, O.; Joutsi-Korhonen, L.; Lassila, R.; Koski, T.; Huhtala, H.; Vaheri, A.; Mäkelä, S.; Mustonen, J. Hantavirus infection-induced thrombocytopenia triggers increased production but associates with impaired aggregation of platelets except for collagen. *Thromb. Res.* **2015**, *136*, 1126–1132. [CrossRef] [PubMed]
153. Lütteke, N.; Raftery, M.J.; Lalwani, P.; Lee, M.H.; Giese, T.; Voigt, S.; Bannert, N.; Schulze, H.; Krüger, D.H.; Schönrich, G. Switch to high-level virus replication and HLA class I upregulation in differentiating megakaryocytic cells after infection with pathogenic hantavirus. *Virology* **2010**, *405*, 70–80. [CrossRef] [PubMed]
154. Goeijenbier, M.; Meijers, J.C.; Anfasa, F.; Roose, J.M.; van de Weg, C.A.; Bakhtiari, K.; Henttonen, H.; Vaheri, A.; Osterhaus, A.D.; van Gorp, E.C.; et al. Effect of Puumala hantavirus infection on human umbilical vein endothelial cell hemostatic function: Platelet interactions, increased tissue factor expression and fibrinolysis regulator release. *Front. Microbiol.* **2015**, *6*, 220. [CrossRef]

155. Miyoshi, Y.; Yoshioka, S.; Gosho, H.; Miyazoe, S.; Suenaga, H.; Aoki, M.; Hashimoto, K. A neonatal case of coxsackievirus B3 vertical infection with symptoms of hemophagocytic lymphohistiocytosis. *IDCases* **2020**, *20*, e00738. [CrossRef] [PubMed]
156. Kaga, A.; Katata, Y.; Suzuki, A.; Otani, K.; Watanabe, H.; Kitaoka, S.; Kumaki, S. Perinatal Coxsackievirus B3 Infection with Transient Thrombocytopenia. *Tohoku J. Exp. Med.* **2016**, *239*, 135–138. [CrossRef]
157. Hara, S.; Kawada, J.; Kawano, Y.; Yamashita, T.; Minagawa, H.; Okumura, N.; Ito, Y. Hyperferritinemia in neonatal and infantile human parechovirus-3 infection in comparison with other infectious diseases. *J. Infect. Chemother.* **2014**, *20*, 15–19. [CrossRef]
158. Negrotto, S.; Jaquenod de Giusti, C.; Rivadeneyra, L.; Ure, A.E.; Mena, H.A.; Schattner, M.; Gomez, R.M. Platelets interact with Cox-sackieviruses B and have a critical role in the pathogenesis of virus-induced myocarditis. *J. Thromb. Haemost.* **2015**, *13*, 271–282. [CrossRef] [PubMed]
159. Troeger, C.; Khalil, I.A.; Rao, P.C.; Cao, S.; Blacker, B.F.; Ahmed, T.; Armah, G.; Bines, J.E.; Brewer, T.G.; Colombara, D.V.; et al. Rotavirus Vaccination and the Global Burden of Rotavirus Diarrhea Among Children Younger Than 5 Years. *JAMA Pediatr.* **2018**, *172*, 958–965. [CrossRef]
160. Mete, E.; Akelma, A.Z.; Cizmeci, M.N.; Bozkaya, D.; Kanburoglu, M.K. Decreased mean platelet volume in children with acute rotavirus gastroenteritis. *Platelets* **2014**, *25*, 51–54. [CrossRef]
161. Plosa, E.J.; Esbenshade, J.C.; Fuller, M.P.; Weitkamp, J.-H. Cytomegalovirus Infection. *Pediatr. Rev.* **2012**, *33*, 156. [CrossRef] [PubMed]
162. Dunmire, S.K.; Hogquist, K.A.; Balfour, H.H. Infectious Mononucleosis. *Curr. Top. Microbiol. Immunol.* **2015**, *390 Pt 1*, 211–240.
163. Freeman, M.L.; Burkum, C.E.; Lanzer, K.G.; Roberts, A.D.; Pinkevych, M.; Itakura, E.; Kummer, L.W.; Szaba, F.M.; Davenport, M.P.; McCarty, O.J.; et al. Gammaherpesvirus latency induces antibody-associated thrombocytopenia in mice. *J. Autoimmun.* **2013**, *42*, 71–79. [CrossRef] [PubMed]
164. Dulery, R.; Salleron, J.; Dewilde, A.; Rossignol, J.; Boyle, E.M.; Gay, J.; de Berranger, E.; Coiteux, V.; Jouet, J.P.; Duhamel, A.; et al. Early human herpesvirus type 6 reactivation after al-logeneic stem cell transplantation: A large-scale clinical study. *Biol. Blood Marrow Transplant.* **2012**, *18*, 1080–1089. [CrossRef]
165. Scotch, A.H.; Hoss, E.; Orenstein, R.; Budavari, A.I. Disseminated Varicella-Zoster Virus After Vaccination in an Immunocompetent Patient. *J. Am. Osteopat. Assoc.* **2016**, *116*, 402–405. [CrossRef]
166. Kim, S.T.; Park, K.H.; Oh, S.C.; Seo, J.H.; Shin, S.W.; Kim, J.S.; Kim, Y.H. Varicella Zoster Virus Infection during Chemotherapy in Solid Cancer Patients. *Oncology* **2012**, *82*, 126–130. [CrossRef] [PubMed]
167. Saitoh, T.; Takahashi, N.; Nanjo, H.; Kawabata, Y.; Hirokawa, M.; Sawada, K. Varicella-Zoster Virus-associated Fulminant Hepatitis Following Allogeneic Hematopoietic Stem Cell Transplantation for Multiple Myeloma. *Intern. Med.* **2013**, *52*, 1727–1730. [CrossRef]
168. Zhang, W.; Ruan, Q.L.; Yan, F.; Hu, Y.K. Fatal hemorrhagic varicella in a patient with abdominal pain: A case report. *BMC Infect. Dis.* **2020**, *20*, 54. [CrossRef] [PubMed]
169. Furuto, Y.; Kawamura, M.; Namikawa, A.; Takahashi, H.; Shibuya, Y. Successful management of visceral disseminated varicella zoster virus infection during treatment of membranous nephropathy: A case report. *BMC Infect. Dis.* **2019**, *19*, 625. [CrossRef]
170. Bollea-Garlatti, M.L.; Bollea-Garlatti, L.A.; Vacas, A.S.; Torre, A.C.; Kowalczuk, A.M.; Galimberti, R.L.; Ferreyro, B.L. Clinical Characteristics and Outcomes in a Population With Disseminated Herpes Zoster: A Retrospective Cohort Study. *Actas Dermo-Sifiliográficas* **2017**, *108*, 145–152. [CrossRef]
171. Nagel, M.A.; Traktinskiy, I.; Azarkh, Y.; Kleinschmidt-DeMasters, B.; Hedley-Whyte, T.; Russman, A.; VanEgmond, E.M.; Stenmark, K.; Frid, M.; Mahalingam, R.; et al. Varicella zoster virus vasculopathy: Analysis of virus-infected arteries. *Neurology* **2011**, *77*, 364–370. [CrossRef]
172. Hoshino, T.; Toi, S.; Toda, K.; Uchiyama, Y.; Yoshizawa, H.; Iijima, M.; Shimizu, Y.; Kitagawa, K. Ischemic Stroke due to Virologically-Confirmed Varicella Zoster Virus Vasculopathy: A Case Series. *J. Stroke Cerebrovasc. Dis.* **2019**, *28*, 338–343. [CrossRef]
173. Uthayakumar, A.; Harrington, D. Spontaneous splenic rupture complicating primary varicella zoster infection: A case report. *BMC Res. Notes* **2018**, *11*, 334. [CrossRef]
174. Tsappa, I.; Missouris, C.; Psarellis, S. Acyclovir-induced thrombocytopaenia in a patient with SLE. *BMJ Case Rep.* **2018**, *2018*, bcr-2018. [CrossRef]
175. Shibusawa, M.; Motomura, S.; Hidai, H.; Tsutsumi, H.; Fujita, A. Varicella infection complicated by marked thrombocytopenia. *Jpn. J. Infect. Dis.* **2014**, *67*, 292–294. [CrossRef]
176. Yoshida, T.; Higuchi, T.; Suzuki, L.; Koyamada, R.; Okada, S. Relapse of Immune Thrombocytopenia Associated with Varicella 20 Years after Splenectomy. *Intern. Med.* **2014**, *53*, 2721–2723. [CrossRef]
177. Diniz, L.M.O.; Maia, M.M.M.; Oliveira, Y.V.; Mourão, M.S.F.; Couto, A.V.; Mota, V.C.; Versiani, C.M.; Silveira, P.; Romanelli, R.M.C. Study of Complications of Varicella-Zoster Virus Infection in Hospitalized Children at a Reference Hospital for Infectious Disease Treatment. *Hosp. Pediatr.* **2018**, *8*, 419–425. [CrossRef] [PubMed]
178. Kim, H.J.; Choi, S.M.; Lee, J.; Park, Y.S.; Lee, C.H.; Yim, J.J.; Yoo, C.G.; Kim, Y.W.; Han, S.K.; Lee, S.M. Respiratory virus of severe pneumonia in South Korea: Prevalence and clinical implications. *PLoS ONE* **2018**, *13*, e0198902. [CrossRef] [PubMed]
179. Shang, X.; Liabsuetrakul, T.; Sangsupawanich, P.; Xia, X.; He, P.; Cao, H.; McNeil, E. Efficacy and safety of Laggera pterodonta in children 3–24 months with acute bronchiolitis: A randomized controlled trial. *Clin. Respir. J.* **2017**, *11*, 296–304. [CrossRef] [PubMed]

180. Al Shibli, A.; Alkuwaiti, N.; Hamie, M.; Abukhater, D.; Noureddin, M.B.; Amri, A.; Al Kaabi, S.; Al Kaabi, A.; Harbi, M.; Narchi, H. Significance of platelet count in children admitted with bronchiolitis. *World J. Clin. Pediatrics* **2017**, *6*, 118–123. [CrossRef]
181. Zheng, S.Y.; Xiao, Q.Y.; Xie, X.H.; Deng, Y.; Ren, L.; Tian, D.Y.; Luo, Z.X.; Luo, J.; Fu, Z.; Huang, A.L.; et al. Association between secondary thrombocytosis and viral respiratory tract infections in children. *Sci. Rep.* **2016**, *6*, 22964. [CrossRef] [PubMed]
182. Chan, C.Y.; Low, J.G.; Wyone, W.; Oon, L.L.; Tan, B.H. Survey of Respiratory Virus in Patients Hospitalised for Acute Exacerbations of Heart Failure—A Prospective Observational Study. *Ann. Acad. Med. Singap.* **2018**, *47*, 445–450.
183. Lefrançais, E.; Ortiz-Muñoz, G.; Caudrillier, A.; Mallavia, B.; Liu, F.; Sayah, D.M.; Thornton, E.E.; Headley, M.B.; David, T.; Coughlin, S.R.; et al. The lung is a site of platelet biogenesis and a reservoir for haematopoietic progenitors. *Nature* **2017**, *544*, 105–109. [CrossRef]
184. Gupalo, E.; Buriachkovskaia, L.; Othman, M. Human platelets express CAR with localization at the sites of intercellular interac-tion. *Virol. J.* **2011**, *8*, 456. [CrossRef] [PubMed]
185. Jin, Y.Y.; Yu, X.N.; Qu, Z.Y.; Zhang, A.A.; Xing, Y.L.; Jiang, L.X.; Shang, L.; Wang, Y.C. Adenovirus type 3 induces platelet activation in vitro. *Mol. Med. Rep.* **2014**, *9*, 370–374. [CrossRef]
186. Gupalo, E.; Kuk, C.; Qadura, M.; Buriachkovskaia, L.; Othman, M. Platelet–adenovirus vs. inert particles interaction: Effect on aggregation and the role of platelet membrane receptors. *Platelets* **2013**, *24*, 383–391. [CrossRef] [PubMed]
187. Escutenaire, S.; Cerullo, V.; Diaconu, I.; Ahtiainen, L.; Hannuksela, P.; Oksanen, M.; Haavisto, E.; Karioja-Kallio, A.; Holm, S.L.; Kangasniemi, L.; et al. In vivo and in vitro distribution of type 5 and fiber-modified oncolytic adenoviruses in human blood compartments. *Ann. Med.* **2011**, *43*, 151–163. [CrossRef]
188. Zhu, R.; Chen, C.; Wang, Q.; Zhang, X.; Lu, C.; Sun, Y. Routine blood parameters are helpful for early identification of influenza infection in children. *BMC Infect. Dis.* **2020**, *20*, 864. [CrossRef]
189. Rose, J.J.; Voora, D.; Cyr, D.D.; Lucas, J.E.; Zaas, A.K.; Woods, C.W.; Newby, L.K.; Kraus, W.E.; Ginsburg, G.S. Gene Expression Profiles Link Respiratory Viral Infection, Platelet Response to Aspirin, and Acute Myocardial Infarction. *PLoS ONE* **2015**, *10*, e0132259. [CrossRef]
190. Sugiyama, M.G.; Gamage, A.; Zyla, R.; Armstrong, S.M.; Advani, S.; Advani, A.; Wang, C.; Lee, W.L. Influenza Virus Infection Induces Plate-let-Endothelial Adhesion Which Contributes to Lung Injury. *J. Virol.* **2016**, *90*, 1812–1823. [CrossRef]
191. Jansen, A.J.G.; Spaan, T.; Low, H.Z.; Di Iorio, D.; van den Brand, J.; Tieke, M.; Barendrecht, A.; Rohn, K.; van Amerongen, G.; Stittelaar, K.; et al. Influenza-induced thrombocytopenia is dependent on the subtype and sialoglycan receptor and increases with virus pathogenicity. *Blood Adv.* **2020**, *4*, 2967–2978. [CrossRef]
192. Koupenova, M.; Corkrey, H.A.; Vitseva, O.; Manni, G.; Pang, C.J.; Clancy, L.; Yao, C.; Rade, J.; Levy, D.; Wang, J.P.; et al. The role of platelets in mediating a response to human influenza infection. *Nat. Commun.* **2019**, *10*, 1780. [CrossRef]
193. Boilard, E.; Paré, G.; Rousseau, M.; Cloutier, N.; Dubuc, I.; Lévesque, T.; Borgeat, P.; Flamand, L. Influenza virus H1N1 activates platelets through FcγRIIA signaling and thrombin generation. *Blood* **2014**, *123*, 2854–2863. [CrossRef]
194. Almohammadi, A.; Lundin, M.S.; Abro, C.; Hrinczenko, B. Epistaxis and gross haematuria with severe thrombocytopaenia asso-ciated with influenza vaccination. *BMJ Case Rep.* **2019**, *12*, e229423. [CrossRef]
195. Hamiel, U.; Kventsel, I.; Youngster, I. Recurrent Immune Thrombocytopenia After Influenza Vaccination: A Case Report. *Pediatrics* **2016**, *138*, e20160124. [CrossRef]
196. Laksono, B.M.; de Vries, R.D.; Verburgh, R.J.; Visser, E.G.; de Jong, A.; Fraaij, P.L.A.; Ruijs, W.L.M.; Nieuwenhuijse, D.F.; van den Ham, H.J.; Koopmans, M.P.G.; et al. Studies into the mechanism of mea-sles-associated immune suppression during a measles outbreak in the Netherlands. *Nat. Commun.* **2018**, *9*, 4944. [CrossRef] [PubMed]
197. Moss, W.J. Measles. *Lancet* **2017**, *390*, 2490–2502. [CrossRef]
198. Premaratna, R.; Luke, N.; Perera, H.; Gunathilake, M.; Amarasena, P.; Chandrasena, T.G. Sporadic cases of adult measles: A research article. *BMC Res. Notes* **2017**, *10*, 38. [CrossRef] [PubMed]
199. Sunnetcioglu, M.; Baran, A.I.; Sunnetcioglu, A.; Mentes, O.; Karadas, S.; Aypak, A. Clinical and laboratory features of adult measles cases detected in Van, Turkey. *J. Pak. Med. Assoc.* **2015**, *65*, 273–276. [PubMed]
200. Celesia, B.M.; Fontana, R.; Pinzone, M.R.; Cuccia, M.; Bellissimo, F.; Rapisarda, L.; Rinnone, S.; Rapisarda, V.; Pavone, P.; Cacopardo, B.; et al. A measles outbreak in Catania, Sicily: The importance of high vaccination coverage and early notification of cases for health and economic reasons. *Le Infezioni Medicina* **2014**, *22*, 222–226. [PubMed]
201. Oncel, I.; Saltik, S.; Anlar, B. Subacute sclerosing panencephalitis and immune thrombocytopenia: More than a coincidence? *Med Hypotheses* **2018**, *111*, 70–72. [CrossRef]
202. Okazaki, N.; Takeguchi, M.; Sonoda, K.; Handa, Y.; Kakiuchi, T.; Miyahara, H.; Akiyoshi, K.; Korematsu, S.; Suenobu, S.; Izumi, T. Detection of platelet-binding anti-measles and anti-rubella virus IgG antibodies in infants with vaccine-induced thrombocytopenic purpura. *Vaccine* **2011**, *29*, 4878–4880. [CrossRef]
203. Agra, I.K.R.; Amorim Filho, A.G.; Lin, L.H.; Biancolin, S.E.; Francisco, R.P.V.; Brizot, M.L. Parameters Associated with Adverse Fetal Outcomes in Parvovirus B19 Congenital Infection. *Revista Brasileira de Ginecologia e Obstetrícia* **2017**, *39*, 596–601. [CrossRef] [PubMed]
204. Melamed, N.; Whittle, W.; Kelly, E.N.; Windrim, R.; Seaward, P.G.; Keunen, J.; Keating, S.; Ryan, G. Fetal thrombocytopenia in pregnancies with fetal human parvovirus-B19 infection. *Am. J. Obstet. Gynecol.* **2015**, *212*, 793.e1–793.e8. [CrossRef]
205. Rajput, R.; Sehgal, A.; Jain, D.; Sen, R.; Gupta, A. Acute Parvovirus B19 Infection Leading to Severe Aplastic Anemia in a Previously Healthy Adult Female. *Indian J. Hematol. Blood Transfus.* **2012**, *28*, 123–126. [CrossRef] [PubMed]

206. Shin, H.; Park, S.; Lee, G.W.; Koh, E.H.; Kim, H.Y. Parvovirus B19 infection presenting with neutropenia and thrombocytopenia: Three case reports. *Medicine* **2019**, *98*, e16993. [CrossRef]
207. Yaguchi, D.; Marui, N.; Matsuo, M. Three Adult Cases of HPV-B19 Infection with Concomitant Leukopenia and Low Platelet Counts. *Clin. Med. Insights Case Rep.* **2015**, *8*, 19–22. [CrossRef]
208. Furkan Demir, B.; Karahan Meteris, A.; Yirgin, G.; Comoglu, M.; Katipoglu, B.; Yılmaz, N.; Ates, I. Parvovırus-induced thrombocy-topenıa. *Hematol. Oncol. Stem Cell Ther.* **2019**, *12*, 226–227. [CrossRef] [PubMed]
209. Jain, A.; Jain, P.; Prakash, S.; Kumar, A.; Khan, D.N.; Seth, A.; Gupta, S.; Kant, R. Genotype 3b of human parvovirus B19 detected from hospitalized children with solid malignancies in a North Indian tertiary care hospital. *J. Med Virol.* **2016**, *88*, 1922–1929. [CrossRef]
210. Jitschin, R.; Peters, O.; Plentz, A.; Turowski, P.; Segerer, H.; Modrow, S. Impact of parvovirus B19 infection on paediatric patients with haematological and/or oncological disorders. *Clin. Microbiol. Infect.* **2011**, *17*, 1336–1342. [CrossRef] [PubMed]
211. Bachelier, K.; Biehl, S.; Schwarz, V.; Kindermann, I.; Kandolf, R.; Sauter, M.; Ukena, C.; Yilmaz, A.; Sliwa, K.; Bock, C.T.; et al. Parvovirus B19-induced vascular damage in the heart is associated with elevated circulating endothelial microparticles. *PLoS ONE* **2017**, *12*, e0176311. [CrossRef]
212. Wurster, T.; Pölzelbauer, C.; Schönberger, T.; Paul, A.; Seizer, P.; Stellos, K.; Schuster, A.; Botnar, R.M.; Gawaz, M.; Bigalke, B. Green Fluorescent Protein (GFP) Color Reporter Gene Visualizes Parvovirus B19 Non-Structural Segment 1 (NS1) Transfected Endothelial Modification. *PLoS ONE* **2012**, *7*, e33502. [CrossRef] [PubMed]
213. Griffiths, C.; Drews, S.J.; Marchant, D.J. Respiratory Syncytial Virus: Infection, Detection, and New Options for Prevention and Treatment. *Clin. Microbiol. Rev.* **2017**, *30*, 277. [CrossRef]
214. Kullaya, V.I.; de Mast, Q.; van der Ven, A.; elMoussaoui, H.; Kibiki, G.; Simonetti, E.; de Jonge, M.I.; Ferwerda, G. Platelets Modulate Innate Immune Response Against Human Respiratory Syncytial Virus In Vitro. *Viral Immunol.* **2017**, *30*, 576–581. [CrossRef]
215. Bels, J.L.M.; van Kuijk, S.M.J.; Ghossein-Doha, C.; Tijssen, F.H.; van Gassel, R.J.J.; Tas, J.; Collaborators, M.; Schnabel, R.M.; Aries, M.J.H.; van de Poll, M.C.G.; et al. Decreased serial scores of severe organ failure assessments are associated with survival in mechanically ventilated patients; the prospective Maastricht Intensive Care COVID cohort. *J. Crit. Care* **2021**, *62*, 38–45. [CrossRef]
216. Kaptein, F.H.J.; Stals, M.A.M.; Grootenboers, M.; Braken, S.J.E.; Burggraaf, J.L.I.; van Bussel, B.C.T.; Cannegieter, S.C.; ten Cate, H.; Endeman, H.; Gommers, D.A.M.P.J.; et al. Incidence of thrombotic compli-cations and overall survival in hospitalized patients with COVID-19 in the second and first wave. *Thromb. Res.* **2020**.
217. Brüggemann, R.A.G.; Spaetgens, B.; Gietema, H.A.; Brouns, S.H.A.; Stassen, P.M.; Magdelijns, F.J.; Rennenberg, R.J.; Henry, R.M.A.; Mulder, M.M.G.; van Bussel, B.C.T.; et al. The prevalence of pulmonary embolism in patients with COVID-19 and respiratory decline: A three-setting comparison. *Thromb. Res.* **2020**, *196*, 486–490. [CrossRef]
218. Levi, M.; Thachil, J.; Iba, T.; Levy, J.H. Coagulation abnormalities and thrombosis in patients with COVID-19. *Lancet Haematol.* **2020**, *7*, e438–e440. [CrossRef]
219. The COVID-19 Autopsy. The first COVID-19 autopsy in Spain performed during the early stages of the pandemic. *Revista Espanola de Patologia* **2020**, *53*, 182–187. [CrossRef] [PubMed]
220. Nicolai, L.; Leunig, A.; Brambs, S.; Kaiser, R.; Weinberger, T.; Weigand, M.; Muenchhoff, M.; Hellmuth, J.C.; Ledderose, S.; Schulz, H.; et al. Immunothrombotic Dysregulation in COVID-19 Pneumonia Is Associated with Respiratory Failure and Coagulopathy. *Circulation* **2020**, *142*, 1176–1189. [CrossRef]
221. Middleton, E.A.; He, X.Y.; Denorme, F.; Campbell, R.A.; Ng, D.; Salvatore, S.P.; Mostyka, M.; Baxter-Stoltzfus, A.; Borczuk, A.C.; Loda, M.; et al. Neutrophil extracellular traps contribute to im-munothrombosis in COVID-19 acute respiratory distress syndrome. *Blood* **2020**, *136*, 1169–1179. [CrossRef]
222. Venter, C.; Bezuidenhout, J.A.; Laubscher, G.J.; Lourens, P.J.; Steenkamp, J.; Kell, D.B.; Pretorius, E. Erythrocyte, Platelet, Serum Ferritin, and P-Selectin Pathophysiology Implicated in Severe Hypercoagulation and Vascular Complications in COVID-19. *Int. J. Mol. Sci.* **2020**, *21*, 8234. [CrossRef]
223. Zhang, S.; Liu, Y.; Wang, X.; Yang, L.; Li, H.; Wang, Y.; Liu, M.; Zhao, X.; Xie, Y.; Yang, Y.; et al. SARS-CoV-2 binds platelet ACE2 to enhance thrombosis in COVID-19. *J. Hematol. Oncol.* **2020**, *13*, 120. [CrossRef]
224. Manne, B.K.; Denorme, F.; Middleton, E.A.; Portier, I.; Rowley, J.W.; Stubben, C.; Petrey, A.C.; Tolley, N.D.; Guo, L.; Cody, M.; et al. Platelet gene expression and function in patients with COVID-19. *Blood* **2020**, *136*, 1317–1329. [CrossRef]
225. Rokni, M.; Ahmadikia, K.; Asghari, S.; Mashaei, S.; Hassanali, F. Comparison of clinical, para-clinical and laboratory findings in survived and deceased patients with COVID-19: Diagnostic role of inflammatory indications in determining the severity of illness. *BMC Infect. Dis.* **2020**, *20*, 869. [CrossRef]
226. Lu, G.; Wang, J. Dynamic changes in routine blood parameters of a severe COVID-19 case. *Clin. Chim. Acta* **2020**, *508*, 98–102. [CrossRef] [PubMed]
227. Ferrari, D.; Motta, A.; Strollo, M.; Banfi, G.; Locatelli, M. Routine blood tests as a potential diagnostic tool for COVID-19. *Clin. Chem. Lab. Med.* **2020**, *58*, 1095–1099. [CrossRef]
228. Zhang, J.; Liu, J.; Yuan, Y.; Huang, F.; Ma, R.; Luo, B.; Xi, Z.; Pan, T.; Liu, B.; Zhang, Y.; et al. Two waves of pro-inflammatory factors are released during the in-fluenza A virus (IAV)-driven pulmonary immunopathogenesis. *PLoS Pathog.* **2020**, *16*, e1008334. [CrossRef] [PubMed]

229. Busch, M.H.; Timmermans, S.; Nagy, M.; Visser, M.; Huckriede, J.; Aendekerk, J.P.; de Vries, F.; Potjewijd, J.; Jallah, B.; Ysermans, R.; et al. Neutrophils and Contact Activation of Co-agulation as Potential Drivers of COVID-19. *Circulation* **2020**, *142*, 1787–1790. [CrossRef] [PubMed]
230. Hottz, E.D.; Azevedo-Quintanilha, I.G.; Palhinha, L.; Teixeira, L.; Barreto, E.A.; Pão, C.R.R.; Righy, C.; Franco, S.; Souza, T.M.L.; Kurtz, P.; et al. Platelet activation and plate-let-monocyte aggregate formation trigger tissue factor expression in patients with severe COVID-19. *Blood* **2020**, *136*, 1330–1341. [CrossRef] [PubMed]
231. Li, M.; Nguyen, C.B.; Yeung, Z.; Sanchez, K.; Rosen, D.; Bushan, S. Evans syndrome in a patient with COVID-19. *Br. J. Haematol.* **2020**, *190*, e59–e61. [CrossRef]
232. Li, H.; Wang, B.; Ning, L.; Luo, Y.; Xiang, S. Transient appearance of EDTA dependent pseudothrombocytopenia in a patient with 2019 novel coronavirus pneumonia. *Platelets* **2020**, *31*, 825–826. [CrossRef]
233. Fausther-Bovendo, H.; Kobinger, G. Vaccine innovation spurred by the long wait for an Ebola virus vaccine. *Lancet Infect. Dis.* **2020**. [CrossRef]
234. Mulangu, S.; Dodd, L.E.; Davey, R.T., Jr.; Tshiani Mbaya, O.; Proschan, M.; Mukadi, D.; Lusakibanza Manzo, M.; Nzolo, D.; Tshomba Oloma, A.; Ibanda, A.; et al. A Randomized, Controlled Trial of Ebola Virus Disease Therapeutics. *N. Engl. J. Med.* **2019**, *381*, 2293–2303. [CrossRef] [PubMed]
235. da Costa, P.S.; Ribeiro, G.M.; Junior, C.S.; da Costa Campos, L. Severe thrombotic events associated with dengue fever, Brazil. *Am. J. Trop. Med. Hyg.* **2012**, *87*, 741–742. [CrossRef]
236. Liu, S.; DeLalio, L.J.; Isakson, B.E.; Wang, T.T. AXL-Mediated Productive Infection of Human Endothelial Cells by Zika Virus. *Circ. Res.* **2016**, *119*, 1183–1189. [CrossRef]
237. Ramacciotti, E.; Agati, L.B.; Aguiar, V.C.R.; Wolosker, N.; Guerra, J.C.; de Almeida, R.P.; Alves, J.C.; Lopes, R.D.; Wakefield, T.W.; Comerota, A.J.; et al. Zika and Chikungunya Virus and Risk for Venous Thromboembolism. *Clin. Appl. Thromb. Hemost.* **2019**, *25*, 1076029618821184. [CrossRef]
238. Guillevin, L.; Mahr, A.; Callard, P.; Godmer, P.; Pagnoux, C.; Leray, E.; Cohen, P. Hepatitis B virus-associated polyarteritis nodosa: Clinical characteristics, outcome, and impact of treatment in 115 patients. *Medicine* **2005**, *84*, 313–322. [CrossRef] [PubMed]
239. Mitchell, O.; Feldman, D.M.; Diakow, M.; Sigal, S.H. The pathophysiology of thrombocytopenia in chronic liver disease. *Hepatic Med. Évid. Res.* **2016**, *8*, 39–50.
240. Wijarnpreecha, K.; Thongprayoon, C.; Panjawatanan, P.; Ungprasert, P. Hepatitis C Virus Infection and Risk of Venous Thromboembolism: A Systematic Review and Meta-Analysis. *Ann. Hepatol.* **2017**, *16*, 514–520. [CrossRef]
241. Nery, F.; Chevret, S.; Condat, B.; de Raucourt, E.; Boudaoud, L.; Rautou, P.E.; Plessier, A.; Roulot, D.; Chaffaut, C.; Bourcier, V.; et al. Causes and consequences of portal vein thrombosis in 1,243 patients with cirrhosis: Results of a longitudinal study. *Hepatology* **2015**, *61*, 660–667. [CrossRef] [PubMed]
242. Wijarnpreecha, K.; Thongprayoon, C.; Panjawatanan, P.; Ungprasert, P. Hepatitis B virus infection and risk of coronary artery disease: A meta-analysis. *Ann. Transl. Med.* **2016**, *4*, 423. [CrossRef] [PubMed]
243. Butt, A.A.; Xiaoqiang, W.; Budoff, M.; Leaf, D.; Kuller, L.H.; Justice, A.C. Hepatitis C Virus Infection and the Risk of Coronary Disease. *Clin. Infect. Dis.* **2009**, *49*, 225–232. [CrossRef] [PubMed]
244. Blüm, P.; Pircher, J.; Merkle, M.; Czermak, T.; Ribeiro, A.; Mannell, H.; Krötz, F.; Hennrich, A.; Spannagl, M.; Köppel, S.; et al. Arterial thrombosis in the context of HCV-associated vascular disease can be prevented by protein C. *Cell. Mol. Immunol.* **2017**, *14*, 986–996. [CrossRef]
245. Baiocchini, A.; Del Nonno, F.; Taibi, C.; Visco-Comandini, U.; D'Offizi, G.; Piacentini, M.; Falasca, L. Liver sinusoidal endothelial cells (LSECs) modifications in patients with chronic hepatitis C. *Sci. Rep.* **2019**, *9*, 8760. [CrossRef]
246. Ragab, G.; Hussein, M.A. Vasculitic syndromes in hepatitis C virus: A review. *J. Adv. Res.* **2017**, *8*, 99–111. [CrossRef] [PubMed]
247. Benjamin, L.A.; Allain, T.J.; Mzinganjira, H.; Connor, M.D.; Smith, C.; Lucas, S.; Joekes, E.; Kampondeni, S.; Chetcuti, K.; Turnbull, I.; et al. The Role of Human Immunodeficiency Vi-rus-Associated Vasculopathy in the Etiology of Stroke. *J. Infect. Dis.* **2017**, *216*, 545–553. [CrossRef] [PubMed]
248. Eugenin, E.A.; Morgello, S.; Klotman, M.E.; Mosoian, A.; Lento, P.A.; Berman, J.W.; Schecter, A.D. Human immunodeficiency virus (HIV) infects human arterial smooth muscle cells in vivo and in vitro: Implications for the pathogenesis of HIV-mediated vascular disease. *Am. J. Pathol.* **2008**, *172*, 1100–1111. [CrossRef]
249. Nixon, C.C.; Vatakis, D.N.; Reichelderfer, S.N.; Dixit, D.; Kim, S.G.; Uittenbogaart, C.H.; Zack, J.A. HIV-1 infection of hematopoietic pro-genitor cells in vivo in humanized mice. *Blood* **2013**, *122*, 2195–2204. [CrossRef]
250. Rokx, C.; Borjas Howard, J.F.; Smit, C.; Wit, F.W.; Pieterman, E.D.; Reiss, P.; Cannegieter, S.C.; Lijfering, W.M.; Meijer, K.; Bierman, W.; et al. Risk of recurrent venous thromboembolism in patients with HIV infection: A nationwide cohort study. *PLoS Med.* **2020**, *17*, e1003101. [CrossRef]
251. Freiberg, M.S.; Chang, C.C.; Kuller, L.H.; Skanderson, M.; Lowy, E.; Kraemer, K.L.; Butt, A.A.; Bidwell Goetz, M.; Leaf, D.; Oursler, K.A.; et al. HIV Infection and the Risk of Acute Myocardial Infarction. *JAMA Intern. Med.* **2013**, *173*, 614–622. [CrossRef] [PubMed]
252. Van Wyk, V.; Kotzé, H.F.; Heyns, A.P. Kinetics of indium-111-labelled platelets in HIV-infected patients with and without asso-ciated thrombocytopaenia. *Eur. J. Haematol.* **1999**, *62*, 332–335. [PubMed]

253. Ambler, K.L.; Vickars, L.M.; Leger, C.S.; Foltz, L.M.; Montaner, J.S.; Harris, M.; Dias Lima, V.; Leitch, H.A. Clinical Features, Treatment, and Outcome of HIV-Associated Immune Thrombocytopenia in the HAART Era. *Adv. Hematol.* **2012**, *2012*, 910954. [CrossRef] [PubMed]
254. Telles, J.P.; de Andrade Perez, M.; Marcusso, R.; Correa, K.; Teixeira, R.F.A.; Tobias, W.M. Hemophagocytic syndrome in patients living with HIV: A retrospective study. *Ann. Hematol.* **2019**, *98*, 67–72. [CrossRef]

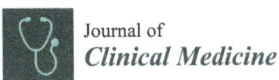

Review

Thrombocytopathies: Not Just Aggregation Defects—The Clinical Relevance of Procoagulant Platelets

Alessandro Aliotta [1,†], Debora Bertaggia Calderara [1,†], Maxime G. Zermatten [1], Matteo Marchetti [1,2] and Lorenzo Alberio [1,*]

1. Hemostasis and Platelet Research Laboratory, Division of Hematology and Central Hematology Laboratory, Lausanne University Hospital (CHUV) and University of Lausanne (UNIL), CH-1010 Lausanne, Switzerland; Alessandro.Aliotta@chuv.ch (A.A.); Debora.Bertaggia-Calderara@chuv.ch (D.B.C.); Maxime.Zermatten@chuv.ch (M.G.Z.); matteo.marchetti@ghol.ch (M.M.)
2. Service de Médecine Interne, Hôpital de Nyon, CH-1260 Nyon, Switzerland
* Correspondence: Lorenzo.Alberio@chuv.ch
† These authors contributed equally to this work.

Abstract: Platelets are active key players in haemostasis. Qualitative platelet dysfunctions result in thrombocytopathies variously characterized by defects of their adhesive and procoagulant activation endpoints. In this review, we summarize the traditional platelet defects in adhesion, secretion, and aggregation. In addition, we review the current knowledge about procoagulant platelets, focusing on their role in bleeding or thrombotic pathologies and their pharmaceutical modulation. Procoagulant activity is an important feature of platelet activation, which should be specifically evaluated during the investigation of a suspected thrombocytopathy.

Keywords: thrombocytopathy; platelet disorders; procoagulant platelets; activation endpoints

1. Introduction

Platelets or thrombocytes are small (2–5 μm) discoid anucleated cells produced by megakaryocytes. They are released in the blood stream where they circulate for 7–10 days to be eventually cleared by the spleen and the liver [1]. Platelets are responsible for maintaining the integrity of the vascular system, are active key players of primary haemostasis and enhance coagulation. Consequently, platelet disorders cause defective clot formation that may induce a bleeding or thrombotic diathesis.

Platelet disorders can be either inherited or acquired and are characterized by (i) quantitative defects, with an abnormal number of circulating platelets, either high (thrombocytosis) or low (thrombocytopenia); and/or (ii) qualitative platelet dysfunctions (thrombocytopathies) [2].

Thrombocytopathies may be induced either by extrinsic (e.g., systemic disease or medication) or by intrinsic factors [3,4]. In this review, we summarize intrinsic platelet anomalies resulting in defects of the various traditional activation endpoints, such as adhesion and aggregation (See Section 2), and we offer an in-depth and complete overview of the accumulating evidence for the physiological and clinical role of procoagulant platelets as an alternative, increasingly recognized critical endpoint of platelet function (see Sections 3 and 4).

2. Platelet Activation End-Points and Related Defects

At the site of vascular damage, platelets interact with exposed adhesive agonists such as von Willebrand factor (VWF) and collagen. VWF binds to the platelet glycoprotein (GP) Ib-IX-V complex tethering platelets at the site of vessel wall injury. Collagen interacts with integrin $\alpha_2\beta_1$ (also named GPIa/IIa) for adhesion and GPVI to initiate platelet activation. Soluble agonists, such as thromboxane A_2 and adenosine diphosphate (ADP) subsequently amplify activation. Endpoints following platelet activation are characterized by: (1) shape change, (2) secretion of soluble agonists and granule content enhancing the activation process, (3) change of GPIIb/IIIa conformation to bind fibrinogen, which sustains platelet aggregation, and/or (4) externalization of negatively charged amino-phospholipids contributing to platelet procoagulant activity (Figure 1) [5–7]. Because of the three-dimensional configuration of the growing thrombus, platelets are differently exposed to agonists resulting in heterogeneous activation profiles [8]. Common examples of the pathophysiology are described below for each activation endpoint.

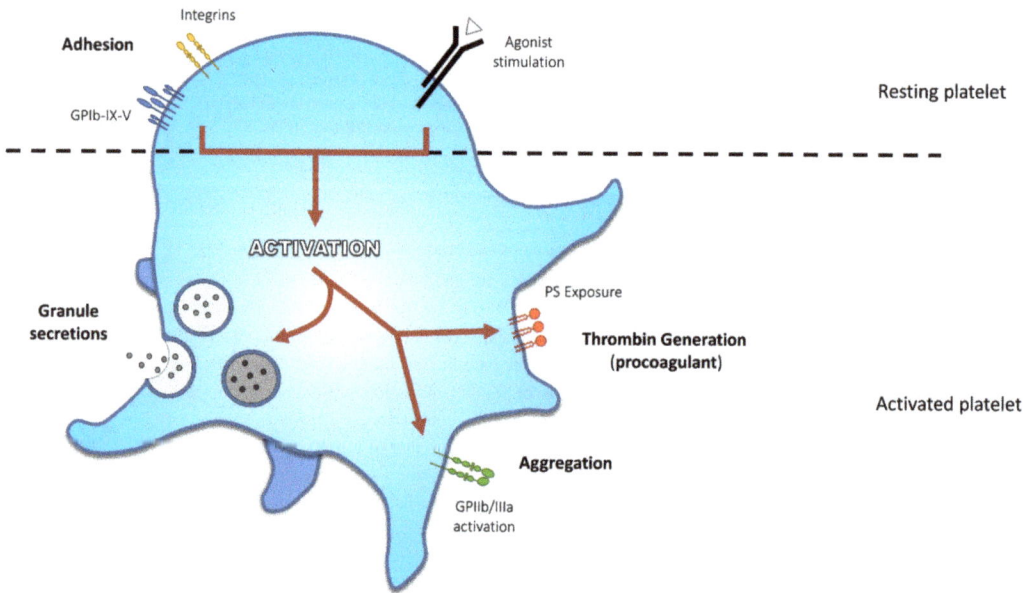

Figure 1. Principal Activation Endpoints During Platelet Activation. At first, platelet receptors interact with adhesive agonists exposed at the site of lesion: von Willebrand factor (VWF) binds to glycoprotein (GP) Ib-IX-V complex and collagen interacts with integrin $\alpha_2\beta_1$ for adhesion and GPVI to mediate platelet activation. These first interactions initiate platelet response. Soluble agonists released by either activated platelets or injured tissue amplify platelet response and activation. These agonists induce proper receptor activation and their signalling converge to activate a core set of intracellular signalling pathways leading to various activation endpoints, such as shape change and formation of pseudopodia, secretion of α-granule and dense granule content, activation of GPIIb/IIIa sustaining platelet aggregation, and externalization of negatively charged amino-phospholipids, contributing to platelet procoagulant activity (thrombin generation).

2.1. Adhesion

Under normal physiological conditions, the endothelium does not provide an adhesive surface for platelets. However, in the presence of vascular damage, the sub-endothelial matrix and/or layer(s) become exposed, revealing collagen and tissue factor, which are powerful haemostatic activators. The main function of platelet receptor GPIb-IX-V is to mediate the initial adhesion of circulating platelets to VWF adhered on the exposed collagen [9]. Four subunits compose the GPIb-IX-V complex: GPIbα, GPIbβ, GPIX, and GPV (encoded by four different genes *GPIBA*, *GPIBB*, *GP9*, and *GP5*) [10,11]. The N-terminal domain of GPIbα subunit has a binding site for VWF, which acts as a bridge between platelets and the fibrils of collagen in the sub-endothelial matrix and/or layer(s). This interaction is particularly important in the presence of high shear stress, in order to: i) slow down platelets in the blood stream, ii) recruit them to the site of the injury and iii) initiate the signalling cascades that will lead to platelet activation [12]. In addition to VWF, the same N-terminal domain of GPIα offers a binding site for multiple ligands, which are critical for normal or pathological haemostasis. For instance, the GPIb-IX-V complex binds to P-selectin [13] (which is present on activated platelets and endothelial cells) and to leukocyte integrin aMB2 [14], thus regulating both the recruitment of leukocytes at the site of vascular injury [15] and the complex interactions between platelets and leukocytes in thrombosis and response to inflammation [16]. In addition, the GPIb-IX-V receptor has procoagulant functions, since it mediates platelet dependent coagulation through the binding of α-thrombin, coagulation factors XI (FXI) and XII (FXII), and high molecular weight kininogen [17]. Finally, The GPIb-IX-V complex is anchored to the actin filaments of the platelets' cytoskeleton through the binding of GPIbα cytoplasmic tail to filamin A [18]. This interaction is important for maintaining platelet shape and stability [19,20]. Defects and/or dysfunctions of this multitasker receptor have major consequences in platelet functions.

2.1.1. Bernard-Soulier Syndrome

Bernard Soulier Syndrome (BSS) is an inherited bleeding disorders characterized by bleeding tendency, macro-thrombocytopenia, and defective ristocetin-induced platelet agglutination [21–23].

Clinical features of patients with BSS are non-specific and characterized by epistaxis, mucocutaneous and post trauma bleedings, and severe menorrhagia in females [17,24].

In most patients, BSS has an autosomal recessive pattern of inheritance, but rare forms with autosomal dominant pattern are also known [25,26]. A large number of mutations (missense, nonsense or deletions) in genes *GPIBA*, *GPIBB*, and *GP9* (but not in *GP5* [27]) have been mapped and found to be causative of BSS [17,24]. In fact, these genes (*GPIBA*, *GPIBB*, and *GP9*) are required to express efficiently the functional GPIb-IX-V complex at the platelets' surface. In BSS platelets, the GPIb-IX-V complex is either low, absent or dysfunctional (i.e., unable to bind VWF). Thus, in BSS platelets, the normal interaction of GPIbα with VWF is abolished and platelets' adhesion to the sub-endothelium is impaired [28]. In addition, BSS platelets show other characteristics, such as an increased membrane deformability, a poor response to low doses of thrombin, and a decreased ability to support thrombin generation [29–31]. All these features can be related to the absence/dysfunction of GPIb-IX-V complex [17].

The clinical suspicion of BSS has to be confirmed by different laboratory investigations. A variable degree of thrombocytopenia (platelet count range: $<30 \times 10^9$/L to normal [22,24]) might be observed, with a blood smear revealing abnormally large or irregularly shaped platelets (even in patients with normal platelet count) [32,33]. The closure time measured by the platelet function analyser (PFA-100/200) is increased and the bleeding time prolonged [34,35]. However, the sensitivity of PFA-100/200 assay depends on the severity of the defect [15,36], which implies further investigations (aggregometry and/or flow cytometry) to establish an accurate diagnosis. The VWF-dependent agglutination measured in the presence of ristocetin by light transmission aggregometry (LTA) is defective in homozygous BSS platelets (but normal in heterozygous form) [33]. Of note, this defect will not be rescued by the addition of normal plasma, which distinguishes BSS from von Willebrand disease (VWD) [35,37]. In vitro aggregation of BSS platelets in response to epinephrine, ADP, collagen, and arachidonic acid is normal, but a slow response is observed with low doses of thrombin [33]. The expression of GPIb-IX-V complex at the platelet surface can be assessed by flow cytometry. The specific antibody anti-CD42b directed against GPIbα is reduced or absent in BSS platelets, while the expression of CD41 (GPIIb) and CD61 (GPIIIa)–the two components of the fibrinogen receptor (also named integrin $\alpha_{IIb}\beta_3$)–is normal [32,38]. Finally, in BSS platelets, the expression of GPIb-IX-V could apparently be normal because of the enlarged surface of the platelets, but the ratio between GPI-IX-V and GPIIb-IIIa will always be decreased compared to normal platelets [33].

2.1.2. Platelet Type von Willebrand's Disease

Platelet type pseudo-von Willebrand's disease (PT-VWD) is a rare autosomal dominant disorder with a mild to moderate bleeding phenotype, intermittent thrombocytopenia, and enlarged platelets.

PT-VWD is characterized by mutations in *GP1BA* [39], which enhance the affinity of the surface glycoprotein GPIbα for the VWF multimers. As a result, spontaneous binding of high molecular weight VWF to platelets occurs in vivo, leading to platelet clumping and increasing platelet clearance [40]. This causes thrombocytopenia and removal from plasma of the largest VWF multimers (which have the greatest haemostatic capacity), leading to an increased bleeding risk.

At laboratory work-up, patients with PT-VWD often have a prolonged bleeding time and platelet clumping can be observed on blood smears. The response of PT-VWD platelets to low doses of ristocetin is enhanced and the VWF multimers analysis (which assesses concentration and distribution of VWF multimers in plasma) shows loss/reduction of the largest VWF forms. PT-VWD phenotype is very similar to type 2B VWD. However, in type 2B VWD, the defect lies in the VWF molecules, which have an increased affinity for platelets. Differential diagnosis is fundamental for the correct therapy of PT-VWF or VWD 2B patients. The two conditions can be distinguished by (i) ristocetin induced platelets agglutination (RIPA) mixing experiments, (ii) cryoprecipitate challenge, and (iii) flow cytometry. In the RIPA assay, washed or gel-filtered platelets from the patient are mixed with normal plasma and vice versa (i.e., normal platelets are mixed with patient plasma) in presence of low dose ristocetin. Washed/gel-filtered platelets from PT-VWD patients (but not VWD 2B platelets) will agglutinate in normal plasma (because of the abnormal GPIbα avidity for VWF characteristic of PT-VWD) and washed/gel-filtered normal platelets will aggregate in the presence of VWD 2B plasma (containing the hyper-adhesive VWF) [41,42]. Of note, in the negative control (washed/gel-filtered platelets + plasma from a healthy donor) there is no aggregation at low doses of ristocetin. The cryoprecipitate challenge [43] consists in the addition of high concentrate normal VWF to platelets, which causes PT-VWF spontaneous aggregation, but not for VWD 2B platelets; however, false positive results have been observed among VWD 2B patients [44] and this test is not included in the diagnostic algorithm proposed for PT-VWD diagnostic work-up [45]. A flow cytometry method able to highlight the increased affinity of VWF for GPIbα and to discriminate between PT-VWD and VWD 2B through mixing tests has also been proposed [46]. Finally, the identification of mutations in the *GP1BA* gene will confirm the diagnosis of PT-VWD [45].

2.2. Secretion

The secretion of bioactive molecules is one of the characteristics of platelet activation. Once a platelet agonist has engaged its corresponding platelet surface receptor, a signal transduction takes place, leading to a short-time increase of intracellular calcium, which promotes platelet shape change, fusion of platelet granules with the plasma membrane and consequent release of platelet contents [47]. Platelets contain three major types of granules, which are in order of abundance, α-granules (50–80/platelet), dense-granules (3–8/platelet), and lysosomes (1–3/platelet) [48]. α- and dense-granules seem to derive, like lysosomes, from multivesicular precursors [49–51]. The content of α-granules consists of a large variety of proteins, such as adhesive molecules (e.g., fibrinogen, VWF, fibronectin, P-selectin), coagulation factors (e.g., FV, FIX, FXIII), anticoagulants (e.g., antithrombin), fibrinolytic proteins (e.g., plasminogen), and growth factors, immune mediators, and integral membrane proteins (e.g., $\alpha_{IIb}\beta_3$, P-selectin) [52,53]. Thus, α-granule proteins can be involved in a large spectrum of physiological functions, such as normal and pathological haemostasis, inflammation, wound healing, antimicrobial response, and cancer metastasis [54,55]. Dense-granules contain small non-protein molecules, such as nucleotides (ADP/ATP), serotonin, histamine, calcium ions (which give the dense appearance on electron microscopy), inorganic polyphosphates, membrane proteins [such as granulophysin (CD63), lysosomal-associated membrane protein 2 (LAMP-2)], [55]); plasma membrane adhesive receptors GPIb and $\alpha_{IIb}\beta_3$ have also been identified on dense-granules by immune-histochemical studies [56]. The main function of dense-granules content is to amplify platelet activation and to sustain platelet aggregation [57]. Lysosomes store digestive enzyme involved in the degradation of proteins, carbohydrates and lipids. Their role in haemostasis and thrombosis is still unknown [55].

Platelet storage pool deficiencies (SPD) refer to a group of inherited heterogeneous disorders in which the number and/or the content of α-granules, dense-granules, or both are reduced and cannot be adequately released during platelet activation [58,59]; as a consequence, a defect mostly in ADP release from activated platelet and in secretion-dependent aggregation is observed [60]. According to the type of granule pool deficiency, the clinical syndrome is called α-SPD, δ-SPD or αδ-SPD [58,61] These anomalies are to be distinguished from secretion defects, in which granules are normally present, but abnormally secreted due to defective signal transduction or granule trafficking defects [62].

2.2.1. α-Storage Pool Disease or Gray Platelet Syndrome

The Gray platelet syndrome (GPS) is a very rare disease characterized by a quantitative and qualitative deficiency of α-granules [63,64]. Patients with GPS have a mild to moderate bleeding diathesis, mild but progressive thrombocytopenia, and presence of larger and vacuolated platelets [65]. The associated phenotype is the presence of bone marrow fibrosis (due to the release of megakaryocytes in the bone marrow environment) and of splenomegaly (due to extramedullary haematopoiesis) [65–67]. Other features of GPS have been linked to immune dysregulation and autoimmune defects [68].

GPS megakaryocytes show a defect in α-granule production and are unable to correctly pack and store endogenous and exogenous proteins into α-granule precursors [69]. The lack of soluble proteins within α-granules, whose content is fundamental for normal haemostasis, leads to a small and unstable platelet plug [70]. The classical GPS is inherited with an autosomal-recessive pattern and it is associated with mutations or splicing alterations in *NBEAL2* gene, involved in granule trafficking [71] and retention of cargo proteins in maturing α-granules [72]. Other GPS forms with autosomal-dominant or X-linked inheritance have been reported (reviewed in [73]).

The absence of α-granules in the cytoplasm of affected platelets results in a characteristic pale or gray appearance, opposite to the purple staining of granules in normal platelets on Wright-Giemsa stained blood smears. Platelet aggregation analysis by LTA is variable: in most of the GPS patients, the responses to ADP, epinephrine, and acid arachidonic are normal, while responses to thrombin and collagen are decreased [65]. Of note, content and surface expression of P-selectin are variable and their assessment is inadequate for diagnostic purposes [65,74–77]. The diagnosis is confirmed by the lack of α-granules observed by electron microscopy and by the absence of α-granule proteins [78,79].

2.2.2. δ-Storage Pool Disease

δ-Storage pool disease (δ-SPD) is a congenital abnormality characterized by a deficiency of dense-granules in megakaryocytes and platelets [79]. δ-SPD can be associated with disorders of others lysosome related organelles leading to syndromic forms, known as Hermansky-Pudlack, Chediak-Higashi, and Grisicelli syndromes, in which albinism and immune deficiency are associated with platelet function defects [80]. Patients with non-syndromic δ-SPD have a mild to moderate bleeding diathesis, mainly mucocutaneous; however life-threatening bleedings can occur after surgery or trauma [81]. Clinical presentation of δ-SPD is highly variable and so far there are no validated recommendations concerning the decisional algorithm to reach an accurate diagnosis [81], nor for δ-SPD management [82].

Patients with δ-SPD usually have normal platelet counts with a prolonged bleeding time [83]. The lack of dense-granules (and thus of ADP/ATP and serotonin) will be reflected by an impaired aggregation response to different agonists in vitro. Typically, LTA curves performed with citrated platelet rich plasma (PRP) are characterized by the absence of a second wave in ADP induced platelet aggregation and a diminished response to collagen induced aggregation (at low concentrations) [79,81]. However, a study reported that δ-SPD patients (23% of the cohort studied) had normal aggregation response [84]. Thus, further specialized tests are sometimes needed to confirm the diagnosis. In particular, whole mount transmission electron microscopy can be used to highlight the absence/reduction of dense-granules [85], while flow cytometry, by the mepacrine test uptake, is useful to evaluate the dense-granule content and secretion capacity of platelets. The mepacrine test is based on the fact that mepacrine binds to adenine nucleotides and accumulates rapidly in dense-granules. The mepacrine taken up by dense-granules is then released after platelet stimulation and fluorescence can be quantified before and after platelet activation [86,87]. δ-SPD platelets will have reduced dense-granules and low uptake and release of mepacrine [79,88,89]. Platelet content of adenine nucleotides and serotonin can be evaluated by chemiluminescence aggregometry and radio-labelled or chemical methods, respectively (reviewed in [59,81]). δ-SPD platelets will be characterized by reduced adenine nucleotides and serotonin content, with an elevated ATP/ADP ratio [90].

2.3. Aggregation

Platelet aggregation is mediated by the GPIIb/IIIa (integrin $\alpha_{IIb}\beta_3$), a major receptor of the platelet surface, whose activated form binds to fibrinogen. Surface expression of GPIIb/IIIa increases after platelet activation. Upon agonist induced platelet activation, a signalling process ("inside-out" signalling) leads to conformational changes of the GPIIb/IIIa receptor, which increases its affinity for fibrinogen. The binding of fibrinogen with platelet GPIIb/IIIa receptors allows platelet aggregation (leading to the primary platelet plug), providing primary haemostasis. Binding of fibrinogen to the GPIIb/IIIa receptor initiates further intracellular signalling ("outside-in") which induces additional granule secretion, platelet spreading, and contraction of the fibrin mesh. This signalling pathway culminates in a stable and irreversible aggregation of platelets [47,91].

Glanzmann Thrombasthenia

Glanzmann thrombasthenia (GT) is a rare autosomal inherited bleeding disorder, characterized by a quantitative or qualitative defect in integrin $\alpha_{IIb}\beta_3$, also known as glycoprotein GPIIb/IIIa, which is essential for platelet aggregation and normal haemostasis.

GT is caused by mutations in the genes *ITGA2B* and *ITGB3*, which encode for subunits α_{IIb} (GPIIb, CD41) and β_3 (GPIIIa, CD61), respectively, of integrin $\alpha_{IIb}\beta_3$. Mutations in these genes compromise the normal function of the GPIIb/IIIa receptor, impairing platelet aggregation and interaction with its adhesive ligands and thus leading to inefficient clot formation/consolidation and to GT bleeding phenotype.

Bleeding tendency in patients with GT is highly variable and poorly correlated with the underlying genetic mutations or $\alpha_{IIb}\beta_3$ expression level [92]. It ranges from a mild to severe haemorrhagic condition [93,94]. Typical bleeding manifestations are purpura, gum bleeding and menorrhagia, while gastrointestinal or central nervous system bleeding are less frequently reported [95]; bleeding after trauma or surgery might be severe [93,96,97]. Most patients are diagnosed in childhood, but heterozygous patients can reach adulthood being asymptomatic [93]; in general, the bleeding tendency in GT decreases with age [98].

GT is divided in three subtypes [93,99] according to the GPIIb/IIIa expression (determined by flow cytometry [100]) on the platelet membrane:
- Type I, the most severe form of GT: the expression of GPIIb/IIIa is absent (<5% of normal); platelet fibrinogen and clot retraction are also absent;
- Type II, a moderate form of the disease: surface GPIIb/IIIa is reduced with a level of expression varying between 10–20% of normal; reduced fibrinogen content and clot retraction;
- Type III, a variant form: the expression of GPIIb/IIIa is near normal or normal (between 50–100%), but the receptor is dysfunctional; variable platelet fibrinogen content and clot retraction.

GT platelets adhere normally to the sub-endothelium, but spreading is abnormal [101–103]. GT platelets have decreased or absent aggregation to physiological agonists, but agglutination in response to ristocetin is normal (because it is mediated by GPIb-IX-V via VWF). Since a functional GPIIb/IIIa is required for efficient dense-granules release, in GT platelets an abnormal release might also be observed [104,105]. Laboratory findings include a normal platelet count, size and granularity, but a prolonged bleeding time [35,98]. PFA-100/200 assay shows a very prolonged closure time (>300 s), which is compatible with GT, but not specific [36,98]. LTA is considered the gold standard method for the clinical diagnosis of GT [98]. GT PRP is analysed before and after the addition of different agonists, such as arachidonic acid, ADP, collagen, and epinephrine. The absence or marked reduced aggregation in response to low or high concentrations of multiple agonists, along with a maintained response to ristocetin, indicates a defect in GPIIb/IIIa and is highly indicative of GT [36,98]. Due to variability of platelet aggregation results, it is recommended that the analysis be confirmed with a second sample [98,106,107] and to use a second round of testing with a larger spectrum of agonists [106,107]. Flow cytometry can be used to assess the quantitative deficiency of GPIIb/IIIa (GT type I and II) in the membrane of resting platelets through the use of fluorescent probes recognizing α_{IIb} (CD41) and/or β_3 (CD61) subunits. The GT variant form, (GPIIb/IIIa expressed but not functional) can be investigated by flow cytometry using the monoclonal antibody PAC-1, which recognizes the activated form of the GPIIb/IIIa receptor after platelets stimulation. GT activated platelets will not bind with the PAC-1 monoclonal antibody, due to the dysfunctional GPIIb/IIIa receptor [107–109]. Finally, the identification of the specific mutation variants in *ITGA2B* and *ITGB3* genes is the key to a complete diagnosis of GT [98,108].

2.4. Procoagulant Activity

Following strong activation, platelets expose negatively charged phospholipids on their outer membrane. This is essential in order to achieve an efficient haemostatic response by generating high amounts of thrombin and subsequent clot stabilization by fibrin. This peculiar platelet feature and its clinical role and relevance will be extensively described in the second part of this review.

3. Expression of Negatively Charged Phospholipids and Their Role in Coagulation

At resting state, the phospholipids of the cell membrane are asymmetrically distributed, thanks to flippase/floppase activity [110]. Neutral phospholipids (e.g., phosphatidylcholine, sphingomyelin, and sugar-linked sphingolipids) are located on the external leaflet of the membrane, while negatively charged phospholipids (phosphatidylserine (PS) and phosphatidylethanolamine) are within the inner surface of the membrane.

Under specific circumstances, such as apoptosis or strong platelet activation, this distribution is altered. During platelet activation, scramblases (such as TMEM16F, also known as anoctamin 6) shuffles the phospholipids between the two layers, resulting in the expression of PS on the external leaflet [110]. Despite similar endpoints, apoptotic-induced and agonist-induced PS exposure are two distinct pathways, both resulting in PS exposure (reviewed in [111]).

Apoptosis is a slow process (taking hours) that results with platelet aging and is mediated through the activation of caspases, pro-apoptotic Bak/Bax-mediated mitochondrial collapse, and PS exposure (mostly TMEM16F-independent) [112]. This slow process leads to platelet clearance.

Strong platelet activation induces a rapid (one–two minutes) necrotic-like phenotype via elevated and sustained cytosolic calcium concentration, mitochondrial depolarization, calpain activation, and TMEM16F-dependent PS exposure [113,114]. Plasma membranes form a small "cap" area enriched in exposed PS [115]. Such micro-domains concentrate blood coagulation factors and accelerate enzymatic reactions.

Indeed, in synchrony with platelet activation and aggregation, fibrin deposition is an important process for the stabilization of the haemostatic clot [116]. This is achieved by thrombin cleaving fibrinogen into fibrin as a consequence of a series of sequential reactions engaging activated coagulation factors, in which calcium and negatively charged phospholipids are critical mediators [117].

Some coagulation factors (factors II, VII, IX, X) experience vitamin-K dependent post-translational γ-carboxylation of C-terminal glutamic acid residues [118,119]. These highly negative domains confer to factors high-affinity binding for calcium, which facilitates their interaction with negatively charged phospholipids. In fact, activated coagulation factors interact poorly with each other in solution. Calcium binding is instrumental for supporting binding of coagulation factors to a membrane of negatively-charge phospholipids, such as the surface of procoagulant platelets [120,121].

In addition to rapid phospholipid membrane remodelling and PS externalization, platelet procoagulant response is accompanied by the release of microparticles from the membrane surface of activated platelets [122,123]. The mechanisms underlying the formation of platelet derived microparticles (PMPs) involve the increase of cytoplasmic calcium affecting the activity of intracellular enzymes, the phospholipid transient mass imbalance between the two leaflets of the membrane, and the proteolytic action of calpain on the cytoskeleton [124]. PMPs shed from activated platelets provide a source of supplementary negatively charged surface on which blood coagulation factors can assemble, thereby enhancing the procoagulant response [122]. Dale et al. [125] showed that the number of PMPs produced by procoagulant platelet was higher than the number of PMPs produced by aggregating platelets but 5.4 times lower than PMPs originating from A23187 calcium ionophore activated platelets. Sinauridze et al. [126] studied the procoagulant properties of A23187-calcium ionophore activated platelets and PMPs. The authors showed that the surface of PMPs originated after A23187 activation is 50- to 100-fold more procoagulant than the surface of activated procoagulant platelets. This stronger procoagulant activity was related to a higher density of procoagulant phospholipids on PMPs' membrane. From a physiological point of view, the observation that procoagulant collagen-and-thrombin (COAT) platelets produce less PMPs than ionophore does [125,127], might indicate that COAT platelet dependent thrombin generation (TG) should be contained at the site of vascular injury to avoid an unnecessary and dangerous systemic spread.

Taken together, the phospholipid surfaces enhance the enzymatic function of coagulation factors [128]. Membrane binding and surface diffusion facilitate and accelerate the encounter of coagulation partners (e.g., the assembly of tenase and prothrombinase complexes) [128]. This facilitates the rate of activation of prothrombin by several orders of magnitude. Therefore, the platelet contribution has a considerable impact on the procoagulant response, by localizing and enhancing thrombin generation directly at the site of vascular wall damage.

4. Procoagulant Platelets

Following strong activation, a fraction of platelets expresses PS on their surface and become highly efficient in sustaining thrombin generation.

Since the first descriptions in the late 1990s, several synonyms have been used (extensively described in recent reviews [129,130]) such as collagen-and-thrombin (COAT)-

activated platelets [87,127,131], COATed platelets [132,133], ballooned and procoagulant platelets (BAPS) [134], sustained calcium-induced platelet morphology (SCIP) platelets [135], super-activated platelets [136], super platelets [137] and even zombie platelets [138,139]. Despite this diverse classification, they all share the very same characteristics of necrotic-like mechanisms [111,140], leading to procoagulant activity through expression of PS [130].

In particular, after strong activation, all platelets display an initial cytosolic calcium increase and GPIIb/IIIa activation [131]. However, after a certain delay (1–2 min), while aggregating, platelets decrease their calcium level, and procoagulant platelets reach higher cytosolic calcium concentration [131,141,142]. In addition to calcium mobilization from intracellular stores and store-operated calcium entry, calcium influx mediated by sodium-calcium exchanger (NCX) reverse mode is critical for achieving the high calcium level required to trigger the formation of the mitochondrial permeability transition pore (mPTP), leading to cyclophilin D-dependent mitochondrial depolarization [141–143]. This results in very high and sustained cytoplasmic calcium, gradual inactivation of GPIIb/IIIa receptors [131,144], activation of TMEM16F [113], and PS externalization [114,134], which eventually induces the procoagulant activity of platelets together with microparticle generation [47,127,134,145].

In addition to the procoagulant activity mediated through PS exposure, procoagulant platelets gain pro-haemostatic function by retaining α-granule proteins on their membranes, such as coagulation factor V/Va, fibrinogen, VWF, thrombospondin, fibronectin, and α2-antiplasmin in a serotonin- and transglutaminase-dependent mechanism [146].

4.1. Clinical Features of Procoagulant Platelets

The potential generation of procoagulant platelets is on average ca. 30% in healthy donors, with a wide range from 15–57% described in the literature [87,132,147,148]. In our laboratory, we have a mean of 38.9% (SD 8.3; range 21.9–59.1%, n = 73) ([149] and Adler et al., manuscript in preparation). However, despite a wide inter-person variability, the individual values are stable over time [132].

Clinical interest in procoagulant platelet potential has largely increased during the last two decades. Especially, stratification of this wide range could associate extreme values to clinically relevant medical situations, such as in haemostatic imbalances (bleeding or thrombotic events) or even in non-haemostatic circumstances.

4.1.1. Low Level of Procoagulant Platelets Is Associated with Impaired Platelet Function and Bleeding Diathesis

The Scott syndrome was the first clinically relevant bleeding disorder associated with impaired platelet procoagulant activity [150]. In this very rare congenital bleeding disorder, patients have impaired phospholipid scrambling and do not expose PS at the membrane surface even after treatment with calcium ionophores [151,152]. Besides this complete absence of PS exposure, a reduced ability to generate procoagulant platelets has been shown to increase bleeding risk. Of note, low levels of procoagulant platelets (<20%) were detectable in about 15% of patients with a clinically relevant bleeding diathesis and an unrevealing standard work-up, including LTA and secretion assays ([87,153] and Adler et al., manuscript in preparation).

Moreover, patients with spontaneous intracerebral haemorrhage have a significantly lower percentage of procoagulant platelets compared to controls (24.8 ± 9.7% vs. 32.9 ± 12.6%) [154]. In a similar cohort of patients, those who generated the lowest levels of procoagulant platelets encountered more severe haemorrhages with increased bleed volumes [155] and, in another study, patients with procoagulant platelet levels lower than 27% had a poor outcome and increased mortality at 30 days [156]. Similarly, patients with subarachnoid haemorrhage that generate procoagulant platelets in the lowest range of the cohort (<36.7%) faced an increased mortality rate after one month [157]. However, these patients had on average a higher level of procoagulant platelets compared to controls (41.8 ± 11.4% vs. 30.7 ± 12.2%). As discussed by the authors, this antithetical observation could be related to the presence of a chronic inflammation in this pathology (but whether inflammatory state amplifies the procoagulant activity or the other way around is difficult to clarify; see below).

Interestingly, even in some cerebral thrombotic pathologies, patients who generated procoagulant platelets in the lowest range of the cohort presented increased bleeding phenotypes, with more microbleeds [158] or early secondary bleeding into the ischemic brain area compared to the other patients from the same cohort [159].

Discordant observations were reported regarding platelet procoagulant potential in two cohorts of haemophilia A patients. Both studies reported a reduced potency in generating procoagulant platelets compared to controls [160,161]. However, while Saxena et al. [160] observed a significant difference of procoagulant platelet levels in relationship to the phenotype severity, this was not replicated by Lastrapes et al. [161].

A single study also reported an impaired ability to generate procoagulant platelet in patients with essential thrombocythemia compared to controls and this was rescued by hydroxyurea treatment [162].

4.1.2. High Level of Procoagulant Platelets Worsens Thrombotic Events

In contrast to the findings in bleeding phenotypes, it was demonstrated that patients with prothrombotic states had a higher potential to generate procoagulant platelets.

Mean levels of procoagulant platelets were elevated in patients with cortical strokes [163] or transient ischemic attack (TIA) [164]. Moreover, the stratification of procoagulant platelet levels increased their prognostic value. Higher levels of procoagulant platelets at the time of the cortical strokes (>34%) or TIA (>51%) were associated in both conditions with an increased incidence of stroke recurrences [165,166]. In patients with symptomatic large-artery disease, procoagulant platelet levels in the highest range of the cohort ($\geq$50%) were associated with a higher risk for early ischemic events [167]. Similarly, for patients with asymptomatic carotid stenosis, higher levels of procoagulant platelets ($\geq$45%) predicted a risk for stroke or TIA [168].

Contrary to the other brain ischemic situations, data showed lower mean levels of procoagulant platelets following lacunar stroke compared to non-lacunar or control levels [163]. Nevertheless, patients with higher procoagulant platelet levels ($\geq$42.6%) experienced more recurrent ischemic events following lacunar stroke [169].

In addition to brain infarction, a high level of procoagulant platelets was also observed in coronary artery disease and heart failures [170–172].

Monitoring of procoagulant platelet potential, following an acute event, may also predict severe outcomes. A significant rise of procoagulant platelet generation after aneurys-mal subarachnoid haemorrhage predicted delayed cerebral ischemia and worsening of cognitive and physical outcomes [173,174].

Higher mean levels of procoagulant platelets were also measured in cigarette smokers compared to non-smokers [147,169,175]. This is of particular interest as smoking is widely associated with an increased risk factor for cardiovascular diseases. Interestingly, smoking cessation was observed to lower the procoagulant platelet levels for individuals who quit smoking after a stroke in comparison to those who continued smoking [176].

4.1.3. Procoagulant Platelets in Non-Haemostatic Pathologies

Massive haemorrhage in trauma is a leading cause of morbidity and mortality. Interestingly, it was recently reported that these patients experienced an increase in circulating procoagulant (balloon-like) platelets, which is in line with an increased ability to generate thrombin and a reduction of platelet aggregation [177]. This work highlights that trauma contributes to the increase of the procoagulant phenotype by the release of histone H4 from injured tissues, and, very interestingly, the authors could identify a platelet procoagulant phenotype that is already present in vivo, in contrast to other studies where the procoagulant ability of platelets is usually appreciated with ex vivo stimulations.

Interestingly, procoagulant platelets are also able to retain full-length amyloid precursor protein on their surface [178]. Further studies related levels of procoagulant platelets with Alzheimer disease severity and progression. Higher levels of procoagulant platelets were measured in early stages of the disease [179], among patients with the most severe decline [180], and among amnesic subtypes of patients with mild cognitive impairment with a progression to Alzheimer disease [181,182].

High levels of procoagulant platelets were observed in patients with end-stage renal failure [183]. Authors associated this with an increased inflammation state, but the role of procoagulant platelets as marker or trigger of thrombosis in this situation needs further investigations. Moreover, the direct influence of inflammation on procoagulant platelets (or vice versa) is not fully understood and dissecting this clearly remains challenging. Of note, inflammation is able to directly activate the haemostatic system [184] and some authors reported a relationship between high levels of procoagulant platelets and inflammation or immune system activation [132,147,183]. However, necrotic-like phenotypes, such as in procoagulant platelets, are also known to activate inflammation and immune cells [111,185].

In transfusion medicine, a low level of procoagulant platelets was observed in platelet concentrates from apheresis (16%) [186], buffy-coat (8%) [187], or cryopreserved platelet concentrates (17%) [188].

4.2. Pharmacological Modulation of Procoagulant Platelets

Platelets play a very important role in arterial thrombosis. Various antiplatelet therapies have been developed to prevent thrombotic events. However, these drugs aim at inhibiting platelet aggregation and, thus far, poor attention has been paid to platelet procoagulant activity.

On the other hand, different clinically relevant pharmacologic molecules have already been shown to modulate generation of procoagulant platelets.

4.2.1. Antiplatelet Drugs

Aspirin (acetyl-salicylic acid) is universally used as a standard for secondary prevention of recurrent arterial ischemic events. It irreversibly acetylates the active site of cyclooxygenase-1 (COX-1), required for the production of the soluble platelet agonist thromboxane A2. Chronic use of aspirin reduces the levels of procoagulant platelets in individuals [140,147,176]. However, intermittent or short-term uses do not relevantly impact potency in generating procoagulant platelets. While long-term use of aspirin appears to have an effect on megakaryocyte physiology inducing impaired platelet function, the direct interference with thromboxane A2 signalling does not seem to have a direct impact on the generation of procoagulant platelets [189].

ADP is able to augment the procoagulant potential induced by combined platelet activation with strong agonists, such as collagen and thrombin [187,189,190]. Accordingly, inhibition of P2Y12 (but not P2Y1) with clopidogrel [176,190] and cangrelor [191] reduces the generation of procoagulant platelets [189]. A similar effect was observed in vitro with the active metabolite of prasugrel [192].

Some of the data is sparse on the in vitro use of antagonists of the GPIIb/IIIa and the effect on procoagulant platelets. One study demonstrated that pre-treatment with either eptifibatide, tirofiban, or abciximab augmented the potential to generate procoagulant platelets [193]. This could explain the failure of long-term use of oral GPIIb/IIIa-antagonists observed in the early 2000s [194]. However, the procoagulant potentiation obtained with GPIIb/IIIa-antagonists was not corroborated by others [149,195–197]. These discordant data were all obtained with in vitro pre-treatment. Directly investigating the ability to generate procoagulant platelets in patients under treatment with GPIIb/IIIa-antagonists would help to clarify these discrepancies.

4.2.2. Off-Target Procoagulant Platelet Modulation

Desmopressin (1-deamino-8-D-arginine vasopressin (DDAVP)), a synthetic analogue of vasopressin initially used to treat diabetes insipidus and enuresis nocturna, improves the haemostatic status of patients by raising plasma levels of VWF and coagulation factor VIII [198]. In addition, it has also been demonstrated in vitro that DDAVP is a weak inducer of procoagulant response of platelets [199] as well as arginine vasopressin [200]. This was corroborated with in vivo treatment of patients with mild platelet disorders [201]. In this study, DDAVP was able to increase generation of procoagulant platelets by enhancing calcium and sodium mobilization. A similar observation was made in cardiac surgery patients receiving DDAVP because of postoperative excessive bleeding [202].

Auranofin, a thioredoxin reductase inhibitor used to treat rheumatoid arthritis was reported to induce calcium overload and increased oxidative stress in platelets, which would contribute to a necrotic PS exposure [203].

Patients using selective serotonin reuptake inhibitors (SSRI) had significantly lower procoagulant platelet levels compared to individuals not taking SSRI [147]. Furthermore, citalopram, a SSRI, was demonstrated to impair GPVI-mediated platelet function [204]. This is supported by the importance of serotonin for the formation of procoagulant platelets [146,205] and the mild bleeding diathesis reported in patients under SSRI treatment [206].

Inhibition of the procoagulant response of platelets was also observed with tyrosine kinase inhibitors used in oncology [207–210]. These pharmaceuticals reduce formation of procoagulant platelets by inhibiting tyrosine signalling downstream of GPVI activation.

4.3. Laboratory Work-Up for Investigating Procoagulant Platelets

Procoagulant platelets can be easily detected and characterized in vitro with fluorescence labelling and therefore by using microscopy or flow cytometry. Flow cytometry assays allow quantification of the ability to generate procoagulant platelets (see above, Sections 4.1 and 4.2) and to analyse phenotypically different platelet subpopulations. Moreover, flow cytometry is an accessible, easy, and rapid diagnostic tool for haematological diagnostic laboratories. Procoagulant activity can be appreciated as well with other assays, such as ex vivo platelet-dependent thrombin generation and flow chambers. However, these latter techniques are for now experimental methods and their diagnostic utility still needs more investigations. Finally, in vivo assays with animal models are also of high interest to study the thrombus distribution of procoagulant platelets and to understand better physiological and pathophysiological thrombus formation.

4.3.1. Quantification and Characterization of Procoagulant Platelets

Table 1 summarizes the main procoagulant activation endpoints and the markers used to detect and to discriminate the procoagulant platelet subpopulation, commonly used for flow cytometry. Surface expression of PS is the major standard activation endpoint widely recognized for procoagulant platelets. The gold standard assay to detect this event resides in the ability of the platelets to bind Annexin V [87,127] or lactadherin [211–213]. Another necrotic-like event that occurs in procoagulant platelets is the loss of the mitochondrial potential. This cytoplasmic event can be detected with mitochondrial probes like rhodamine derivatives, such as tetra-methyl-rhodamine methyl ester (TMRM) or tetra-methylrhodamine ethyl ester (TMRE) [131,142,214] or the carbocyanine JC-1 [140]. Rhodamine probes accumulate into intact mitochondria, but once platelets experience loss of the mitochondrial membrane potential, they escape and fluorescence decreases [215]. The JC-1 probe naturally exhibits green fluorescence. Its accumulation into intact mitochondria induces formation of probe aggregates that induce a fluorescence emission shift from green to red. Therefore, the red/green fluorescence intensity ratio is an indicator of the mitochondrial potential allowing the detection of mitochondrial depolarization by a decrease in the red/green fluorescence ratio [215].

Table 1. Activation endpoints of procoagulant platelets and common flow cytometry markers to detect and discriminate them.

Endpoint	Description	Common Markers	Phenotype in Procoagulant Platelets	Phenotype in Non-Procoagulant Platelets
Necrotic-like Phosphatidylserine	Negatively charged amino-phospholipids of platelet membrane bilayer, contribute to the procoagulant activity	Annexin V, lactadherin	Positive	Negative
Mitochondrial membrane depolarization	Mitochondrial events (depolarization) are implicated in platelet procoagulant activity process	Rhodamine (such as TMRM) JC-1	Low TMRM staining Lower JC-1 fluorescence ratio (red/green)	High TMRM staining Higher JC-1 fluorescence ratio (red/green)
Fibrinogen receptor GPIIb/IIIa (integrin $\alpha_{IIb}\beta_3$)	Platelet membrane glycoprotein; in its activated conformation binds to fibrinogen and mediates platelet aggregation	Anti-CD41/CD61 IgM antibody recognizing the activated conformation (PAC-1)	Negative	Positive
Platelet surface coating by α-granule proteins	Proteins present in α-granule secreted upon platelet activation and retained on the platelet surface by a serotonin- and transglutaminase mechanism	Specific antibodies against α-granule proteins, such as FV/Va, fibrinogen, VWF, fibronectin, thrombospondin, and α2-antiplasmin	Positive	Negative

Legend: FV, coagulation factor V; FVa, activated coagulation factor V; TMRM, tetra-methyl-rhodamine methyl ester; VWF, von Willebrand factor.

Because procoagulant platelets lose their properties to aggregate, the PAC-1 binding assay is another interesting approach to discriminate procoagulant platelets from non-coagulant aggregating platelets [131,142,216,217].

Last but not least, procoagulant endpoint is the coating of α-granule proteins on the surface of procoagulant COAT platelets [127,146,218,219]. This approach relies on the analysis of the surface retention of α-granule proteins with specific monoclonal antibodies. This technique is not often employed by clinical diagnostic laboratories, but can be performed in research laboratories, as it requires a specialized method and technical expertise to detect it properly.

4.3.2. Assessment of the Overall Coagulation Potential and Procoagulant Activity of Platelets

An arsenal of different complementary methods, which we have briefly summarized in Table 2, are available to assess the procoagulant potential in biological samples. The procoagulant activity of PS expressed by platelets and PMPs can be directly measured in plasma by functional tests (clot or chromogenic based assays), which take advantage of the anionic phospholipid dependent acceleration exerted by PS on prothrombin activation by the FXa-FVa complex [220,221].

Thrombin generation assay (TGA) is a sophisticated technique capable of assessing the delicate balance of procoagulant and anticoagulant pathways involved in the haemostatic process, thus providing a global view of the coagulation potential of an individual. The standard reference method for measuring thrombin generation (TG) is the calibrated automated thrombogram (CAT) developed by Hemker [222]. TGA can be performed using various types of biological material: most commonly, the assay is performed in PRP or platelet poor plasma (PPP). PRP is useful to study the interaction of platelets with coagulation factors in the coagulation process. Working with PPP requires the addition of artificial phospholipids to the sample (as substitute for platelets in order to provide the negatively charged surface that sustains TG); PPP investigation focuses on the action of coagulation factors. A particular advantage of PPP is that the sample can be frozen (thus allowing storage) and thawed just before analysis. The measurement is performed in the presence of defined concentrations of tissue factor (low, normal or high), allowing the modulation of the sensitivity of the test (e.g., high concentration of tissue factor will make the test less sensitive to the intrinsic pathway). Thrombomodulin-modified TGA is a novel variant of the classical TGA, which allows the highlighting of the role of the protein C system in downregulating the coagulation process [223]. This might be of interest for investigating platelet-dependent TG because it has been demonstrated that platelet-derived activated coagulation factor Va (FVa) bound on the surface of procoagulant platelets is protected from inactivation catalysed by activated protein C [224]. Finally, interesting and innovative technologies based on a spatio-temporal model of haemostasis, have been used to measure the contribution of procoagulant platelets or PMPs to the growth of the fibrin clot [126].

A step closer to physiological coagulation is represented by ex vivo TG measurement in whole blood. However, this method is challenging due to the interference of erythrocytes on the stability of fluorescence signal and requires expert operators. An alternative method to overcome the problem of the turbidity or colour of the blood sample is based on monitoring TG by electrochemistry. Such a method was developed by Thuerlemann et al. [225] using a single-use electrochemical biosensor sensible to the electric variations produced by an amperogenic substrate cleaved by thrombin. The variation of electric signal is recorded and the raw data values used to build a TG curve.

To exclude the effect of plasmatic factors, platelets can be isolated by gel filtration [201] or washing steps [131]. The specific contribution of procoagulant platelets to TG can be assessed by modified TG assays [126,201]. Gel filtered/washed platelets, once activated with specific agonists to the procoagulant phenotype, also generate procoagulant PMPs. The latter can be directly identified and investigated by flow cytometry based on their size (FSC) and specific fluorescent dye binding to exposed PS [125]. Flow cytometry is a powerful and preferred technique for investigating PMPs [226], since it allows counting, identifying their origin, and determining PS exposure by Annexin V binding [227]. Drawbacks of PMP measurements with flow cytometry are the small and heterogeneous size (0.1 to 1 μm) of PMPs, which can be very close to the instrument background and the difficult of calibration. It is possible to overcome these limitations by using fluorochrome tagging PMPs (e.g., molecules incorporating the phospholipid bilayer) and size-calibrated fluorescent beads together with background noise reduction (through 0.1 μm liquid filtration). Nevertheless a good expertise and high resolution flow cytometers are required [227]. PMPs generated from procoagulant platelets can be further processed to obtain a pure PMP preparation by subsequent centrifugation steps and used to measure PMP-dependent TG [126].

Table 2. A non-exhaustive list of techniques to assess coagulation potential and procoagulant activity.

Type of Sample	Assay What Does It Measure?	Assay Name and Principle	Advantages	Disadvantages	References
WB	Coagulation potential (subsampling TG measurement)	TGA chromogenic	Presence of all blood cells and coagulation factors	Tedious subsampling at interval points; Time consuming; Only a snapshot picture of TG is available	[228]
WB	Coagulation potential (continuous TG measurement)	TGA Paper based WB-TG assay Fluorogenic (rhodamine 110-based thrombin substrate)	Close to physiological haemostasis; Presence of all blood cells and coagulation factors	Potential of procoagulant platelets is not specifically targeted; Calibration is difficult because of haemolysis and/or haematocrit might vary in WB sample; Interference of contact activation; Needs experienced operator	[229,230]
WB	Coagulation potential (continuous TG measurement)	TGA Novel WB-TG assay Fluorogenic (rhodamine 110-based thrombin substrate)	Close to physiological haemostasis; Presence of all blood cells and coagulation factors; Stable light transmission achieved by continuous mixing of the assay plate	Potential of procoagulant platelets is not specifically targeted;	[231]
PRP	Coagulation potential (continuous TG measurement)	TGA e.g., Thrombinoscope (Stago), Techno-thrombin (Techno-clone) Fluorogenic	Mimics in vivo condition; Consider the interaction of platelets and coagulation factors	Potential of procoagulant platelets is not specifically targeted; Standardization is difficult; Reactivity of platelets: easy to provoke unwanted activation	[232]
PRP	Coagulation potential (continuous TG measurement)	TGA e.g., Thrombinoscope (Stago), ST Genesia (Stago) Fluorogenic	Defined concentration of tissue factor and artificial phospholipids; Standardization possible in automated version; Possible to store frozen samples	Potential of procoagulant platelets is not specifically targeted; Do not consider the interaction of platelets with coagulation factors; Loss of sensitivity for the intrinsic pathway if high amount of TF is used	[222,233]
PPP		TM-TGA ST Genesia (Stago), Fluorogenic	To study the role of protein C system by comparison of TM− and TM+ samples	TGA automated version: exact tissue factor concentration is not communicated	[223,234]
PPP	Spatio-temporal dynamics of coagulation (real time TG and fibrin clot formation)	Thrombodynamics Video microscopy system based on measurements of light scattering images intensity	Pre-analytics is standardized; TG and fibrin formation measured at the same time; Allows to investigate separately TF-dependent and TF-independent coagulation; PRP can be added to the mix	Problematic with lipemic samples; Available only in specialized laboratory	[235,236]

Table 2. Cont.

Type of Sample	Assay What Does It Measure?	Assay Name and Principle	Advantages	Disadvantages	References
Gel filtered or washed platelets	Coagulation potential (continuous TG)	Modified TGA assay fluorogenic	Targets specific procoagulant populations	Preparation is laborious; Requires experienced operator	[126,201]
	Quantifies the number of procoagulant platelets	Flow cytometry fluorescence	Targets procoagulant platelet formation and associated markers		[131]
	Measures the rate of clot growth	Experimental video microscopy Based on intensity of light scattering images	Specifically assess the contribution of activated platelets to clot growth	Requires experienced operator	[126]
PMPs	Quantifies procoagulant potential of PMPs expressing PS.	Zymuphen MP Activity assay (Hyphen BioMed) ELISA, chromogenic	Easy to perform; High speed of sample analysis	Size of the PMPs can affect binding to Annexin V, thus lower detection of PS; No information on count, size or origin	[220,221,237,238]
	Procoagulant potential of PMPs expressing PS added to phospholipid free plasma	Procoag PPL (Stago) Clotting time Number of PMPs is inversely proportional to clotting time	Can be used also on WB, PRP, PPP; Easy to perform	No information on count, size or origin	[239–241]
	Quantifies PMPs derived from gel filtered/washed platelets	Flow cytometry fluorescence Identification of PMPs by size (FSC) and fluorescence (e.g., bodily-label)	Target PMPs derived specifically from procoagulant platelets; Gel filtration/washing remove plasmatic components	PMPs are close to electronic noise and debris, part of the population might be below the threshold Require expertise and sensitive cytometer	[125,242]
	Coagulation potential (continuous TG)	Modified TGA Fluorogenic Isolation of PMPs by centrifugation	Specifically assess contribution of PMPs derived from procoagulant platelets to TG	Preparation is laborious	[126]
	Measures the rate of clot growth	Experimental video microscopy system Based on intensity of light scattering images	Specifically assess the contribution of PMPs isolated from activated platelets to clot growth	Require experienced operator	[126]

Legend: ELISA, enzyme linked immunosorbent assay; FSC, forward scatter; PMPs, platelet derived microparticles; PPL, procoagulant phospholipid; PPP, platelet poor plasma; PRP, platelet rich plasma; PS, phosphatidylserine; TGA, thrombin generation assay; TG, thrombin generation; UFP, ultra-centrifuged plasma; WB, whole blood.

4.3.3. In-Vivo Investigations of Procoagulant Platelets

Intravital microscopy permits the study of physiological haemostasis and the appreciation the heterogeneous structure of a growing thrombus [243,244]. More and more publications are present in the literature assessing the heterogeneous platelet activation status with a particular focus on the role of procoagulant platelets [134,245,246]. Very recently, Nechipurenko et al. demonstrated that, during the in vivo formation of the thrombus, the procoagulant platelets are located at the periphery of the clot, which is driven by their mechanical extrusion as a result of the clot contraction [247]. These increasing new data provided by intravital microscopy and future experimentation with genetically-engineered mouse models, such as TMEM16F-deficient mice [246], will increase our knowledge on the in vivo role of procoagulant platelets. Obviously, this can be extended to other thrombocytopathies, where we can also obtain a real time monitoring of thrombus formation in pathophysiological conditions [248–250].

Nevertheless, one should be aware that such experiments still lack standardization, and inter-laboratory replicability is laborious. We should also keep in mind that even though this technique allows a step closer in studying haemostasis and thrombosis, experiments have thus far been performed with non-physiological injuries and in murine models.

5. Thrombocytopathy Associated to COVID-19

The current ongoing outbreak of coronavirus disease 2019 (COVID-19) is caused by a viral infection from severe acute respiratory syndrome coronavirus 2 (SARS-CoV-2) [251]. Even though SARS-CoV-2 infection initially results in excessive inflammation and mild to acute respiratory distress syndrome, patients also experience a hypercoagulable state characterized by immuno-thrombosis [252,253]. Therefore, venous and arterial thrombotic complications are an important cause of morbidity and mortality in COVID-19 patients [254].

Although the research on mechanisms implicated on platelet dysfunction in COVID-19 is still ongoing, at the time of this review there is some emerging evidence of COVID-19-associated thrombocytopathy [255–258]. In addition to a mild thrombocytopenia, which is frequent among COVID-19 patients, studies have described altered platelet function and reactivity [257,259–261].

Platelets seem to circulate in an activated state as demonstrated by a higher expression of specific platelet activation markers, such as P-selectin (CD62P), LAMP-3, and GPIIb/IIIa in unstimulated platelets from COVID-19 patients compared to healthy controls [259,261,262]. Platelets from SARS-CoV-2 infected patients increased basal reactive oxygen species (ROS), but basal surface expression of PS was not altered [261,263].

In addition, platelets from COVID-19 patients are hyper-responsive. Platelets had increased aggregation response to subthreshold concentrations of agonists, as well as increased adhesion and spreading [259–261]. This could be linked to the observed increased expression of adhesive receptors, such as VWF- and fibrinogen-receptors, respectively GPIbα/GPIX and GPIIb/IIIa [259]. Of note, COVID-19 patients had a reduced procoagulant platelet response ex vivo [263]. This was observed with a reduced mitochondrial depolarization and externalization of PS, compared to controls.

Mechanisms leading to thrombocytopathy in COVID-19 still need to be understood. However, based on the literature, platelet hyper-responsiveness may be induced by increased circulating VWF (endothelial injury) [264], hypoxia [265–267], and/or a hyper-inflammatory environment with high cytokine levels [268–270], and increased oxidative stress [271].

On current observations, it seems that procoagulant platelets should not contribute to the pathophysiology of COVID-19 patients, but the hyperreactive adhesion and aggregation may be implicated.

6. Conclusions

Thrombocytopathies are a diagnostic challenge. The introduction of flow cytometry, as an extension to routine diagnostic work-up by LTA and secretion assays, greatly improved management of patients with a bleeding diathesis in whom previous laboratory analysis could not identify a cause [87]. Moreover, in addition to the traditional platelet aggregation assays, flow cytometry has the advantage of rapidly acquiring intrinsic properties from thousands of single platelets, of requiring small blood volumes thus enabling the analysis of samples from thrombocytopenic patients, and the exploration of more than only one endpoint of the heterogeneous profiles, as performed with traditional aggregation assays. Flow cytometry is therefore able to point out surface membrane receptor deficiencies, such as BSS (adhesion endpoint) or GT (aggregation endpoint), as well as secretion endpoint defects (dense granule content and secretion by means of mepacrine, or alpha-granules, by investigating e.g., VWF content or surface expression of P-selectin). Finally, as highlighted in this review, flow cytometry is also able to cover the important procoagulant aspect of the pleomorphic platelet activation endpoints.

Wide systematic investigation of the procoagulant activity of platelets is increasingly described in the literature. This accumulating evidence indicates that the ability to generate procoagulant platelets at and beyond the extremes of the wide normal reference range [87] is associated with clinically relevant bleeding or thrombotic disease. Specifically, the generation of procoagulant platelets at levels <20% or >50% seems to worsen bleeding or thrombotic episodes, respectively. Moreover, the individual potential to generate procoagulant platelets at the time of the clinical event (e.g., stroke) seems to be strongly related to prognosis. It remains to be investigated whether an individual baseline potential to generate high or low level procoagulant platelets would also be a risk stratification for cardiovascular diseases before their clinical manifestation.

However, most of the publications were monocentric pilot studies and/or performed with relatively small cohort sizes and/or with short follow-up timeframes. The flow cytometric investigation of procoagulant platelets still needs standardization to allow proper meta-analysis and generalization of its use. In parallel, future research and experimentation on the procoagulant status of platelets and in vivo thrombus formation models will help to better appreciate the crucial role of procoagulant platelets in haemostatic diseases. These approaches will help to dissect the role of procoagulant platelets in thrombotic and haemorrhagic events.

Author Contributions: Conceptualization, A.A., D.B.C. and L.A.; Funding acquisition, A.A. and L.A.; Supervision, L.A.; Writing—original draft, A.A., D.B.C. and L.A.; Writing—review & editing, A.A., D.B.C., M.G.Z., M.M. and L.A. All authors have read and agreed to the published version of the manuscript.

Funding: Our research is supported by grants from Dr. Henri Dubois-Ferrière Dinu Lipatti Foundation, Novartis Foundation for Medical-Biological Research (Grant #18B074), Swiss Heart Foundation (Grant FF19117), and the Swiss National Science Foundation (SNSF grant 320030-197392).

Conflicts of Interest: The authors declare no conflict of interest.

References

1. Quach, M.E.; Chen, W.; Li, R. Mechanisms of platelet clearance and translation to improve platelet storage. *Blood* **2018**, *131*, 1512–1521. [CrossRef] [PubMed]
2. Jobe, S.M.; Di Paola, J. Congenital and acquired disorders of platelet function and number. In *Consultative Hemostasis and Thrombosis*; Elsevier: Amsterdam, The Netherlands, 2019; pp. 145–166.
3. Shen, Y.M.; Frenkel, E.P. Acquired platelet dysfunction. *Hematol. Oncol. Clin. North. Am.* **2007**, *21*, 647–661. [CrossRef] [PubMed]
4. Cherry-Bukowiec, J.; Napolitano, L. What platelet disorders occur in the intensive care unit and how should they be treated? In *Evidence-Based Practice of Critical Care*; Elsevier: Amsterdam, The Netherlands, 2010; pp. 645–660.
5. Bye, A.P.; Unsworth, A.J.; Gibbins, J.M. Platelet signaling: A complex interplay between inhibitory and activatory networks. *J. Thromb. Haemost.* **2016**, *14*, 918–930. [CrossRef]
6. Stegner, D.; Nieswandt, B. Platelet receptor signaling in thrombus formation. *J. Mol. Med.* **2011**, *89*, 109–121. [CrossRef] [PubMed]

7. Heemskerk, J.W.; Bevers, E.M.; Lindhout, T. Platelet activation and blood coagulation. *Thromb. Haemost.* **2002**, *88*, 186–193. [CrossRef] [PubMed]
8. van der Meijden, P.E.J.; Heemskerk, J.W.M. Platelet biology and functions: New concepts and clinical perspectives. *Nat. Rev. Cardiol.* **2019**, *16*, 166–179. [CrossRef]
9. Andrews, R.K.; Lopez, J.A.; Berndt, M.C. Molecular mechanisms of platelet adhesion and activation. *Int. J. Biochem. Cell Biol.* **1997**, *29*, 91–105. [CrossRef]
10. Lopez, J.A.; Dong, J.F. Structure and function of the glycoprotein ib-ix-v complex. *Curr. Opin. Hematol.* **1997**, *4*, 323–329. [CrossRef]
11. Li, R.; Emsley, J. The organizing principle of the platelet glycoprotein ib-ix-v complex. *J. Thromb. Haemost.* **2013**, *11*, 605–614. [CrossRef]
12. Andrews, R.K.; Berndt, M.C. The gpib-ix-v complex. In *Platelets*; Michelson, A.D., Ed.; Academic Press: Cambridge, MA, USA, 2013; pp. 195–213.
13. Romo, G.M.; Dong, J.F.; Schade, A.J.; Gardiner, E.E.; Kansas, G.S.; Li, C.Q.; McIntire, L.V.; Berndt, M.C.; Lopez, J.A. The glycoprotein ib-ix-v complex is a platelet counterreceptor for p-selectin. *J. Exp. Med.* **1999**, *190*, 803–814. [CrossRef] [PubMed]
14. Simon, D.I.; Chen, Z.; Xu, H.; Li, C.Q.; Dong, J.; McIntire, L.V.; Ballantyne, C.M.; Zhang, L.; Furman, M.I.; Berndt, M.C.; et al. Platelet glycoprotein ibalpha is a counterreceptor for the leukocyte integrin mac-1 (cd11b/cd18). *J. Exp. Med.* **2000**, *192*, 193–204. [CrossRef]
15. Wang, Y.; Sakuma, M.; Chen, Z.; Ustinov, V.; Shi, C.; Croce, K.; Zago, A.C.; Lopez, J.; Andre, P.; Plow, E.; et al. Leukocyte engagement of platelet glycoprotein ibalpha via the integrin mac-1 is critical for the biological response to vascular injury. *Circulation* **2005**, *112*, 2993–3000. [CrossRef] [PubMed]
16. Libby, P.; Simon, D.I. Inflammation and thrombosis: The clot thickens. *Circulation* **2001**, *103*, 1718–1720. [CrossRef]
17. Berndt, M.C.; Andrews, R.K. Bernard-soulier syndrome. *Haematologica* **2011**, *96*, 355–359. [CrossRef] [PubMed]
18. Nakamura, F.; Pudas, R.; Heikkinen, O.; Permi, P.; Kilpelainen, I.; Munday, A.D.; Hartwig, J.H.; Stossel, T.P.; Ylanne, J. The structure of the gpib-filamin a complex. *Blood* **2006**, *107*, 1925–1932. [CrossRef] [PubMed]
19. Kanaji, T.; Russell, S.; Ware, J. Amelioration of the macrothrombocytopenia associated with the murine bernard-soulier syndrome. *Blood* **2002**, *100*, 2102–2107. [CrossRef]
20. Cranmer, S.L.; Pikovski, I.; Mangin, P.; Thompson, P.E.; Domagala, T.; Frazzetto, M.; Salem, H.H.; Jackson, S.P. Identification of a unique filamin a binding region within the cytoplasmic domain of glycoprotein ibalpha. *Biochem. J.* **2005**, *387*, 849–858. [CrossRef]
21. Nurden, A.T. Qualitative disorders of platelets and megakaryocytes. *J. Thromb. Haemost.* **2005**, *3*, 1773–1782. [CrossRef]
22. Lopez, J.A.; Andrews, R.K.; Afshar-Kharghan, V.; Berndt, M.C. Bernard-soulier syndrome. *Blood* **1998**, *91*, 4397–4418. [CrossRef]
23. Bernard, J.; Soulier, J.P. On a new variety of congenital thrombocytary hemo-ragiparous dystrophy. *Sem. Hop.* **1948**, *24*, 3217–3223. [PubMed]
24. Lanza, F. Bernard-soulier syndrome (hemorrhagiparous thrombocytic dystrophy). *Orphanet J. Rare Dis.* **2006**, *1*, 46. [CrossRef]
25. Savoia, A.; Kunishima, S.; De Rocco, D.; Zieger, B.; Rand, M.L.; Pujol-Moix, N.; Caliskan, U.; Tokgoz, H.; Pecci, A.; Noris, P.; et al. Spectrum of the mutations in bernard-soulier syndrome. *Hum. Mutat.* **2014**, *35*, 1033–1045. [CrossRef] [PubMed]
26. Miller, J.L.; Lyle, V.A.; Cunningham, D. Mutation of leucine-57 to phenylalanine in a platelet glycoprotein ib alpha leucine tandem repeat occurring in patients with an autosomal dominant variant of bernard-soulier disease. *Blood* **1992**, *79*, 439–446. [CrossRef] [PubMed]
27. Kahn, M.L.; Diacovo, T.G.; Bainton, D.F.; Lanza, F.; Trejo, J.; Coughlin, S.R. Glycoprotein v-deficient platelets have undiminished thrombin responsiveness and do not exhibit a bernard-soulier phenotype. *Blood* **1999**, *94*, 4112–4121. [CrossRef]
28. Weiss, H.J.; Tschopp, T.B.; Baumgartner, H.R.; Sussman, II.; Johnson, M.M.; Egan, J.J. Decreased adhesion of giant (bernard-soulier) platelets to subendothelium: Further implications on the role of the von willebrand factor in hemostasis. *Am. J. Med.* **1974**, *57*, 920–925. [CrossRef]
29. Jamieson, G.A.; Okumura, T. Reduced thrombin binding and aggregation in bernard-soulier platelets. *J. Clin. Investig.* **1978**, *61*, 861–864. [CrossRef]
30. Dormann, D.; Clemetson, K.J.; Kehrel, B.E. The gpib thrombin-binding site is essential for thrombin-induced platelet procoagulant activity. *Blood* **2000**, *96*, 2469–2478. [CrossRef]
31. Bevers, E.M.; Comfurius, P.; Nieuwenhuis, H.K.; Levy-Toledano, S.; Enouf, J.; Belluci, S.; Caen, J.P.; Zwaal, R.F. Platelet prothrombin converting activity in hereditary disorders of platelet function. *Br. J. Haematol.* **1986**, *63*, 335–345. [CrossRef]
32. Pham, A.; Wang, J. Bernard-soulier syndrome: An inherited platelet disorder. *Arch. Pathol. Lab. Med.* **2007**, *131*, 1834–1836. [CrossRef] [PubMed]
33. Balduini, C.L.; Iolascon, A.; Savoia, A. Inherited thrombocytopenias: From genes to therapy. *Haematologica* **2002**, *87*, 860–880.
34. Harrison, P.; Robinson, M.; Liesner, R.; Khair, K.; Cohen, H.; Mackie, I.; Machin, S. The pfa-100: A potential rapid screening tool for the assessment of platelet dysfunction. *Clin. Lab. Haematol.* **2002**, *24*, 225–232. [CrossRef] [PubMed]
35. Bolton-Maggs, P.H.; Chalmers, E.A.; Collins, P.W.; Harrison, P.; Kitchen, S.; Liesner, R.J.; Minford, A.; Mumford, A.D.; Parapia, L.A.; Perry, D.J.; et al. A review of inherited platelet disorders with guidelines for their management on behalf of the ukhcdo. *Br. J. Haematol.* **2006**, *135*, 603–633. [CrossRef] [PubMed]
36. Ibrahim-Kosta, M.; Alessi, M.C.; Hezard, N. Laboratory techniques used to diagnose constitutional platelet dysfunction. *Hämostaseologie* **2020**, *40*, 444–459. [CrossRef] [PubMed]

37. Andrews, R.K.; Berndt, M.C. Bernard-soulier syndrome: An update. *Semin. Thromb. Hemost.* **2013**, *39*, 656–662. [CrossRef] [PubMed]
38. Cohn, R.J.; Sherman, G.G.; Glencross, D.K. Flow cytometric analysis of platelet surface glycoproteins in the diagnosis of bernard-soulier syndrome. *Pediatr. Hematol. Oncol.* **1997**, *14*, 43–50. [CrossRef]
39. Othman, M.; Emsley, J. Gene of the issue: Gp1ba gene mutations associated with bleeding. *Platelets* **2017**, *28*, 832–836. [CrossRef]
40. Tait, A.S.; Cranmer, S.L.; Jackson, S.P.; Dawes, I.W.; Chong, B.H. Phenotype changes resulting in high-affinity binding of von willebrand factor to recombinant glycoprotein ib-ix: Analysis of the platelet-type von willebrand disease mutations. *Blood* **2001**, *98*, 1812–1818. [CrossRef] [PubMed]
41. Othman, M. Platelet-type von willebrand disease: Three decades in the life of a rare bleeding disorder. *Blood Rev.* **2011**, *25*, 147–153. [CrossRef]
42. Franchini, M.; Montagnana, M.; Lippi, G. Clinical, laboratory and therapeutic aspects of platelet-type von willebrand disease. *Int. J. Lab. Hematol.* **2008**, *30*, 91–94. [CrossRef] [PubMed]
43. Miller, J.L.; Boselli, B.D.; Kupinski, J.M. In vivo interaction of von willebrand factor with platelets following cryoprecipitate transfusion in platelet-type von willebrand's disease. *Blood* **1984**, *63*, 226–230. [CrossRef] [PubMed]
44. Favaloro, E.J. 2b or not 2b? What is the role of vwf in platelet-matrix interactions? And what is the role of the vwf:Cb in vwd diagnostics? These are the questions. *J. Thromb. Haemost.* **2006**, *4*, 892–894. [CrossRef]
45. Othman, M.; Gresele, P. Guidance on the diagnosis and management of platelet-type von willebrand disease: A communication from the platelet physiology subcommittee of the isth. *J. Thromb. Haemost.* **2020**, *18*, 1855–1858. [CrossRef]
46. Giannini, S.; Cecchetti, L.; Mezzasoma, A.M.; Gresele, P. Diagnosis of platelet-type von willebrand disease by flow cytometry. *Haematologica* **2010**, *95*, 1021–1024. [CrossRef] [PubMed]
47. Versteeg, H.H.; Heemskerk, J.W.; Levi, M.; Reitsma, P.H. New fundamentals in hemostasis. *Physiol Rev.* **2013**, *93*, 327–358. [CrossRef]
48. Sharda, A.; Flaumenhaft, R. The life cycle of platelet granules. *F1000Research* **2018**, *7*, 236. [CrossRef] [PubMed]
49. Marks, M.S.; Heijnen, H.F.; Raposo, G. Lysosome-related organelles: Unusual compartments become mainstream. *Curr. Opin. Cell Biol.* **2013**, *25*, 495–505. [CrossRef]
50. Heijnen, H.F.; Debili, N.; Vainchencker, W.; Breton-Gorius, J.; Geuze, H.J.; Sixma, J.J. Multivesicular bodies are an intermediate stage in the formation of platelet alpha-granules. *Blood* **1998**, *91*, 2313–2325. [CrossRef]
51. Youssefian, T.; Cramer, E.M. Megakaryocyte dense granule components are sorted in multivesicular bodies. *Blood* **2000**, *95*, 4004–4007. [CrossRef] [PubMed]
52. Maynard, D.M.; Heijnen, H.F.; Horne, M.K.; White, J.G.; Gahl, W.A. Proteomic analysis of platelet alpha-granules using mass spectrometry. *J. Thromb. Haemost.* **2007**, *5*, 1945–1955. [CrossRef] [PubMed]
53. Coppinger, J.A.; Cagney, G.; Toomey, S.; Kislinger, T.; Belton, O.; McRedmond, J.P.; Cahill, D.J.; Emili, A.; Fitzgerald, D.J.; Maguire, P.B. Characterization of the proteins released from activated platelets leads to localization of novel platelet proteins in human atherosclerotic lesions. *Blood* **2004**, *103*, 2096–2104. [CrossRef] [PubMed]
54. Golebiewska, E.M.; Poole, A.W. Platelet secretion: From haemostasis to wound healing and beyond. *Blood Rev.* **2015**, *29*, 153–162. [CrossRef]
55. Flaumenhaft, R. Platelet secretion. In *Platelets in Thrombotic and Non-Thrombotic Disorders*; Gresele, P., Kleiman, N.S., Lopez, J.A., Page, C.P., Eds.; Springer International Publishing: Cham, Switzerland, 2017; pp. 353–366.
56. Youssefian, T.; Massé, J.-M.; Rendu, F.; Guichard, J.; Cramer, E.M. Platelet and megakaryocyte dense-granules contain glycoproteins ib and iib-iiia. *Blood* **1997**, *89*, 4047–4057. [CrossRef] [PubMed]
57. Rendu, F.; Brohard-Bohn, B. The platelet release reaction: Granules' constituents, secretion and functions. *Platelets* **2001**, *12*, 261–273. [CrossRef]
58. Weiss, H.J.; Witte, L.D.; Kaplan, K.L.; Lages, B.A.; Chernoff, A.; Nossel, H.L.; Goodman, D.S.; Baumgartner, H.R. Heterogeneity in storage pool deficiency: Studies on granule-bound substances in 18 patients including variants deficient in alpha-granules, platelet factor 4, beta-thromboglobulin, and platelet-derived growth factor. *Blood* **1979**, *54*, 1296–1319. [CrossRef]
59. Mumford, A.D.; Frelinger, A.L., 3rd; Gachet, C.; Gresele, P.; Noris, P.; Harrison, P.; Mezzano, D. A review of platelet secretion assays for the diagnosis of inherited platelet secretion disorders. *Thromb. Haemost.* **2015**, *114*, 14–25. [CrossRef]
60. Nurden, A.; Nurden, P. Advances in our understanding of the molecular basis of disorders of platelet function. *J. Thromb. Haemost.* **2011**, *9* (Suppl. S1), 76–91. [CrossRef] [PubMed]
61. Sandrock, K.; Zieger, B. Current strategies in diagnosis of inherited storage pool defects. *Transfus. Med. Hemother.* **2010**, *37*, 248–258. [CrossRef] [PubMed]
62. Heijnen, H.; van der Sluijs, P. Platelet secretory behaviour: As diverse as the granules... or not? *J. Thromb. Haemost.* **2015**, *13*, 2141–2151. [CrossRef] [PubMed]
63. Raccuglia, G. Gray platelet syndrome. A variety of qualitative platelet disorder. *Am. J. Med.* **1971**, *51*, 818–828. [CrossRef]
64. Gerrard, J.M.; Phillips, D.R.; Rao, G.H.; Plow, E.F.; Walz, D.A.; Ross, R.; Harker, L.A.; White, J.G. Biochemical studies of two patients with the gray platelet syndrome. Selective deficiency of platelet alpha granules. *J. Clin. Investig.* **1980**, *66*, 102–109. [CrossRef] [PubMed]
65. Nurden, A.T.; Nurden, P. The gray platelet syndrome: Clinical spectrum of the disease. *Blood Rev.* **2007**, *21*, 21–36. [CrossRef] [PubMed]

66. Jantunen, E.; Hanninen, A.; Naukkarinen, A.; Vornanen, M.; Lahtinen, R. Gray platelet syndrome with splenomegaly and signs of extramedullary hematopoiesis: A case report with review of the literature. *Am. J. Hematol.* **1994**, *46*, 218–224. [CrossRef]
67. Caen, J.P.; Deschamps, J.F.; Bodevin, E.; Bryckaert, M.C.; Dupuy, E.; Wasteson, A. Megakaryocytes and myelofibrosis in gray platelet syndrome. *Nouv. Rev. Fr. Hematol.* **1987**, *29*, 109–114. [PubMed]
68. Sims, M.C.; Mayer, L.; Collins, J.H.; Bariana, T.K.; Megy, K.; Lavenu-Bombled, C.; Seyres, D.; Kollipara, L.; Burden, F.S.; Greene, D.; et al. Novel manifestations of immune dysregulation and granule defects in gray platelet syndrome. *Blood* **2020**, *136*, 1956–1967. [CrossRef] [PubMed]
69. Breton-Gorius, J.; Vainchenker, W.; Nurden, A.; Levy-Toledano, S.; Caen, J. Defective alpha-granule production in megakaryocytes from gray platelet syndrome: Ultrastructural studies of bone marrow cells and megakaryocytes growing in culture from blood precursors. *Am. J. Pathol.* **1981**, *102*, 10–19. [PubMed]
70. Simon, D.; Kunicki, T.; Nugent, D. Platelet function defects. *Haemophilia* **2008**, *14*, 1240–1249. [CrossRef] [PubMed]
71. Mayer, L.; Jasztal, M.; Pardo, M.; Aguera de Haro, S.; Collins, J.; Bariana, T.K.; Smethurst, P.A.; Grassi, L.; Petersen, R.; Nurden, P.; et al. Nbeal2 interacts with dock7, sec16a, and vac14. *Blood* **2018**, *131*, 1000–1011. [CrossRef]
72. Lo, R.W.; Li, L.; Leung, R.; Pluthero, F.G.; Kahr, W.H.A. Nbeal2 (neurobeachin-like 2) is required for retention of cargo proteins by -granules during their production by megakaryocytes. *Arter. Thromb. Vasc. Biol.* **2018**, *38*, 2435–2447. [CrossRef]
73. Nurden, A.T.; Nurden, P. Should any genetic defect affecting alpha-granules in platelets be classified as gray platelet syndrome? *Am. J. Hematol.* **2016**, *91*, 714–718. [CrossRef]
74. Villeneuve, J.; Block, A.; Le Bousse-Kerdiles, M.C.; Lepreux, S.; Nurden, P.; Ripoche, J.; Nurden, A.T. Tissue inhibitors of matrix metalloproteinases in platelets and megakaryocytes: A novel organization for these secreted proteins. *Exp. Hematol.* **2009**, *37*, 849–856. [CrossRef]
75. Rosa, J.P.; George, J.N.; Bainton, D.F.; Nurden, A.T.; Caen, J.P.; McEver, R.P. Gray platelet syndrome. Demonstration of alpha granule membranes that can fuse with the cell surface. *J. Clin. Investig.* **1987**, *80*, 1138–1146. [CrossRef]
76. Drouin, A.; Favier, R.; Masse, J.M.; Debili, N.; Schmitt, A.; Elbim, C.; Guichard, J.; Adam, M.; Gougerot-Pocidalo, M.A.; Cramer, E.M. Newly recognized cellular abnormalities in the gray platelet syndrome. *Blood* **2001**, *98*, 1382–1391. [CrossRef]
77. Lages, B.; Sussman, I.I.; Levine, S.P.; Coletti, D.; Weiss, H.J. Platelet alpha granule deficiency associated with decreased p-selectin and selective impairment of thrombin-induced activation in a new patient with gray platelet syndrome (alpha-storage pool deficiency). *J. Lab. Clin. Med.* **1997**, *129*, 364–375. [CrossRef]
78. Shahraki, H.; Dorgalaleh, A.; Bain, B.J. Gray platelet syndrome (gps). In *Congenital Bleeding Disorders: Diagnosis and Management*; Dorgalaleh, A., Ed.; Springer International Publishing: Cham, Switzerland, 2018; pp. 379–396.
79. Podda, G.; Femia, E.A.; Pugliano, M.; Cattaneo, M. Congenital defects of platelet function. *Platelets* **2012**, *23*, 552–563. [CrossRef] [PubMed]
80. Huizing, M.; Helip-Wooley, A.; Westbroek, W.; Gunay-Aygun, M.; Gahl, W.A. Disorders of lysosome-related organelle biogenesis: Clinical and molecular genetics. *Annu Rev. Genom. Hum. Genet.* **2008**, *9*, 359–386. [CrossRef] [PubMed]
81. Dupuis, A.; Bordet, J.C.; Eckly, A.; Gachet, C. Platelet delta-storage pool disease: An update. *J. Clin. Med.* **2020**, *9*, 2508. [CrossRef] [PubMed]
82. Woldie, I.; Guo, R.; Ososki, R.; Dyson, G.; Mohamad, S.; Raval, K.K.; Gabali, A.M. *Clinical Characteristics of Patients Diagnosed with Delta Granule Platelet Storage Pool Deficiency (Δ-PSPD)*; The Detroit Medical Center (DMC): Detroit, MI, USA, 2017.
83. Masliah-Planchon, J.; Darnige, L.; Bellucci, S. Molecular determinants of platelet delta storage pool deficiencies: An update. *Br. J. Haematol.* **2013**, *160*, 5–11. [CrossRef]
84. Nieuwenhuis, H.K.; Akkerman, J.W.; Sixma, J.J. Patients with a prolonged bleeding time and normal aggregation tests may have storage pool deficiency: Studies on one hundred six patients. *Blood* **1987**, *70*, 620–623. [CrossRef]
85. White, J.G. Use of the electron microscope for diagnosis of platelet disorders. *Semin. Thromb. Hemost.* **1998**, *24*, 163–168. [CrossRef]
86. Wall, J.E.; Buijswilts, M.; Arnold, J.T.; Wang, W.; White, M.M.; Jennings, L.K.; Jackson, C.W. A flow cytometric assay using mepacrine for study of uptake and release of platelet dense granule contents. *Br. J. Haematol.* **1995**, *89*, 380–385. [CrossRef]
87. Daskalakis, M.; Colucci, G.; Keller, P.; Rochat, S.; Silzle, T.; Biasiutti, F.D.; Barizzi, G.; Alberio, L. Decreased generation of procoagulant platelets detected by flow cytometric analysis in patients with bleeding diathesis. *Cytometry B Clin. Cytom* **2014**, *86*, 397–409. [CrossRef]
88. Gordon, N.; Thom, J.; Cole, C.; Baker, R. Rapid detection of hereditary and acquired platelet storage pool deficiency by flow cytometry. *Br. J. Haematol.* **1995**, *89*, 117–123. [CrossRef] [PubMed]
89. Cai, H.; Mullier, F.; Frotscher, B.; Briquel, M.E.; Toussaint, M.; Massin, F.; Lecompte, T.; Latger-Cannard, V. Usefulness of flow cytometric mepacrine uptake/release combined with cd63 assay in diagnosis of patients with suspected platelet dense granule disorder. *Semin. Thromb. Hemost.* **2016**, *42*, 282–291. [CrossRef] [PubMed]
90. Holmsen, H.; Weiss, H.J. Secretable storage pools in platelets. *Annu. Rev. Med.* **1979**, *30*, 119–134. [CrossRef] [PubMed]
91. Shattil, S.J.; Kashiwagi, H.; Pampori, N. Integrin signaling: The platelet paradigm. *Blood* **1998**, *91*, 2645–2657. [CrossRef]
92. Poon, M.C.; Di Minno, G.; d'Oiron, R.; Zotz, R. New insights into the treatment of glanzmann thrombasthenia. *Transfus. Med. Rev.* **2016**, *30*, 92–99. [CrossRef]
93. George, J.N.; Caen, J.P.; Nurden, A.T. Glanzmann's thrombasthenia: The spectrum of clinical disease. *Blood* **1990**, *75*, 1383–1395. [CrossRef]

94. D'Andrea, G.; Margaglione, M.; Glansmann's Thrombasthemia Italian T. Glanzmann's thrombasthenia: Modulation of clinical phenotype by alpha2c807t gene polymorphism. *Haematologica* **2003**, *88*, 1378–1382. [CrossRef]
95. Di Minno, G.; Zotz, R.B.; d'Oiron, R.; Bindslev, N.; Di Minno, M.N.; Poon, M.C.; Glanzmann Thrombasthenia Registry Investigators. The international, prospective glanzmann thrombasthenia registry: Treatment modalities and outcomes of non-surgical bleeding episodes in patients with glanzmann thrombasthenia. *Haematologica* **2015**, *100*, 1031–1037. [CrossRef]
96. Nurden, A.T. Glanzmann thrombasthenia. *Orphanet J. Rare Dis.* **2006**, *1*, 10. [CrossRef]
97. Bellucci, S.; Caen, J. Molecular basis of glanzmann's thrombasthenia and current strategies in treatment. *Blood Rev.* **2002**, *16*, 193–202. [CrossRef]
98. Botero, J.P.; Lee, K.; Branchford, B.R.; Bray, P.F.; Freson, K.; Lambert, M.P.; Luo, M.; Mohan, S.; Ross, J.E.; Bergmeier, W.; et al. Glanzmann thrombasthenia: Genetic basis and clinical correlates. *Haematologica* **2020**, *105*, 888–894. [CrossRef] [PubMed]
99. Caen, J.P. Glanzmann's thrombasthenia. *Baillieres Clin. Haematol.* **1989**, *2*, 609–625. [CrossRef]
100. Linden, M.D.; Frelinger, A.L., 3rd; Barnard, M.R.; Przyklenk, K.; Furman, M.I.; Michelson, A.D. Application of flow cytometry to platelet disorders. *Semin. Thromb. Hemost.* **2004**, *30*, 501–511. [CrossRef] [PubMed]
101. Weiss, H.J.; Turitto, V.T.; Baumgartner, H.R. Further evidence that glycoprotein iib-iiia mediates platelet spreading on subendothelium. *Thromb. Haemost.* **1991**, *65*, 202–205. [CrossRef]
102. Weiss, H.J.; Turitto, V.T.; Baumgartner, H.R. Platelet adhesion and thrombus formation on subendothelium in platelets deficient in glycoproteins iib-iiia, ib, and storage granules. *Blood* **1986**, *67*, 322–330. [CrossRef]
103. Jurk, K.; Kehrel, B.E. Inherited and acquired disorders of platelet function. *Transfus. Med. Hemotherapy* **2007**, *34*, 6–19. [CrossRef]
104. Gobbi, G.; Sponzilli, I.; Mirandola, P.; Tazzari, P.L.; Caimi, L.; Cacchioli, A.; Matteucci, A.; Giuliani Piccari, G.; Cocco, L.; Vitale, M. Efficient platelet delta-granule release induced by [Ca2+]i elevation is modulated by gpiibiiia. *Int. J. Mol. Med.* **2006**, *18*, 309–313.
105. Dorgalaleh, A.; Poon, M.; Shiravand, Y. Glanzmann thrombasthenia. In *Congenital Bleeding Disorders*; Dorgalaleh, A., Ed.; Springer: Cham, Switzerland, 2018.
106. Gresele, P.; Subcommittee on Platelet Physiology of the International Society on T. Hemostasis. Diagnosis of inherited platelet function disorders: Guidance from the ssc of the isth. *J. Thromb. Haemost.* **2015**, *13*, 314–322. [CrossRef]
107. Alessi, M.C.; Sie, P.; Payrastre, B. Strengths and weaknesses of light transmission aggregometry in diagnosing hereditary platelet function disorders. *J. Clin. Med.* **2020**, *9*, 763. [CrossRef]
108. Nurden, A.T.; Pillois, X.; Wilcox, D.A. Glanzmann thrombasthenia: State of the art and future directions. *Semin Thromb. Hemost.* **2013**, *39*, 642–655. [CrossRef] [PubMed]
109. Lanza, F.; Stierle, A.; Fournier, D.; Morales, M.; Andre, G.; Nurden, A.T.; Cazenave, J.P. A new variant of glanzmann's thrombasthenia (strasbourg i). Platelets with functionally defective glycoprotein iib-iiia complexes and a glycoprotein iiia 214arg—214trp mutation. *J. Clin. Investig.* **1992**, *89*, 1995–2004. [CrossRef]
110. Nagata, S.; Sakuragi, T.; Segawa, K. Flippase and scramblase for phosphatidylserine exposure. *Curr. Opin. Immunol.* **2020**, *62*, 31–38. [CrossRef] [PubMed]
111. Jackson, S.P.; Schoenwaelder, S.M. Procoagulant platelets: Are they necrotic? *Blood* **2010**, *116*, 2011–2018. [CrossRef] [PubMed]
112. van Kruchten, R.; Mattheij, N.J.; Saunders, C.; Feijge, M.A.; Swieringa, F.; Wolfs, J.L.; Collins, P.W.; Heemskerk, J.W.; Bevers, E.M. Both tmem16f-dependent and tmem16f-independent pathways contribute to phosphatidylserine exposure in platelet apoptosis and platelet activation. *Blood* **2013**, *121*, 1850–1857. [CrossRef] [PubMed]
113. Suzuki, J.; Umeda, M.; Sims, P.J.; Nagata, S. Calcium-dependent phospholipid scrambling by tmem16f. *Nature* **2010**, *468*, 834–838. [CrossRef] [PubMed]
114. Yang, H.; Kim, A.; David, T.; Palmer, D.; Jin, T.; Tien, J.; Huang, F.; Cheng, T.; Coughlin, S.R.; Jan, Y.N.; et al. Tmem16f forms a ca2+-activated cation channel required for lipid scrambling in platelets during blood coagulation. *Cell* **2012**, *151*, 111–122. [CrossRef]
115. Podoplelova, N.A.; Sveshnikova, A.N.; Kotova, Y.N.; Eckly, A.; Receveur, N.; Nechipurenko, D.Y.; Obydennyi, S.I.; Kireev, II.; Gachet, C.; Ataullakhanov, F.I.; et al. Coagulation factors bound to procoagulant platelets concentrate in cap structures to promote clotting. *Blood* **2016**, *128*, 1745–1755. [CrossRef]
116. Swieringa, F.; Spronk, H.M.H.; Heemskerk, J.W.M.; van der Meijden, P.E.J. Integrating platelet and coagulation activation in fibrin clot formation. *Res. Pract. Thromb. Haemost.* **2018**, *2*, 450–460. [CrossRef]
117. Zwaal, R.F.; Comfurius, P.; Bevers, E.M. Lipid-protein interactions in blood coagulation. *Biochim. Biophys. Acta* **1998**, *1376*, 433–453. [CrossRef]
118. Stenflo, J.; Fernlund, P.; Egan, W.; Roepstorff, P. Vitamin k dependent modifications of glutamic acid residues in prothrombin. *Proc. Natl. Acad. Sci. USA* **1974**, *71*, 2730–2733. [CrossRef] [PubMed]
119. Vermeer, C. Gamma-carboxyglutamate-containing proteins and the vitamin k-dependent carboxylase. *Biochem. J.* **1990**, *266*, 625–636. [CrossRef] [PubMed]
120. Ohkubo, Y.Z.; Tajkhorshid, E. Distinct structural and adhesive roles of ca2+ in membrane binding of blood coagulation factors. *Structure* **2008**, *16*, 72–81. [CrossRef] [PubMed]
121. Huang, M.; Rigby, A.C.; Morelli, X.; Grant, M.A.; Huang, G.; Furie, B.; Seaton, B.; Furie, B.C. Structural basis of membrane binding by gla domains of vitamin k-dependent proteins. *Nat. Struct. Biol.* **2003**, *10*, 751–756. [CrossRef]
122. Morel, O.; Toti, F.; Hugel, B.; Bakouboula, B.; Camoin-Jau, L.; Dignat-George, F.; Freyssinet, J.M. Procoagulant microparticles: Disrupting the vascular homeostasis equation? *Arterioscler. Thromb. Vasc. Biol.* **2006**, *26*, 2594–2604. [CrossRef] [PubMed]

123. Owens, A.P., 3rd; Mackman, N. Microparticles in hemostasis and thrombosis. *Circ. Res.* **2011**, *108*, 1284–1297. [CrossRef] [PubMed]
124. Morel, O.; Jesel, L.; Freyssinet, J.M.; Toti, F. Cellular mechanisms underlying the formation of circulating microparticles. *Arterioscler. Thromb. Vasc. Biol.* **2011**, *31*, 15–26. [CrossRef]
125. Dale, G.L.; Remenyi, G.; Friese, P. Quantitation of microparticles released from coated-platelets. *J. Thromb. Haemost.* **2005**, *3*, 2081–2088. [CrossRef] [PubMed]
126. Sinauridze, E.I.; Kireev, D.A.; Popenko, N.Y.; Pichugin, A.V.; Panteleev, M.A.; Krymskaya, O.V.; Ataullakhanov, F.I. Platelet microparticle membranes have 50- to 100-fold higher specific procoagulant activity than activated platelets. *Thromb. Haemost.* **2007**, *97*, 425–434. [CrossRef] [PubMed]
127. Alberio, L.; Safa, O.; Clemetson, K.J.; Esmon, C.T.; Dale, G.L. Surface expression and functional characterization of alpha-granule factor v in human platelets: Effects of ionophore a23187, thrombin, collagen, and convulxin. *Blood* **2000**, *95*, 1694–1702. [CrossRef]
128. Shaw, A.W.; Pureza, V.S.; Sligar, S.G.; Morrissey, J.H. The local phospholipid environment modulates the activation of blood clotting. *J. Biol. Chem.* **2007**, *282*, 6556–6563. [CrossRef] [PubMed]
129. Reddy, E.C.; Rand, M.L. Procoagulant phosphatidylserine-exposing platelets in vitro and in vivo. *Front. Cardiovasc. Med.* **2020**, *7*, 15. [CrossRef]
130. Agbani, E.O.; Poole, A.W. Procoagulant platelets: Generation, function, and therapeutic targeting in thrombosis. *Blood* **2017**, *130*, 2171–2179. [CrossRef] [PubMed]
131. Alberio, L.; Ravanat, C.; Hechler, B.; Mangin, P.H.; Lanza, F.; Gachet, C. Delayed-onset of procoagulant signalling revealed by kinetic analysis of coat platelet formation. *Thromb. Haemost.* **2017**, *117*, 1101–1114. [CrossRef] [PubMed]
132. Dale, G.L. Coated-platelets: An emerging component of the procoagulant response. *J. Thromb. Haemost.* **2005**, *3*, 2185–2192. [CrossRef] [PubMed]
133. Kirkpatrick, A.C.; Stoner, J.A.; Dale, G.L.; Rabadi, M.; Prodan, C.I. Higher coated-platelet levels in acute stroke are associated with lower cognitive scores at three months post infarction. *J. Stroke Cerebrovasc. Dis.* **2019**, *28*, 2398–2406. [CrossRef]
134. Agbani, E.O.; van den Bosch, M.T.; Brown, E.; Williams, C.M.; Mattheij, N.J.; Cosemans, J.M.; Collins, P.W.; Heemskerk, J.W.; Hers, I.; Poole, A.W. Coordinated membrane ballooning and procoagulant spreading in human platelets. *Circulation* **2015**, *132*, 1414–1424. [CrossRef]
135. Kulkarni, S.; Jackson, S.P. Platelet factor xiii and calpain negatively regulate integrin alphaiibbeta3 adhesive function and thrombus growth. *J. Biol. Chem.* **2004**, *279*, 30697–30706. [CrossRef] [PubMed]
136. Mazepa, M.; Hoffman, M.; Monroe, D. Superactivated platelets: Thrombus regulators, thrombin generators, and potential clinical targets. *Arterioscler Thromb. Vasc. Biol.* **2013**, *33*, 1747–1752. [CrossRef]
137. Pecci, A.; Balduini, C.L. Desmopressin and super platelets. *Blood* **2014**, *123*, 1779–1780. [CrossRef]
138. Storrie, B. A tip of the cap to procoagulant platelets. *Blood* **2016**, *128*, 1668–1669. [CrossRef]
139. Heemskerk, J.W. Procoagulant 'Zombie' Platelets. Available online: https://academy.isth.org/isth/2017/berlin/186727/johan.heemskerk.procoagulant.zombie.platelets.html (accessed on 25 January 2021).
140. Hua, V.M.; Abeynaike, L.; Glaros, E.; Campbell, H.; Pasalic, L.; Hogg, P.J.; Chen, V.M. Necrotic platelets provide a procoagulant surface during thrombosis. *Blood* **2015**, *126*, 2852–2862. [CrossRef] [PubMed]
141. Obydennyy, S.I.; Sveshnikova, A.N.; Ataullakhanov, F.I.; Panteleev, M.A. Dynamics of calcium spiking, mitochondrial collapse and phosphatidylserine exposure in platelet subpopulations during activation. *J. Thromb. Haemost.* **2016**, *14*, 1867–1881. [CrossRef]
142. Aliotta, A.; Bertaggia Calderara, D.; Zermatten, M.G.; Alberio, L. Sodium-calcium exchanger reverse mode sustains dichotomous ion fluxes required for procoagulant coat platelet formation. *Thromb. Haemost.* **2020**, *121*, 309–321. [CrossRef]
143. Kholmukhamedov, A.; Janecke, R.; Choo, H.J.; Jobe, S.M. The mitochondrial calcium uniporter regulates procoagulant platelet formation. *J. Thromb. Haemost* **2018**, *16*, 2315–2321. [CrossRef] [PubMed]
144. Mattheij, N.J.; Gilio, K.; van Kruchten, R.; Jobe, S.M.; Wieschhaus, A.J.; Chishti, A.H.; Collins, P.; Heemskerk, J.W.; Cosemans, J.M. Dual mechanism of integrin alphaiibbeta3 closure in procoagulant platelets. *J. Biol. Chem.* **2013**, *288*, 13325–13336. [CrossRef] [PubMed]
145. London, F.S.; Marcinkiewicz, M.; Walsh, P.N. Par-1-stimulated factor ixa binding to a small platelet subpopulation requires a pronounced and sustained increase of cytoplasmic calcium. *Biochemistry* **2006**, *45*, 7289–7298. [CrossRef]
146. Dale, G.L.; Friese, P.; Batar, P.; Hamilton, S.F.; Reed, G.L.; Jackson, K.W.; Clemetson, K.J.; Alberio, L. Stimulated platelets use serotonin to enhance their retention of procoagulant proteins on the cell surface. *Nature* **2002**, *415*, 175–179. [CrossRef] [PubMed]
147. Prodan, C.I.; Joseph, P.M.; Vincent, A.S.; Dale, G.L. Coated-platelet levels are influenced by smoking, aspirin, and selective serotonin reuptake inhibitors. *J. Thromb. Haemost.* **2007**, *5*, 2149–2151. [CrossRef] [PubMed]
148. Dale, G.L. Procoagulant platelets: Further details but many more questions. *Arterioscler. Thromb. Vasc. Biol.* **2017**, *37*, 1596–1597. [CrossRef]
149. Aliotta, A.; Krusi, M.; Bertaggia Calderara, D.; Zermatten, M.G.; Gomez, F.J.; Batista Mesquita Sauvage, A.P.; Alberio, L. Characterization of procoagulant coat platelets in patients with glanzmann thrombasthenia. *Int. J. Mol. Sci.* **2020**, *21*, 9515. [CrossRef] [PubMed]
150. Weiss, H.J.; Vicic, W.J.; Lages, B.A.; Rogers, J. Isolated deficiency of platelet procoagulant activity. *Am. J. Med.* **1979**, *67*, 206–213. [CrossRef]
151. Zwaal, R.F.; Comfurius, P.; Bevers, E.M. Scott syndrome, a bleeding disorder caused by defective scrambling of membrane phospholipids. *Biochim. Biophys. Acta* **2004**, *1636*, 119–128. [CrossRef] [PubMed]

152. van Geffen, J.P.; Swieringa, F.; Heemskerk, J.W. Platelets and coagulation in thrombus formation: Aberrations in the scott syndrome. *Thromb. Res.* **2016**, *141* (Suppl. S2), S12–S16. [CrossRef]
153. Adler, M.; Kaufmann, J.; Alberio, L.; Nagler, M. Diagnostic utility of the isth bleeding assessment tool in patients with suspected platelet function disorders. *J. Thromb. Haemost.* **2019**, *17*, 1104–1112. [CrossRef] [PubMed]
154. Prodan, C.I.; Vincent, A.S.; Padmanabhan, R.; Dale, G.L. Coated-platelet levels are low in patients with spontaneous intracerebral hemorrhage. *Stroke* **2009**, *40*, 2578–2580. [CrossRef]
155. Prodan, C.I.; Vincent, A.S.; Dale, G.L. Coated platelet levels correlate with bleed volume in patients with spontaneous intracerebral hemorrhage. *Stroke* **2010**, *41*, 1301–1303. [CrossRef]
156. Prodan, C.I.; Stoner, J.A.; Dale, G.L. Lower coated-platelet levels are associated with increased mortality after spontaneous intracerebral hemorrhage. *Stroke* **2015**, *46*, 1819–1825. [CrossRef]
157. Prodan, C.I.; Vincent, A.S.; Kirkpatrick, A.C.; Hoover, S.L.; Dale, G.L. Higher levels of coated-platelets are observed in patients with subarachnoid hemorrhage but lower levels are associated with increased mortality at 30 days. *J. Neurol. Sci.* **2013**, *334*, 126–129. [CrossRef] [PubMed]
158. Prodan, C.I.; Stoner, J.A.; Gordon, D.L.; Dale, G.L. Cerebral microbleeds in nonlacunar brain infarction are associated with lower coated-platelet levels. *J. Stroke Cerebrovasc. Dis.* **2014**, *23*, e325–e330. [CrossRef] [PubMed]
159. Prodan, C.I.; Stoner, J.A.; Cowan, L.D.; Dale, G.L. Lower coated-platelet levels are associated with early hemorrhagic transformation in patients with non-lacunar brain infarction. *J. Thromb. Haemost.* **2010**, *8*, 1185–1190. [CrossRef] [PubMed]
160. Saxena, K.; Pethe, K.; Dale, G.L. Coated-platelet levels may explain some variability in clinical phenotypes observed with severe hemophilia. *J. Thromb. Haemost.* **2010**, *8*, 1140–1142. [CrossRef]
161. Lastrapes, K.K.; Mohammed, B.M.; Mazepa, M.A.; Martin, E.J.; Barrett, J.C.; Massey, G.V.; Kuhn, J.G.; Nolte, M.E.; Hoffman, M.; Monroe, D.M.; et al. Coated platelets and severe haemophilia a bleeding phenotype: Is there a connection? *Haemophilia* **2016**, *22*, 148–151. [CrossRef] [PubMed]
162. Remenyi, G.; Szasz, R.; Debreceni, I.B.; Szarvas, M.; Batar, P.; Nagy, B., Jr.; Kappelmayer, J.; Udvardy, M. Comparison of coated-platelet levels in patients with essential thrombocythemia with and without hydroxyurea treatment. *Platelets* **2013**, *24*, 486–492. [CrossRef]
163. Prodan, C.I.; Joseph, P.M.; Vincent, A.S.; Dale, G.L. Coated-platelets in ischemic stroke: Differences between lacunar and cortical stroke. *J. Thromb. Haemost.* **2008**, *6*, 609–614. [CrossRef] [PubMed]
164. Prodan, C.I.; Vincent, A.S.; Dale, G.L. Coated-platelet levels are elevated in patients with transient ischemic attack. *Transl. Res.* **2011**, *158*, 71–75. [CrossRef] [PubMed]
165. Prodan, C.I.; Stoner, J.A.; Cowan, L.D.; Dale, G.L. Higher coated-platelet levels are associated with stroke recurrence following nonlacunar brain infarction. *J. Cereb. Blood Flow Metab.* **2013**, *33*, 287–292. [CrossRef] [PubMed]
166. Kirkpatrick, A.C.; Vincent, A.S.; Dale, G.L.; Prodan, C.I. Coated-platelets predict stroke at 30 days following tia. *Neurology* **2017**, *89*, 125–128. [CrossRef] [PubMed]
167. Kirkpatrick, A.C.; Stoner, J.A.; Dale, G.L.; Prodan, C.I. Elevated coated-platelets in symptomatic large-artery stenosis patients are associated with early stroke recurrence. *Platelets* **2014**, *25*, 93–96. [CrossRef]
168. Kirkpatrick, A.C.; Tafur, A.J.; Vincent, A.S.; Dale, G.L.; Prodan, C.I. Coated-platelets improve prediction of stroke and transient ischemic attack in asymptomatic internal carotid artery stenosis. *Stroke* **2014**, *45*, 2995–3001. [CrossRef]
169. Kirkpatrick, A.C.; Vincent, A.S.; Dale, G.L.; Prodan, C.I. Increased platelet procoagulant potential predicts recurrent stroke and tia after lacunar infarction. *J. Thromb. Haemost.* **2020**, *18*, 660–668. [CrossRef]
170. Wang, L.; Bi, Y.; Yu, M.; Li, T.; Tong, D.; Yang, X.; Zhang, C.; Guo, L.; Wang, C.; Kou, Y.; et al. Phosphatidylserine-exposing blood cells and microparticles induce procoagulant activity in non-valvular atrial fibrillation. *Int. J. Cardiol.* **2018**, *258*, 138–143. [CrossRef] [PubMed]
171. Pasalic, L.; Wing-Lun, E.; Lau, J.K.; Campbell, H.; Pennings, G.J.; Lau, E.; Connor, D.; Liang, H.P.; Muller, D.; Kritharides, L.; et al. Novel assay demonstrates that coronary artery disease patients have heightened procoagulant platelet response. *J. Thromb. Haemost.* **2018**, *16*, 1198–1210. [CrossRef]
172. Kou, Y.; Zou, L.; Liu, R.; Zhao, X.; Wang, Y.; Zhang, C.; Dong, Z.; Kou, J.; Bi, Y.; Fu, L.; et al. Intravascular cells and circulating microparticles induce procoagulant activity via phosphatidylserine exposure in heart failure. *J. Thromb. Thrombolysis* **2019**, *48*, 187–194. [CrossRef]
173. Ray, B.; Pandav, V.M.; Mathews, E.A.; Thompson, D.M.; Ford, L.; Yearout, L.K.; Bohnstedt, B.N.; Chaudhary, S.; Dale, G.L.; Prodan, C.I. Coated-platelet trends predict short-term clinical outcomeafter subarachnoid hemorrhage. *Transl. Stroke Res.* **2017**, *9*, 459–470. [CrossRef]
174. Ray, B.; Ross, S.R.; Danala, G.; Aghaei, F.; Nouh, C.D.; Ford, L.; Hollabaugh, K.M.; Karfonta, B.N.; Santucci, J.A.; Cornwell, B.O.; et al. Systemic response of coated-platelet and peripheral blood inflammatory cell indices after aneurysmal subarachnoid hemorrhage and long-term clinical outcome. *J. Crit. Care* **2019**, *52*, 1–9. [CrossRef]
175. Jenkins, A.J.; Gosmanova, A.K.; Lyons, T.J.; May, K.D.; Dashti, A.; Baker, M.Z.; Olansky, L.; Aston, C.E.; Dale, G.L. Coated-platelet levels in patients with type 1 and with type 2 diabetes mellitus. *Diabetes Res. Clin. Pract.* **2008**, *81*, e8–e10. [CrossRef] [PubMed]
176. Kirkpatrick, A.C.; Vincent, A.S.; Dale, G.L.; Prodan, C.I. Clopidogrel use and smoking cessation result in lower coated-platelet levels after stroke. *Platelets* **2019**, *31*, 236–241. [CrossRef] [PubMed]

177. Vulliamy, P.; Gillespie, S.; Armstrong, P.C.; Allan, H.E.; Warner, T.D.; Brohi, K. Histone h4 induces platelet ballooning and microparticle release during trauma hemorrhage. *Proc. Natl. Acad. Sci. USA* **2019**, *116*, 17444–17449. [CrossRef]
178. Prodan, C.I.; Szasz, R.; Vincent, A.S.; Ross, E.D.; Dale, G.L. Coated-platelets retain amyloid precursor protein on their surface. *Platelets* **2006**, *17*, 56–60. [CrossRef]
179. Prodan, C.I.; Ross, E.D.; Vincent, A.S.; Dale, G.L. Coated-platelets correlate with disease progression in alzheimer disease. *J. Neurol.* **2007**, *254*, 548–549. [CrossRef] [PubMed]
180. Prodan, C.I.; Ross, E.D.; Vincent, A.S.; Dale, G.L. Rate of progression in alzheimer's disease correlates with coated-platelet levels–a longitudinal study. *Transl. Res.* **2008**, *152*, 99–102. [CrossRef]
181. Prodan, C.I.; Ross, E.D.; Vincent, A.S.; Dale, G.L. Coated-platelets are higher in amnestic versus nonamnestic patients with mild cognitive impairment. *Alzheimer Dis. Assoc. Disord.* **2007**, *21*, 259–261. [CrossRef]
182. Prodan, C.I.; Ross, E.D.; Stoner, J.A.; Cowan, L.D.; Vincent, A.S.; Dale, G.L. Coated-platelet levels and progression from mild cognitive impairment to alzheimer disease. *Neurology* **2011**, *76*, 247–252. [CrossRef] [PubMed]
183. Valaydon, Z.S.; Lee, P.; Dale, G.L.; Januszewski, A.S.; Rowley, K.G.; Nandurkar, H.; Karschimkus, C.; Best, J.D.; Lyons, T.J.; Jenkins, A.J. Increased coated-platelet levels in chronic haemodialysis patients. *Nephrology* **2009**, *14*, 148–154. [CrossRef]
184. Foley, J.H.; Conway, E.M. Cross talk pathways between coagulation and inflammation. *Circ. Res.* **2016**, *118*, 1392–1408. [CrossRef]
185. Kulkarni, S.; Woollard, K.J.; Thomas, S.; Oxley, D.; Jackson, S.P. Conversion of platelets from a proaggregatory to a proinflammatory adhesive phenotype: Role of paf in spatially regulating neutrophil adhesion and spreading. *Blood* **2007**, *110*, 1879–1886. [CrossRef]
186. Charania, R.; Smith, J.; Vesely, S.K.; Dale, G.L.; Holter, J. Quantitation of coated platelet potential during collection, storage, and transfusion of apheresis platelets. *Transfusion* **2011**, *51*, 2690–2694. [CrossRef] [PubMed]
187. Bertaggia Calderara, D.; Crettaz, D.; Aliotta, A.; Barelli, S.; Tissot, J.D.; Prudent, M.; Alberio, L. Generation of procoagulant collagen- and thrombin-activated platelets in platelet concentrates derived from buffy coat: The role of processing, pathogen inactivation, and storage. *Transfusion* **2018**, *58*, 2395–2406. [CrossRef]
188. Gerber, B.; Alberio, L.; Rochat, S.; Stenner, F.; Manz, M.G.; Buser, A.; Schanz, U.; Stussi, G. Safety and efficacy of cryopreserved autologous platelet concentrates in hla-alloimmunized patients with hematologic malignancies. *Transfusion* **2016**, *56*, 2426–2437. [CrossRef]
189. Kotova, Y.N.; Ataullakhanov, F.I.; Panteleev, M.A. Formation of coated platelets is regulated by the dense granule secretion of adenosine 5'diphosphate acting via the p2y12 receptor. *J. Thromb. Haemost.* **2008**, *6*, 1603–1605. [CrossRef]
190. Norgard, N.B.; Saya, S.; Hann, C.L.; Hennebry, T.A.; Schechter, E.; Dale, G.L. Clopidogrel attenuates coated-platelet production in patients undergoing elective coronary catheterization. *J. Cardiovasc. Pharmacol.* **2008**, *52*, 536–539. [CrossRef] [PubMed]
191. Norgard, N.B.; Hann, C.L.; Dale, G.L. Cangrelor attenuates coated-platelet formation. *Clin. Appl. Thromb. Hemost.* **2009**, *15*, 177–182. [CrossRef] [PubMed]
192. Judge, H.M.; Buckland, R.J.; Sugidachi, A.; Jakubowski, J.A.; Storey, R.F. The active metabolite of prasugrel effectively blocks the platelet p2y12 receptor and inhibits procoagulant and pro-inflammatory platelet responses. *Platelets* **2008**, *19*, 125–133. [CrossRef]
193. Hamilton, S.F.; Miller, M.W.; Thompson, C.A.; Dale, G.L. Glycoprotein iib/iiia inhibitors increase coat-platelet production in vitro. *J. Lab. Clin. Med.* **2004**, *143*, 320–326. [CrossRef] [PubMed]
194. Vermylen, J.; Hoylaerts, M.; Arnout, J. Increased mortality with long-term platelet glycoprotein iib/iiia antagonists: An explanation? *Circulation* **2001**, *104*, E109. [CrossRef] [PubMed]
195. Topalov, N.N.; Kotova, Y.N.; Vasil'ev, S.A.; Panteleev, M.A. Identification of signal transduction pathways involved in the formation of platelet subpopulations upon activation. *Br. J. Haematol.* **2012**, *157*, 105–115. [CrossRef]
196. van der Meijden, P.E.; Feijge, M.A.; Swieringa, F.; Gilio, K.; Nergiz-Unal, R.; Hamulyak, K.; Heemskerk, J.W. Key role of integrin alpha(iib)beta (3) signaling to syk kinase in tissue factor-induced thrombin generation. *Cell. Mol. Life Sci.* **2012**, *69*, 3481–3492. [CrossRef]
197. Razmara, M.; Hu, H.; Masquelier, M.; Li, N. Glycoprotein iib/iiia blockade inhibits platelet aminophospholipid exposure by potentiating translocase and attenuating scramblase activity. *Cell. Mol. Life Sci.* **2007**, *64*, 999–1008. [CrossRef]
198. Mannucci, P.M.; Ruggeri, Z.M.; Pareti, F.I.; Capitanio, A. 1-deamino-8-d-arginine vasopressin: A new pharmacological approach to the management of haemophilia and von willebrands' diseases. *Lancet* **1977**, *1*, 869–872. [CrossRef]
199. Tomasiak, M.M.; Stelmach, H.; Bodzenta-Lukaszyk, A.; Tomasiak, M. Involvement of na+/h+ exchanger in desmopressin-induced platelet procoagulant response. *Acta Biochim. Pol.* **2004**, *51*, 773–788. [CrossRef]
200. Tomasiak, M.; Stelmach, H.; Rusak, T.; Ciborowski, M.; Radziwon, P. Vasopressin acts on platelets to generate procoagulant activity. *Blood Coagul. Fibrinolysis* **2008**, *19*, 615–624. [CrossRef] [PubMed]
201. Colucci, G.; Stutz, M.; Rochat, S.; Conte, T.; Pavicic, M.; Reusser, M.; Giabbani, E.; Huynh, A.; Thurlemann, C.; Keller, P.; et al. The effect of desmopressin on platelet function: A selective enhancement of procoagulant coat platelets in patients with primary platelet function defects. *Blood* **2014**, *123*, 1905–1916. [CrossRef] [PubMed]
202. Swieringa, F.; Lance, M.D.; Fuchs, B.; Feijge, M.A.; Solecka, B.A.; Verheijen, L.P.; Hughes, K.R.; van Oerle, R.; Deckmyn, H.; Kannicht, C.; et al. Desmopressin treatment improves platelet function under flow in patients with postoperative bleeding. *J. Thromb. Haemost.* **2015**, *13*, 1503–1513. [CrossRef] [PubMed]
203. Harper, M.T. Auranofin, a thioredoxin reductase inhibitor, causes platelet death through calcium overload. *Platelets* **2019**, *30*, 98–104. [CrossRef]

204. Tseng, Y.L.; Braun, A.; Chang, J.P.; Chiang, M.L.; Tseng, C.Y.; Chen, W. Micromolar concentrations of citalopram or escitalopram inhibit glycoprotein vi-mediated and integrin alphaiibbeta3-mediated signaling in human platelets. *Toxicol. Appl. Pharmacol.* **2019**, *364*, 106–113. [CrossRef]
205. Galan, A.M.; Lopez-Vilchez, I.; Diaz-Ricart, M.; Navalon, F.; Gomez, E.; Gasto, C.; Escolar, G. Serotonergic mechanisms enhance platelet-mediated thrombogenicity. *Thromb. Haemost.* **2009**, *102*, 511–519. [CrossRef]
206. Laporte, S.; Chapelle, C.; Caillet, P.; Beyens, M.N.; Bellet, F.; Delavenne, X.; Mismetti, P.; Bertoletti, L. Bleeding risk under selective serotonin reuptake inhibitor (ssri) antidepressants: A meta-analysis of observational studies. *Pharmacol. Res.* **2017**, *118*, 19–32. [CrossRef] [PubMed]
207. Mezei, G.; Debreceni, I.B.; Kerenyi, A.; Remenyi, G.; Szasz, R.; Illes, A.; Kappelmayer, J.; Batar, P. Dasatinib inhibits coated-platelet generation in patients with chronic myeloid leukemia. *Platelets* **2019**, *30*, 836–843. [CrossRef]
208. Deb, S.; Boknas, N.; Sjostrom, C.; Tharmakulanathan, A.; Lotfi, K.; Ramstrom, S. Varying effects of tyrosine kinase inhibitors on platelet function-a need for individualized cml treatment to minimize the risk for hemostatic and thrombotic complications? *Cancer Med.* **2020**, *9*, 313–323. [CrossRef]
209. Tullemans, B.M.E.; Nagy, M.; Sabrkhany, S.; Griffioen, A.W.; Oude Egbrink, M.G.A.; Aarts, M.; Heemskerk, J.W.M.; Kuijpers, M.J.E. Tyrosine kinase inhibitor pazopanib inhibits platelet procoagulant activity in renal cell carcinoma patients. *Front. Cardiovasc. Med.* **2018**, *5*, 142. [CrossRef]
210. Cao, H.; Umbach, A.T.; Bissinger, R.; Gawaz, M.; Lang, F. Inhibition of collagen related peptide induced platelet activation and apoptosis by ceritinib. *Cell Physiol. Biochem.* **2018**, *45*, 1707–1716. [CrossRef] [PubMed]
211. Keuren, J.F.; Wielders, S.J.; Ulrichts, H.; Hackeng, T.; Heemskerk, J.W.; Deckmyn, H.; Bevers, E.M.; Lindhout, T. Synergistic effect of thrombin on collagen-induced platelet procoagulant activity is mediated through protease-activated receptor-1. *Arterioscler. Thromb. Vasc. Biol.* **2005**, *25*, 1499–1505. [CrossRef]
212. Agbani, E.O.; Williams, C.M.; Hers, I.; Poole, A.W. Membrane ballooning in aggregated platelets is synchronised and mediates a surge in microvesiculation. *Sci. Rep.* **2017**, *7*, 2770. [CrossRef]
213. Denorme, F.; Manne, B.K.; Portier, I.; Eustes, A.S.; Kosaka, Y.; Kile, B.T.; Rondina, M.T.; Campbell, R.A. Platelet necrosis mediates ischemic stroke outcome in mice. *Blood* **2020**, *135*, 429–440. [CrossRef]
214. Choo, H.J.; Saafir, T.B.; Mkumba, L.; Wagner, M.B.; Jobe, S.M. Mitochondrial calcium and reactive oxygen species regulate agonist-initiated platelet phosphatidylserine exposure. *Arterioscler. Thromb. Vasc. Biol.* **2012**, *32*, 2946–2955. [CrossRef] [PubMed]
215. Perry, S.W.; Norman, J.P.; Barbieri, J.; Brown, E.B.; Gelbard, H.A. Mitochondrial membrane potential probes and the proton gradient: A practical usage guide. *Biotechniques* **2011**, *50*, 98–115. [CrossRef] [PubMed]
216. Sodergren, A.L.; Ramstrom, S. Platelet subpopulations remain despite strong dual agonist stimulation and can be characterised using a novel six-colour flow cytometry protocol. *Sci. Rep.* **2018**, *8*, 1441. [CrossRef]
217. Topalov, N.N.; Yakimenko, A.O.; Canault, M.; Artemenko, E.O.; Zakharova, N.V.; Abaeva, A.A.; Loosveld, M.; Ataullakhanov, F.I.; Nurden, A.T.; Alessi, M.C.; et al. Two types of procoagulant platelets are formed upon physiological activation and are controlled by integrin alpha(iib)beta(3). *Arterioscler. Thromb. Vasc. Biol.* **2012**, *32*, 2475–2483. [CrossRef]
218. Szasz, R.; Dale, G.L. Coat platelets. *Curr. Opin. Hematol.* **2003**, *10*, 351–355. [CrossRef] [PubMed]
219. Abaeva, A.A.; Canault, M.; Kotova, Y.N.; Obydennyy, S.I.; Yakimenko, A.O.; Podoplelova, N.A.; Kolyadko, V.N.; Chambost, H.; Mazurov, A.V.; Ataullakhanov, F.I.; et al. Procoagulant platelets form an alpha-granule protein-covered "cap" on their surface that promotes their attachment to aggregates. *J. Biol. Chem.* **2013**, *288*, 29621–29632. [CrossRef]
220. Aupeix, K.; Hugel, B.; Martin, T.; Bischoff, P.; Lill, H.; Pasquali, J.L.; Freyssinet, J.M. The significance of shed membrane particles during programmed cell death in vitro, and in vivo, in hiv-1 infection. *J. Clin. Investig.* **1997**, *99*, 1546–1554. [CrossRef] [PubMed]
221. Bohling, S.D.; Pagano, M.B.; Stitzel, M.R.; Ferrell, C.; Yeung, W.; Chandler, W.L. Comparison of clot-based vs chromogenic factor xa procoagulant phospholipid activity assays. *Am. J. Clin. Pathol.* **2012**, *137*, 185–192. [CrossRef] [PubMed]
222. Hemker, H.C.; Wielders, S.; Kessels, H.; Beguin, S. Continuous registration of thrombin generation in plasma, its use for the determination of the thrombin potential. *Thromb. Haemost.* **1993**, *70*, 617–624. [CrossRef]
223. Zermatten, M.G.; Fraga, M.; Calderara, D.B.; Aliotta, A.; Moradpour, D.; Alberio, L. Biomarkers of liver dysfunction correlate with a prothrombotic and not with a prohaemorrhagic profile in patients with cirrhosis. *JHEP Rep. Innov. Hepatol.* **2020**, *2*, 100120. [CrossRef] [PubMed]
224. Camire, R.M.; Kalafatis, M.; Simioni, P.; Girolami, A.; Tracy, P.B. Platelet-derived factor va/va leiden cofactor activities are sustained on the surface of activated platelets despite the presence of activated protein c. *Blood* **1998**, *91*, 2818–2829. [CrossRef]
225. Thuerlemann, C.; Haeberli, A.; Alberio, L. Monitoring thrombin generation by electrochemistry: Development of an amperometric biosensor screening test for plasma and whole blood. *Clin. Chem.* **2009**, *55*, 505–512. [CrossRef]
226. Jy, W.; Horstman, L.L.; Jimenez, J.J.; Ahn, Y.S.; Biro, E.; Nieuwland, R.; Sturk, A.; Dignat-George, F.; Sabatier, F.; Camoin-Jau, L.; et al. Measuring circulating cell-derived microparticles. *J. Thromb. Haemost.* **2004**, *2*, 1842–1851. [CrossRef] [PubMed]
227. Lacroix, R.; Robert, S.; Poncelet, P.; Dignat-George, F. Overcoming limitations of microparticle measurement by flow cytometry. *Semin. Thromb. Hemost.* **2010**, *36*, 807–818. [CrossRef] [PubMed]
228. Kessels, H.; Beguin, S.; Andree, H.; Hemker, H.C. Measurement of thrombin generation in whole blood–the effect of heparin and aspirin. *Thromb. Haemost.* **1994**, *72*, 78–83. [CrossRef]
229. Ninivaggi, M.; Apitz-Castro, R.; Dargaud, Y.; de Laat, B.; Hemker, H.C.; Lindhout, T. Whole-blood thrombin generation monitored with a calibrated automated thrombogram-based assay. *Clin. Chem.* **2012**, *58*, 1252–1259. [CrossRef]

230. Prior, S.M.; Mann, K.G.; Freeman, K.; Butenas, S. Continuous thrombin generation in whole blood: New applications for assessing activators and inhibitors of coagulation. *Anal. Biochem.* **2018**, *551*, 19–25. [CrossRef] [PubMed]
231. Wan, J.; Konings, J.; Yan, Q.; Kelchtermans, H.; Kremers, R.; de Laat, B.; Roest, M. A novel assay for studying the involvement of blood cells in whole blood thrombin generation. *J. Thromb. Haemost.* **2020**, *18*, 1291–1301. [CrossRef]
232. Hemker, H.C.; Giesen, P.L.; Ramjee, M.; Wagenvoord, R.; Beguin, S. The thrombogram: Monitoring thrombin generation in platelet-rich plasma. *Thromb. Haemost.* **2000**, *83*, 589–591. [CrossRef]
233. Douxfils, J.; Morimont, L.; Bouvy, C.; de Saint-Hubert, M.; Devalet, B.; Devroye, C.; Dincq, A.S.; Dogne, J.M.; Guldenpfennig, M.; Baudar, J.; et al. Assessment of the analytical performances and sample stability on st genesia system using the stg-drugscreen application. *J. Thromb. Haemost.* **2019**, *17*, 1273–1287. [CrossRef]
234. Talon, L.; Sinegre, T.; Lecompte, T.; Pereira, B.; Massoulie, S.; Abergel, A.; Lebreton, A. Hypercoagulability (thrombin generation) in patients with cirrhosis is detected with st-genesia. *J. Thromb. Haemost.* **2020**, *18*, 2177–2190. [CrossRef] [PubMed]
235. Bertaggia Calderara, D.; Zermatten, M.G.; Aliotta, A.; Batista Mesquita Sauvage, A.P.; Carle, V.; Heinis, C.; Alberio, L. Tissue factor-independent coagulation correlates with clinical phenotype in factor xi deficiency and replacement therapy. *Thromb. Haemost.* **2021**, *121*, 150–163. [CrossRef] [PubMed]
236. Koltsova, E.M.; Kuprash, A.D.; Dashkevich, N.M.; Vardanyan, D.M.; Chernyakov, A.V.; Kumskova, M.A.; Nair, S.C.; Srivastava, A.; Ataullakhanov, F.I.; Panteleev, M.A.; et al. Determination of fibrin clot growth and spatial thrombin propagation in the presence of different types of phospholipid surfaces. *Platelets* **2020**, 1–7. [CrossRef] [PubMed]
237. Aswad, M.H.; Kissova, J.; Rihova, L.; Zavrelova, J.; Ovesna, P.; Penka, M. High level of circulating microparticles in patients with bcr/abl negative myeloproliferative neoplasm—A pilot study. *Klein. Onkol.* **2019**, *32*, 109–116. [CrossRef] [PubMed]
238. Mooberry, M.J.; Bradford, R.; Hobl, E.L.; Lin, F.C.; Jilma, B.; Key, N.S. Procoagulant microparticles promote coagulation in a factor xi-dependent manner in human endotoxemia. *J. Thromb. Haemost.* **2016**, *14*, 1031–1042. [CrossRef] [PubMed]
239. Exner, T.; Joseph, J.E.; Connor, D.; Low, J.; Ma, D.D. Increased procoagulant phospholipid activity in blood from patients with suspected acute coronary syndromes: A pilot study. *Blood Coagul. Fibrinolysis* **2005**, *16*, 375–379. [CrossRef]
240. Marchetti, M.; Tartari, C.J.; Russo, L.; Panova-Noeva, M.; Leuzzi, A.; Rambaldi, A.; Finazzi, G.; Woodhams, B.; Falanga, A. Phospholipid-dependent procoagulant activity is highly expressed by circulating microparticles in patients with essential thrombocythemia. *Am. J. Hematol.* **2014**, *89*, 68–73. [CrossRef]
241. van Dreden, P.; Rousseau, A.; Fontaine, S.; Woodhams, B.J.; Exner, T. Clinical evaluation of a new functional test for detection of plasma procoagulant phospholipids. *Blood Coagul. Fibrinolysis* **2009**, *20*, 494–502. [CrossRef] [PubMed]
242. Dasgupta, S.K.; Abdel-Monem, H.; Niravath, P.; Le, A.; Bellera, R.V.; Langlois, K.; Nagata, S.; Rumbaut, R.E.; Thiagarajan, P. Lactadherin and clearance of platelet-derived microvesicles. *Blood* **2009**, *113*, 1332–1339. [CrossRef] [PubMed]
243. Polak, D.; Talar, M.; Watala, C.; Przygodzki, T. Intravital assessment of blood platelet function. A review of the methodological approaches with examples of studies of selected aspects of blood platelet function. *Int. J. Mol. Sci.* **2020**, *21*, 8334. [CrossRef] [PubMed]
244. Montague, S.J.; Lim, Y.J.; Lee, W.M.; Gardiner, E.E. Imaging platelet processes and function-current and emerging approaches for imaging in vitro and in vivo. *Front. Immunol.* **2020**, *11*, 78. [CrossRef] [PubMed]
245. Marcinczyk, N.; Golaszewska, A.; Misztal, T.; Gromotowicz-Poplawska, A.; Rusak, T.; Chabielska, E. New approaches for the assessment of platelet activation status in thrombus under flow condition using confocal microscopy. *Naunyn Schmiedebergs Arch. Pharmacol.* **2020**, *393*, 727–738. [CrossRef] [PubMed]
246. Fujii, T.; Sakata, A.; Nishimura, S.; Eto, K.; Nagata, S. Tmem16f is required for phosphatidylserine exposure and microparticle release in activated mouse platelets. *Proc. Natl. Acad. Sci. USA* **2015**, *112*, 12800–12805. [CrossRef]
247. Nechipurenko, D.Y.; Receveur, N.; Yakimenko, A.O.; Shepelyuk, T.O.; Yakusheva, A.A.; Kerimov, R.R.; Obydennyy, S.I.; Eckly, A.; Leon, C.; Gachet, C.; et al. Clot contraction drives the translocation of procoagulant platelets to thrombus surface. *Arter. Thromb. Vasc. Biol.* **2019**, *39*, 37–47. [CrossRef] [PubMed]
248. Cho, J.; Kennedy, D.R.; Lin, L.; Huang, M.; Merrill-Skoloff, G.; Furie, B.C.; Furie, B. Protein disulfide isomerase capture during thrombus formation in vivo depends on the presence of beta3 integrins. *Blood* **2012**, *120*, 647–655. [CrossRef] [PubMed]
249. Denis, C.; Methia, N.; Frenette, P.S.; Rayburn, H.; Ullman-Cullere, M.; Hynes, R.O.; Wagner, D.D. A mouse model of severe von willebrand disease: Defects in hemostasis and thrombosis. *Proc. Natl. Acad. Sci. USA* **1998**, *95*, 9524–9529. [CrossRef] [PubMed]
250. Deppermann, C.; Cherpokova, D.; Nurden, P.; Schulz, J.N.; Thielmann, I.; Kraft, P.; Vogtle, T.; Kleinschnitz, C.; Dutting, S.; Krohne, G.; et al. Gray platelet syndrome and defective thrombo-inflammation in nbeal2-deficient mice. *J. Clin. Investig.* **2013**, *123*, 3331–3342. [CrossRef]
251. Guan, W.J.; Ni, Z.Y.; Hu, Y.; Liang, W.H.; Ou, C.Q.; He, J.X.; Liu, L.; Shan, H.; Lei, C.L.; Hui, D.S.C.; et al. Clinical characteristics of coronavirus disease 2019 in China. *N. Engl. J. Med.* **2020**, *382*, 1708–1720. [CrossRef] [PubMed]
252. Helms, J.; Tacquard, C.; Severac, F.; Leonard-Lorant, I.; Ohana, M.; Delabranche, X.; Merdji, H.; Clere-Jehl, R.; Schenck, M.; Fagot Gandet, F.; et al. High risk of thrombosis in patients with severe sars-cov-2 infection: A multicenter prospective cohort study. *Intensive Care Med.* **2020**, *46*, 1089–1098. [CrossRef] [PubMed]
253. Engelmann, B.; Massberg, S. Thrombosis as an intravascular effector of innate immunity. *Nat. Rev. Immunol.* **2013**, *13*, 34–45. [CrossRef]

254. Gasecka, A.; Borovac, J.A.; Guerreiro, R.A.; Giustozzi, M.; Parker, W.; Caldeira, D.; Chiva-Blanch, G. Thrombotic complications in patients with covid-19: Pathophysiological mechanisms, diagnosis, and treatment. *Cardiovasc. Drugs Ther.* **2020**, 1–15. [CrossRef] [PubMed]
255. Gu, S.X.; Tyagi, T.; Jain, K.; Gu, V.W.; Lee, S.H.; Hwa, J.M.; Kwan, J.M.; Krause, D.S.; Lee, A.I.; Halene, S.; et al. Thrombocytopathy and endotheliopathy: Crucial contributors to covid-19 thromboinflammation. *Nat. Rev. Cardiol.* **2020**, 1–16. [CrossRef]
256. Larsen, J.B.; Pasalic, L.; Hvas, A.M. Platelets in coronavirus disease 2019. *Semin. Thromb. Hemost.* **2020**, *46*, 823–825. [CrossRef] [PubMed]
257. Koupenova, M.; Freedman, J.E. Platelets and covid-19: Inflammation, hyperactivation and additional questions. *Circ. Res.* **2020**, *127*, 1419–1421. [CrossRef] [PubMed]
258. Koupenova, M. Potential role of platelets in covid-19: Implications for thrombosis. *Res. Pract. Thromb. Haemost.* **2020**, *4*, 737–740. [CrossRef]
259. Bongiovanni, D.; Klug, M.; Lazareva, O.; Weidlich, S.; Biasi, M.; Ursu, S.; Warth, S.; Buske, C.; Lukas, M.; Spinner, C.D.; et al. Sars-cov-2 infection is associated with a pro-thrombotic platelet phenotype. *Cell Death. Dis.* **2021**, *12*, 50. [CrossRef] [PubMed]
260. Zaid, Y.; Puhm, F.; Allaeys, I.; Naya, A.; Oudghiri, M.; Khalki, L.; Limami, Y.; Zaid, N.; Sadki, K.; Ben El Haj, R.; et al. Platelets can associate with sars-cov-2 rna and are hyperactivated in covid-19. *Circ. Res.* **2020**, *127*, 1404–1418. [CrossRef]
261. Manne, B.K.; Denorme, F.; Middleton, E.A.; Portier, I.; Rowley, J.W.; Stubben, C.; Petrey, A.C.; Tolley, N.D.; Guo, L.; Cody, M.; et al. Platelet gene expression and function in patients with covid-19. *Blood* **2020**, *136*, 1317–1329. [CrossRef] [PubMed]
262. Hottz, E.D.; Azevedo-Quintanilha, I.G.; Palhinha, L.; Teixeira, L.; Barreto, E.A.; Pao, C.R.R.; Righy, C.; Franco, S.; Souza, T.M.L.; Kurtz, P.; et al. Platelet activation and platelet-monocyte aggregate formation trigger tissue factor expression in patients with severe covid-19. *Blood* **2020**, *136*, 1330–1341. [CrossRef] [PubMed]
263. Denorme, F.; Manne, B.K.; Portier, I.; Petrey, A.C.; Middleton, E.A.; Kile, B.T.; Rondina, M.T.; Campbell, R.A. Covid-19 patients exhibit reduced procoagulant platelet responses. *J. Thromb. Haemost.* **2020**, *18*, 3067–3073. [CrossRef] [PubMed]
264. Goshua, G.; Pine, A.B.; Meizlish, M.L.; Chang, C.H.; Zhang, H.; Bahel, P.; Baluha, A.; Bar, N.; Bona, R.D.; Burns, A.J.; et al. Endotheliopathy in covid-19-associated coagulopathy: Evidence from a single-centre, cross-sectional study. *Lancet Haematol.* **2020**, *7*, e575–e582. [CrossRef]
265. Maclay, J.D.; McAllister, D.A.; Johnston, S.; Raftis, J.; McGuinnes, C.; Deans, A.; Newby, D.E.; Mills, N.L.; MacNee, W. Increased platelet activation in patients with stable and acute exacerbation of copd. *Thorax* **2011**, *66*, 769–774. [CrossRef] [PubMed]
266. Lehmann, T.; Mairbaurl, H.; Pleisch, B.; Maggiorini, M.; Bartsch, P.; Reinhart, W.H. Platelet count and function at high altitude and in high-altitude pulmonary edema. *J. Appl. Physiol.* **2006**, *100*, 690–694. [CrossRef] [PubMed]
267. Tyagi, T.; Ahmad, S.; Gupta, N.; Sahu, A.; Ahmad, Y.; Nair, V.; Chatterjee, T.; Bajaj, N.; Sengupta, S.; Ganju, L.; et al. Altered expression of platelet proteins and calpain activity mediate hypoxia-induced prothrombotic phenotype. *Blood* **2014**, *123*, 1250–1260. [CrossRef]
268. Yan, S.L.; Russell, J.; Granger, D.N. Platelet activation and platelet-leukocyte aggregation elicited in experimental colitis are mediated by interleukin-6. *Inflamm. Bowel Dis.* **2014**, *20*, 353–362. [CrossRef]
269. Senchenkova, E.Y.; Komoto, S.; Russell, J.; Almeida-Paula, L.D.; Yan, L.S.; Zhang, S.; Granger, D.N. Interleukin-6 mediates the platelet abnormalities and thrombogenesis associated with experimental colitis. *Am. J. Pathol.* **2013**, *183*, 173–181. [CrossRef] [PubMed]
270. Burstein, S.A.; Peng, J.; Friese, P.; Wolf, R.F.; Harrison, P.; Downs, T.; Hamilton, K.; Comp, P.; Dale, G.L. Cytokine-induced alteration of platelet and hemostatic function. *Stem Cells* **1996**, *14* (Suppl. S1), 154–162. [CrossRef] [PubMed]
271. Masselli, E.; Pozzi, G.; Vaccarezza, M.; Mirandola, P.; Galli, D.; Vitale, M.; Carubbi, C.; Gobbi, G. Ros in platelet biology: Functional aspects and methodological insights. *Int. J. Mol. Sci.* **2020**, *21*, 4866. [CrossRef] [PubMed]

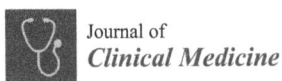

Review

When Should We Think of Myelodysplasia or Bone Marrow Failure in a Thrombocytopenic Patient? A Practical Approach to Diagnosis

Nicolas Bonadies [1,2,†], Alicia Rovó [1,†], Naomi Porret [1] and Ulrike Bacher [1,*]

1. Department of Hematology and Central Hematology Laboratory, Inselspital Bern, University of Bern, 3010 Bern, Switzerland; nicolas.bonadies@insel.ch (N.B.); alicia.rovo@insel.ch (A.R.); NaomiAzur.Porret@insel.ch (N.P.)
2. Department for BioMedical Research, University of Bern, 3008 Bern, Switzerland
* Correspondence: veraulrike.bacher@insel.ch; Tel.: +41-31-632-1390; Fax: +41-31-632-3406
† Equal contribution.

Abstract: Thrombocytopenia can arise from various conditions, including myelodysplastic syndromes (MDS) and bone marrow failure (BMF) syndromes. Meticulous assessment of the peripheral blood smear, identification of accompanying clinical conditions, and characterization of the clinical course are important for initial assessment of unexplained thrombocytopenia. Increased awareness is required to identify patients with suspected MDS or BMF, who are in need of further investigations by a step-wise approach. Bone marrow cytomorphology, histopathology, and cytogenetics are complemented by myeloid next-generation sequencing (NGS) panels. Such panels are helpful to distinguish reactive cytopenia from clonal conditions. MDS are caused by mutations in the hematopoietic stem/progenitor cells, characterized by cytopenia and dysplasia, and an inherent risk of leukemic progression. Aplastic anemia (AA), the most frequent acquired BMF, is immunologically driven and characterized by an empty bone marrow. Diagnosis remains challenging due to overlaps with other hematological disorders. Congenital BMF, certainly rare in adulthood, can present atypically with thrombocytopenia and can be misdiagnosed. Analyses for chromosome fragility, telomere length, and germline gene sequencing are needed. Interdisciplinary expert teams contribute to diagnosis, prognostication, and choice of therapy for patients with suspected MDS and BMF. With this review we aim to increase the awareness and provide practical approaches for diagnosis of these conditions in suspicious cases presenting with thrombocytopenia.

Keywords: thrombocytopenia; myelodysplastic syndromes (MDS); bone marrow failure (BMF) syndromes; aplastic anemia (AA); next-generation sequencing (NGS)

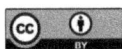

1. Introduction

Thrombocytopenia can be associated with a variety of benign and malignant hematological and non-hematological conditions and the investigation of potential causes is a challenge for clinicians and involved laboratory specialists. Mild and isolated thrombocytopenia (platelet count (PLT) 100–150 G/L) is frequently neglected and not further investigated. In contrast, isolated severe thrombocytopenia (PLT <50 G/L) is often considered as immune-mediated thrombocytopenia (ITP) and treated with steroids without further investigations, in accordance with current guidelines [1]. However, more severe underlying diseases can be potentially missed and the correct diagnosis, consequently, reached with delay. With the currently available diagnostic modalities, the correct and timely identification of myelodysplastic syndromes (MDS) and bone marrow failure (BMF) syndromes can be efficiently done, which is the mainstay for offering patients the most appropriate treatment. With this review we aim to increase the awareness for MDS and BMF, providing practical approaches in suspicious cases presenting with thrombocytopenia.

2. Clinical Presentations and Symptoms of MDS and BMF

General practitioners are commonly involved in the initial diagnostic assessment of patients with unclear thrombocytopenia. Thus, their role is crucial in identifying suspicious cases of both MDS and BMF and initiate the correct diagnostic assessments timely. Knowledge on the characteristic clinical features for MDS or BMF are therefore helpful.

2.1. Myelodysplastic Syndromes

With ageing of the general population, and the introduction of next-generation sequencing (NGS) into clinical practice, patients with clonal hematological conditions are increasingly identified. Therefore, in elderly patients with unexplained cytopenia, including isolated thrombocytopenia, clonal disorders, such as MDS and other related myeloid neoplasms, should always be considered as potential differential diagnosis.

2.1.1. Definition and Pathogenesis of MDS

Patients with unexplained chronic thrombocytopenia should direct awareness towards a potentially underlying myeloid neoplasm, especially in elderly patients with worsening bi- or pancytopenia, or in individuals with previous exposure to chemo- or radiotherapy [2]. MDS are heterogeneous hematopoietic stem and progenitor cell (HSPC) disorders characterized by cytopenia, dysplasia, inflammation, and a propensity to evolve towards secondary acute myeloid leukemia (AML) [3,4]. MDS originate from HSPCs affected by somatic mutations in leukemia-associated genes (SM-LAGs). These mutated HSPC are selected through a stochastic drift that is influenced by a variety of cell-intrinsic and cell-extrinsic mechanisms over a variable duration of time [5].

2.1.2. Epidemiology of MDS and Risk Factors

As in many other cancers, MDS and related myeloid disorders are diseases of elderly patients with a median age at presentation above 70 years and male predominance. The exposure to mutagenic agents, such as chemotherapy, radiotherapy, pesticides, insecticides, benzoyl, and solvents, are recognized risk factors [6–9]. The age-adjusted incidence rate of MDS is between 3–4 per 100,000 patient-years in western countries, with an increase of the age-specific incidence rate to more than ten-fold for individuals >70 years of age [2,10,11]. Incident cases of MDS are assumed to rise substantially in the forthcoming years, due to population ageing, increased cancer survivorship, and improvements in diagnostic accuracy for the detection of clonal hematopoiesis. MDS can also occur in children and younger to middle-aged adults (aged <50 years), in whom an underlying germline predisposition has to be actively explored [12].

2.1.3. Presentation and Symptoms of Patients with MDS

Depending on the cell lineages affected by cytopenia, MDS patients suffer from a variety of symptoms at presentation, which comprise fatigue, dyspnea, tachycardia, bacterial infections, or mucocutaneous bleeding [3]. A substantial number of patients with chronic and mild cytopenia can be asymptomatic. In MDS patients, anemia (usually macrocytic) is the predominant abnormality in the peripheral blood (80–85%), followed by thrombocytopenia (30–65%) and neutropenia (40–50%) [13]. Sometimes, patients present with overlapping features of myelodysplasia with cytopenia as well as myeloproliferation. In such cases, patients can present with splenomegaly and accompanying monocytosis ($\geq$1.0 G/L and $\geq$10% of all leukocytes) in chronic myelomonocytic leukemia (CMML), granulocytosis, or even thrombocytosis in other rare MDS/MPN (myelodysplastic syndrome/myeloproliferative neoplasm) overlap conditions [14]. The association of clonal hematopoiesis with a broad range of autoinflammatory and autoimmune manifestations is generally underestimated. These manifestations may be of paraneoplastic origin and should direct further investigations for an underlying myeloid or lymphatic malignancy [15,16].

2.2. Bone Marrow Failure Syndromes

BMF can be separated in acquired and inherited BMF (iBMF) forms. While acquired forms can affect children and adults, congenital forms are particularly more frequent in children less than five years of age, but also in adolescents and young adults. Unusual presentation of congenital forms may show a late presentation even after the fourth decade of life, may be oligosymptomatic, and can be therefore particularly difficult to diagnose.

2.2.1. Definition and Pathogenesis of BMF

Aplastic anemia (AA) is a rare BMF. This non-malignant disease is characterized by pancytopenia and bone marrow hypoplasia of varying severity. Aplastic anemia will be considered idiopathic when no underlying cause can be identified. Idiopathic AA results from autoimmune mediated destruction of early precursors of hematopoietic cells [17,18]. AA can be related to paroxysmal nocturnal hemoglobinuria (PNH), which is a clonal hematopoietic stem cell disorder with various features including hemolytic anemia, bone marrow failure, and thrombosis. Other pathophysiologic mechanisms may also be involved in secondary forms of AA. Direct damage of hematopoietic cells may occur in patients exposed to irradiation, drugs or chemicals, and may represent an underlying cause of AA. Different viral infections including cytomegalovirus (CMV), Epstein–Barr virus (EBV), dengue virus, parvovirus b19, human herpes virus 6 (HHV6), human immunodeficiency virus (HIV), and disseminated adenovirus infections [19] can be associated with the development of AA. Seronegative hepatitis has been reported in 5–10% of patients with AA [20–22]. Accelerated attrition of telomeres [23–25] and acquired somatic mutations of genes related to myeloid diseases [26–28] are associated with an increased risk of MDS, AML, and early death.

iBMF represent a relevant cause of AA in children and are frequently related to germline mutations (Supplemental Table S1). Evidence of such syndromes may be obvious in patients with BMF. On the other hand, the clinical changes can be subtle and the syndrome can only be diagnosed when the hematological picture becomes manifest with severe cytopenias. In this regard, various syndromes exist. Fanconi anemia (FA) [29] is caused by a defect in the DNA repair mechanisms, predisposing to various tumors. Telomeropathies involve a wide variation of genetic disorders caused by mutations in genes of the telomerase or the DNA damage response complexes. The most characteristic syndrome is dyskeratosis congenita (DC) [25]. Shwachman–Diamond syndrome (SDS) [30] is caused by variants of pathogenic genes that affect the biogenesis and mitosis of ribosomes. Congenital amegakaryocytic thrombocytopenia (CAMT) [31] results mainly from mutations in the oncogene of the virus myeloproliferative leukemia (MPL) responsible for encoding the thrombopoietin receptor.

2.2.2. Epidemiology of BMF and Risk Factors

AA has a variable geographic distribution, the global incidence ranging from 0.7 to 7.4 cases per million inhabitants per year, with 2- to 3-fold higher rates in Asia than in Europe and the U.S. The disease can present at any age, but the presentation is bimodal with a peak in young adults and the elderly. AA affects both sexes in similar proportions [32,33]. Ethnicity and some specific human leukocyte antigen (HLA) characteristics have been associated with higher predisposition to develop AA, higher frequency of small PNH clones and response to immunosuppression [34–38]. Environmental factors may be relevant, such as frequent exposure to benzene-based products [39]. Clonal hematopoiesis is prevalent in AA, and some mutations impact on clinical outcomes. At present, however, prediction of clinical significance is often difficult [40]. The iBMF appear mainly between 2 and 5 years of life, but can manifest at any age during childhood or adolescence. More rarely, diagnosis will be reached later in life [41].

2.2.3. General Presentation and Symptoms of Patients with BMF

Patients with AA usually refer symptoms of onset in the previous weeks that are related to the type and number of cytopenias. Symptoms are frequently related to anemia, mainly fatigue, and dyspnea on exertion. Bleeding symptoms are also common including easy bruising, menorrhagia, skin or oronal petechiae typically occurring when thrombocytopenia is significant. Although less frequent, infections can be life-threatening, mainly affecting patients with profound neutropenia [18,42]. Other than that, the clinical examination is classically negative, with absence of lymphadenopathy, splenomegaly or hepatomegaly.

In AA patients, a positive family history including other members affected with cytopenia or malignancy suggests an iBMF. The presence of abnormal clinical features, such as short stature, thumb, or radial ray and/or skeletal abnormalities, microcephaly, hypo- or hyperpigmentation (café au lait spots), eye, renal, or gonadal malformations are changes related to FA [29]. The presence of abnormal pigmentation of the skin, nail dystrophy affecting hands and feet, and oral leukoplakia is considered to be the classic presentation of DC. In addition, premature gray hair and pulmonary fibrosis have been reported [43]. SDS can have a broad clinical phenotype with skeletal abnormalities, steatorrhea consequently to exocrine pancreatic dysfunction, and recurrent infections [30]. CAMT presents with isolated thrombocytopenia and reduced megakaryocytes in the bone marrow without birth defects characteristic of other iBMF [31].

3. Diagnostic Approach for MDS and BMF

In the following, we will describe our suggest stepwise diagnostic approach, as summarized in Figure 1.

3.1. Primary Diagnostic Work-Up

The exclusion of other conditions associated with thrombocytopenia is the mainstay for the primary work up (Table 1). Complete blood counts (CBC) including white blood count (WBC) with a full differential, red blood cell (RBC) analysis of hemoglobin, hematocrit, and RBC indices (including mean cellular volume, MCV) and reticulocyte counts are essential. In patients with MDS or BMF, peripheral blood parameters reveal evidence of different combinations of cytopenia. Anemia is frequently macrocytic (increased MCV), and reticulocytes are usually significantly reduced [44]. The immature platelet fraction (IPF) can be helpful to identify younger platelets and is increased in peripheral consumption. Microscopic cytomorphologic examination of the peripheral blood smear has to be done in cases with unexplained cytopenia to identify morphological RBC abnormalities (schistocytes, anisocytosis, and poikilocytosis), dysplasia, or the presence of cell line precursors and blasts.

Substrate deficiency should be excluded by determination of serum folate, transcobalamin, iron, total iron binding capacity (TIBC), and ferritin. Parameters that may be indicative for hemolysis, such an increased rate of reticulocytes, lactate dehydrogenase (LDH), and bilirubin combined with decreased haptoglobin, with or without a positive direct antiglobulin test (DAT/direct Coombs test), should cast suspicion on hemolytic anemia (PNH, autoimmune hemolytic anemia). Viral infections such as HIV, Parvovirus B19, CMV, EBV, hepatitis B (HBV), and C virus (HCV) should be excluded. Lymphoid neoplasms or plasma cell neoplasms can be identified with protein electrophoresis, immunofixation and free light chain assays. Thyroid-stimulating hormone (TSH), antinuclear antibodies (ANA), antineutrophil cytoplasmic antibodies (ANCA) and rheumatoid factor (RF) direct towards a potential rheumatological disorder and abdominal ultrasound might identify an underlying liver disease, splenomegaly, or lymphoma. Thalassemia and other forms of hereditary hemoglobinopathies should be excluded according to ethnicity as well as personal and family history.

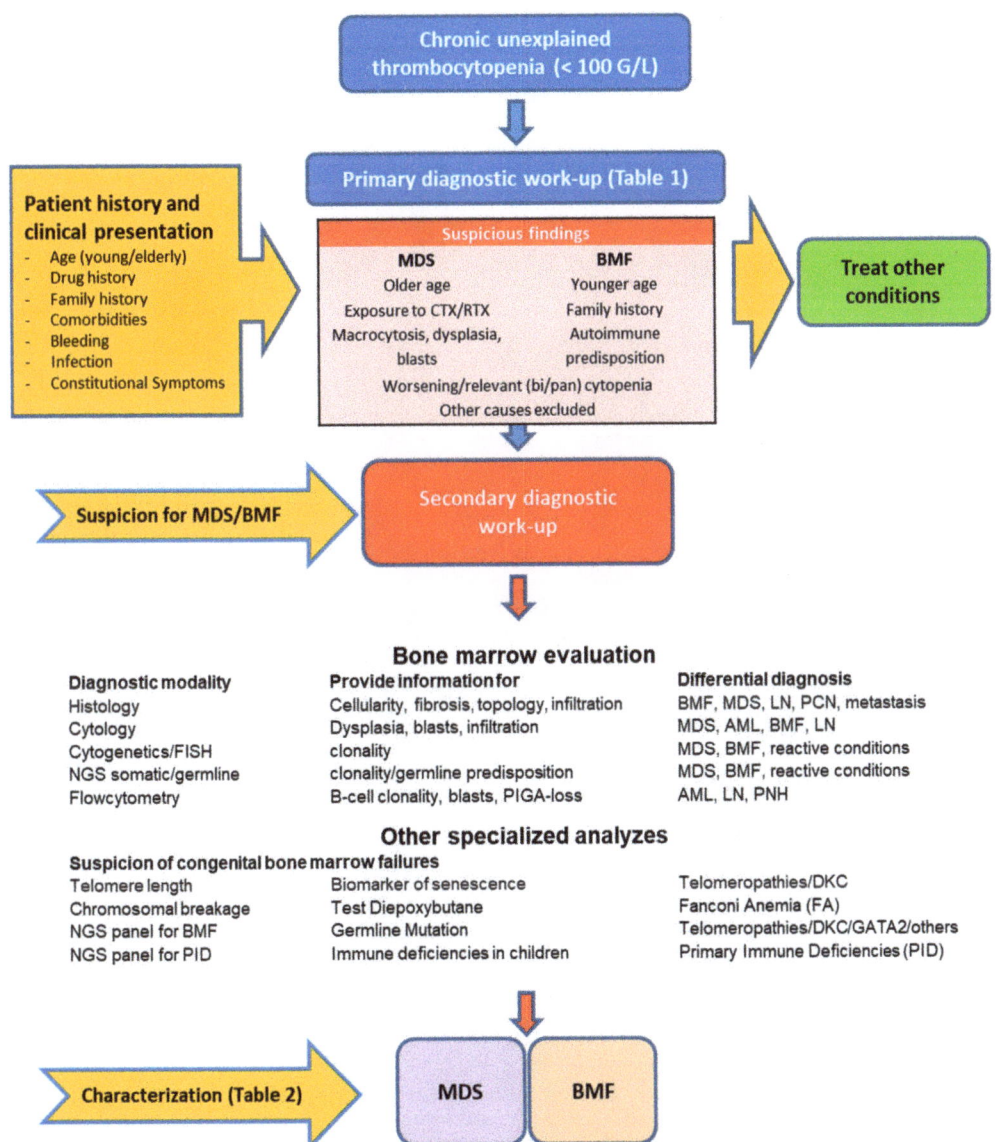

Figure 1. Stepwise diagnostic approach to thrombocytopenia in patients with suspected myelodysplastic syndromes (MDS) or bone marrow failure (BMF) syndromes.

Table 1. Primary laboratory evaluation in patients with unexplained thrombocytopenia.

Laboratory Test	Provide Information on
Automated blood count (MPV, IPF), reticulocytes	CBC. Quantitative values. Platelet size and production capacity of the bone marrow.
Blood smear	Pseudothrombocytopenia, schistocytes, dysplasia, blasts, general cell line; changes and maturation
Substrates (folate, Vitamin B12/holoTC, iron tests)	Substrate deficiency
PT, INR, aPTT, Fibrinogen	Coagulopathy (DIC, TTP)
Liver and kidney tests function	Liver or kidney disease
Infections (HIV, HCV, HBV, CMV, EBV, Parvo B19)	Viral infection
Protein electrophoresis with immunofixation	Lymphoid neoplasms, plasma cell neoplasms
Free light chains	plasma cell neoplasms
LDH, bilirubin, haptoglobin, DAT	Hemolysis
TSH (ANA, ANCA, RF)	Autoimmunity
Abdominal ultrasound	Liver disease, splenomegaly, lymph nodes enlargement

CBC: complete blood count; DAT: direct antiglobulin test; DIC: disseminated intravascular coagulation; holoTC: holotranscobalamin; IPF: immature platelet fraction; LDH: Lactate dehydrogenase; MPV: mean platelet volume; TTP: thrombotic thrombocytopenic purpura.

3.2. Secondary Diagnostic Work-Up

Patients with suspicious findings with worsening/relevant cytopenia and exclusion of other causes in the primary work-up should be referred to specialized centers for more detailed investigations. Morphological evaluation of peripheral blood (PB), bone marrow (BM) histology, and cytology with iron staining/assessment as well as cytogenetic analysis are mandatory for the assessment of MDS and BMF. Cytogenetics is indispensable to determine clonality and assess the disease-based risk in case of MDS [45,46]. Currently, asservation of bone-marrow samples for eventual molecular diagnostics with NGS is also advisable. NGS with myeloid panels is instrumental in all patients with unclear cytopenia as well as MDS with normal cytogenetics since it might prove clonality, refine prognosis, contribute to predicting treatment response, and serve as measurable residual disease (MRD) marker after allogeneic hematopoietic stem cell transplantation (allo HSCT) [47].

3.3. Peripheral Blood Smear

Bi- or pancytopenia is common in both MDS and BMF; however, at their onset, single cell lineages can also be affected. Non-regenerative anemia is almost a constant finding, with suppression of reticulocyte production. RBC macrocytosis is a common feature for MDS and BMF; however, relevant anisocytosis and/or poikilocytosis is predominantly found in MDS [42]. The observation of iron deficiency in the presence of pancytopenia should direct the investigations towards PNH. A normal WBC does not exclude an abnormal differentiation with neutropenia. Neutropenia can occur in varying degrees of severity. Lymphocyte count is generally decreased in MDS but normal in BMF [48]. In some cases, an expansion of large granular lymphocyte (LGL) can accompany AA. Its clinical relevance remains frequently unclear and it can be difficult to distinguish from LGL leukemia [41,49,50]. Monocytopenia may expand the differential diagnosis to hairy cell leukemia. Cytomorphologic examination of the peripheral blood smear has to be done microscopically to assess for morphologic abnormalities of RBC, dysgranulopoiesis and abnormal platelets. The presence of hematopoietic precursors with or without blasts is suggestive for an underling chronic myeloid neoplasm, whereas blasts without hematopoietic precursors (hiatus leucaemicus) is characteristic of acute leukemia. Atypical lymphocytes, e.g., hairy cells, suggest a lymphoproliferative disorder [42,51].

3.4. Bone Marrow Cytomorphology

Bone marrow cyto- (aspirate) and histomorphology (biopsy) are essential and complementary for the diagnosis of MDS and BMF. The examination of bone marrow smears reveals quantitative information about cellularity, assessment of the different hematopoietic lineages (granulopoiesis, erythropoiesis, megakaryopoiesis), and the maturation stages.

Increase of blasts or infiltrations of pathologic cell populations may be identified. Scant amount of bone marrow particles can be found in BMF and sometimes in MDS; however, a dry tap is unusual in BMF and suggests other diagnoses [52]. Quantitative and qualitative dysplastic morphological alterations of bone marrow precursors and peripheral blood cells are still fundamental for classification of MDS [44]. According to the 2016 World Health Organization (WHO) update, the presence of at least 10% of dysplastic cells in at least one hematopoietic lineage in the bone marrow is sufficient for a diagnosis of MDS [53]. Nevertheless, dysplastic features of hematopoiesis occur also in healthy individuals. On the other hand, substantial clonal hematopoiesis may exist in cases with less than 10% dysplasia. Following iron staining of the bone marrow smears, evidence of more than 15% ring sideroblasts (that result from mitochondrial iron accumulation) [44] or, in the presence of characteristic *SF3B1* mutations, more than 5%, is a diagnostic criterion for MDS with ring sideroblasts). Increase of marrow myeloblasts to 5% to 19% assign cases to advanced MDS with excess of blasts 1 and 2 (EB-1 or EB-2).

3.5. Bone Marrow Histopathology

Bone marrow trephine biopsies reveal information on cellularity, lineage distribution within the marrow space, and stroma fibrosis. In addition, bone marrow biopsy improves the characterization of megakaryocytes, blast quantification, and characterization of clusters of blasts: this phenomenon is known as "atypical localization of immature precursors" (ALIP). Identification of MDS with fibrosis and also hypoplastic MDS (hMDS) is rendered possible [44]. Likewise, histopathology is essential for the discrimination of MDS cases from overlapping disorders. For better discrimination of MDS from CMML, monocytic cells can be identified by immunohistochemistry, e.g., staining for CD68. Histopathology is crucial for the diagnosis of BMF and requires representative and sometimes repetitive sampling [54]. Aplastic and hypocellular BM is defined by a cellularity below 10% or 30%, respectively. The quality of the trephine biopsy is particularly important in the elderly, who have physiologically hypocellular marrow [55]. A typical AA marrow presents with variable amounts of residual hematopoietic cells with large fat spaces. Abundant plasma cells, lymphocyte and mast cell hyperplasia accompany the picture. Stromal cell hyperplasia can simulate normal cellularity and the increase in lymphocytes and/or mast cells sometimes pretend an infiltrative character. In such cases, immunohistochemistry or flow cytometry may be required to rule out a lymphoid neoplasms or mastocytosis [56]. Erythropoiesis nests forming "hot spots" are characteristic as well [51]. A certain degree of dyserythropoiesis with megaloblastic changes is frequently found in AA and needs to be carefully distinguished from MDS. Granulopoiesis and megakaryocytes are usually severely diminished or absent, without relevant dysplastic changes. Immunohistological staining allows the identification, quantification as well as topographic distribution of blasts, megakaryocytes, abnormal cells and infiltrates. Not infrequently, AA can be associated with lymphoproliferative disorders [56–58].

3.6. Multiparameter Flow Cytometry

For MDS, flow cytometric scores have been developed to contribute to the diagnostic process [59]. Dysplastic changes can be identified, e.g., by sophisticated interpretation of surface marker abnormalities in the myeloid compartment, and immature progenitor compartments can be identified. However, NGS seems to replace flow cytometry increasingly for the detection of clonality in MDS [60]. Nonetheless, flow cytometry remains essential to exclude other diagnoses, such as hairy cell leukemia. In patients with AA or hypoplastic MDS, subclones of PNH may be identified, which contribute in confirming the diagnosis. PNH clones are characterized by absence or severe deficiency of glycosylphosphatidylinositol (GPI)-anchored proteins, CD55, and CD59. Loss of the respective antigens is detected by staining with monoclonal antibodies and a reagent known as fluorescent aerolysin (FLAER) [61].

3.7. Cytogenetics

In around 50% of patients with de novo MDS and in around 80% of patients with therapy-associated MDS (t-MDS), clonal cytogenetic aberrations can be identified by chromosome banding analyses. Entities, such as MDS with isolated 5q deletion according to the WHO classification, can only be defined by karyotyping. Other examples of typical clonal cytogenetic alterations in MDS are abnormalities of chromosomes 7 or 17p. It should be considered that loss of the Y chromosome can be either clonal or age-related in male patients, depending on the proportion of aberrant metaphases [53]. Additionally, the karyotype has a central role for the revised International Prognostic Scoring System (IPSS-R) that discriminates five cytogenetic risk groups [46,62]. In AA, cytogenetic abnormalities can be present in up to 15% of patients [63]. Frequent anomalies include trisomy 8, uniparental disomy of 6p, 5q-, anomalies of chromosome 7 and 13. While abnormalities of chromosome 5 and 7 are very consistent with an underlying MDS, the finding of other abnormalities is not diagnostic. AA patients with del(13q) were reported with favorable response to immunosuppression [64,65]. Fluorescence in situ hybridization (FISH) allows detecting chromosome abnormalities of interphase nuclei also in the case of insufficient chromosome banding analysis. Vital cells are not required for interphase FISH. For patients with suspected or proven MDS, comprehensive interphase probe panels detecting frequent cytogenetic alterations, e.g., of chromosomes 7/7q, 5q, or 17p, may be used. Besides the detection of relevant cytogenetic alterations, FISH allows to confirm or further clarify doubtful results of chromosome banding analysis. At follow-up, the percentage of aberrant interphase nuclei in the case of a previously detected abnormality can be monitored at a sensitive level. Single nucleotide polymorphism (SNP) array analysis allows capturing both DNA copy number and SNP based genotype at a submegabase resolution. This facilitates the detection of small areas of loss of heterozygosity (LOH) of uniparental disomy (UPD) [66] and submicroscopic changes on a cryptic level [60,67]. However, array analyses are increasingly loosing relevance since the introduction of NGS for diagnosis of MDS.

3.8. Next-Generation Sequencing

The detection of SM-LAGs by NGS has gained increasing importance in hematological molecular diagnostics laboratories. NGS allows high-throughput screening for variants that are relevant for diagnosis, classification, risk stratification and, treatment monitoring in patients with hematologic malignancies [68]. At present, targeted sequencing using specific panels covering hotspots of a selection of relevant genes is the method of choice for hematologic diagnostics [69,70]. Examples for commercially available myeloid NGS panels include the Illumina TruSight Myeloid panel (Illumina Switzerland GmBH, Zürich, Switzerland), the Oncomine Myeloid panel (Thermo Fisher Scientific, Reinach, Switzerland), and the Human Myeloid Neoplasms QiaSeq DNA Panel (Qiagen, Rotkreuz, Switzerland). These panels cover hotspots in 25 to more than 50 genes. NGS-targeted sequencing shows a sensitivity between 1% and 5–10%, depending on allele coverage and type of NGS. Each NGS platform has its own technical limitation calling for caution to avoid false positive and negative results. Interpretation of genetic variants relies on thorough assessment using appropriate databases, and the differentiation of a MDS associated mutation from a germline variant needs to be addressed whenever a variant is close to 50% variant allele frequency (VAF). The knowledge on MDS-related markers and the information collected in variant databases are undergoing constant changes, so that variant interpretation can change over time.

3.9. Role of Next-Generation Sequencing in BMF

BMF have a high complexity on the molecular level. The molecular profile may show overlaps with myeloid disorders, rendering the discrimination from MDS difficult. In children and young adults with BMF, it will be necessary to rule out congenital forms by molecular methods, while in older adults, the focus will be more likely on somatic mutations. NGS allows investigating both relevant germline and somatic mutations. The choice of the most appropriate NGS gene panel is of utmost importance. Users of NGS technology should be aware that new pathogenic relevant genes or non-coding regions, like promoter or intronic regions, can be discovered after the design of the gene panel. For this reason, whole exome sequencing is a method of choice for germline panels, allowing a re-analysis of further genes without repetition of the analysis (caveat: non-coding regions are usually missing). Copy number variation (CNV) is a phenomenon frequently observed in BMF where large sections of DNA can be deleted or duplicated; sometimes whole genes are missing. CNV can be detected by array-based comparative genomic hybridization (Array-CGH) technology, which covers large parts of the genome, or multiplex ligation-dependent probe amplification (MLPA) analysis, which focuses on specific genes or genomic regions. Cytogenetic analysis is applied for detection of large chromosomal rearrangements, either by karyotyping (for large rearrangements) or by FISH (for specific rearrangements).

The molecular diagnosis of some iBMF can be straightforward, while others are very complex and heterogeneous [43,71–74]. DC is heterogeneous and shows complex clinical criteria in concordance with complex genetic findings [75]. For suspected iBMF without a specific clinical pattern, more and more heterogeneous clinical and molecular findings are identified, resulting in newly recognized disease entities [76]. In addition to germline variants, patients with different BMF entities may carry somatic mutations.

3.10. Discrimination of Germline from Somatic Mutations

Somatic NGS analysis in MDS yields a variety of different genetic variants in numerous genes. Most of these variants can be assigned to two groups: first, clonal alterations in relation to the hematologic disorder, and, second, benign germline variants. The first group comprises driver mutations, contributing to the malignant development, and additional passenger mutations. By now, numerous driver mutations are known, including RNA splicing, DNA methylation, transcription, chromatin modification, signal transduction, DNA repair, cohesin complex and associated proteins, RAS pathway, a variety of other signaling molecules, and pathways such as *TP53* [77]. The second group, the benign variants, show always either 50 or 100% VAF, as they are germline variants, unless a somatic deletion at this specific locus has happened, and they are usually listed in databases (UCSC, gnomAD, others). However, there can be variants with a VAF close to 50%, or sometimes distinctly above 50%, which are neither clearly benign nor clonal. Loss of heterozygosity (LOH) needs to be considered in such cases (variant clearly over 50% VAF). Alterations in the *DX41*, *RUNX1*, *GATA2*, and *TP53* genes are potentially present in the germline and can cause a predisposition to AML or MDS. For solid tumors, the American College of Medical Genetics (ACMG) developed recommendations for the reporting of presumed germline pathogenic variants (PGPVs) [78]. Confirmatory germline testing should be performed in a specialized laboratory, and positive results have to be explained to the patient by clinicians with genetic expertise.

4. Characterization of MDS and BMF

4.1. Challenges in Finding the Diagnosis of MDS and BMF

The approach to suspected MDS of BMF is work-intensive and requires expertise in the interpretation and integration of the laboratory results from various diagnostic modalities, which is best achieved within an interdisciplinary pathological review board.

The conditio sine qua non for MDS is the presence of unexplained cytopenia accompanied by signs of dysplasia in the peripheral blood or bone marrow and, at later stages, increase of immature myeloid blasts. In many instances, cytomorphology alone is not sufficient to confirm or exclude MDS. In such cases, bone marrow cytogenetic analyses can help to identify clonality with chromosome abnormalities in ~50% of all affected patients. NGS has increased the diagnostic sensitivity for the identification of clonal markers of hematopoietic cells in most MDS patients. However, SM-LAGs may also be present in AA, showing some overlap between AA and hMDS, and the distinction may be challenging (Table 2).

Table 2. Common findings and differences between hypoplastic myelodysplastic syndrome (hMDS) and aplastic anemia (AA) [52].

Parameters	Hypoplastic MDS	Aplastic Anemia
Cytopenia	Present	Present
BM cellularity	Hypocellular	Aplastic (<10% cellularity or significantly hypocellular)
BM hematopoiesis		
Erythropoiesis	Present	Present in nests, "hot spots"
Granulopoiesis	Present	Typically decreased
Megakaryopoiesis	Present	Decreased or absent
BM fat replacement	Possible	Typical
Dysplasia		
Erythroid dysplasia	Frequent	Possible
Granulocytic dysplasia	Frequent	Normal morphology
Megakaryocytic dysplasia	Frequent	Normal morphology
Ring sideroblasts	Possible	Absent
Blasts	Variable	Absent
CD34+ or CD117+ immunohistochemistry	Normal or increased	No increase
Marrow fibrosis	Possible	Absent
PNH clone	Unusual	Frequent
Splenomegaly at diagnosis	Possible	Absent
Karyotype	Abnormal ~50%	Clonal abnormality possible (~12%)
Recurrent cytogenetic abnormalities	-Y, del(11q), -5/del(5q), del(12p), del(20q), -7/del(7q), +8, +19, i(17q), inv(3)/t(3q)/del(3q)	At Diagnosis: del(13q), +8 Evolution: -7, -5/del(5q), del(20q)
Complex cytogenetics (≥3 abnormalities)	Possible	Absent
Acquired CN-LOH	Possible	Possible (<20%)
Somatic mutated genes	SF3B1, SRSF2, U2AF1, ZRSR2, TET2, DNMT3A, IDH1, IDH2, ASXL1, EZH2, RUNX1, NRAS, BCOR, TP53, STAG2	Particularly PIGA, ASXL1, BCOR, BCORL1; 5–52% of patients will present MDS-associated mutations
Germline mutations	Should be investigated in patients with suspicion of underlying germline predisposition.	Should be investigated in patients with suspicion of underlying congenital BMF.

BM: bone marrow; PNH: paroxysmal nocturnal hemoglobinuria CN-LOH: copy number-neutral loos of heterozygosity.

AA has phenotypic overlaps with many other hematological disorders, including hypoplastic forms of MDS, AML, and lymphoblastic leukemia (ALL). Moreover, LGL, PNH, and iBMF can manifest with a hypocellular BM. The diagnostic discrimination of these entities is demanding, as AA can occur at any age, lacks specific diagnostic markers, and remains a diagnosis of exclusion. For iBMF, such as telomeropathies and FA, assessment of telomere lengths and chromosome fragility, respectively, are required. (Figure 1). An integrated cyto-histologic/genetic score (hg-score) has been shown to be useful to distinguish hMDS from AA [26,79] (Table 3). The correct diagnosis is especially challenging in asymptomatic patients with moderate thrombocytopenia (PLT 50–100 G/L) and otherwise unsuspicious peripheral blood values. The distinction from immunological, infectious and toxic-reactive causes is critical, as the prognosis and evolution can differ substantially depending on the underlying cause.

Table 3. Integrated cyto-histologic/genetic score (hg-score) for distinction of hypoplastic myelodysplastic syndrome (hMDS) and aplastic anemia (AA) [26].

Cytological/Histological Variables	
Requisite criteria	**Scoring points**
Bone marrow blasts AND/OR CD34 + cells $\geq$5%	2
Bone marrow blasts AND/OR CD34 + cells 2–4%	1
Fibrosis grade 2–3	1
Dysmegakaryopoiesis	1
Co-criteria	
Ring sideroblasts $\geq$15%	2
Ring sideroblasts 5–14% *	1
Severe dysgranulopoiesis	1
Karyotype (co-criterion)	
Presumptive cytogenetic abnormality *	2
Somatic mutation (co-criterion)	
Specific high-risk mutation pattern **	1

* According to World Health Organization (WHO) criteria [53] ** According to Malcovati et al. [79] Receiver Operating Characteristic (ROC) analysis confirmed that a cutoff hg-score of 2 is associated with the highest percentage of correctly classified (Area Under the Curve, (AUC) 0.89, $p < 0.001$).

Etiologies can also be multifactoral in elderly patients, i.e., transient aggravation of thrombocytopenia can be observed during infections or drug-exposure in patients with chronic, border-line thrombocytopenia. Delay in recovery after these intercurrences may suggest deficiencies at the HSPC level.

4.2. Characterization of MDS

The challenge to distinguish reactive conditions from early stages of MDS has led an international working group of MDS experts to define minimal diagnostic criteria required for diagnosis of MDS (Table 4) [80]. MDS can develop either primarily or secondarily, after previous radio- or chemotherapy, and are sub-classified according to the 2016 WHO update (Table 5) [53]. Correct MDS sub-classification should be followed by appropriate disease-based and patient-based risk stratification. The International Prognostic Scoring System (IPSS), the revised IPSS (IPSS-R) as well as the WHO Prognostic Scoring System (WPSS) can determine the risk for progression to AML and overall survival [45,46,81]. In order to optimize efficacy against tolerability, patient-derived risk stratification is particularly important for elderly and frail MDS patients. Karnofsky and Eastern Cooperative Oncology Group (ECOG) scores allow assessing the performance status but should be complemented by assessment of comorbidity and frailty. The Charlson Comorbidity Index

(CCI) was adapted by Sorror [82,83] and validated for MDS-patients that are sufficiently fit for undergoing allo HSCT (hematopoietic stem cell transplantation comorbidity index: HCT-CI) [84]. A simplified scoring system can be used for elderly MDS patients that considers cardiac, pulmonary, renal and hepatic comorbidities as well as prior treatment for solid tumors as most relevant factors (myelodysplastic syndromes comorbidity index: MDS-CI) [85].

Table 4. Minimal diagnostic criteria for myelodysplastic syndromes (MDS) [80].

Criteria	Major Diagnostic Tests
Prerequisite criteria (both must be fulfilled)	
Constant cytopenia	Blood counts (over 6 months)
Exclusion of all other diseases as primary cause of cytopenia/dysplasia	BM smear and BM histology, cytogenetics, flow cytometry, molecular markers, other relevant investigations *
MDS-related criteria (one of these must be fulfilled)	
Morphological dysplasia in one of the three major lineages	BM and PB smear, in certain situations BM histology
Blast count ≥5%	BM smear and histology
Ring sideroblasts ≥15% or ≥5% and SF3B1 mutation	Iron staining
Typical karyotype anomaly	Conventional karyotyping and/or FISH
Co-criteria	
Monoclonality of myeloid cells	Molecular markers and mutations
BM stem cell function	Circulating CFC, reticulocytes
Abnormal immunophenotype of BM cells	Multicolor flow cytometry, immunohistochemistry
Abnormal gene expression profile	mRNA profiling assays

BM, bone marrow; PB, peripheral blood; FISH, fluorescence in situ hybridization; CFC, colony-forming progenitor cells. * Investigations depend on the case history and overall situation in each case, and should always include a complete chemistry profile with inflammation parameters, immunoglobulins, a serum erythropoietin level, and a serum tryptase level.

Table 5. WHO 2016 classification for Myelodysplastic Syndromes (MDS) [53].

Subtype [1]	No. of Dysplastic Lineages	No. of Cytopenic Lineages [2]	% RS of all Erythroid Cells in BM		% Blasts in PB or BM AR: Auer Rods			Conventional Cytogenetics
			wt$SF3B1$	m$SF3B1$	BM	PB	AR	
MDS-SLD	1	1 or 2	<15	<5	<5	<1	-	
MDS-MLD	2 or 3	1–3	<15	<5	<5	<1	-	
MDS RS-SLD	1	1 or 2	≥15	≥5	<5	<1	-	
MDS RS-MLD	2 or 3	1–3	≥15	≥5	<5	<1	-	
MDS del(5q)	1–3	1 or 2	n.a.	n.a.	<5	<1	-	Isolated del(5q) +/− 1 add. aberration without del(7q)/−7
MDS EB-1	0–3	1–3	n.a.	n.a.	5–9	2–4	-	
MDS EB-2	0–3	1–3	n.a.	n.a.	10–19	5–19	+	
MDS-U			<15	<5	<5	<1	-	
(a) 1% blasts in PB	1–3	1–3	n.a.	n.a.	<5	1 [3]	-	
(b) SLD with pancytopenia	1	3	n.a.	n.a.	<5	<1	-	
(c) defining cytogenetic aberration	0	1–3	<15 [4]	n.a.	<5	<1	-	MDS defining cytogenetic aberration
RCC	1–3	1–3	<15	≤5	<5	<1	-	

SLD: single-lineage dysplasia; MLD: multilineage dysplasia; RS: ring sideroblasts; EB: excess of blasts; RCC: refractory cytopenia of the childhood; wt/m$SF3B1$: wild type or mutated $SF3B1$; PB: peripheral blood; BM: bone marrow; AR: Auer rods. [1] Without previous cytotoxic treatment or germline predisposition for myeloid neoplasms. [2] Cytopenias: hemoglobin <100 g/L, thrombocytes <100 G/L, neutrophils <1.8 G/L, monocytes <1 G/L. [3] 1% blasts in PB must be confirmed with a 2nd analysis. [4] ≥15% RS corresponds to MDS-RS-SLD. CAVE: If ≥50% are erythroid precursors and ≥20% blast cells of non-erythroid-lineage but <20% of all cells, this corresponds now to MDS (MDS-SLD/MLD or EB) and not any more to AML M6 erythroid/myeloid.

4.3. Relevance of Thrombocytopenia in the Context of MDS Patients

Thrombocytopenia in MDS patients is mainly caused by insufficient or ineffective thrombopoiesis, but some patients may have additional immunological mechanisms targeting the mature platelets as well as the megakaryocytic progenitor cells in the bone marrow [86]. In these circumstances, the morphological differential diagnosis between MDS and immune thrombocytopenia (ITP) and the amegakaryocytic form of AA requires identification of characteristic genetic lesions. In retrospective studies, 12% of MDS patients had isolated thrombocytopenia as first presentation [87] and 20% of patients, who were initially classified as ITP, were reclassified with an unusual presentation of MDS [88]. In a review of MDS patients referred to the MD Anderson Cancer Center, 67% of patients were thrombocytopenic (PLT < 100 G/L), of which 26% had moderate (PLT 20–50 G/L) and 17% severe (PLT < 20 G/L) thrombocytopenia [89]. Thrombocytopenia and severe thrombocytopenia were more prominent in higher risk (77% and 20%) compared to lower risk disease (51% and 12%) [89]. The impact of thrombocytopenia on morbidity and mortality is relevant, as half of all MDS patients experience bleeding and a quarter experience even serious bleedings during the course of disease [89,90]. Bleeding episodes can be triggered by treatments with antiplatelet agents or anticoagulants for cardiovascular or thromboembolic comorbidities. Bleeding can be related to quantitative thrombocytopenia (PLT < 10–20 G/L) but also qualitative platelet defects (dysfunctional platelets) [91], caused by somatic or germ-line mutations (i.e., *ETV6, RUNX1, ANKR1*) [92]. Isolated chronic thrombocytopenia is rare in MDS patients as other lineages are frequently affected either by mild cytopenia or dysplasia [93]. Based on the increased awareness of MDS, earlier hematological assessment of mild cytopenias, and increased use of NGS panels, we and others are currently observing an increasing number of patients with isolated thrombocytopenia as initial manifestation of MDS. Other than that, primary myelofibrosis (PMF) may also present with isolated thrombocytopenia. In such cases, splenomegaly may be detected, accompanied by circulating dakryocytes, myeloid, or erythroid precursors and thrombocyte anisocytosis [53].

4.4. Characterization of BMF

The rarity of AA, the difficulties in establishing the correct diagnosis due to the lack of specific markers, and the overlaps with other disorders can delay its diagnosis. When AA occurs in children, congenital forms should be considered. iBMF should be considered in patients with a family history of cytopenias, tendency to cancer, or certain unexplained liver or lung conditions independent of their age. In older adults, the discrimination from hMDS is mandatory and particularly difficult (Tables 2 and 3).

Identifying the correct underlying disease has implications on the type of treatment. For example, in patients with AA resulting from a nuclear accident as in Chernobyl, allo HSCT is the only option [94], as damage of the hematopoietic cells will not respond to immunosuppressive treatment. Following confirmation of AA and identification of the underlying pathomechanism, its severity must be defined as basis for further therapeutic decisions [95,96].

4.5. Isolated Thrombocytopenia as First Presentation of a BMF

Isolated thrombocytopenia will be interpreted and treated as ITP in some patients and only in the course of the disease, a BMF will be finally diagnosed [97]. Nowadays, in accordance with international guidelines, patients with suspected ITP do not necessarily undergo bone marrow investigation [1], and marrow investigations will be done only after failure of standard therapy. Some reports suggested that acquired amegakaryocytic thrombocytopenia may precede AA [98–100]. In cases of isolated thrombocytopenia, a detailed personal and family medical history is mandatory, evaluating history of cytopenias, hematological diseases, or a tendency to certain tumors. In a patient with thrombocytopenia, the finding of dysmorphic nails, a history of gray hair early in life, café au lait spots, or any type of physical dysmorphia may suggest an underlying iBMF. Likewise, a history of fibrotic lung disease, liver, or skeletal changes are reasons to consider a consultation in a specialized center [41].

4.6. Aplastic Anemia and PNH

PNH is a rare bone marrow failure disorder that manifests with hemolytic anemia, thrombosis, and peripheral blood cytopenias. The absence of two glycosylphosphatidylinositol (GPI)-anchored proteins, CD55 and CD59, leads to uncontrolled complement activation that accounts for hemolysis and other PNH manifestations [61]. PNH and AA are related entities [101]. Patients with the typical hemolytic form of PNH can develop AA and around 50% of patients with the acquired form of AA typically have PNH clones [102]. PNH clones accompanying AA are smaller than they are in the PNH hemolytic form. Flow cytometry is the gold standard method for detection and diagnosis of PNH [103]. In AA, PNH clones should be quantified at presentation and at follow-up by serial monitoring every 6 to 12 months, even when the initial result was negative.

4.7. Inherited Bone Marrow Failures (iBMF)

In patients with BMF, a positive family history that includes other affected members with cytopenia or malignancy suggests an iBMF. The presence of unusual clinical features (skin, liver, lung, skeletal disease) should alert to the possibility of a congenital form of BMF. A normal clinical examination does not definitively rule out asymptomatic forms of telomeropathies or non-classical presentations of FA. If FA is suspected, investigations that may demonstrate higher sensitivity to chromosomal breakage with mitomycin C or diepoxybutane are necessary [104]. These investigations should be carried out in patients with suspicion of an underlying iBMF. If the mitomycin C or diepoxybutane test is positive, all family candidates to be donors for allo HSCT should also be investigated to rule out asymptomatic forms of FA. In patients with FA, the correct diagnosis is of urgent importance, as less toxic conditioning regimens are mandatory in the case of allo HSCT due to defective DNA repair mechanisms.

Measurement of the telomere length of peripheral blood leukocytes can be performed as a screening test in case of suspected telomeropathy. A variable percentage of patients without telomeropathies will also show telomere attrition [23,24]. Mutations in the *TERC* and *TERT* genes for example can cause telomeropathies in both children and adults [25]. When telomeropathies occur in adult patients they are more subtle in their clinical presentation, which renders their detection difficult.

4.8. Future Challenges: Unexplained Thrombocytopenia with Clonal Hematopoiesis

After thorough diagnostic assessment, patients with unexplained thrombocytopenia may show insufficient dysplastic morphological changes and lack MDS-defining cytogenetic alterations or sufficient criteria for BMF. These disease forms can be assigned to Idiopathic Cytopenia of Unknown Significance (ICUS), if other clinical conditions are insufficient to explain the cytopenia [80]. In the case that the severity of thrombocytopenia imposes the need of therapeutic intervention, a steroid trial may be justified, whereas in mild to moderate cases observation for 3–6 months is sufficient [105]. As shown in recent years by numerous large studies, SM-LAGs can be identified by NGS in the peripheral blood in an age-dependent, increasing frequency in the elderly population, in up to 20–40% of individuals aged more than 80 years. These mutations are per se not indicative for a hematological neoplasia [106–110], and the affected individuals have generally normal peripheral blood values or only mild cytopenia that do not otherwise fulfill the diagnostic criteria for a hematological malignancy [111]. In case that the variant allele frequency (VAF) of the respective mutations is 2% or more, the condition is termed clonal hematopoiesis with indeterminate potential (CHIP) in otherwise healthy individuals with normal blood values, or clonal cytopenia with unknown significance (CCUS) in individuals with cytopenia, respectively [79,109]. CHIP and CCUS can be considered facultative precanceroses as they are at an increased risk for transformation to overt hematological neoplasms in a rate of 0.5–1% per year [111]. If SM-LAGs present with a VAF level $\geq$10% or with evidence of two or more somatic associated mutations, a myeloid neoplasm can be diagnosed in patients with unexplained cytopenia with a positive predictive value of >85% [79]. However, with the exception of mutations in spliceosome genes, single mutations in *DNMT3A*, *ASXL1* and *TET2* (DAT mutations) with a VAF <10% are not sufficiently predictive for the diagnosis of a myeloid malignancy, especially in elderly individuals [109]. On the contrary, a negative analysis with a panel of ≥40 genes can exclude a myeloid malignancy with a negative predictive value of >80% [79]. In summary, the advent of NGS has substantially increased the diagnostic sensitivity for detecting clonality and poses some novel challenges in the correct interpretation of these results. Some of those patients will fulfill the criteria for overt myeloid neoplasm as specified above, which will inevitably contribute to steadily increasing incident cases of MDS and associated disorders.

5. Conclusions

- Unexplained chronic thrombocytopenia has to be considered as an early and unusual presentation in MDS or BMF.
- Patient's history remains crucial to identify suspicious cases and for the correct interpretation of primary laboratory values.
- Various diagnostic modalities are required to confirm or exclude MDS or BMF and an interdisciplinary workup is frequently required, especially in difficult cases.
- Meticulous assessment of the PB smear, BM cyto- and histomorphology, as well as cytogenetics are the mainstay of diagnostic evaluation, and is nowadays complemented by NGS and other specialized analyses (telomere length, DNA breakage).
- Repeated bone marrow investigation may be necessary, especially in cases with hypocellular BM for the distinction of sampling errors, reactive-toxic conditions, BMF, and hypoplastic MDS.
- In some occasions, conclusive diagnosis is only possible after follow-up. However, NGS has substantially contributed in identifying early conditions of clonal hematopoiesis, but additional challenges arise for classification and prognostication.

Supplementary Materials: The following are available online at https://www.mdpi.com/2077-0383/10/5/1026/s1, Table S1: Overview of some of the typical germline mutations in different bone marrow failure entities.

Author Contributions: Design of review manuscript: U.B.; literature search, interpretation of literature, writing of manuscript: N.B., A.R., N.P., U.B.; critical review of manuscript and final approval: all authors. All authors have read and agreed to the published version of the manuscript.

Funding: No funding was received.

Institutional Review Board Statement: Not applicable.

Informed Consent Statement: Not applicable.

Data Availability Statement: Not applicable.

Conflicts of Interest: U.B. and N.P.: nothing to declare. Potentially perceived conflicts of interests: N.B.: *Amgen*: travel support; *Astellas*: research funding to institution; *Celgene*: travel support, research funding to institution; *Janssen*: financial support for travel; *Novartis*: travel support, research funding to institution; *Roche*: travel support, research funding to institution; *Sandoz*: research funding to institution; *Servier*: research funding to institution; *Takeda*: research funding to institution; A.R.: Novartis: Consultancy, Honoraria, Advisory Board, Research Funding; CSL Behring: research funding; Alexion: research funding; Orphaswiss: advisory board; Celgene/BMS: advisory board; AstraZeneca: advisory board.

References

1. Neunert, C.; Terrell, D.R.; Arnold, D.M.; Buchanan, G.; Cines, D.B.; Cooper, N.; Cuker, A.; Despotovic, J.M.; George, J.N.; Grace, R.F.; et al. American Society of Hematology 2019 guidelines for immune thrombocytopenia. *Blood Adv.* **2019**, *3*, 3829–3866. [CrossRef]
2. Roman, E.; Smith, A.; Appleton, S.; Crouch, S.; Kelly, R.; Kinsey, S.; Cargo, C.; Patmore, R. Myeloid malignancies in the real-world: Occurrence, progression and survival in the UK's population-based Haematological Malignancy Research Network 2004–15. *Cancer Epidemiol.* **2016**, *42*, 186–198. [CrossRef]
3. Hellström-Lindberg, E.; Tobiasson, M.; Greenberg, P. Myelodysplastic syndromes: Moving towards personalized management. *Haematologica* **2020**, *105*, 1765–1779. [CrossRef]
4. Corey, S.J.; Minden, M.D.; Barber, D.L.; Kantarjian, H.; Wang, J.C.Y.; Schimmer, A.D. Myelodysplastic syndromes: The complexity of stem-cell diseases. *Nat. Rev. Cancer* **2007**, *7*, 118–129. [CrossRef] [PubMed]

5. Steensma, D.P. Clinical Implications of Clonal Hematopoiesis. *Mayo Clin. Proc.* **2018**, *93*, 1122–1130. [CrossRef]
6. Steensma, D.P. Predicting therapy-related myeloid neoplasms-and preventing them? *Lancet Oncol.* **2017**, *18*, 11–13. [CrossRef]
7. Neukirchen, J.; Schoonen, W.M.; Strupp, C.; Gattermann, N.; Aul, C.; Haas, R.; Germing, U. Incidence and prevalence of myelodysplastic syndromes: Data from the Düsseldorf MDS-registry. *Leuk. Res.* **2011**, *35*, 1591–1596. [CrossRef] [PubMed]
8. Foran, J.M.; Shammo, J.M. Clinical Presentation, Diagnosis, and Prognosis of Myelodysplastic Syndromes. *Am. J. Med.* **2012**, *125* (Suppl. S7), S6–S13. [CrossRef]
9. Strom, S.S.; Gu, Y.; Gruschkus, S.K.; Pierce, S.; Estey, E.H. Risk factors of myelodysplastic syndromes: A case–control study. *Leukemia* **2005**, *19*, 1912–1918. [CrossRef]
10. Bonadies, N.; Feller, A.; Rovo, A.; Ruefer, A.; Blum, S.; Gerber, B.; Stuessi, G.; Benz, R.; Cantoni, N.; Holbro, A.; et al. Trends of classification, incidence, mortality, and survival of MDS patients in Switzerland between 2001 and 2012. *Cancer Epidemiol.* **2017**, *46*, 85–92. [CrossRef]
11. Rollison, D.E.; Howlader, N.; Smith, M.T.; Strom, S.S.; Merritt, W.D.; Ries, L.A.; Edwards, B.K.; List, A.F. Epidemiology of myelodysplastic syndromes and chronic myeloproliferative disorders in the United States, 2001–2004, using data from the NAACCR and SEER programs. *Blood* **2008**, *112*, 45–52. [CrossRef]
12. Babushok, D.V.; Bessler, M. Genetic predisposition syndromes: When should they be considered in the work-up of MDS? *Best Pract. Res. Clin. Haematol.* **2015**, *28*, 55–68. [CrossRef]
13. Steensma, D.P.; Bennett, J.M. The Myelodysplastic Syndromes: Diagnosis and Treatment. *Mayo Clin. Proc.* **2006**, *81*, 104–130. [CrossRef]
14. Thota, S.; Gerds, A.T. Myelodysplastic and myeloproliferative neoplasms: Updates on the overlap syndromes. *Leuk. Lymphoma* **2017**, *59*, 803–812. [CrossRef]
15. Kipfer, B.; Daikeler, T.; Kuchen, S.; Hallal, M.; Andina, N.; Allam, R.; Bonadies, N. Increased cardiovascular comorbidities in patients with myelodysplastic syndromes and chronic myelomonocytic leukemia presenting with systemic inflammatory and autoimmune manifestations. *Semin. Hematol.* **2018**, *55*, 242–247. [CrossRef]
16. Mekinian, A.; Grignano, E.; Braun, T.; Decaux, O.; Liozon, E.; Costedoat-Chalumeau, N.; Kahn, J.-E.; Hamidou, M.; Park, S.; Puéchal, X.; et al. Systemic inflammatory and autoimmune manifestations associated with myelodysplastic syndromes and chronic myelomonocytic leukaemia: A French multicentre retrospective study. *Rheumatology* **2016**, *55*, 291–300. [CrossRef]
17. Risitano, A.M.; Maciejewski, J.P.; Green, S.; Plasilova, M.; Zeng, W.; Young, N.S. In-vivo dominant immune responses in aplastic anaemia: Molecular tracking of putatively pathogenetic T-cell clones by TCR beta-CDR3 sequencing. *Lancet* **2004**, *364*, 355–364. [CrossRef]
18. Young, N.S. Current concepts in the pathophysiology and treatment of aplastic anemia. *Hematol. Am. Soc. Hematol. Educ. Program* **2013**, *2013*, 76–81. [CrossRef]
19. Min, K.-W.; Jung, H.Y.; Han, H.S.; Hwang, T.S.; Kim, S.-Y.; Kim, W.S.; Lim, S.D.; Kim, W.Y. Ileal mass-like lesion induced by Epstein-Barr virus-associated hemophagocytic lymphohistiocytosis in a patient with aplastic anemia. *APMIS* **2014**, *123*, 81–86. [CrossRef]
20. Brown, K.E.; Idrees, M.; Shah, S.A.; Butt, S.; Butt, A.M.; Ali, L.; Hussain, A.; Rehman, I.U.; Ali, M. Hepatitis-associated aplastic anemia. *N. Engl. J. Med.* **1997**, *336*, 1059–1064. [CrossRef]
21. Young, N.S. Flaviviruses and bone marrow failure. *JAMA* **1990**, *263*, 3065–3068. [CrossRef] [PubMed]
22. Locasciulli, A.; Bacigalupo, A.; Bruno, B.; Montante, B.; Marsh, J.; Tichelli, A.; Socié, G.; Passweg, J. Hepatitis-associated aplastic anaemia: Epidemiology and treatment results obtained in Europe. A report of The EBMT aplastic anaemia working party. *Br. J. Haematol.* **2010**, *149*, 890–895. [CrossRef] [PubMed]
23. Calado, R.T.; Cooper, J.N.; Padilla-Nash, H.M.; Sloand, E.M.; Wu, C.O.; Scheinberg, P.; Ried, T.; Young, N.S. Short telomeres result in chromosomal instability in hematopoietic cells and precede malignant evolution in human aplastic anemia. *Leukemmia* **2011**, *26*, 700–707. [CrossRef]
24. Dumitriu, B.; Feng, X.; Townsley, D.M.; Ueda, Y.; Yoshizato, T.; Calado, R.T.; Yang, Y.; Wakabayashi, Y.; Kajigaya, S.; Ogawa, S.; et al. Telomere attrition and candidate gene mutations preceding monosomy 7 in aplastic anemia. *Blood* **2015**, *125*, 706–709. [CrossRef]
25. Townsley, D.M.; Dumitriu, B.; Young, N.S. Bone marrow failure and the telomeropathies. *Blood* **2014**, *124*, 2775–2783. [CrossRef]
26. Bono, E.; McLornan, D.; Travaglino, E.; Gandhi, S.; Gallì, A.; Khan, A.A.; Kulasekararaj, A.G.; Boveri, E.; Raj, K.; Elena, C.; et al. Clinical, histopathological and molecular characterization of hypoplastic myelodysplastic syndrome. *Leukemia* **2019**, *33*, 2495–2505. [CrossRef]
27. Stanley, N.; Olson, T.S.; Babushok, D.V. Recent advances in understanding clonal haematopoiesis in aplastic anaemia. *Br. J. Haematol.* **2017**, *177*, 509–525. [CrossRef]
28. Kulasekararaj, A.G.; Jiang, J.; Smith, A.E.; Mohamedali, A.M.; Mian, S.; Gandhi, S.; Gaken, J.; Czepulkowski, B.; Marsh, J.C.; Mufti, G.J. Somatic mutations identify a subgroup of aplastic anemia patients who progress to myelodysplastic syndrome. *Blood* **2014**, *124*, 2698–2704. [CrossRef]
29. Triemstra, J.; Pham, A.; Rhodes, L.; Waggoner, D.J.; Onel, K. A Review of Fanconi Anemia for the Practicing Pediatrician. *Pediatr. Ann.* **2015**, *44*, 444–452. [CrossRef]
30. Farooqui, S.M.; Ward, R.; Aziz, M. Shwachman-Diamond Syndrome. In *StatPearls*; StatPearls Publishing: Treasure Island, FL, USA, 2020.

31. Geddis, A.E. Inherited Thrombocytopenia: Congenital Amegakaryocytic Thrombocytopenia and Thrombocytopenia with Absent Radii. *Semin. Hematol.* **2006**, *43*, 196–203. [CrossRef]
32. Kojima, S. Why is the incidence of aplastic anemia higher in Asia? *Expert Rev. Hematol.* **2017**, *10*, 277–279. [CrossRef]
33. Young, N.S.; Kaufman, D.W. The epidemiology of acquired aplastic anemia. *Haematologica* **2008**, *93*, 489–492. [CrossRef] [PubMed]
34. Song, E.Y.; Kang, H.J.; Shin, H.Y.; Ahn, H.S.; Kim, I.; Yoon, S.-S.; Park, S.; Kim, B.K.; Park, M.H. Association of human leukocyte antigen class II alleles with response to immunosuppressive therapy in Korean aplastic anemia patients. *Hum. Immunol.* **2010**, *71*, 88–92. [CrossRef]
35. Sugimori, C.; Yamazaki, H.; Feng, X.; Mochizuki, K.; Kondo, Y.; Takami, A.; Chuhjo, T.; Kimura, A.; Teramura, M.; Mizoguchi, H.; et al. Roles of DRB1 *1501 and DRB1 *1502 in the pathogenesis of aplastic anemia. *Exp. Hematol.* **2007**, *35*, 13–20. [CrossRef]
36. Yoshida, N.; Yagasaki, H.; Takahashi, Y.; Yamamoto, T.; Liang, J.; Wang, Y.; Tanaka, M.; Hama, A.; Nishio, N.; Kobayashi, R.; et al. Clinical impact of HLA-DR15, a minor population of paroxysmal nocturnal haemoglobinuria-type cells, and an aplastic anaemia-associated autoantibody in children with acquired aplastic anaemia. *Br. J. Haematol.* **2008**, *142*, 427–435. [CrossRef]
37. Wang, M.; Nie, N.; Feng, S.; Shi, J.; Ge, M.; Li, X.; Shao, Y.; Huang, J.; Zheng, Y. The polymorphisms of human leukocyte antigen loci may contribute to the susceptibility and severity of severe aplastic anemia in Chinese patients. *Hum. Immunol.* **2014**, *75*, 867–872. [CrossRef]
38. Jeong, T.-D.; Mun, Y.-C.; Chung, H.-S.; Seo, D.; Im, J.; Huh, J. Novel deletion mutation of HLA-B*40:02 gene in acquired aplastic anemia. *HLA* **2016**, *89*, 47–51. [CrossRef]
39. Maluf, E.; Hamerschlak, N.; Cavalcanti, A.B.; Júnior, Á.A.; Eluf-Neto, J.; Falcão, R.P.; Lorand-Metze, I.G.; Goldenberg, D.; Santana, C.L.; Rodrigues, D.D.O.W.; et al. Incidence and risk factors of aplastic anemia in Latin American countries: The LATIN case-control study. *Haematology* **2009**, *94*, 1220–1226. [CrossRef]
40. Yoshizato, T.; Dumitriu, B.; Hosokawa, K.; Makishima, H.; Yoshida, K.; Townsley, D.; Sato-Otsubo, A.; Sato, Y.; Liu, D.; Suzuki, H.; et al. Somatic Mutations and Clonal Hematopoiesis in Aplastic Anemia. *N. Engl. J. Med.* **2015**, *373*, 35–47. [CrossRef]
41. Kallen, M.E.; Dulau-Florea, A.; Wang, W.; Calvo, K.R. Acquired and germline predisposition to bone marrow failure: Diagnostic features and clinical implications. *Semin. Hematol.* **2019**, *56*, 69–82. [CrossRef]
42. Killick, S.B.; Bown, N.; Cavenagh, J.; Dokal, I.; Foukaneli, T.; Hill, A.; Hillmen, P.; Ireland, R.; Kulasekararaj, A.G.; Mufti, G.J.; et al. Guidelines for the diagnosis and management of adult aplastic anaemia. *Br. J. Haematol.* **2016**, *172*, 187–207. [CrossRef]
43. Shimamura, A.; Alter, B.P. Pathophysiology and management of inherited bone marrow failure syndromes. *Blood Rev.* **2010**, *24*, 101–122. [CrossRef]
44. Invernizzi, R.; Quaglia, F.; Della Porta, M.G. Importance of classical morphology in the diagnosis of myelodysplastic syndrome. *Mediterr. J. Hematol. Infect. Dis.* **2015**, *7*, e2015035. [CrossRef] [PubMed]
45. Greenberg, P.; Cox, C.; Lebeau, M.M.; Fenaux, P.; Morel, P.; Sanz, G.; Sanz, M.; Vallespi, T.; Hamblin, T.; Oscier, D.; et al. International scoring system for evaluating prognosis in myelodysplastic syndromes. *Blood* **1997**, *89*, 2079–2088. [CrossRef] [PubMed]
46. Greenberg, P.L.; Tuechler, H.; Schanz, J.; Sanz, G.F.; Garcia-Manero, G.; Solé, F.; Bennett, J.M.; Bowen, D.; Fenaux, P.; Dreyfus, F.; et al. Revised International Prognostic Scoring System for Myelodysplastic Syndromes. *Blood* **2012**, *120*, 2454–2465. [CrossRef]
47. Bonadies, N.; Bacher, V.U. What role can next-generation sequencing play in myelodysplastic syndrome care? *Expert Rev. Hematol.* **2019**, *12*, 379–382. [CrossRef] [PubMed]
48. Silzle, T.; Blum, S.; Schuler, E.; Kaivers, J.; Rudelius, M.; Hildebrandt, B.; Gattermann, N.; Haas, R.; Germing, U. Lymphopenia at diagnosis is highly prevalent in myelodysplastic syndromes and has an independent negative prog-nostic value in IPSS-R-low-risk patients. *Blood Cancer J.* **2019**, *9*, 63. [CrossRef] [PubMed]
49. Go, R.S.; Lust, J.A.; Phyliky, R.L. Aplastic anemia and pure red cell aplasia associated with large granular lymphocyte leukemia. *Semin. Hematol.* **2003**, *40*, 196–200. [CrossRef]
50. Wang, L.; Zhou, Y.; Tang, J.; Zhan, Q.; Liao, Y. CD4(−)/CD8(−)/CD56(+)/TCRgammadelta(+) T-cell large granular lymphocyte leukemia presenting as aplastic ane-mia: A case report and literature review. *Zhonghua Xue Ye Xue Za Zhi* **2019**, *40*, 525–527.
51. Tichelli, A.; Gratwohl, A.; Nissen, C.; Signer, E.; Gysi, C.S.; Speck, B. Morphology in patients with severe aplastic anemia treated with antilymphocyte globulin. *Blood* **1992**, *80*, 337–345. [CrossRef]
52. Rovó, A.; Ebmt, O.B.O.T.S.-W.; Tichelli, A.; Dufour, C. Diagnosis of acquired aplastic anemia. *Bone Marrow Transplant.* **2012**, *48*, 162–167. [CrossRef]
53. Arber, D.A.; Orazi, A.; Hasserjian, R.; Thiele, J.; Borowitz, M.J.; Le Beau, M.M.; Bloomfield, C.D.; Cazzola, M.; Vardiman, J.W. The 2016 revision to the World Health Organization classification of myeloid neoplasms and acute leukemia. *Blood* **2016**, *127*, 2391–2405. [CrossRef]
54. Bain, B.J.; Clark, D.M.; Wilkins, B.S. *Bone Marrow Pathology*, 4th ed.; Wiley-Blackwell: Hoboken, NJ, USA, 2009.
55. Bain, B.J. Bone marrow trephine biopsy. *J. Clin. Pathol.* **2001**, *54*, 737–742. [CrossRef]
56. Rovo, A.; Kulasekararaj, A.; Medinger, M.; Chevallier, P.; Ribera, J.M.; Peffault de Latour, R.; Knol, C.; Iacobelli, S.; Kanfer, E.; Bruno, B.; et al. Association of aplastic anaemia and lymphoma: A report from the severe aplastic anaemia working party of the Euro-pean Society of Blood and Bone Marrow Transplantation. *Br. J. Haematol.* **2019**, *184*, 294–298. [CrossRef]
57. Medinger, M.; Buser, A.; Stern, M.; Heim, D.; Halter, J.; Rovó, A.; Tzankov, A.; Tichelli, A.; Passweg, J. Aplastic anemia in association with a lymphoproliferative neoplasm: Coincidence or causality? *Leuk. Res.* **2012**, *36*, 250–251. [CrossRef]

58. Zonder, J.A.; Keating, M.; Schiffer, C.A. Chronic lymphocytic leukemia presenting in association with aplastic anemia. *Am. J. Hematol.* **2002**, *71*, 323–327. [CrossRef]
59. Westers, T.M.; Ireland, R.; Kern, W.; Alhan, C.C.; Balleisen, J.S.; Bettelheim, P.; Burbury, K.; Cullen, M.; Cutler, J.; Della Porta, M.G.; et al. Standardization of flow cytometry in myelodysplastic syndromes: A report from an international consortium and the European LeukemiaNet Working Group. *Leukemia* **2012**, *26*, 1730–1741. [CrossRef] [PubMed]
60. Stojkov, K.; Silzle, T.; Stussi, G.; Schwappach, D.; Bernhard, J.; Bowen, D.; Čermák, J.; Dinmohamed, A.G.; Eeltink, C.; Eggmann, S.; et al. Guideline-based indicators for adult patients with myelodysplastic syndromes. *Blood Adv.* **2020**, *4*, 4029–4044. [CrossRef]
61. Brodsky, R.A. Paroxysmal nocturnal hemoglobinuria. *Blood* **2014**, *124*, 2804–2811. [CrossRef]
62. Schanz, J.; Tüchler, H.; Solé, F.; Mallo, M.; Luño, E.; Cervera, J.; Granada, I.; Hildebrandt, B.; Slovak, M.L.; Ohyashiki, K.; et al. New Comprehensive Cytogenetic Scoring System for Primary Myelodysplastic Syndromes (MDS) and Oligoblastic Acute Myeloid Leukemia After MDS Derived from an International Database Merge. *J. Clin. Oncol.* **2012**, *30*, 820–829. [CrossRef]
63. Gupta, V.; Brooker, C.; Tooze, J.A.; Yi, Q.-L.; Sage, D.; Turner, D.; Kangasabapathy, P.; Marsh, J.C.W. Clinical relevance of cytogenetic abnormalities at diagnosis of acquired aplastic anaemia in adults. *Br. J. Haematol.* **2006**, *134*, 95–99. [CrossRef] [PubMed]
64. Hosokawa, K.; Katagiri, T.; Sugimori, N.; Ishiyama, K.; Sasaki, Y.; Seiki, Y.; Sato-Otsubo, A.; Sanada, M.; Ogawa, S.; Nakao, S. Favorable outcome of patients who have 13q deletion: A suggestion for revision of the WHO 'MDS-U' designation. *Haematologica* **2012**, *97*, 1845–1849. [CrossRef] [PubMed]
65. Holbro, A.; Jotterand, M.; Passweg, J.R.; Buser, A.; Tichelli, A.; Rovó, A. Comment to "Favorable outcome of patients who have 13q deletion: A suggestion for revision of the WHO 'MDS-U' designation". *Haematologica* **2013**, *98*, e46–e47. [CrossRef]
66. Heinrichs, S.; Li, C.; Look, A.T. SNP array analysis in hematologic malignancies: Avoiding false discoveries. *Blood* **2010**, *115*, 4157–4161. [CrossRef]
67. Ouahchi, I.; Zhang, L.; Brito, R.B.; Benz, R.; Müller, R.; Bonadies, N.; Tchinda, J. Microarray-based comparative genomic hybridisation reveals additional recurrent aberrations in adult patients evaluated for myelodysplastic syndrome with normal karyotype. *Br. J. Haematol.* **2019**, *184*, 282–287. [CrossRef]
68. Kamps, R.; Brandão, R.D.; Bosch, B.J.V.D.; Paulussen, A.D.C.; Xanthoulea, S.; Blok, M.J.; Romano, A. Next-Generation Sequencing in Oncology: Genetic Diagnosis, Risk Prediction and Cancer Classification. *Int. J. Mol. Sci.* **2017**, *18*, 308. [CrossRef] [PubMed]
69. Braggio, E.; Egan, J.B.; Fonseca, R.; Stewart, A.K. Lessons from next-generation sequencing analysis in hematological malignancies. *Blood Cancer J.* **2013**, *3*, e127. [CrossRef]
70. Merker, J.D.; Valouev, A.; Gotlib, J. Next-generation sequencing in hematologic malignancies: What will be the dividends? *Ther. Adv. Hematol.* **2012**, *3*, 333–339. [CrossRef]
71. Chirnomas, S.D.; Kupfer, G.M. The Inherited Bone Marrow Failure Syndromes. *Pediatr. Clin. N. Am.* **2013**, *60*, 1291–1310. [CrossRef]
72. Mangaonkar, A.A.; Patnaik, M.M. Hereditary Predisposition to Hematopoietic Neoplasms: When Bloodline Matters for Blood Cancers. *Mayo Clin. Proc.* **2020**, *95*, 1482–1498. [CrossRef]
73. Wegman-Ostrosky, T.; Savage, S.A. The genomics of inherited bone marrow failure: From mechanism to the clinic. *Br. J. Haematol.* **2017**, *177*, 526–542. [CrossRef]
74. Alter, B.P. Diagnosis, Genetics, and Management of Inherited Bone Marrow Failure Syndromes. *Hematol. Am. Soc. Hematol. Educ. Program.* **2007**, 29–39. [CrossRef] [PubMed]
75. Walne, A.J.; Collopy, L.; Cardoso, S.; Ellison, A.; Plagnol, V.; Albayrak, C.; Albayrak, D.; Kilic, S.S.; Patıroglu, T.; Akar, H.; et al. Marked overlap of four genetic syndromes with dyskeratosis congenita confounds clinical diagnosis. *Haematologica* **2016**, *101*, 1180–1189. [CrossRef] [PubMed]
76. Bluteau, O.; Sebert, M.; Leblanc, T.; De Latour, R.P.; Quentin, S.; Lainey, E.; Hernandez, L.; Dalle, J.-H.; De Fontbrune, F.S.; Lengline, E.; et al. A landscape of germ line mutations in a cohort of inherited bone marrow failure patients. *Blood* **2018**, *131*, 717–732. [CrossRef]
77. Ogawa, S. Genetics of MDS. *Blood* **2019**, *133*, 1049–1059. [CrossRef]
78. Li, M.M.; Chao, E.; Esplin, E.D.; Miller, D.T.; Nathanson, K.L.; Plon, S.E.; Scheuner, M.T.; Stewart, D.R.; ACMG Professional Practice and Guidelines Committee. Points to consider for reporting of germline variation in patients undergoing tumor testing: A statement of the Ameri-can College of Medical Genetics and Genomics (ACMG). *Genet. Med.* **2020**, *22*, 1142–1148. [CrossRef]
79. Malcovati, L.; Gallì, A.; Travaglino, E.; Ambaglio, I.; Rizzo, E.; Molteni, E.; Elena, C.; Ferretti, V.V.; Catricalà, S.; Bono, E.; et al. Clinical significance of somatic mutation in unexplained blood cytopenia. *Blood* **2017**, *129*, 3371–3378. [CrossRef]
80. Valent, P.; Orazi, A.; Steensma, D.P.; Ebert, B.L.; Haase, D.; Malcovati, L.; Van De Loosdrecht, A.A.; Haferlach, T.; Westers, T.M.; Wells, D.A.; et al. Proposed minimal diagnostic criteria for myelodysplastic syndromes (MDS) and potential pre-MDS conditions. *Oncotarget* **2017**, *8*, 73483–73500. [CrossRef]
81. Malcovati, L.; Germing, U.; Kuendgen, A.; Della Porta, M.G.; Pascutto, C.; Invernizzi, R.; Giagounidis, A.; Hildebrandt, B.; Bernasconi, P.; Knipp, S.; et al. Time-Dependent Prognostic Scoring System for Predicting Survival and Leukemic Evolution in Myelodysplastic Syndromes. *J. Clin. Oncol.* **2007**, *25*, 3503–3510. [CrossRef]
82. Charlson, M.E.; Pompei, P.; Ales, K.L.; MacKenzie, C. A new method of classifying prognostic comorbidity in longitudinal studies: Development and validation. *J. Chronic Dis.* **1987**, *40*, 373–383. [CrossRef]

83. Sorror, M.L.; Maris, M.B.; Storb, R.; Baron, F.; Sandmaier, B.M.; Maloney, D.G.; Storer, B. Hematopoietic cell transplantation (HCT)-specific comorbidity index: A new tool for risk assessment before alloge-neic HCT. *Blood* **2005**, *106*, 2912–2919. [CrossRef]
84. Sorror, M.L.; Storb, R.F.; Sandmaier, B.M.; Maziarz, R.T.; Pulsipher, M.A.; Maris, M.B.; Bhatia, S.; Ostronoff, F.; Deeg, H.J.; Syrjala, K.L.; et al. Comorbidity-Age Index: A Clinical Measure of Biologic Age Before Allogeneic Hematopoietic Cell Transplantation. *J. Clin. Oncol.* **2014**, *32*, 3249–3256. [CrossRef]
85. Della Porta, M.G.; Malcovati, L.; Strupp, C.; Ambaglio, I.; Kuendgen, A.; Zipperer, E.; Travaglino, E.; Invernizzi, R.; Pascutto, C.; Lazzarino, M.; et al. Risk stratification based on both disease status and extra-hematologic comorbidities in patients with myelo-dysplastic syndrome. *Haematologica* **2011**, *96*, 441–449. [CrossRef]
86. Swinkels, M.; Rijkers, M.; Voorberg, J.; Vidarsson, G.; Leebeek, F.W.G.; Jansen, A.J.G. Emerging Concepts in Immune Thrombocytopenia. *Front. Immunol.* **2018**, *9*, 880. [CrossRef]
87. Waisbren, J.; Dinner, S.; Altman, J.; Frankfurt, O.; Helenowski, I.; Gao, J.; McMahon, B.J.; Stein, B.L. Disease characteristics and prognosis of myelodysplastic syndrome presenting with isolated thrombocytopenia. *Int. J. Hematol.* **2016**, *105*, 44–51. [CrossRef]
88. Kuroda, J.; Kimura, S.; Kobayashi, Y.; Wada, K.; Uoshima, N.; Yoshikawa, T. Unusual myelodysplastic syndrome with the initial presentation mimicking idiopathic thrombocytopenic purpura. *Acta Haematol.* **2002**, *108*, 139–143. [CrossRef] [PubMed]
89. Bryan, J.; Jabbour, E.; Prescott, H.; Kantarjian, H. Thrombocytopenia in patients with myelodysplastic syndromes. *Semin. Hematol.* **2010**, *47*, 274–280. [CrossRef] [PubMed]
90. Mittelman, M. Good news for patients with myelodysplastic syndromes and thrombocytopenia. *Lancet Haematol.* **2018**, *5*, e100–e101. [CrossRef]
91. Manoharan, A.; Brighton, T.; Gemmell, R.; Lopez, K.; Moran, S.; Kyle, P. Platelet Dysfunction in Myelodysplastic Syndromes: A Clinicopathological Study. *Int. J. Hematol.* **2002**, *76*, 272–278. [CrossRef]
92. Galera, P.; Dulau-Florea, A.; Calvo, K.R. Inherited thrombocytopenia and platelet disorders with germline predisposition to myeloid neoplasia. *Int. J. Lab. Hematol.* **2019**, *41* (Suppl. S1), 131–141. [CrossRef]
93. Sekeres, M.A.; Schoonen, W.M.; Kantarjian, H.; List, A.; Fryzek, J.; Paquette, R.; Maciejewski, J.P. Characteristics of US Patients with Myelodysplastic Syndromes: Results of Six Cross-sectional Physician Surveys. *J. Natl. Cancer Inst.* **2008**, *100*, 1542–1551. [CrossRef]
94. Klymenko, S.V.; Belyi, D.A.; Ross, J.R.; Owzar, K.; Jiang, C.; Li, Z.; Minchenko, J.N.; Kovalenko, A.N.; Bebeshko, V.G.; Chao, N.J. Hematopoietic cell infusion for the treatment of nuclear disaster victims: New data from the Chernobyl accident. *Int. J. Radiat. Biol.* **2011**, *87*, 846–850. [CrossRef]
95. Camitta, B.M.; Rappeport, J.M.; Parkman, R.; Nathan, D.G. Selection of patients for bone marrow transplantation in severe aplastic anemia. *Blood* **1975**, *45*, 355–363. [CrossRef]
96. Bacigalupo, A.; Hows, J.; Gluckman, E.; Nissen, C.; Marsh, J.; Van Lint, M.T.; Congiu, M.; De Planque, M.M.; Ernst, P.; McCann, S.; et al. Bone marrow transplantation (BMT) versus immunosuppression for the treatment of severe aplastic anaemia (SAA): A report of the EBMT SAA Working Party. *Br. J. Haematol.* **1988**, *70*, 177–182. [CrossRef]
97. Gross, S.; Kiwanuka, J. Chronic ITP terminating in aplastic anemia. *Am. J. Pediatr. Hematol. Oncol.* **1981**, *3*, 446–448.
98. Yun, G.-W.; Yang, Y.-J.; Song, I.-C.; Baek, S.-W.; Lee, K.-S.; Lee, H.-J.; Yun, H.-J.; Kwon, K.-C.; Kim, S.; Jo, D.-Y. Long-term outcome of isolated thrombocytopenia accompanied by hypocellular marrow. *Korean J. Hematol.* **2011**, *46*, 128–134. [CrossRef]
99. Levy, I.; Laor, R.; Jiries, N.; Bejar, J.; Polliack, A.; Tadmor, T. Amegakaryocytic Thrombocytopenia and Subsequent Aplastic Anemia Associated with Apparent Epstein-Barr Virus Infection. *Acta Haematol.* **2018**, *139*, 7–11. [CrossRef]
100. King, J.A.C.; ElKhalifa, M.Y.; Latour, L.F. Rapid Progression of Acquired Amegakaryocytic Thrombocytopenia to Aplastic Anemia. *South. Med. J.* **1997**, *90*, 91–94. [CrossRef]
101. Young, N.S.; Maciejewski, J.P.; Sloand, E.; Chen, G.; Zeng, W.; Risitano, A.; Miyazato, A. The relationship of aplastic anemia and PNH. *Int. J. Hematol.* **2002**, *76*, 168–172. [CrossRef]
102. Pu, J.J.; Mukhina, G.; Wang, H.; Savage, W.J.; Brodsky, R.A. Natural history of paroxysmal nocturnal hemoglobinuria clones in patients presenting as aplastic anemia. *Eur. J. Haematol.* **2011**, *87*, 37–45. [CrossRef]
103. Sutherland, D.R.; Illingworth, A.; Marinov, I.; Ortiz, F.; Andrea, I.; Payne, D.; Wallace, P.K.; Keeney, M. ICCS/ESCCA Consensus Guidelines to detect GPI-deficient cells in Paroxysmal Nocturnal Hemoglobinuria (PNH) and related Disorders Part 2—Reagent Selection and Assay Optimization for High-Sensitivity Testing. *Cytom. Part B Clin. Cytom.* **2018**, *94*, 23–48. [CrossRef]
104. Auerbach, A.D. Fanconi anemia and its diagnosis. *Mutat. Res. Mol. Mech. Mutagen.* **2009**, *668*, 4–10. [CrossRef]
105. Malcovati, L.; Hellström-Lindberg, E.; Bowen, D.; Adès, L.; Cermak, J.; Del Cañizo, C.; Della Porta, M.G.; Fenaux, P.; Gattermann, N.; Germing, U.; et al. Diagnosis and treatment of primary myelodysplastic syndromes in adults: Recommendations from the European LeukemiaNet. *Blood* **2013**, *122*, 2943–2964. [CrossRef] [PubMed]
106. Abdel-Wahab, O.; Figueroa, M.E. Interpreting new molecular genetics in myelodysplastic syndromes. *Haematology* **2012**, *2012*, 56–64. [CrossRef]
107. Heuser, M.; Thol, F.; Ganser, A. Clonal Hematopoiesis of Indeterminate Potential. *Dtsch. Aerzteblatt Int.* **2016**, *113*, 317–322. [CrossRef]
108. Jaiswal, S.; Fontanillas, P.; Flannick, J.; Manning, A.; Grauman, P.V.; Mar, B.G.; Lindsley, R.C.; Mermel, C.H.; Burtt, N.; Chavez, A.; et al. Age-Related Clonal Hematopoiesis Associated with Adverse Outcomes. *N. Engl. J. Med.* **2014**, *371*, 2488–2498. [CrossRef] [PubMed]

109. Genovese, G.; Kähler, A.K.; Handsaker, R.E.; Lindberg, J.; Rose, S.A.; Bakhoum, S.F.; Chambert, K.; Mick, E.; Neale, B.M.; Fromer, M.; et al. Clonal Hematopoiesis and Blood-Cancer Risk Inferred from Blood DNA Sequence. *N. Engl. J. Med.* **2014**, *371*, 2477–2487. [CrossRef] [PubMed]
110. Xie, M.; Lu, C.; Wang, J.; McLellan, M.D.; Johnson, K.J.; Wendl, M.C.; McMichael, J.F.; Schmidt, H.K.; Yellapantula, V.; Miller, C.A.; et al. Age-related mutations associated with clonal hematopoietic expansion and malignancies. *Nat. Med.* **2014**, *20*, 1472–1478. [CrossRef]
111. Steensma, D.P.; Bejar, R.; Jaiswal, S.; Lindsley, R.C.; Sekeres, M.A.; Hasserjian, R.P.; Ebert, B.L. Clonal hematopoiesis of indeterminate potential and its distinction from myelodysplastic syndromes. *Blood* **2015**, *126*, 9–16. [CrossRef] [PubMed]

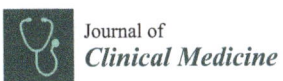

Review

Platelet Phenotyping and Function Testing in Thrombocytopenia

Kerstin Jurk [1,*] and Yavar Shiravand [2]

[1] Center for Thrombosis and Hemostasis (CTH), University Medical Center of the Johannes Gutenberg University Mainz, 55131 Mainz, Germany
[2] Department of Molecular Medicine and Medical Biotechnology, University of Naples Federico II, 80131 Naples, Italy; shiravandy@gmail.com
* Correspondence: kerstin.jurk@unimedizin-mainz.de; Tel.: +49-6131-178278

Abstract: Patients who suffer from inherited or acquired thrombocytopenia can be also affected by platelet function defects, which potentially increase the risk of severe and life-threatening bleeding complications. A plethora of tests and assays for platelet phenotyping and function analysis are available, which are, in part, feasible in clinical practice due to adequate point-of-care qualities. However, most of them are time-consuming, require experienced and skilled personnel for platelet handling and processing, and are therefore well-established only in specialized laboratories. This review summarizes major indications, methods/assays for platelet phenotyping, and in vitro function testing in blood samples with reduced platelet count in relation to their clinical practicability. In addition, the diagnostic significance, difficulties, and challenges of selected tests to evaluate the hemostatic capacity and specific defects of platelets with reduced number are addressed.

Keywords: thrombocytopenia; bleeding; platelet function tests; platelet disorders; platelet count; flow cytometry

1. Introduction

Platelet bleeding disorders are a heterogeneous group in terms of frequency and bleeding severity. They are characterized by qualitative/function and/or quantitative/number platelet defects. Patients with a platelet count of less than 150×10^9/L in whole blood present with thrombocytopenia, which is caused by inadequate megakaryopoiesis and platelet production or enhanced platelet clearance due to platelet destruction or pathological platelet activation. Rare gene defects cause inherited thrombocytopenia, but thrombocytopenia is more frequently acquired in response to systemic disease manifestations (e.g., uremia, liver disease, and myeloproliferative disorders), autoimmune diseases (e.g., idiopathic thrombocytopenic purpura (ITP), heparin-induced thrombocytopenia (HIT), thrombotic thrombocytopenic purpura (TTP), and antiphospholipid syndrome), infection, pregnancy, surgery, transfusion, and certain drugs (e.g., heparin, thiazide diuretics, and tamoxifen). Severe thrombocytopenia with a platelet count of less than 50×10^9/L increases the risk of spontaneous skin and mucocutaneous bleeding diathesis, such as petechiae, ecchymoses, epistaxis, menorrhagia, and gastrointestinal bleeding. However, bleeding due to major hemostatic challenges (e.g., surgery and trauma) is especially frequently observed when moderate (50–100 $\times 10^9$ platelets/L) and even mild thrombocytopenia (>100–<150 $\times 10^9$ platelets/L) is associated with inherited or acquired platelet dysfunction [1].

Though inherited platelet function disorders are rare, their prevalence is underestimated due to limited diagnostic potential. Multiple platelet phenotype and functional tests are recommended by different laboratory guidelines for the diagnosis of platelet function disorders [2–4]. Recently, the Scientific and Standardization Committee (SSC) "Platelet Physiology" of the International Society on Thrombosis and Haemostasis (ISTH) established a three-step algorithm of platelet function tests for the identification of well-known and complex entities of inherited platelet function disorders, which are commonly associated with mild-to-moderate bleeding diathesis [3,5]. However, only a couple of tests allow for a standardized and easy-to-use analysis of platelet function in clinical routine practice. Indeed, most platelet function tests require skilled personnel and are restricted to specialized platelet laboratories, which have to ensure intra-laboratory standardization and validated reference values. Furthermore, platelet function testing in thrombocytopenia requires expertise and experience about sensitivity and the limitations of reduced platelet counts for each test. This review addresses major indications, methods/assays for platelet phenotyping, and in vitro function testing in blood samples with reduced platelet count in relation to their clinical practicability. In addition, the diagnostic significance, difficulties, and challenges of selected tests to evaluate the hemostatic capacity and specific defects of platelets in reduced number are summarized.

2. Indications for Testing Platelet Phenotype and Function in Thrombocytopenia

Though a low platelet count significantly increases the risk for hemorrhagic complications, many patients with thrombocytopenia, even with a severe reduction of the platelet count, do not suffer from spontaneous, clinically relevant bleeding. Previous studies have not provided much evidence that bleeding risk is associated with platelet count in patients with acquired thrombocytopenia caused by hematological malignancies, non-hematological cancer, sepsis, and chronic liver and renal disease [6–8], and impaired platelet function has been demonstrated in these disease entities [9–12]. However, the molecular mechanisms responsible for platelet dysfunction in acquired thrombocytopenias are only marginally understood. There is evidence that alterations in megakaryopoiesis and platelet production leads to defective platelet activation/aggregation and granule storage pool deficiency (SPD) in patients with acute leukemia and myelodysplastic syndromes [9]. Patients with advanced chronic liver, e.g., cirrhosis, and kidney disease, e.g., uremia, are known to show impaired platelet activation induced by several agonists, as determined by flow cytometry (see Section 5.3) and aggregation tests (see Section 5.1). Acquired storage pool defects, defective transmembrane signaling associated with the reduced surface expression of integrin αIIbβ3 and proteolytically cleaved glycoprotein (GP) Ibα, dysregulated arachidonic and thromboxane A_2 (TxA_2) metabolism, diminished cytosolic Ca^{2+} release/entry, and elevated cytosolic levels of inhibitory second messengers, i.e., cyclic adenosine monophosphate (cAMP) and guanosine monophosphate (cGMP), have been observed for both systemic diseases. On the one hand, it has been suggested that the hyporeactive platelet phenotype in vitro is caused by in vivo activation and "exhaustion" during intravascular activation. On the other hand, increased levels of different plasma factors, e.g., fibrin(ogen) degradation products, bile salts, ethanol, and uremic toxins (like phenol, phenolic acid, and guanidine succinic acid), may interfere with platelets, thus leading to hyporeactivity [10,12,13]. An increased in vivo activation status of platelets, leading to platelet exhaustion and impaired platelet reactivity in vitro, is observed in patients with sepsis when bacterial and viral infections are dysregulated. Here, platelet activation is mediated by direct interactions with pathogens via pattern recognition receptors, the release of inflammatory mediators from leukocytes and endothelial cells, and complement activation [11]. The enhanced formation of pathogen-coated and -stimulated platelets drives platelet clearance and turnover, leading to thrombocytopenia and increased levels of more reactive immature/reticulated platelets, respectively (see Section 3.3). The immature platelet fraction has been suggested to predict sepsis severity [14].

In addition, platelet dysfunction associated with acquired thrombocytopenia is frequently observed in hospitalized patients to be caused by iatrogenic etiologies, including drug-induced immune thrombocytopenia [15,16], major surgery, and extracorporeal/mechanical circulatory support. Ventricular assist devices (VADs) and the extracorporeal membrane oxygenation (ECMO) device induce pathological hemodynamics associated with high shear stress and contact of platelets with non-physiological mechanical surfaces. Acquired von Willebrand disease (VWD) may result from elevated shear stress conditions and is characterized by the loss of high-molecular-weight multimers of the von Willebrand factor (VWF), leading to impaired VWF-mediated platelet functions. Furthermore, platelets become activated by interacting with non-physiological mechanical surfaces, leading to the pronounced platelet consumption and impaired capacity of granule secretion and aggregation in vitro [17].

Inherited thrombocytopenias are commonly caused by pathogenic variants of genes encoding for proteins involved in megakaryopoiesis (e.g., thrombopoietin (THPO)/ myeloproliferative leukemia virus (MPL) signaling and transcription regulation), megakaryocyte maturation (i.e., granulopoiesis and trafficking), and platelet production/release (i.e., cytoskeleton regulation and glycoprotein receptor signaling). For a detailed overview of inherited thrombocytopenias, the reader is referred to the review about inherited thrombocytopenias by Paolo Gresele in this special issue on "The Latest Clinical Advances of Thrombocytopenia." Recent studies have shown that a significant proportion of defective genes causing thrombocytopenia also affect platelet function. Figure 1 and Table S1 present an overview of important disease-causing genes related to thrombocytopenia that are associated with platelet function defects. Biallelic Bernard–Soulier syndrome (BSS), gray platelet syndrome (GPS), platelet type VWD, and Wiskott–Aldrich syndrome (WAS) are well-known platelet number and function disorders that are additionally characterized by abnormal platelet volume. Thus, the intrinsic hemostatic capacity of platelets needs to be viewed as reflection of platelet count, size/volume (platelet mass), and function.

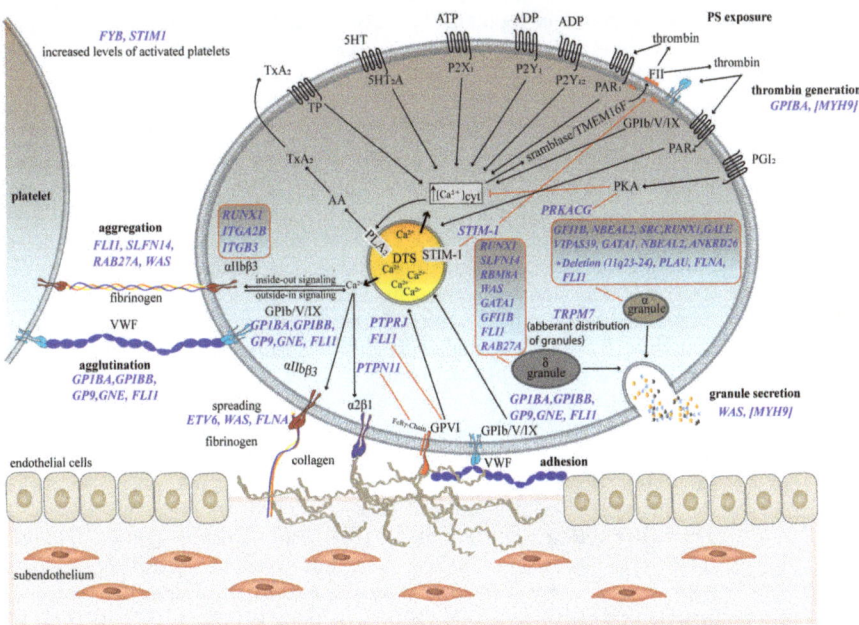

Figure 1. Current view of important thrombocytopenia-causing genes associated with platelet function defects. Gene names (blue italic font), activating responses (black arrow), inhibitory effects (red blunted arrow), and gene mutation consequences (red line) are indicated, and further details are listed in Table S1 [18–22]. *MYH9*-associated platelet dysfunction according to a case report [23]. VWF: Von Willebrand factor; ADP: adenosine diphosphate; PAR: proteinase-activated receptor; PLA$_2$: phospholipase A$_2$; PKA: protein kinase A; STIM-1: stromal interaction molecule-1; TMEM16F: transmembrane protein 16F; TxA$_2$: thromboxane A$_2$; TP: TxA$_2$ receptor; AA: arachidonic acid; PGI$_2$: prostacyclin; DTS: dense tubular system; GP: glycoprotein; PS: phosphatidylserine.

Overall, platelet function testing in thrombocytopenia is essential (1) if the level of platelet count reduction cannot explain the bleeding tendency and (2) to complement the diagnosis of known and novel thrombocytopenic diseases with potential bleeding risk, even when pathogenic or likely-pathogenic mutation(s) could be identified by next generation sequencing (NGS). Platelet function tests allow for, depending on the technique, (1) the evaluation of the overall hemostatic platelet activity and (2) the identification of specific platelet function defects and their molecular targets. It is noteworthy to recapitulate the strengths and limitations of each platelet function test with regard to the sensitivity and specificity for different platelet function parameters and their utility for the analysis of the global hemostatic capacity of whole blood, the intrinsic hemostatic capacity of platelets, and specific platelet responses/molecular targets. Platelet function testing may only contribute to the evaluation of the potential bleeding risk in thrombocytopenia, as other hemostatic factors of other blood and vascular cells could impair overall hemostatic capacity. In addition, prospective clinical cohort studies, which are yet very limited, are necessary for the evaluation of the predictive value of platelet function tests for bleeding, especially in case of thrombocytopenic diseases. Thus far, there is a lack of evidence for most platelet function assays to predict prophylactic platelet transfusions or other "pro"-platelet therapies.

3. Platelet Phenotyping in Thrombocytopenia

Before platelet function testing should be applied, an extensive clinical evaluation of the patient's and family's bleeding history; an examination of other disease manifestations, medication and/or food affecting platelet function; a laboratory assessment of platelet count, size, morphology, as well as of plasma coagulation/fibrinolysis and VWF parameters, are essential.

3.1. Bleeding Assessment Tool (BAT)

The use of a standardized bleeding assessment tool (BAT) is recommended to calculate a bleeding score for the accurate evaluation of the bleeding tendency. In addition to the bleeding score of the World Health Organization (WHO), several BATs have been established, especially for type 1 VWD [24]. More recently, the SSC "Platelet Physiology" of the ISTH performed a validation study to test the diagnostic utility of the type 1 VWD ISTH-BAT for inherited platelet function and number disorders in a large cohort with more than of 1000 patients across 17 countries worldwide [25]. Inherited platelet function disorders (IPFDs), including major disorders with 40% Glanzmann thrombasthenia, 11% δ-SPD, and about 10% primary secretion defect, as well as 10% thrombocytopenic patients with biallelic BSS, showed a median bleeding score of 9 and an excellent discrimination power between IPFD (bleeding score > 6) and age/sex-matched healthy controls compared to the WHO bleeding score. In contrast, inherited platelet number disorders (IPNDs), including major disorders with about 41% *MYH9*-related disorders, 22% *ANKRD26*-related thrombocytopenia, 19% monoallelic BSS, and 8% *ETV6*-related thrombocytopenia, had a median bleeding score of 2, and ISTH-BAT had a poor discrimination power between IPND and healthy controls. This study also confirmed that patients with IPFD have a higher number of bleeding symptoms and a higher percentage with clinically relevant symptoms than patients with IPND. However, a specific comparison of the ISTH bleeding score between thrombocytopenic patients without and with associated platelet dysfunction has not been performed yet.

3.2. Laboratory Assessment of Platelet Count, Size and Global Morphology

Platelet counting in ethylenediaminetetraacetic acid (EDTA)-anticoagulated whole blood is the first step of platelet phenotyping, especially to exclude thrombocytopenia. Automatic impedance-based cell counters enable the discrimination of low platelet counts when the mean platelet volume is calculated within normal ranges. However, enlarged or giant platelets are not detected as platelets, and sometimes conjugation between platelets and with leukocytes occur (pseudo-thrombocytopenia in EDTA-anticoagulated whole blood), leading to artificially lower platelet counts. In case of an automatically calculated reduced platelet count, the analysis of a May–Grünwald–Giemsa-stained blood smear of EDTA- and non-EDTA- (e.g., 3.2%/109 mM tri-sodium-citrate) anticoagulated whole blood is recommended by light microscopy for the calculation of the count of normal and abnormal sized platelets (e.g., microplatelets detected in WAS and giant platelets observed in biallelic BSS), as well as to exclude pseudo-thrombocytopenia. This method also allows for the assessment of the first morphological alterations of platelets. A pale phenotype of large platelets is indicative of a deficiency of α-granules, as observed for the classical GPS caused by pathogenic *NBEAL-2*-variants, *GFI1b*-related thrombocytopenia caused by *GFI1b*-mutations, and the arthrogryposis—renal dysfunction—cholestasis (ARC)-syndrome caused by pathogenic gene variants in *VPS33B* or *VIPAS39*. *GATA1*-related diseases are typically characterized by a subpopulation of large and vacuolated platelets, and they could be associated with a decreased number of α-granules or a combined α-/δ-storage pool defect [26,27]. In contrast, alterations in the phenotype of neutrophils with "Döhle-like" bodies associated with giant platelet populations are typical for *MYH9*-related diseases such as the May–Hegglin anomaly [18,28] (Table S1 and Figure 1). However, platelet δ-granule defects are not detectable on a conventionally stained blood smear.

3.3. Blood Smear Analysis by Immunofluorescence Microscopy

Recently, advanced immunofluorescence microscopy was used to analyze dried blood films stained with fluorochrome-labeled monoclonal antibodies detecting platelet-specific, surface receptor-related proteins (e.g., GPIb and GPIX of the VWF-receptor complex), α-granule membrane and cargo proteins (P-selectin, thrombospondin-1 (TSP-1), and VWF), and cytoskeletal proteins (i.e., β1-tubulin and filamin-A). This technique facilitates the phenotypic diagnosis of a BSS, α-granule deficiency-related macrothrombocytopenias (e.g., GPS and *GFBI1*-related thrombocytopenia), and *TUBB1*- and *FLNA*-related thrombocytopenia [29,30] (Table S1 and Figure 1).

3.4. Quantitation of Immature/Reticulated Platelets

On the other hand, increased thrombopoiesis in acquired thrombocytopenia, as observed in immune thrombocytopenia or after severe infection, leads to an increased number of young/immature circulating platelets that are larger and enriched in messenger RNA— so-called "reticulated" platelets [31]. There is evidence that reticulated platelets are more reactive than "mature" platelets, and reticulated platelets have been suggested to have the potential to partly compensate for impaired hemostasis in thrombocytopenic ITP patients [32]. However, the use of immature platelet levels as predictive markers for bleeding in thrombocytopenic patients needs further validation in large prospective clinical studies. Some types of fully automated hematology analyzers used in clinical routine laboratories are based on light scatter and fluorescence detection, which allows for the quantification of large(r) and reticulated platelets stained with RNA-specific fluorescent dyes (immature platelet count or fraction in percent). Though automated hematology analyzers offer standardization for different labs, results obtained from laboratories of different companies are not yet comparable [31].

3.5. Flow Cytometry

The flow cytometric analysis of platelet count, size, and immature platelets (RNA stained by thiazole orange or SYTO-13) serves as alternative technique, but skilled personnel is required to permit intra-laboratory standardization and validation [33,34]. The quantitation of platelet surface receptors in citrated whole blood or the assessment of mepacrine uptake in isolated platelets ex vivo at resting conditions by flow cytometry is recommended to support the diagnosis of receptor-linked thrombocytopenias (e.g., BSS) [3] or δ-SPD [35] (see Section 5.3).

3.6. Phenotyping of Platelet Granule Defects by Electron Microscopy and ELISA

Sophisticated transmission electron microscopy techniques allow for the detailed analysis of the altered ultrastructure and morphology of platelets, even at low platelet count [36,37]. In specialized laboratories, a reduced number or deficiency of platelet α- and δ-granules can be validated by transmission electron microscopy and whole mount electron microscopy, respectively [38]. Advanced focused ion beam-scanning electron microscopy enables the visualization of the spatial distribution of platelet α- and δ-granules but is also restricted to specialized laboratories [39]. Commercially available ELISA-based tests allow for the quantitation of specific α-granule proteins, e.g., platelet factor 4 (PF4), β-thromboglobulin, and TSP-1, in the lysates of resting platelets, which are separated from plasma proteins. The sensitivity of such ELISAs determines the cut-off for the platelet count in isolated platelet samples. Granule defects are frequently observed for distinct syndromic thrombocytopenias such as WAS, GPS, and ARC (reduced number or deficiency of α-granules), as well as Paris-Trousseau and Jacobsen syndromes (alterations in α-granule phenotype and δ-SPD) (Table S1 and Figure 1).

4. Point-of-Care-Related Platelet Function Tests

The practicability of platelet function tests in clinical routine is defined by point-of-care (POC) attributes, e.g., near patient usage, simple and easy use, automatization, and rapid read outs. These attributes prefer analysis in whole blood without sample processing. The spectrum of platelet function tests is remarkable [40]. However, only a few tests share the POC criteria. This section summarizes the limitations and challenges of thrombocytopenia for a selection of frequently clinically used platelet function tests.

4.1. Impedance-Based Aggregometry—Multiplate® Analyzer

Platelet aggregation responses induced by a variety of platelet agonists are widely used read-out parameters for screening platelet function in primary hemostasis (Figure 1). Impedance-based multiple electrode aggregometers allow for the quantitation of platelet aggregation in anticoagulated whole blood through the detection of increased electrode coating by aggregated platelets over time under stirring conditions at 37 °C. These global devices allow for the assessment of the hemostatic capacity of platelets determined by platelet count, size, and function, but they also represent the overall hemostatic capacity of whole blood, which is further affected by red blood cells (hematocrit) and leukocytes (count and function) [2,41].

The Multiplate analyzer® serves as clinical pioneer of multiple electrode aggregometry, which was originally developed as semi-automated POC monitoring test for antiplatelet drugs (e.g., aspirin, purinergic adenosine diphosphate (ADP) receptor $P2Y_{12}$ blockers, and GPIIb/IIIa antagonists) in diluted hirudin-anticoagulated whole blood [42,43]. However, its utility for the diagnosis of platelet dysfunction is quite limited. This test showed a good correlation with light transmission aggregometry according to Born (see Section 5.1) in detecting impaired platelet aggregation from patients with severe platelet function disorders and normal platelet count, such as Glanzmann thrombasthenia [44,45]. Conversely, it lacks sensitivity and specificity for the diagnosing of mild platelet disorders [46,47], which are frequently observed in thrombocytopenias [18] (Table S1). In addition, multiple electrode aggregometry shows a high sensitivity for platelet count in samples from thrombocytopenic patients [48], as well as from healthy donors after the adjustment of platelets in vitro to low and even to normal (150–450 × 10^9/L) counts [49]. Notably, the platelet count is recommended to be adjusted with a buffer (e.g., Tyrode's buffer at pH 7.4) and not with platelet-poor plasma (PPP) due to the potential inhibitory effects of PPP on platelet function [49,50]. Thus, the Multiplate device is able to screen the hemostatic capacity of the whole blood environment and antiplatelet drugs, but it is not recommended for the specific detection of platelet dysfunction in thrombocytopenia [3,49]. Alternatively, control samples with adjusted platelet count have the potential to serve as references [32,49,51]. However, the preparation of such standardized and validated control samples is very time-consuming and requires expertise in platelet handling, which is commonly not feasible in clinical practice.

4.2. Platelet Function Analyzer (PFA)

The platelet function analyzer (PFA-100®, INNOVANCE® PFA-200) was originally developed as rapid and standardized technique to assess bleeding time in vitro. This test measured the occlusion time in seconds of a collagen/ADP or collagen/epinephrine-coated aperture when platelets adhere and aggregate under high arterial shear rate (>5000/s) in buffered citrated (3.8%) whole blood [52]. Thus, global VWF-dependent primary hemostasis is screened, and the pathological prolongation of the closure time may be indicative of a moderate-to-severe VWD or platelet function defects [47,53,54] but not for mild platelet disorders (e.g., storage pool defects and primary secretion defects) due to the lack of specificity and sensitivity [55,56]. In addition to VWF levels, important determinants are low hematocrit and platelet count. Therefore, samples from thrombocytopenic patients with a platelet count <100 × 10^9/L and/or a hematocrit measurement of less than 30% should not be analyzed. Due to all these limitations, the PFA device is no longer recommended by the ISTH and others for the diagnosis of platelet function defects [3,57].

4.3. Impact-R™ System

The Impact-R™ system represents a semi-automated cone and plate(let) analyzer (CPA). Platelet adhesion and aggregation are determined on a polystyrene surface immobilized by plasma proteins (e.g., VWF) in citrated whole blood under arterial shear rate (1800/s), which is induced by a rotating cone. May–Grünwald-stained platelets are quantified as the percent surface coverage and average size in μm by an image analyzer [58]. Similar to the PFA device, the CPA is sensitive to VWF plasma levels, hematocrit, and platelet count, but it could be used as a supportive platelet function test for the diagnosis of biallelic BSS [59] and for the analysis of the effect of low plasma a disintegrin and metalloprotease with thrombospondin type 1 motif 13 (ADAMTS-13) activity on VWF-mediated platelet adhesion and aggregation in patients with TTP [60]. The CPA device even allows for the analysis of blood samples from patients with severe acquired thrombocytopenia such as ITP [61]. However, previous studies with thrombocytopenic patients have been very limited and did not adjust for platelet count and hematocrit in control samples [62].

4.4. Thromboelastography/Metry

The viscoelastic-based methods, thromboelastography (TEG®) and thromboelastometry (ROTEM®) quantify different parameters of global coagulation and fibrinolysis, respectively, in anticoagulated whole blood, characterized by clot initiation, formation, strength/stiffness, and clot resolution/lysis. Both devices were primarily developed for the peri-/post-operative coagulation and transfusion management [63]. Platelet reactivity in vitro significantly contributes to thrombin generation, clot retraction, and the activation of fibrinolysis [64,65], and the interaction between platelets, fibrin, and its stabilization by activated factor XIII are important determinants for clot strength. However, thromboelastography/metry is not sufficiently sensitive to alterations in platelet function induced by antiplatelet drugs such as aspirin and $P2Y_{12}$ blockers [66]. Therefore, the TEG system has been updated to the Platelet Mapping™ system, which is more sensitive to the platelet-induced increase of clot strength in response to arachidonic acid and ADP. However, sensitivity to platelet dysfunction is still limited and only valid for severe platelet function defects, as observed for the non-thrombocytopenic inherited disorder Glanzmann thrombasthenia [67]. Strikingly, clot strength is also affected by low platelet count in thrombocytopenic samples, so it is not surprising that a lower clot strength is observed in samples from severe and moderate thrombocytopenic patients with BSS and immune thrombocytopenia [67–69]. A prospective observational study, ATHENA (risk factors for bleeding in haematology patients with low platelet counts), including 50 patients with hematological malignancies and moderate-to-severe thrombocytopenia, showed a significant association between the ROTEM parameter "maximum clot firmness (MCF)" and bleeding among these patients, which was lost after the statistical adjustment for platelet count [70]. This study demonstrated that the observed low MCF exclusively depends on a low platelet count and was not further affected by potentially additional platelet dysfunction. Thus, TEG and ROTEM devices quantify the overall coagulation and fibrinolysis capacity of blood, but they cannot discriminate between the effects of platelet count and function and therefore should not be used for the diagnosis of platelet function defects in thrombocytopenic samples [66,71].

In summary, most of the clinically used whole blood platelet function tests, which share POC attributes, are recommended to screen global processes of primary and secondary hemostasis. These overall hemostatic activities depend on platelet function, count, and size/volume—in addition to hematocrit, leukocyte count/function and plasma coagulation/fibrinolysis factors—and are not sensitive to evaluate platelet function defects in samples with low platelet counts. The establishment of standardized control samples with adjusted platelet count or platelet mass may solve this limitation, but that requires skilled personnel and represents a great challenge for clinical routine laboratories. The impact of thrombocytopenia on POC-related platelet function tests, described here, is summarized in Table S2.

5. Specialized Platelet Function Tests

Light transmission aggregometry according to Born [72] still represents the gold standard test for platelet function, as well as for the diagnosis of platelet function disorders in clinical routine laboratories. In addition, the lumi-aggregometry has also gained more and more clinical feasibility for the diagnosis of defects in platelet δ-granule secretion, which are associated with inherited (Figure 1) and acquired thrombocytopenias. Though LTA and lumi-aggregometry are being introduced more and more in clinical centers, they require skilled personnel and time-consuming standardization, which is already established in specialized platelet laboratories. Additional important assays predominantly developed for research proposes have been implemented in a panel of tests for the diagnosis of platelet function disorders.

Specific tests allowing for platelet function analysis in anticoagulated whole blood are preferable if only small blood volumes from patients are available or if specific platelet functions require testing in a more physiological environment. For the analysis of platelet-specific activation responses, platelets are isolated as platelet-rich plasma (PRP) or depleted from plasma proteins and leukocytes by advanced washing procedures [73] or gel-filtration [74], which also allow for a concentration process for platelets and thereby platelet analysis for patients with severe thrombocytopenia. The latter techniques are time-consuming and require skilled personnel with extensive expertise in platelet handling and processing.

This section focuses on advantages, options, and clinical utility, as well as the limitations and challenges, of specialized tests for the evaluation of platelet function defects from thrombocytopenic patients. Table S2 summarizes the impact of thrombocytopenia on specialized platelet function tests, as described in the following sections.

5.1. Light Transmission Aggregometry in Platelet-Rich Plasma (LTA)

The turbidimetric-based LTA according to Born [72] photometrically detects an increase in light transmittance over time at 37 °C, which results from the agonist-induced aggregation (fibrinogen-dependent) or agglutination (VWF-dependent) of stirred platelets in platelet-rich plasma. In contrast to impedance-based aggregometry, LTA requires a centrifugation step of citrated whole blood to obtain PRP and a further centrifugation step of the buffy coat to obtain PPP, which serves as a reference [75]. In addition, LTA allows for a more precise analysis of the platelet aggregation process, which includes shape change properties and the detection of reversible platelet aggregation (disaggregation) indicative of a used threshold agonist concentrations and for defects in the platelet release of amplification agonists such as ADP/ATP from the δ-granules and TxA_2.

Multiple platelet agonists are commercially available to evaluate platelet aggregability in vitro. The SSC "platelet physiology" of the ISTH recommends LTA as a first-line screening assay for the diagnosis of inherited platelet function disorders by using classical platelet agonists, e.g., ADP (targeting the purinergic ADP receptors $P2Y_1$ and $P2Y_{12}$), arachidonic acid (targeting Cox-1-related pathways for synthesis and release of TxA2 and TxA2 receptor (TP receptor)), collagen (targeting the collagen receptors integrin α2β1 and GPVI), epinephrine (targeting α2A receptor), and ristocetin (targeting VWF-mediated crosslinking of platelets via the GPIb/V/IX receptor complex (agglutination)) [3]. Further platelet agonists are recommended for extended analysis, including selective GPVI agonists, e.g., collagen-related peptide (cross-linked collagen-related peptide (CRP-XL)) and convulxin), α-thrombin (targeting the thrombin receptors GPIbα, proteinase-activated receptor (PAR)-1, and PAR-4), PAR-1 activating peptide (i.e., thrombin receptor activating peptide-6 (TRAP-6)), PAR-4 activating peptide, TxA2 mimetics (e.g., U46619), Ca^{2+}-ionophore, and phorbol 12-myristate 13-acetate (PMA). International guidelines refer to pre-analytical considerations and pitfalls, as well as standardized procedures, which also include recommendations for standardized agonist concentrations [76,77].

Recently, an inter-laboratory external quality assessment was performed by the THROMKID-Plus Study Group of the German Society of Thrombosis and Haemostais Reasearch (GTH) and German Society for Pediatric Oncology and Hematology (GPOH) in Germany and Austria for the standardization of light transmission aggregometry. Five different agonists were selected according to the guidelines of the SSC/ISTH [75] and shipped to 15 specialized laboratories, which used two different types of light transmission aggregometers [78]. Three sets of agonists were chosen to simulate a healthy subject and inherited or acquired platelet function disorders. This trial showed very consistent data for the maximum percentage of aggregation induced by the same agonists and concentrations, demonstrating the feasibility of agonist shipment for an inter-laboratory survey of LTA. However, this trial also confirmed the results of other international surveys in that there is still a high variability in laboratory-internal agonists in terms of reagent type, concentration, and pathological cut-off values, which significantly limits the exchange of LTA results between different clinical centers [79–81]. The automatization of LTA has been developed to increase standardized operation, which was reviewed by Le Blanc et al. [82].

LTA measurements with a normal platelet count (150–600 × 10^9/L) in PRP have been shown to be stable. Low platelet counts of less than 150 × 10^9/L and at least ≤100 × 10^9/L in PRP are insensitive for the valid evaluation of platelet aggregation defects [75]. Compared to whole blood assays, the platelet count here is relevant in PRP and not in whole blood, which often allows for the extension of LTA application to patients with mild and even moderate thrombocytopenia. Optional control samples from healthy donors with comparably low platelet counts adjusted with a buffer and not with PPP (>100–<150 × 10^9/L) [50,75] and that are measured within the same day of analysis may serve as intra-laboratory references. For platelet samples from patients with macrothrombocytopenia, PRP can be generated by very low centrifugation force or by sedimentation. Here, the platelet mass has to be adjusted in control samples.

Normal platelet aggregation responses to physiological platelet agonists—with the exception of ristocetin, which induces platelet agglutination by the VWF-mediated crosslinking of the GPIb/V/IX receptor complex—are indicative of biallelic BSS when observed with macrothrombocytopenia and when VWD could be excluded. Conversely, platelets with platelet-type VWD show increased agglutination responses induced by a subthreshold concentration of ristocetin (≤0.6 mg/mL) similar to type 2B VWD. Platelet–plasma exchange experiments with blood from patient and healthy donors are recommended to discriminate these two bleeding disorders. The differential impairment of agonist-induced platelet aggregation has been shown to be indicative of further hereditary thrombocytopenias associated with platelet function defects, including WAS, GPS, *GFI1*-related thrombocytopenia, ARC syndrome, and Stormorken syndrome [5,40,77]. Reversible aggregation characterized by an unstable second wave may be indicative for δ-granule or TxA_2 release disorders when the agonist concentrations are titrated in a standardized manner. Notably, LTA alone is not sensitive enough for a definite diagnosis of platelet function disorders associated with thrombocytopenia, especially for mild forms such as storage pool deficiencies [83], and it therefore needs to be complemented by other specific tests of platelet phenotyping and function.

5.2. Lumi-Aggregometry in Platelet-Rich Plasma

Lumi-aggregometry is a further development of light transmission (PRP) and impedance-based aggregometry (whole blood) for the simultaneous detection of agonist-induced platelet aggregation and the release of ADP/ATP from δ-granules. The luciferase-catalyzed conversion of luciferin in the presence of ATP generates bioluminescence, which is detected and quantified. ADP is measured by its conversion to ATP catalyzed by pyruvate kinase in the presence of phosphoenolpyruvate. This approach can be performed in anticoagulated whole blood, but as described for other whole blood tests, analysis in PRP provides platelet-specific results [84]. Similar to LTA, lumi-aggregometry in PRP requires time and expertise for the generation of PRP and PPP. In contrast to LTA, lumi-aggregometry clearly indicates the impairment of platelet δ-granule release capacity in vitro [83] but shows a higher variability and less reproducibility than LTA [85]. This might be due to additional variables regarding the preparation and incubation of the luciferin/luciferase reagent. The secretion of δ-granules is also triggered by integrin αIIbβ3 outside-in signaling, thereby facilitating the irreversible aggregation response [86]. Thus, it should be considered that impaired platelet aggregation may affect ATP release from δ-granules in this assay. A further limitation is that δ-SPD cannot be distinguished from granule release defects (primary secretion defects), which are commonly caused by impaired signal transduction. Therefore, complementary assays have to be performed, either to validate a δ-SPD by transmission electron microscopy, the bioluminescence-/HPLC-based quantification of ATP in lysates of resting platelets, and the flow cytometric quantitation of mepacrine uptake in resting platelets (Sections 3.5 and 5.3) or to confirm a δ-granule secretion defect by the same assays using lysates and intact platelets treated by strong agonists. The advantages and limitations for the analysis of thrombocytopenic samples are similar as described for LTA. The intra-laboratory standardization of operation and establishment of normal reference ranges are therefore also essential for LTA and lumi-aggregometry.

5.3. Flow Cytometry (Whole Blood, Platelet-Rich Plasma)

Flow cytometry is recommended to be used for first-line screening assays, as well as for the evaluation of specific defects in platelet phenotype and function attributes [3,87,88]. Flow cytometry represents the standard technique to quantify receptors and distinct platelet activation markers on the surface of platelets in citrated whole blood for the evaluation of quantitative receptor defects and increased platelet activation status in vivo, including the shedding of surface membrane receptors. The in vitro assessment of platelet reactivity in response to a variety of agonists (see Section 5.1, with the exception of the use of commercially available collagen types with large fibrils), especially in low amounts of whole blood, demonstrates further strengths [43,89]. A large spectrum of different fluorochrome-conjugated monoclonal antibodies, proteins, and fluorescent dyes are commercially available, which allow for a comprehensive phenotyping of single platelets and platelet populations [89,90]. The tracking of intracellular Ca^{2+} release and protein phosphorylation by using phosphosite-specific antibodies are powerful tools to evaluate signal transduction defects in platelets [91,92]. Imaging flow cytometry and mass cytometry are promising new flow cytometric developments of flow cytometry to identify platelet subpopulations [40,93]. Though there is a high variability of protocols and standard operation procedures (SOPs) between different laboratories, intra-laboratory standardization, the validation of assays, and laboratory internal reference ranges are essential and need to be established in diagnosis laboratories. Advanced protocols for platelet antibody labeling and fixation in whole blood enable the remote platelet function testing of shipped blood samples [94]. Flow cytometry-based single cell analysis provides platelet assays, which are largely independent of platelet count and thereby feasible in blood from patients even with severe thrombocytopenia [95,96]. However, a recent study indicated that a platelet count of $\leq 10 \times 10^9$/mL might influence in vitro platelet activation assays due to the platelet count-related decreased release of ADP, which serves as important amplifier of platelet activation [97]. Figure 2 gives an overview of important platelet phenotype and activation markers, which are determined by flow cytometry for the diagnostic purposes of platelet function defects potentially associated with thrombocytopenia.

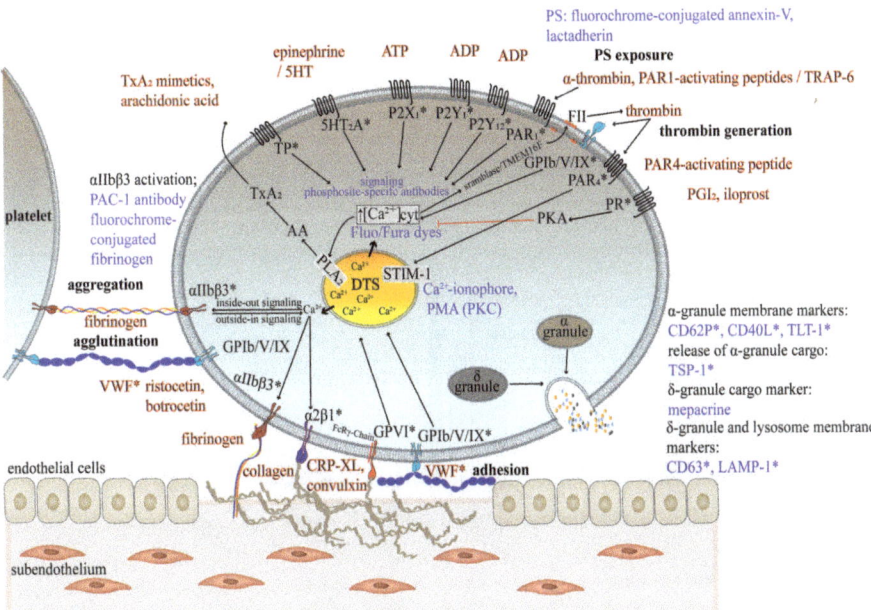

Figure 2. Flow cytometric analysis of the human platelet phenotype ex vivo and functional capacity in vitro in thrombocytopenia. Flow cytometry allows for a comprehensive analysis of common platelet phenotype and function defects in samples of whole blood and platelet-rich plasma, even with a very low platelet count. Commonly observed platelet granule defects (e.g., storage pool deficiency and primary secretion defects) in inherited and acquired thrombocytopenias can be detected by the surface expression of granule membrane markers stained by fluorochrome-conjugated antibodies (*) or by the antibody staining of the α-granule cargo protein TSP-1 and δ-granule cargo molecules ADP and ATP with mepacrine. Quantitative defects in platelet surface receptors, as prominently observed in acquired thrombocytopenias, are detected by staining with fluorochrome-conjugated antibodies (*), too. The use of different platelet agonists enables the detection of activated integrin αIIbβ3 (antibody PAC-1 (*) or the binding of fluorochrome-conjugated fibrinogen, indicative of platelet aggregation), VWF-binding (anti-VWF antibody staining (*), indicative of VWF-mediated platelet agglutination and biallelic BSS, platelet type VWD, and acquired VWD), and the exocytosis of granules by staining of granule membrane proteins with fluorochrome-conjugated antibodies (*). *Antigens of platelet receptors and granule membranes detected by fluorochrome-conjugated antibodies. Fluorochrome-conjugated annexin-V or lactadherin is used to quantify anionic phospholipid exposure ex vivo or in response to agonists, which determines the recruitment of coagulation factors, leading to platelet-based thrombin generation. Distinct signaling defects are detected by phospho-specific antibodies after permeabilization of the platelet surface membrane. Phospho-specific antibodies against phosphorylated VASP at S239 detect a cytosolic increase in levels of inhibitory cAMP, leading to the activation of PKA. A defective release of Ca^{2+} ions from intracellular Ca^{2+} stores (e.g., dense tubular system (DTS)) can be detected by Ca^{2+}-sensitive fluorescent Fluo and Fura dyes. VWF: Von Willebrand factor; cAMP: cyclic adenosine monophosphate; ADP: adenosine diphosphate; CRP-XL: cross-linked collagen-related peptide; PAR: proteinase-activated receptor; PKA: protein kinase A; TxA_2: thromboxane A_2; TP: TxA_2 receptor; AA: arachidonic acid; PLA_2: phospholipase A_2; PKA: protein kinase A; STIM-1: stromal interaction molecule-1; PGI_2: prostacyclin; DTS: dense tubular system; GP: glycoprotein; PS: phosphatidylserine; TRAP-6: thrombin receptor activating peptide-6; TLT-1: trem-like transcript-1; TMEM16F: transmembrane protein 16F; TSP-1: thrombospondin-1; LAMP-1: lysosome-associated membrane glycoprotein-1; PMA: phorbol 12-myristate 13-acetate; VASP: vasodilator-stimulated phosphoprotein; PKC: protein kinase C. PKA and PKC are some examples of protein kinases, but there are many more protein kinases involved.

The flow cytometric quantification of antigen binding sites of fluorochrome-conjugated monoclonal antibodies against platelet receptors is important to identify inherited platelet receptor defects [98], as demonstrated for the detected loss of the platelet VWF receptor complex GPIb/V/IX in a patient with biallelic BSS and a platelet count of 21×10^9/L and a mean platelet volume of >13 fl (Figure 3a). The absence or severe impairment of VWF binding to platelets induced by the antibiotic ristocetin confirmed the typical functional platelet defect in BSS, especially when LTA could not be applied due to severe thrombocytopenia (Figure 3b).

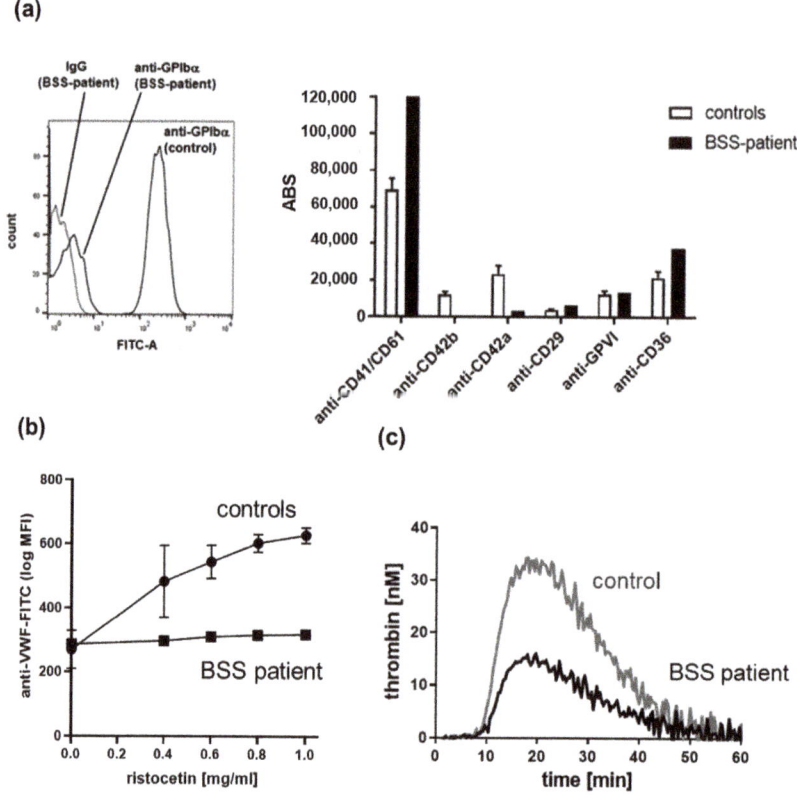

Figure 3. Platelet phenotype and function analysis of a patient with biallelic Bernard–Soulier syndrome (BSS) by flow cytometry and calibrated automated thrombography. (**a**) Representative flow cytometry histogram of platelets labelled with anti-GPIbα antibody SZ2-fluorescein isothiocyanate (FITC) from a donor with GPIbα-deficiency (biallelic Bernard-Soulier syndrome (BSS)) in comparison to platelets from a day control and to platelets labelled with immunoglobulin G1 (IgG1)-FITC as negative control and flow cytometric detection of antigen binding sites (ABSs) of fluorochrome-labelled antibodies against major receptors on platelets in citrated whole blood compared to healthy controls (n = 10, means ± SD). (**b**) Flow cytometric analysis of ristocetin-induced VWF-binding (labeling with anti-VWF-FITC antibody) to platelets from BSS patient compared to controls (n = 10, means ± SD). (**c**) Thrombogram (calibrated automated thrombography) of thrombin-induced thrombin generation in platelet-rich plasma from a BSS patient compared to a day control with adjusted platelet mass. MFI: mean fluorescence intensity.

Notably, in the case of macrothrombocytopenias, platelets have to be gated among their size properties to enable comparisons with control references from healthy controls. Several studies have demonstrated the clinical utility of flow cytometry for the evaluation of platelet dysfunction in acquired thrombocytopenias, such as ITP [99,100] and hematological malignancies [9,101].

Distinct flow cytometric platelet activation assays are recommended for use in buffer-diluted PRP when the detection of distinct fluorescent markers may be influenced by the hemoglobin of red blood cells, or the determination of platelet activation responses should be specifically induced by agonists without potential interference with red blood cells and leukocytes. The flow cytometric assessment of the agonist-induced release/exocytosis of platelet granules is important to complement the diagnosis of SPD. Platelets from patients with the inherited α-SPD GPS show impaired or lacking P-selectin surface expression and TSP-1 binding induced by several platelet agonists [102]. The mepacrine assay allows one to discriminate between platelet δ-SPD and a δ-granule release defect. In resting platelets, mepacrine is loaded to the δ-granules by specific binding to adenosine nucleotides such as ADP or ATP. The decreased uptake of mepacrine in resting platelets is indicative of a δ-SPD with a moderate specificity and sensitivity [103,104]. Interestingly, we observed that platelets from a patient with the *MYH*-9-related thrombocytopenia May–Hegglin anomaly, caused by the frequent *MYH9* mutation E1841K in the C-terminal exon 38 encoding for the tail part of non-muscle myosin heavy chain-IIA, showed normal mepacrine uptake but impaired release in response to increasing concentrations of thrombin and the GPVI agonist convulxin. These data were confirmed by the impaired surface expression of the δ-granule/lysosome membrane marker CD63 (Figures 1 and 4a,b, Table S1). A similar release defect was observed for the α-granules expressed by impaired P-selectin surface expression, whereas the thrombin- and convulxin-induced activation of the integrin αIIbβ3 was normal [23].

This granule release defect may explain the moderated bleeding symptoms of the patient since birth, as his platelet mass was found to be relatively normal and only distributed to a smaller number of giant platelets (35–60×10^9/L, variable MPV > 12 fl). Thus, the flow cytometric application of a panel of activation markers offers a comprehensive evaluation of platelet function defects in inherited and acquired thrombocytopenias.

5.4. Platelet-Based Thrombin Generation Tests (Platelet-Rich Plasma)

Activated platelets significantly contribute to the amplification of thrombin generation, which is essential for thrombus stabilization and for crosstalk between platelets, leukocytes, and endothelial cells [105,106] (Figures 1 and 2). Platelet-dependent thrombin generation tests are offered as commercially available techniques such as the frequently used calibrated automated thrombography (CAT). Active recombinant tissue factor (TF) serves as trigger in the presence of a high Ca^{2+} concentration to induce a strong activation response of platelets in PRP (platelet count adjusted to 150×10^9/L with PPP), leading to the exposure of anionic phospholipids and the subsequent formation of the tenase and prothrombinase complex. This assay allows for the continuous monitoring of fluorescence traces (which are generated through the cleavage of a fluorogenic peptide substrate by thrombin and which directly reflect the in vitro capacity of thrombin generation by platelets) over time in a 96-well plate format by a fluorescence reader [107]. This device complements flow cytometric analysis of platelet procoagulant activity for the identification of causative platelet dysfunction in platelet-based coagulation and secondary hemostasis. A recent review by Panova-Noeva, van der Meijden, and Ten Cate gave a comprehensive overview about clinical applications, pitfalls, and uncertainties of thrombin generation tests performed with PRP [108].

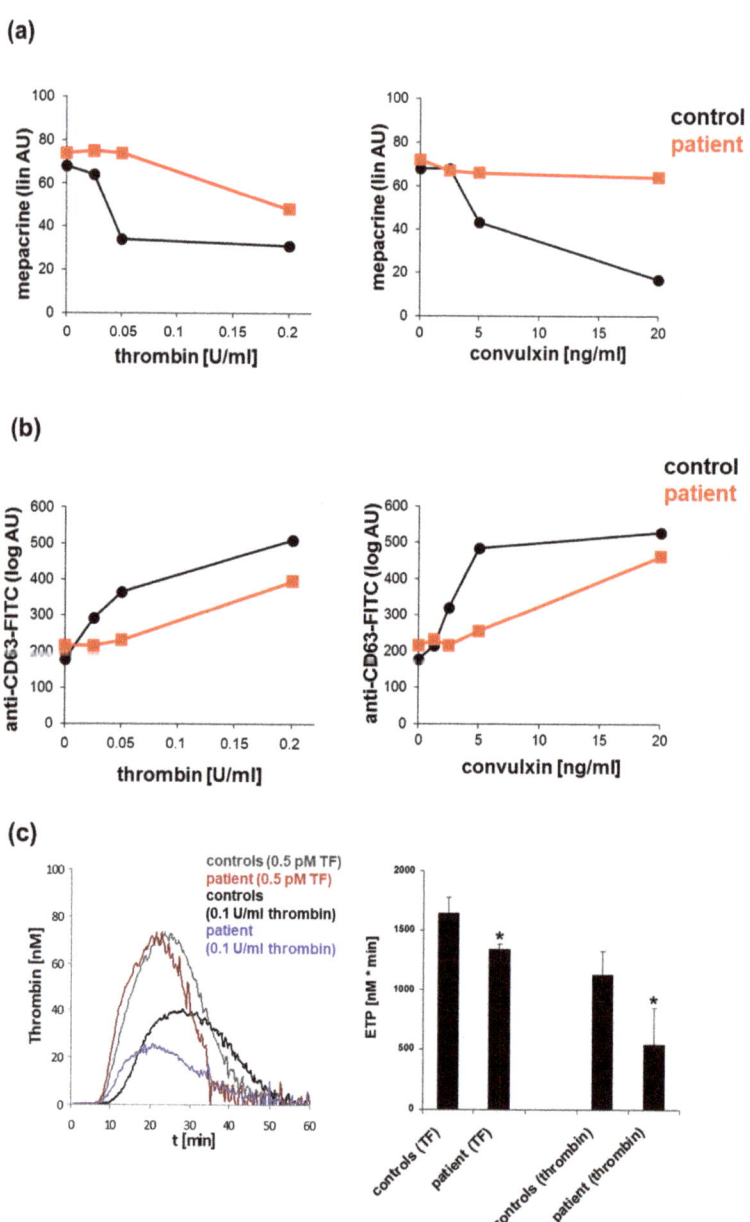

Figure 4. Platelet function analysis of a patient with the May–Hegglin anomaly (pathogenic *MYH9* variant E1841K) by flow cytometry and calibrated automated thrombography. (**a**) Flow cytometric analysis of mepacrine uptake in resting patient platelets and thrombin- or convulxin (GPVI-agonist)-induced mepacrine release compared to a day control. (**b**) Flow cytometric analysis δ-granule/lysosome exocytosis expressed as CD63 surface expression of patient and day control platelets in response to increasing concentrations of thrombin and convulxin, respectively. (**c**) Thrombogram (calibrated automated thrombography) and quantitation of the endogenous thrombin potential (ETP) of tissue factor (TF) or thrombin-stimulated patient and control platelets in platelet-rich plasma; three replicates; n = 3; * $p < 0.05$ versus corresponding controls. AU: arbitrary units.

The knowledge about exclusive defects of platelet procoagulant activity is limited, as observed for the very rare inherited platelet function disorder Scott syndrome caused by pathogenic variants in *ANO6*, which is not usually associated with thrombocytopenia [109]. Indeed, impaired thrombin generation can be also affected by defective primary platelet responses, e.g., deficiency or decreased levels of integrin αIIbβ3 or ADP signaling [110,111]. Using thrombin as direct platelet agonist in the CAT assay, we recently confirmed impaired thrombin generation, expressed by decreased thrombin peak and endogenous thrombin potential (ETP), in PRP from a patient with δ-SPD characterized by decreased release of the feedback agonists ADP and ATP [112]. Similar results were observed for platelets from a biallelic BBS patient, when the platelet mass was adjusted in a control platelet sample from a healthy donor [112] (Figure 3c). This phenomenon can be explained by the impaired binding of thrombin to the GPIb/V/IX complex, which serves as co-receptor for PAR-mediated thrombin signaling [113]. Interestingly, we detected a decreased ETP in PRP from the already described patient with a May–Hegglin anomaly (macrothrombocytopenia, but normal platelet mass) who showed a primary secretion defect of platelet α- and δ-granules (Figure 4c). It is likely that the impaired thrombin generation resulted from a secondary granule secretion defect. Therefore, this test is very helpful to evaluate the impact of primary platelet function defects on thrombin generation and coagulation, but this technique also requires intra- and inter-laboratory standardization [114]. Samples from patients with mild-to-moderate thrombocytopenia allow for a valid analysis in a platelet count range of 50–150 $\times$ 10^9/L in PRP [115], though preferably in direct comparison to control samples with adjusted platelet count/mass (Figures 3c and 4c).

5.5. Microfluidics (Whole Blood)

Flow chamber devices are used to measure platelet adhesion, aggregation and thrombus formation, embolization on subendothelial matrix and plasma proteins under controlled arterial or venous shear stress, and non-coagulant or coagulant conditions in anticoagulated whole blood by advanced bright-field and fluorescence microscopy [116,117]. In comparison to the whole blood PFA and cone and plate(let) analyzer systems, parallel flow chambers have been further developed for systems biology approaches to assess in real-time multiple parameters in an integrated and time-resolving manner by multicolor imaging. Different fluorochrome-conjugated antibodies, proteins, and fluorescent dyes, which are also used for flow cytometry (Figure 2), enable the simultaneous detection of platelet activation markers, e.g., integrin αIIbβ3 activation, P-selectin surface expression, the exposure of anionic phospholipids (e.g., phosphatidylserine), intraplatelet Ca^{2+} release, and the generation of fibrin within a forming platelet aggregate/thrombus [118,119]. Multi-parameter and multi-microspot-based flow assays were recently used for the comprehensive characterization of platelet dysfunction and impaired thrombus formation from patients with inherited platelet function disorders, including the inherited thrombocytopenias GPS, May–Hegglin anomaly, and Stormorken syndrome [120,121]. Thrombus parameters are stable from healthy blood donors within normal platelet count ranges [122], but they are sensitive to low platelet counts. The establishment of reference ranges of reconstituted whole blood samples from healthy subjects with adjusted platelet count/mass is promising to distinguish between platelet count and function-related effects on thrombus formation in thrombocytopenic blood samples. Thus far, the clinical utility of microfluidics is limited for the diagnosis of platelet function and number disorders due to the lack of standardization [116] and validation in prospective cohort studies.

The integration of cultured endothelial within microfluidic devices extends the analysis of the patho(physiological) crosstalk between platelets and the vasculature, which also includes crosstalk with leukocytes [123,124]. A recent proof-of-concept study revealed that distinct components of human umbilical vein endothelial cells (i.e., glycocalyx and thrombomodulin) delay platelet adhesion and fibrin formation on endothelial cells cultured as patches on collagen/tissue factor surfaces under flow in a "vessel-on-a-chip" system [125]. Such advances are currently restricted to research purposes.

6. Conclusions

Whole blood platelet function tests with POC attributes, e.g., impedance aggregometry, platelet function analyzers, cone and plate(let) analyzers, and thromboelastometry/graphy, are commonly used in clinical practice. These tests provide information about the global activity of primary and/or secondary hemostasis in vitro, which are dependent on platelet count, size, and function, as well as determinants including hematocrit, leukocyte count/function, and plasma factors. Due to their sensitivity to low platelet counts, these tests should not be used in clinical centers for the diagnosis of platelet function disorders from thrombocytopenic patients. Light transmission aggregometry and lumi-aggregometry are well-established platelet function tests in specialized platelet laboratories and have become more and more attractive to be used in clinical centers. Centrifugation steps of whole blood to obtain platelet-rich and poor plasma are necessary for the analysis of distinct platelet aggregation parameters with the option of the simultaneous quantitation of ATP/ADP release from platelet δ-granules. These tests are reliable for the screening of primary platelet functions, but they have to be complemented by specialized platelet function assays and phenotyping approaches for diagnostic utility. The analysis of platelet function in samples with a low platelet count is limited but feasible and requires a comparison with control samples from healthy donors, where the platelet count (in the case of thrombocytopenia) or platelet mass (in the case of macro-/micro-thrombocytopenia) is adjusted.

Flow cytometry represents the most powerful technique for a comprehensive characterization of the platelet phenotype and activation capacity in samples from thrombocytopenic patients. It enables the analysis of samples from patients with severe thrombocytopenia and is feasible in both whole blood and platelet-rich plasma. Advanced specialized microfluidic-based tests performed in whole blood are very valuable for the evaluation of specific platelet function parameters under flow and variable coagulant conditions. Thrombin generation assays performed with platelet-rich plasma allow for the assessment of the impact of platelet function defects on coagulation/secondary hemostasis. Nevertheless, a comparison of samples from thrombocytopenic patients with platelet count/mass-adjusted reference samples from healthy donors are necessary for all these tests to distinguish between platelet function and count effects. The predictive value of platelet function testing for the estimation of the bleeding risk of thrombocytopenic patients is promising but currently limited based on only few data from prospective clinical cohort studies.

Supplementary Materials: The following are available online at https://www.mdpi.com/2077-0383/10/5/1114/s1, Table S1: Thrombocytopenia-causing genes associated with platelet function defects; Table S2: Impact of thrombocytopenia on selected point-of-care and specialized platelet function tests.

Author Contributions: Conceptualization, K.J. and Y.S.; resources, K.J.; writing—original draft preparation, K.J. and Y.S.; writing—review and editing, K.J. and Y.S.; visualization, Y.S. All authors have read and agreed to the published version of the manuscript.

Funding: K.J. is supported by the German Federal Ministry of Education and Research (BMBF 01EO1003/01EO1503).

Institutional Review Board Statement: Studies of the authors presented in Figures 3 and 4 were conducted according to the guidelines of the Declaration of Helsinki, and approved by the local Ethics Committee of the University Medical Center Mainz (Study No. 837.302.12/25.07.2012; 2018-13290_1/27.07.2018).

Informed Consent Statement: Informed consent was obtained from all subjects involved in studies of the authors presented in Figures 3 and 4.

Data Availability Statement: Not applicable.

Conflicts of Interest: The authors declare no conflict of interest.

References

1. Mazzano, D.; Pereira, J. Approach to the patient with platelet-related bleeding. In *Platelets in Thrombotic and Non-Thrombotic Disorders: Pathophysiology, Pharmacology and Therapeutics: An Update*; Gresele, P., Kleiman, N.S., Lopez, J.A., Page, C.P., Eds.; Springer International Publishing: Cham, Switzerland, 2017; pp. 717–725.
2. Harrison, P.; Mackie, I.; Mumford, A.; Briggs, C.; Liesner, R.; Winter, M.; Machin, S.; British Committee for Standards in Haematology. Guidelines for the laboratory investigation of heritable disorders of platelet function. *Br. J. Haematol.* **2011**, *155*, 30–44. [CrossRef] [PubMed]
3. Gresele, P.; Subcommittee on Platelet Physiology of the International Society on Thrombosis and Hemostasis. Diagnosis of inherited platelet function disorders: Guidance from the SSC of the ISTH. *J. Thromb. Haemost.* **2015**, *13*, 314–322. [CrossRef] [PubMed]
4. Hayward, C.P.M.; Moffat, K.A.; Brunet, J.; Carlino, S.A.; Plumhoff, E.; Meijer, P.; Zehnder, J.L. Update on diagnostic testing for platelet function disorders: What is practical and useful? *Int. J. Lab. Hematol.* **2019**, *41* (Suppl. 1), 26–32. [CrossRef] [PubMed]
5. Gresele, P.; Bury, L.; Falcinelli, E. Inherited Platelet Function Disorders: Algorithms for Phenotypic and Genetic Investigation. *Semin. Thromb. Hemost.* **2016**, *42*, 292–305. [CrossRef]
6. Slichter, S.J.; Kaufman, R.M.; Assmann, S.F.; McCullough, J.; Triulzi, D.J.; Strauss, R.G.; Gernsheimer, T.B.; Ness, P.M.; Brecher, M.E.; Josephson, C.D.; et al. Dose of prophylactic platelet transfusions and prevention of hemorrhage. *N. Engl. J. Med.* **2010**, *362*, 600–613. [CrossRef] [PubMed]
7. Lambert, M.P. Platelets in liver and renal disease. *Hematol. Am. Soc. Hematol. Educ. Program.* **2016**, *2016*, 251–255. [CrossRef] [PubMed]
8. Hui, P.; Cook, D.J.; Lim, W.; Fraser, G.A.; Arnold, D.M. The frequency and clinical significance of thrombocytopenia complicating critical illness: A systematic review. *Chest* **2011**, *139*, 271–278. [CrossRef]
9. Vinholt, P.J. The role of platelets in bleeding in patients with thrombocytopenia and hematological disease. *Clin. Chem. Lab. Med.* **2019**, *57*, 1808–1817. [CrossRef]
10. Witters, P.; Freson, K.; Verslype, C.; Peerlinck, K.; Hoylaerts, M.; Nevens, F.; Van Geet, C.; Cassiman, D. Review article: Blood platelet number and function in chronic liver disease and cirrhosis. *Aliment. Pharmacol. Ther.* **2008**, *27*, 1017–1029. [CrossRef] [PubMed]
11. Assinger, A.; Schrottmaier, W.C.; Salzmann, M.; Rayes, J. Platelets in Sepsis: An Update on Experimental Models and Clinical Data. *Front. Immunol.* **2019**, *10*, 1687. [CrossRef]
12. Lutz, P.; Jurk, P. Platelets in Advanced Chronic Kidney Disease: Two Sides of the Coin. *Semin. Thromb. Hemost.* **2020**, *46*, 342–356. [CrossRef]
13. Scharf, R.E. Acquired disorders of platelet function. In *Platelets in Thrombotic and Non-Thrombotic Disorders: Pathophysiology, Pharmacology and Therapeutics: An Update*; Gresele, P., Kleiman, N.S., Lopez, J.A., Page, C.P., Eds.; Springer International Publishing: Cham, Switzerland, 2017; pp. 951–973.
14. Thorup, C.V.; Christensen, S.; Hvas, A.M. Immature Platelets As a Predictor of Disease Severity and Mortality in Sepsis and Septic Shock: A Systematic Review. *Semin. Thromb. Hemost.* **2020**, *46*, 320–327. [CrossRef] [PubMed]
15. Danese, E.; Montagnana, M.; Favaloro, E.J.; Lippi, G. Drug-Induced Thrombocytopenia: Mechanisms and Laboratory Diagnostics. *Semin. Thromb. Hemost.* **2020**, *46*, 264–274. [CrossRef] [PubMed]
16. Bakchoul, T.; Marini, I. Drug-associated thrombocytopenia. *Hematol. Am. Soc. Hematol. Educ. Program.* **2018**, *2018*, 576–583. [CrossRef]
17. Schlagenhauf, A.; Kalbhenn, J.; Geisen, U.; Beyersdorf, F.; Zieger, B. Acquired von Willebrand Syndrome and Platelet Function Defects during Extracorporeal Life Support (Mechanical Circulatory Support). *Hamostaseologie* **2020**, *40*, 221–225. [CrossRef] [PubMed]
18. Balduini, C.L.; Pecci, A. Inherited thrombocytopenias. In *Platelets in Thrombotic and Non-Thrombotic Disorders: Pathophysiology, Pharmacology and Therapeutics: An Update*; Gresele, P., Kleiman, N.S., Lopez, J.A., Page, C.P., Eds.; Springer International Publishing: Cham, Switzerland, 2017; pp. 727–747.
19. Pecci, A.; Balduini, C.L. Inherited thrombocytopenias: An updated guide for clinicians. *Blood Rev.* **2020**, 100784. [CrossRef] [PubMed]
20. Ibrahim-Kosta, M.; Alessi, M.C.; Hezard, N. Laboratory Techniques Used to Diagnose Constitutional Platelet Dysfunction. *Hamostaseologie* **2020**, *40*, 444–459. [CrossRef] [PubMed]
21. Almazni, I.; Stapley, R.; Morgan, N.V. Inherited Thrombocytopenia: Update on Genes and Genetic Variants Which may be Associated With Bleeding. *Front. Cardiovasc. Med.* **2019**, *6*, 80. [CrossRef]
22. Johnson, B.; Lowe, G.C.; Futterer, J.; Lordkipanidze, M.; MacDonald, D.; Simpson, M.A.; Sanchez-Guiu, I.; Drake, S.; Bem, D.; Leo, V.; et al. Whole exome sequencing identifies genetic variants in inherited thrombocytopenia with secondary qualitative function defects. *Haematologica* **2016**, *101*, 1170–1179. [CrossRef]
23. Jurk, K.; Greinacher, A.; Walter, U.; Scharrer, I. May-Hegglin anomaly with MYH9 gene E1841K mutation is associated with major platelet defects in granule secretion and thrombin generation. In Proceedings of the 57th Annual Meeting of the Society of Thrombosis and Haemostasis Research, Munich, Germany; P-2-61.
24. Elbaz, C.; Sholzberg, M. An illustrated review of bleeding assessment tools and common coagulation tests. *Res. Pract. Thromb. Haemost.* **2020**, *4*, 761–773. [CrossRef] [PubMed]

25. Gresele, P.; Orsini, S.; Noris, P.; Falcinelli, E.; Alessi, M.C.; Bury, L.; Borhany, M.; Santoro, C.; Glembotsky, A.C.; Cid, A.R.; et al. Validation of the ISTH/SSC bleeding assessment tool for inherited platelet disorders: A communication from the Platelet Physiology SSC. *J. Thromb. Haemost.* **2020**, *18*, 732–739. [CrossRef]
26. Nurden, A.T.; Nurden, P. Should any genetic defect affecting alpha-granules in platelets be classified as gray platelet syndrome? *Am. J. Hematol.* **2016**, *91*, 714–718. [CrossRef] [PubMed]
27. Abdulhay, N.J.; Fiorini, C.; Verboon, J.M.; Ludwig, L.S.; Ulirsch, J.C.; Zieger, B.; Lareau, C.A.; Mi, X.; Roy, A.; Obeng, E.A.; et al. Impaired human hematopoiesis due to a cryptic intronic GATA1 splicing mutation. *J. Exp. Med.* **2019**, *216*, 1050–1060. [CrossRef] [PubMed]
28. Althaus, K.; Greinacher, A. MYH9-related platelet disorders. *Semin. Thromb. Hemost.* **2009**, *35*, 189–203. [CrossRef]
29. Greinacher, A.; Pecci, A.; Kunishima, S.; Althaus, K.; Nurden, P.; Balduini, C.L.; Bakchoul, T. Diagnosis of inherited platelet disorders on a blood smear: A tool to facilitate worldwide diagnosis of platelet disorders. *J. Thromb. Haemost.* **2017**, *15*, 1511–1521. [CrossRef]
30. Zaninetti, C.; Greinacher, A. Diagnosis of Inherited Platelet Disorders on a Blood Smear. *J. Clin. Med.* **2020**, *9*, 539. [CrossRef] [PubMed]
31. Corpataux, N.; Franke, K.; Kille, A.; Valina, C.M.; Neumann, F.J.; Nuhrenberg, T.; Hochholzer, W. Reticulated Platelets in Medicine: Current Evidence and Further Perspectives. *J. Clin. Med.* **2020**, *9*, 3737. [CrossRef] [PubMed]
32. Skipper, M.T.; Rubak, P.; Stentoft, J.; Hvas, A.M.; Larsen, O.H. Evaluation of platelet function in thrombocytopenia. *Platelets* **2018**, *29*, 270–276. [CrossRef]
33. Hedley, B.D.; Llewellyn-Smith, N.; Lang, S.; Hsia, C.C.; MacNamara, N.; Rosenfeld, D.; Keeney, M. Combined accurate platelet enumeration and reticulated platelet determination by flow cytometry. *Cytom. B Clin. Cytom.* **2015**, *88*, 330–337. [CrossRef]
34. Hille, L.; Cederqvist, M.; Hromek, J.; Stratz, C.; Trenk, D.; Nuhrenberg, T.G. Evaluation of an Alternative Staining Method Using SYTO 13 to Determine Reticulated Platelets. *Thromb. Haemost.* **2019**, *119*, 779–785. [CrossRef]
35. Dupuis, A.; Bordet, J.C.; Eckly, A.; Gachet, C. Platelet delta-Storage Pool Disease: An Update. *J. Clin. Med.* **2020**, *9*, 2508. [CrossRef] [PubMed]
36. Heijnen, H.F.; Korporaal, S.J. Platelet morphology and Ultrastructure. In *Platelets in Thrombotic and Non-Thrombotic Disorders: Pathophysiology, Pharmacology and Therapeutics: An Update*; Gresele, P., Kleiman, N.S., Lopez, J.A., Page, C.P., Eds.; Springer International Publishing: Cham, Switzerland, 2017; pp. 21–37.
37. Hayward, C.P.; Moffat, K.A.; Spitzer, E.; Timleck, M.; Plumhoff, E.; Israels, S.J.; White, J.; NASCOLA Working Group on Platelet Dense Granule Deficiency. Results of an external proficiency testing exercise on platelet dense-granule deficiency testing by whole mount electron microscopy. *Am. J. Clin. Pathol.* **2009**, *131*, 671–675. [CrossRef]
38. Brunet, J.G.; Iyer, J.K.; Badin, M.S.; Graf, L.; Moffat, K.A.; Timleck, M.; Spitzer, E.; Hayward, C.P.M. Electron microscopy examination of platelet whole mount preparations to quantitate platelet dense granule numbers: Implications for diagnosing suspected platelet function disorders due to dense granule deficiency. *Int. J. Lab. Hematol.* **2018**, *40*, 400–407. [CrossRef]
39. Eckly, A.; Rinckel, J.Y.; Proamer, F.; Ulas, N.; Joshi, S.; Whiteheart, S.W.; Gachet, C. Respective contributions of single and compound granule fusion to secretion by activated platelets. *Blood* **2016**, *128*, 2538–2549. [CrossRef]
40. Gresele, P.; Bury, L.; Mezzasoma, A.M.; Falcinelli, E. Platelet function assays in diagnosis: An update. *Expert Rev. Hematol.* **2019**, *12*, 29–46. [CrossRef]
41. Rubak, P.; Villadsen, K.; Hvas, A.M. Reference intervals for platelet aggregation assessed by multiple electrode platelet aggregometry. *Thromb. Res.* **2012**, *130*, 420–423. [CrossRef] [PubMed]
42. Toth, O.; Calatzis, A.; Penz, S.; Losonczy, H.; Siess, W. Multiple electrode aggregometry: A new device to measure platelet aggregation in whole blood. *Thromb. Haemost.* **2006**, *96*, 781–788. [PubMed]
43. Michelson, A.D. Methods for the measurement of platelet function. *Am. J. Cardiol.* **2009**, *103*, 20A–26A. [CrossRef]
44. Awidi, A.; Maqablah, A.; Dweik, M.; Bsoul, N.; Abu-Khader, A. Comparison of platelet aggregation using light transmission and multiple electrode aggregometry in Glanzmann thrombasthenia. *Platelets* **2009**, *20*, 297–301. [CrossRef]
45. Albanyan, A.; Al-Musa, A.; AlNounou, R.; Al Zahrani, H.; Nasr, R.; AlJefri, A.; Saleh, M.; Malik, A.; Masmali, H.; Owaidah, T. Diagnosis of Glanzmann thrombasthenia by whole blood impedance analyzer (MEA) vs. light transmission aggregometry. *Int. J. Lab. Hematol.* **2015**, *37*, 503–508. [CrossRef]
46. Al Ghaithi, R.; Drake, S.; Watson, S.P.; Morgan, N.V.; Harrison, P. Comparison of multiple electrode aggregometry with lumi-aggregometry for the diagnosis of patients with mild bleeding disorders. *J. Thromb. Haemost.* **2017**, *15*, 2045–2052. [CrossRef]
47. Moenen, F.; Vries, M.J.A.; Nelemans, P.J.; van Rooy, K.J.M.; Vranken, J.; Verhezen, P.W.M.; Wetzels, R.J.H.; Ten Cate, H.; Schouten, H.C.; Beckers, E.A.M.; et al. Screening for platelet function disorders with Multiplate and platelet function analyzer. *Platelets* **2019**, *30*, 81–87. [CrossRef] [PubMed]
48. Seyfert, U.T.; Haubelt, H.; Vogt, A.; Hellstern, P. Variables influencing Multiplate(TM) whole blood impedance platelet aggregometry and turbidimetric platelet aggregation in healthy individuals. *Platelets* **2007**, *18*, 199–206. [CrossRef] [PubMed]
49. Femia, E.A.; Scavone, M.; Lecchi, A.; Cattaneo, M. Effect of platelet count on platelet aggregation measured with impedance aggregometry (Multiplate analyzer) and with light transmission aggregometry. *J. Thromb. Haemost.* **2013**, *11*, 2193–2196. [CrossRef] [PubMed]
50. Cattaneo, M.; Lecchi, A.; Zighetti, M.L.; Lussana, F. Platelet aggregation studies: Autologous platelet-poor plasma inhibits platelet aggregation when added to platelet-rich plasma to normalize platelet count. *Haematologica* **2007**, *92*, 694–697. [CrossRef]

51. Tiedemann Skipper, M.; Rubak, P.; Halfdan Larsen, O.; Hvas, A.M. Thrombocytopenia model with minimal manipulation of blood cells allowing whole blood assessment of platelet function. *Platelets* **2016**, *27*, 295–300. [CrossRef]
52. Franchini, M. The platelet function analyzer (PFA-100): An update on its clinical use. *Clin. Lab.* **2005**, *51*, 367–372.
53. Favaloro, E.J. Clinical utility of closure times using the platelet function analyzer-100/200. *Am. J. Hematol.* **2017**, *92*, 398–404. [CrossRef]
54. Hayward, C.P.; Harrison, P.; Cattaneo, M.; Ortel, T.L.; Rao, A.K.; Platelet Physiology Subcommittee of the SSC; Standardization Committee of the International Society Society on Thrombosis and Hemostasis. Platelet function analyzer (PFA)-100 closure time in the evaluation of platelet disorders and platelet function. *J. Thromb. Haemost.* **2006**, *4*, 312–319. [CrossRef]
55. Quiroga, T.; Goycoolea, M.; Munoz, B.; Morales, M.; Aranda, E.; Panes, O.; Pereira, J.; Mezzano, D. Template bleeding time and PFA-100 have low sensitivity to screen patients with hereditary mucocutaneous hemorrhages: Comparative study in 148 patients. *J. Thromb. Haemost.* **2004**, *2*, 892–898. [CrossRef]
56. Sladky, J.L.; Klima, J.; Grooms, L.; Kerlin, B.A.; O'Brien, S.H. The PFA-100 (R) does not predict delta-granule platelet storage pool deficiencies. *Haemoph. Off. J. World Fed. Hemoph.* **2012**, *18*, 626–629. [CrossRef]
57. Kaufmann, J.; Adler, M.; Alberio, L.; Nagler, M. Utility of the Platelet Function Analyzer in Patients with Suspected Platelet Function Disorders: Diagnostic Accuracy Study. *TH Open* **2020**, *4*, e427–e436. [CrossRef] [PubMed]
58. Savion, N.; Varon, D. Impact–the cone and plate(let) analyzer: Testing platelet function and anti-platelet drug response. *Pathophysiol. Haemost. Thromb.* **2006**, *35*, 83–88. [CrossRef]
59. Panzer, S.; Eichelberger, B.; Koren, D.; Kaufmann, K.; Male, C. Monitoring survival and function of transfused platelets in Bernard-Soulier syndrome by flow cytometry and a cone and plate(let) analyzer (Impact-R). *Transfusion* **2007**, *47*, 103–106. [CrossRef]
60. Shenkman, B.; Budde, U.; Angerhaus, D.; Lubetsky, A.; Savion, N.; Seligsohn, U.; Varon, D. ADAMTS-13 regulates platelet adhesion under flow. A new method for differentiation between inherited and acquired thrombotic thrombocytopenic purpura. *Thromb. Haemost.* **2006**, *96*, 160–166.
61. Kenet, G.; Lubetsky, A.; Shenkman, B.; Tamarin, I.; Dardik, R.; Rechavi, G.; Barzilai, A.; Martinowitz, U.; Savion, N.; Varon, D. Cone and platelet analyser (CPA): A new test for the prediction of bleeding among thrombocytopenic patients. *Br. J. Haematol.* **1998**, *101*, 255–259. [CrossRef]
62. Vinholt, P.J.; Hvas, A.M.; Nybo, M. An overview of platelet indices and methods for evaluating platelet function in thrombocytopenic patients. *Eur. J. Haematol.* **2014**, *92*, 367–376. [CrossRef] [PubMed]
63. Bolliger, D.; Seeberger, M.D.; Tanaka, K.A. Principles and practice of thromboelastography in clinical coagulation management and transfusion practice. *Transfus. Med. Rev.* **2012**, *26*, 1–13. [CrossRef] [PubMed]
64. Versteeg, H.H.; Heemskerk, J.W.; Levi, M.; Reitsma, P.H. New fundamentals in hemostasis. *Physiol. Rev.* **2013**, *93*, 327–358. [CrossRef] [PubMed]
65. Colucci, M.; Semeraro, N.; Semerao, F. Platelets and fibrinolysis. In *Platelets in Thrombotic and Non-Thrombotic Disorders: Pathophysiology, Pharmacology and Therapeutics: An Update*; Gresele, P., Kleiman, N.S., Lopez, J.A., Page, C.P., Eds.; Springer International Publishing: Cham, Switzerland, 2017; pp. 463–487.
66. Ranucci, M.; Baryshnikova, E. Sensitivity of Viscoelastic Tests to Platelet Function. *J. Clin. Med.* **2020**, *9*, 189. [CrossRef]
67. Castellino, F.J.; Liang, Z.; Davis, P.K.; Balsara, R.D.; Musunuru, H.; Donahue, D.L.; Smith, D.L.; Sandoval-Cooper, M.J.; Ploplis, V.A.; Walsh, M. Abnormal whole blood thrombi in humans with inherited platelet receptor defects. *PLoS ONE* **2012**, *7*, e52878. [CrossRef] [PubMed]
68. Gunduz, E.; Akay, O.M.; Bal, C.; Gulbas, Z. Can thrombelastography be a new tool to assess bleeding risk in patients with idiopathic thrombocytopenic purpura? *Platelets* **2011**, *22*, 516–520. [CrossRef]
69. Greene, L.A.; Chen, S.; Seery, C.; Imahiyerobo, A.M.; Bussel, J.B. Beyond the platelet count: Immature platelet fraction and thromboelastometry correlate with bleeding in patients with immune thrombocytopenia. *Br. J. Haematol.* **2014**, *166*, 592–600. [CrossRef]
70. Estcourt, L.J.; Stanworth, S.J.; Harrison, P.; Powter, G.; McClure, M.; Murphy, M.F.; Mumford, A.D. Prospective observational cohort study of the association between thromboelastometry, coagulation and platelet parameters and bleeding in patients with haematological malignancies- the ATHENA study. *Br. J. Haematol.* **2014**, *166*, 581–591. [CrossRef] [PubMed]
71. Dias, J.D.; Lopez-Espina, C.G.; Bliden, K.; Gurbel, P.; Hartmann, J.; Achneck, H.E. TEG(R)6s system measures the contributions of both platelet count and platelet function to clot formation at the site-of-care. *Platelets* **2020**, *31*, 932–938. [CrossRef] [PubMed]
72. Born, G.V. Aggregation of blood platelets by adenosine diphosphate and its reversal. *Nature* **1962**, *194*, 927–929. [CrossRef] [PubMed]
73. Beck, F.; Geiger, J.; Gambaryan, S.; Solari, F.A.; Dell'Aica, M.; Loroch, S.; Mattheij, N.J.; Mindukshev, I.; Potz, O.; Jurk, K.; et al. Temporal quantitative phosphoproteomics of ADP stimulation reveals novel central nodes in platelet activation and inhibition. *Blood* **2017**, *129*, e1–e12. [CrossRef] [PubMed]
74. Pielsticker, C.; Brodde, M.F.; Raum, L.; Jurk, K.; Kehrel, B.E. Plasmin-Induced Activation of Human Platelets Is Modulated by Thrombospondin-1, Bona Fide Misfolded Proteins and Thiol Isomerases. *Int. J. Mol. Sci.* **2020**, *21*, 8851. [CrossRef] [PubMed]
75. Cattaneo, M.; Cerletti, C.; Harrison, P.; Hayward, C.P.; Kenny, D.; Nugent, D.; Nurden, P.; Rao, A.K.; Schmaier, A.H.; Watson, S.P.; et al. Recommendations for the Standardization of Light Transmission Aggregometry: A Consensus of the Working Party from the Platelet Physiology Subcommittee of SSC/ISTH. *J. Thromb. Haemost.* **2013**, [CrossRef] [PubMed]

76. Hayward, C.P.; Moffat, K.A.; Raby, A.; Israels, S.; Plumhoff, E.; Flynn, G.; Zehnder, J.L. Development of North American consensus guidelines for medical laboratories that perform and interpret platelet function testing using light transmission aggregometry. *Am. J. Clin. Pathol.* **2010**, *134*, 955–963. [CrossRef]
77. Alessi, M.C.; Sie, P.; Payrastre, B. Strengths and Weaknesses of Light Transmission Aggregometry in Diagnosing Hereditary Platelet Function Disorders. *J. Clin. Med.* **2020**, *9*, 763. [CrossRef]
78. Althaus, K.; Zieger, B.; Bakchoul, T.; Jurk, K.; THROMKID-Plus Studiengruppe der Gesellschaft für Thrombose- und Hämostaseforschung (GTH) und der Gesellschaft für Pädiatrische Onkologie und Hämatologie (GPOH). Standardization of Light Transmission Aggregometry for Diagnosis of Platelet Disorders: An Inter-Laboratory External Quality Assessment. *Thromb. Haemost.* **2019**, *119*, 1154–1161. [CrossRef] [PubMed]
79. Gresele, P.; Harrison, P.; Bury, L.; Falcinelli, E.; Gachet, C.; Hayward, C.P.; Kenny, D.; Mezzano, D.; Mumford, A.D.; Nugent, D.; et al. Diagnosis of suspected inherited platelet function disorders: Results of a worldwide survey. *J. Thromb. Haemost.* **2014**, *12*, 1562–1569. [CrossRef]
80. Cattaneo, M.; Hayward, C.P.; Moffat, K.A.; Pugliano, M.T.; Liu, Y.; Michelson, A.D. Results of a worldwide survey on the assessment of platelet function by light transmission aggregometry: A report from the platelet physiology subcommittee of the SSC of the ISTH. *J. Thromb. Haemost.* **2009**, *7*, 1029. [CrossRef] [PubMed]
81. Hayward, C.P.; Pai, M.; Liu, Y.; Moffat, K.A.; Seecharan, J.; Webert, K.E.; Cook, R.J.; Heddle, N.M. Diagnostic utility of light transmission platelet aggregometry: Results from a prospective study of individuals referred for bleeding disorder assessments. *J. Thromb. Haemost.* **2009**, *7*, 676–684. [CrossRef] [PubMed]
82. Le Blanc, J.; Mullier, F.; Vayne, C.; Lordkipanidze, M. Advances in Platelet Function Testing-Light Transmission Aggregometry and Beyond. *J. Clin. Med.* **2020**, *9*, 2636. [CrossRef]
83. Dawood, B.B.; Lowe, G.C.; Lordkipanidze, M.; Bem, D.; Daly, M.E.; Makris, M.; Mumford, A.; Wilde, J.T.; Watson, S.P. Evaluation of participants with suspected heritable platelet function disorders including recommendation and validation of a streamlined agonist panel. *Blood* **2012**, *120*, 5041–5049. [CrossRef] [PubMed]
84. Cattaneo, M. Light transmission aggregometry and ATP release for the diagnostic assessment of platelet function. *Semin. Thromb. Hemost.* **2009**, *35*, 158–167. [CrossRef] [PubMed]
85. Badin, M.S.; Graf, L.; Iyer, J.K.; Moffat, K.A.; Seecharan, J.L.; Hayward, C.P. Variability in platelet dense granule adenosine triphosphate release findings amongst patients tested multiple times as part of an assessment for a bleeding disorder. *Int. J. Lab. Hematol.* **2016**, *38*, 648–657. [CrossRef]
86. Durrant, T.N.; van den Bosch, M.T.; Hers, I. Integrin alphaIIbbeta3 outside-in signaling. *Blood* **2017**, *130*, 1607–1619. [CrossRef] [PubMed]
87. van Asten, I.; Schutgens, R.E.G.; Baaij, M.; Zandstra, J.; Roest, M.; Pasterkamp, G.; Huisman, A.; Korporaal, S.J.A.; Urbanus, R.T. Validation of flow cytometric analysis of platelet function in patients with a suspected platelet function defect. *J. Thromb. Haemost.* **2018**, *16*, 689–698. [CrossRef]
88. Navred, K.; Martin, M.; Ekdahl, L.; Zetterberg, E.; Andersson, N.G.; Strandberg, K.; Norstrom, E. A simplified flow cytometric method for detection of inherited platelet disorders-A comparison to the gold standard light transmission aggregometry. *PLoS ONE* **2019**, *14*, e0211130. [CrossRef] [PubMed]
89. Jurk, K. Analysis of platelet function and dysfunction. *Hamostaseologie* **2015**, *35*, 60–72. [CrossRef]
90. Baaten, C.; Ten Cate, H.; van der Meijden, P.E.J.; Heemskerk, J.W.M. Platelet populations and priming in hematological diseases. *Blood Rev.* **2017**, *31*, 389–399. [CrossRef]
91. Schwarz, U.R.; Geiger, J.; Walter, U.; Eigenthaler, M. Flow cytometry analysis of intracellular VASP phosphorylation for the assessment of activating and inhibitory signal transduction pathways in human platelets–definition and detection of ticlopidine/clopidogrel effects. *Thromb. Haemost.* **1999**, *82*, 1145–1152. [CrossRef] [PubMed]
92. Spurgeon, B.E.J.; Naseem, K.M. Phosphoflow cytometry and barcoding in blood platelets: Technical and analytical considerations. *Cytom. B Clin. Cytom.* **2020**, *98*, 123–130. [CrossRef] [PubMed]
93. Blair, T.A.; Michelson, A.D.; Frelinger, A.L., 3rd. Mass Cytometry Reveals Distinct Platelet Subtypes in Healthy Subjects and Novel Alterations in Surface Glycoproteins in Glanzmann Thrombasthenia. *Sci. Rep.* **2018**, *8*, 10300. [CrossRef]
94. Dovlatova, N.; Lordkipanidze, M.; Lowe, G.C.; Dawood, B.; May, J.; Heptinstall, S.; Watson, S.P.; Fox, S.C.; Group, U.G.S. Evaluation of a whole blood remote platelet function test for the diagnosis of mild bleeding disorders. *J. Thromb. Haemost.* **2014**, *12*, 660–665. [CrossRef]
95. Linden, M.D.; Frelinger, A.L., 3rd; Barnard, M.R.; Przyklenk, K.; Furman, M.I.; Michelson, A.D. Application of flow cytometry to platelet disorders. *Semin. Thromb. Hemost.* **2004**, *30*, 501–511. [CrossRef]
96. van Asten, I.; Schutgens, R.E.G.; Urbanus, R.T. Toward Flow Cytometry Based Platelet Function Diagnostics. *Semin. Thromb. Hemost.* **2018**, *44*, 197–205. [CrossRef]
97. Boknas, N.; Macwan, A.S.; Sodergren, A.L.; Ramstrom, S. Platelet function testing at low platelet counts: When can you trust your analysis? *Res. Pract. Thromb. Haemost.* **2019**, *3*, 285–290. [CrossRef]
98. Loroch, S.; Trabold, K.; Gambaryan, S.; Reiss, C.; Schwierczek, K.; Fleming, I.; Sickmann, A.; Behnisch, W.; Zieger, B.; Zahedi, R.P.; et al. Alterations of the platelet proteome in type I Glanzmann thrombasthenia caused by different homozygous delG frameshift mutations in ITGA2B. *Thromb. Haemost.* **2017**, *117*, 556–569. [CrossRef] [PubMed]

99. van Bladel, E.R.; Laarhoven, A.G.; van der Heijden, L.B.; Heitink-Polle, K.M.; Porcelijn, L.; van der Schoot, C.E.; de Haas, M.; Roest, M.; Vidarsson, G.; de Groot, P.G.; et al. Functional platelet defects in children with severe chronic ITP as tested with 2 novel assays applicable for low platelet counts. *Blood* **2014**, *123*, 1556–1563. [CrossRef]
100. Frelinger, A.L., 3rd; Grace, R.F.; Gerrits, A.J.; Berny-Lang, M.A.; Brown, T.; Carmichael, S.L.; Neufeld, E.J.; Michelson, A.D. Platelet function tests, independent of platelet count, are associated with bleeding severity in ITP. *Blood* **2015**, *126*, 873–879. [CrossRef]
101. Leinoe, E.B.; Hoffmann, M.H.; Kjaersgaard, E.; Nielsen, J.D.; Bergmann, O.J.; Klausen, T.W.; Johnsen, H.E. Prediction of haemorrhage in the early stage of acute myeloid leukaemia by flow cytometric analysis of platelet function. *Br. J. Haematol.* **2005**, *128*, 526–532. [CrossRef]
102. Gunay-Aygun, M.; Falik-Zaccai, T.C.; Vilboux, T.; Zivony-Elboum, Y.; Gumruk, F.; Cetin, M.; Khayat, M.; Boerkoel, C.F.; Kfir, N.; Huang, Y.; et al. NBEAL2 is mutated in gray platelet syndrome and is required for biogenesis of platelet alpha-granules. *Nat. Genet.* **2011**, *43*, 732–734. [CrossRef]
103. Cai, H.; Mullier, F.; Frotscher, B.; Briquel, M.E.; Toussaint, M.; Massin, F.; Lecompte, T.; Latger-Cannard, V. Usefulness of Flow Cytometric Mepacrine Uptake/Release Combined with CD63 Assay in Diagnosis of Patients with Suspected Platelet Dense Granule Disorder. *Semin. Thromb. Hemost.* **2016**, *42*, 282–291. [CrossRef]
104. van Asten, I.; Blaauwgeers, M.; Granneman, L.; Heijnen, H.F.G.; Kruip, M.; Beckers, E.A.M.; Coppens, M.; Eikenboom, J.; Tamminga, R.Y.J.; Pasterkamp, G.; et al. Flow cytometric mepacrine fluorescence can be used for the exclusion of platelet dense granule deficiency. *J. Thromb. Haemost.* **2020**, *18*, 706–713. [CrossRef] [PubMed]
105. Monroe, D.M.; Hoffman, M.; Roberts, H.R. Platelets and thrombin generation. *Arterioscler. Thromb. Vasc. Biol.* **2002**, *22*, 1381–1389. [CrossRef] [PubMed]
106. Tomaiuolo, M.; Brass, L.F.; Stalker, T.J. Regulation of Platelet Activation and Coagulation and Its Role in Vascular Injury and Arterial Thrombosis. *Interv. Cardiol. Clin.* **2017**, *6*, 1–12. [CrossRef] [PubMed]
107. Hemker, H.C.; Giesen, P.; Al Dieri, R.; Regnault, V.; de Smedt, E.; Wagenvoord, R.; Lecompte, T.; Beguin, S. Calibrated automated thrombin generation measurement in clotting plasma. *Pathophysiol. Haemost. Thromb.* **2003**, *33*, 4–15. [CrossRef]
108. Panova-Noeva, M.; van der Meijden, P.E.J.; Ten Cate, H. Clinical Applications, Pitfalls, and Uncertainties of Thrombin Generation in the Presence of Platelets. *J. Clin. Med.* **2019**, *9*, 92. [CrossRef] [PubMed]
109. Weiss, H.J. Impaired platelet procoagulant mechanisms in patients with bleeding disorders. *Semin. Thromb. Hemost.* **2009**, *35*, 233–241. [CrossRef]
110. Hemker, H.C.; Al Dieri, R.; De Smedt, E.; Beguin, S. Thrombin generation, a function test of the haemostatic-thrombotic system. *Thromb. Haemost.* **2006**, *96*, 553–561. [PubMed]
111. van der Meijden, P.E.; Feijge, M.A.; Swieringa, F.; Gilio, K.; Nergiz-Unal, R.; Hamulyak, K.; Heemskerk, J.W. Key role of integrin alpha(IIb)beta (3) signaling to Syk kinase in tissue factor-induced thrombin generation. *Cell. Mol. Life Sci. CMLS* **2012**, *69*, 3481–3492. [CrossRef]
112. Dohrmann, M.; Makhoul, S.; Gross, K.; Krause, M.; Pillitteri, D.; von Auer, C.; Walter, U.; Lutz, J.; Volf, I.; Kehrel, B.E.; et al. CD36-fibrin interaction propagates FXI-dependent thrombin generation of human platelets. *FASEB J.* **2020**, *34*, 9337–9357. [CrossRef] [PubMed]
113. Estevez, B.; Kim, K.; Delaney, M.K.; Stojanovic-Terpo, A.; Shen, B.; Ruan, C.; Cho, J.; Ruggeri, Z.M.; Du, X. Signaling-mediated cooperativity between glycoprotein Ib-IX and protease-activated receptors in thrombin-induced platelet activation. *Blood* **2016**, *127*, 626–636. [CrossRef] [PubMed]
114. Subcommittee on Control of Anticoagulation of the SSC of the ISTHTowards a recommendation for the standardization of the measurement of platelet-dependent thrombin generation. *J. Thromb. Haemost.* **2011**, *9*, 1859–1861. [CrossRef]
115. Vanschoonbeek, K.; Feijge, M.A.; Van Kampen, R.J.; Kenis, H.; Hemker, H.C.; Giesen, P.L.; Heemskerk, J.W. Initiating and potentiating role of platelets in tissue factor-induced thrombin generation in the presence of plasma: Subject-dependent variation in thrombogram characteristics. *J. Thromb. Haemost.* **2004**, *2*, 476–484. [CrossRef] [PubMed]
116. Roest, M.; Reininger, A.; Zwaginga, J.J.; King, M.R.; Heemskerk, J.W. Flow chamber-based assays to measure thrombus formation in vitro: Requirements for standardization. *J. Thromb. Haemost.* **2011**, *9*, 2322–2324. [CrossRef]
117. Neeves, K.B.; McCarty, O.J.; Reininger, A.J.; Sugimoto, M.; King, M.R. Biorheology Subcommittee of the SSC of the ISTHFlow-dependent thrombin and fibrin generation in vitro: Opportunities for standardization: Communication from SSC of the ISTH. *J. Thromb. Haemost.* **2014**, *12*, 418–420. [CrossRef]
118. Diamond, S.L. Systems Analysis of Thrombus Formation. *Circ. Res.* **2016**, *118*, 1348–1362. [CrossRef] [PubMed]
119. Nagy, M.; Heemskerk, J.W.M.; Swieringa, F. Use of microfluidics to assess the platelet-based control of coagulation. *Platelets* **2017**, *28*, 441–448. [CrossRef]
120. de Witt, S.M.; Swieringa, F.; Cavill, R.; Lamers, M.M.; van Kruchten, R.; Mastenbroek, T.; Baaten, C.; Coort, S.; Pugh, N.; Schulz, A.; et al. Identification of platelet function defects by multi-parameter assessment of thrombus formation. *Nat. Commun.* **2014**, *5*, 4257. [CrossRef]
121. Nagy, M.; Mastenbroek, T.G.; Mattheij, N.J.A.; de Witt, S.; Clemetson, K.J.; Kirschner, J.; Schulz, A.S.; Vraetz, T.; Speckmann, C.; Braun, A.; et al. Variable impairment of platelet functions in patients with severe, genetically linked immune deficiencies. *Haematologica* **2018**, *103*, 540–549. [CrossRef] [PubMed]

122. van Geffen, J.P.; Brouns, S.L.N.; Batista, J.; McKinney, H.; Kempster, C.; Nagy, M.; Sivapalaratnam, S.; Baaten, C.; Bourry, N.; Frontini, M.; et al. High-throughput elucidation of thrombus formation reveals sources of platelet function variability. *Haematologica* **2019**, *104*, 1256–1267. [CrossRef]
123. Coenen, D.M.; Mastenbroek, T.G.; Cosemans, J. Platelet interaction with activated endothelium: Mechanistic insights from microfluidics. *Blood* **2017**, *130*, 2819–2828. [CrossRef] [PubMed]
124. Jurk, K.; Kehrel, B.E. Pathophysiology and biochemistry of platelets. *Der Internist* **2010**, *51*, 1086, 1088–1092, 1094. [CrossRef] [PubMed]
125. Brouns, S.L.N.; Provenzale, I.; van Geffen, J.P.; van der Meijden, P.E.J.; Heemskerk, J.W.M. Localized endothelial-based control of platelet aggregation and coagulation under flow: A proof-of-principle vessel-on-a-chip study. *J. Thromb. Haemost.* **2020**, *18*, 931–941. [CrossRef]

Review

Challenges and Advances in Managing Thrombocytopenic Cancer Patients

Avi Leader [1,2,3,*], Liron Hofstetter [1,2] and Galia Spectre [1,2]

1. Institute of Hematology, Davidoff Cancer Center, Rabin Medical Center, Petah Tikva 4941492, Israel; lironho@clalit.org.il (L.H.); galiasp1@clalit.org.il (G.S.)
2. Sackler School of Medicine, Tel Aviv University, Tel Aviv 6997801, Israel
3. Cardiovascular Research Institute Maastricht (CARIM), Maastricht University, 6229 ER Maastricht, The Netherlands
* Correspondence: avileader@yahoo.com; Tel.: +972-3-9377906

Abstract: Cancer patients have varying incidence, depth and duration of thrombocytopenia. The mainstay of managing severe chemotherapy-induced thrombocytopenia (CIT) in cancer is the use of platelet transfusions. While prophylactic platelet transfusions reduce the bleeding rate, multiple unmet needs remain, such as high residual rates of bleeding, and anticancer treatment dose reductions/delays. Accordingly, the following promising results in other settings, antifibrinolytic drugs have been evaluated for prevention and treatment of bleeding in patients with hematological malignancies and solid tumors. In addition, Thrombopoeitin receptor agonists have been studied for two major implications in cancer: treatment of severe thrombocytopenia associated with myelodysplastic syndrome and acute myeloid leukemia; primary and secondary prevention of CIT in solid tumors in order to maintain dose density and intensity of anti-cancer treatment. Furthermore, thrombocytopenic cancer patients are often prescribed antithrombotic medication for indications arising prior or post cancer diagnosis. Balancing the bleeding and thrombotic risks in such patients represents a unique clinical challenge. This review focuses upon non-transfusion-based approaches to managing thrombocytopenia and the associated bleeding risk in cancer, and also addresses the management of antithrombotic therapy in thrombocytopenic cancer patients.

Keywords: anticoagulation; antifibrinolytic; antiplatelet; cancer; thrombocytopenia; thrombopoietin receptor agonist; tranexamic acid

1. Introduction

Cancer patients have varying incidence, depth and duration of thrombocytopenia, depending on cancer type, anticancer treatment, bone marrow involvement and comorbidities [1]. For example, patients with hematological malignancies and those receiving carboplatin or oxaliplatin based chemotherapy regimens, have a higher risk of severe thrombocytopenia. Anticancer drugs can cause thrombocytopenia via various mechanisms [2–15], as previously reviewed [1] and as shown in Figure 1. While pancytopenia due to general bone marrow suppression is most common, some antineoplastic drugs, such as proteosome inhibitors used primarily in multiple myeloma, can cause isolated thrombocytopenia. Bortezomib, a first-generation proteasome inhibitor, was found to reduce the mean platelet number by approximately 60%, independent of the baseline platelet count [9]. Proteosome inhibitor associated thrombocytopenia has a cyclic, transient pattern [16,17]. The mechanism was first suggested to be related to the prevention of the activation of NF-κB which may potentially prevent platelet budding from megakaryocytes. Further studies found that the pharmacologic inhibition of proteasome activity blocks proplatelet formation, due to the upregulation and hyperactivation of the small GTPase RhoA, rather than NF-κB [18]. Although thrombocytopenia is commonly observed, there are only a few reports of serious bleeding complications with proteosome inhibitors [17,19].

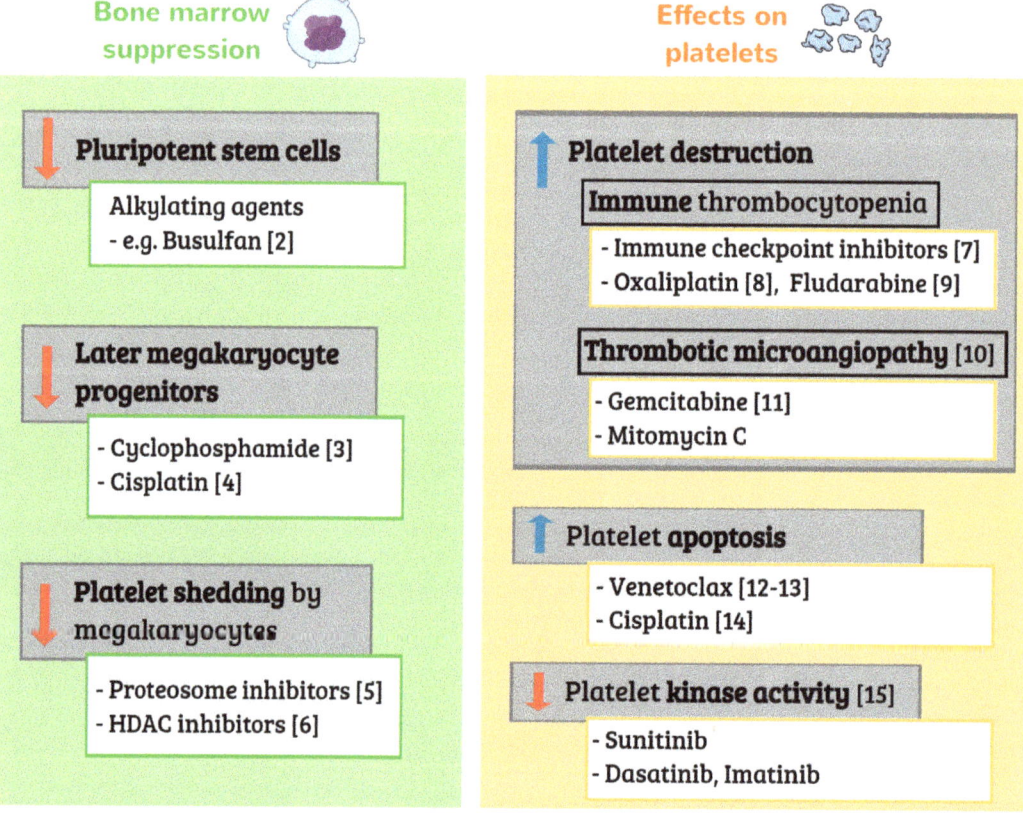

Figure 1. Selected mechanisms of drug induced thrombocytopenia in cancer. Examples of implicated drugs are given for each mechanism. *HDAC*, histone deacetylase.

Severe thrombocytopenia ($<10 \times 10^9$/L) is associated with an increased risk of bleeding in cancer [20,21]. However, individual platelet counts between 10 and 50×10^9/L do not clearly predict bleeding [22–24]. Multiple other factors affect the bleeding risk, such as fever, sex, renal failure, liver dysfunction, hematocrit $\leq 25\%$ and use of antithrombotic drugs [21,24,25]. These factors should be considered when assessing bleeding risk and addressed when modifiable. In addition, emerging data show that patients with cancer-associated thrombocytopenia have additional hemostatic defects, such as platelet and endothelial dysfunction, as well as coagulation abnormalities, such as hyperfibrinolysis [26–28].

The mainstay of managing severe chemotherapy-induced thrombocytopenia (CIT) in cancer is the use of platelet transfusions. In most cancer settings, platelet transfusions are indicated prophylactically when platelets counts are $<10 \times 10^9$/L or therapeutically when bleeding occurs with platelets below 50×10^9/L [29]. Different platelet transfusion thresholds may be warranted in the context of invasive procedures, sepsis, autologous stem cell transplantation and chronic stable disease-related thrombocytopenia, among other scenarios [21,29]. While prophylactic platelet transfusions reduce the rate of WHO grade ≥ 2 bleeding [22,23], multiple unmet needs remain in patients with cancer and thrombocytopenia, including the following: high rates of bleeding despite platelet transfusion [22]; thrombocytopenia-driven anticancer treatment dose reductions or delay; platelet-transfusion refractoriness [30]; managing antithrombotic drugs when indicated.

This review focuses upon non-transfusion-based approaches to managing thrombocytopenia and the associated bleeding risk in cancer, and also addresses the management of antithrombotic therapy in thrombocytopenic cancer patients. The topic of platelet transfusions in cancer patients has been previously reviewed [29] and is covered elsewhere in this issue of the Journal.

2. Managing Thrombocytopenia in Cancer

2.1. Antifibrinolytic Therapy

Tranexamic acid (TXA) and aminocaproic acid (EACA) are synthetic antifibrinolytic drugs that lead to the inhibition of the conversion of plasminogen to plasmin and to the decrease in the lysis of fibrin clots [31]. Antifibrinolytic therapy has been shown to aid in the management of bleeding in multiple clinical scenarios such as trauma, postpartum hemorrhage, menorrhagia, and surgical bleeding [32]. On the other hand, recent negative findings of a randomized controlled trial (RCT) of TXA in acute gastrointestinal bleeding and a higher rate venous thromboembolism (VTE) in the TXA arm, serve as a reminder that setting-specific evidence is needed [33]. In light of this, the utility of antifibrinolytic drugs in solid tumors and hematological malignancies has also been evaluated. This review focuses on CIT or cancer-related thrombocytopenia, outside the context of disseminated intravascular coagulation (DIC) [34,35].

2.1.1. Solid Tumors

A number of small RCTs and retrospective cohort studies were performed to assess the effect of perioperative antifibrinolytics on bleeding during and after cancer surgery, in a variety of solid malignancies. The studies including patients with liver, prostate and gynecological cancer found a reduction in blood transfusion requirements during and after surgery in the TXA arms [36–41]. In contrast, antifibrinolytics did not influence bleeding outcomes in major orthopedic cancer surgery or in oncologic spinal canal, head and neck and neurosurgeries [42–45].

Data on the use of antifibrinolytics for the treatment of active bleeding in solid cancer is scarce and limited to case reports and series. Several case reports showed favorable bleeding outcomes with TXA in the management of bleeding from malignant mesothelioma with hemothorax [46], hemoptysis due to bronchogenic carcinoma [47] and DIC after a prostatic biopsy [48]. One small case series (n = 16) demonstrated high rates of bleeding control with TXA and EACA for cancer associated bleeding in the palliative care setting [49].

2.1.2. Hematological Malignancies with Thrombocytopenia

EACA and TXA have been studied over the years in patients with hematological malignancies and thrombocytopenia (generally <50 × 10^9/L) with or without bleeding. However, most of the studies are small, non-controlled and retrospective with various treatment protocols and doses. Since EACA and TXA have not been compared directly, the evidence on each of these drugs is presented separately, first as treatment and then as prophylaxis.

Treatment of Bleeding

Two studies published in 1980 and 1985 evaluated the use of EACA for the control of bleeding in patients with various hematological malignancies and thrombocytopenia (<20 × 10^9/L) and reported the improvement in bleeding control and a reduction in platelet transfusions [50,51]. An additional study published in 1998 evaluated 15 patients with bleeding and severe thrombocytopenia (platelets <20 × 10^9/L) and showed a positive effect with a maximum EACA dose of 6 g/day [52]. In 2006, a retrospective study from the Cleveland clinic reviewed the use of EACA in 77 patients with thrombocytopenic (median platelet count = 7 × 10^9/L) hemorrhage (mostly mucosal and gastrointestinal). The majority of patients had hematological malignancies, predominantly acute leukemia and non-Hodgkin lymphoma, and the remainder had solid tumors. The median average dose was also 6 g/day. Complete (i.e., cessation of bleeding at all sites) and partial response were achieved in 51 (66%) and 13 (17%) patients, respectively, resulting in a decrease in platelet and red blood cell transfusions [53]. In 2008, a retrospective study evaluating EACA in acute promyelocytic leukemia (APL) patients with coagulopathy defined as low alpha-2-antiplasmin levels suggested a lower incidence of severe hemorrhagic events [54].

A recent Dutch survey indicated that TXA is more commonly used for the control of bleeding in hematological malignancies than as prophylaxis [55], even though most studies of TXA were in the context of prophylaxis. There is currently scarce evidence supporting the use of this specific agent in this context.

Prophylaxis of Bleeding

EACA as prophylactic treatment was evaluated in 1983 in a randomized controlled trial versus placebo in patients undergoing remission induction for acute leukemia. There was no difference in major bleeding between the two groups; however, there was a non-significant reduction in platelet transfusions in the EACA group [56]. A subsequent retrospective study in 2013 reported on EACA treatment in 44 chronically and severely thrombocytopenic patients with hematological malignancies and median platelet counts of $8 \times 10^9/L$. EACA was associated with a low risk of major spontaneous bleeding and was well tolerated [57]. Two additional retrospective studies (2016, 2018) provided additional safety data by demonstrating no increase in VTE rates with EACA as prophylactic therapy in thrombocytopenic patients with hematological malignancy [58,59]. The PROBLEMA Trial, a phase II control trial study evaluating the effectiveness and safety of EACA versus prophylactic platelet transfusions to prevent bleeding in thrombocytopenic patients with hematological malignancies, is still ongoing [60]. Table 1 details the ongoing studies of antifibrinolytics in thrombocytopenic cancer patients.

Table 1. Ongoing and planned clinical trials of antifibrinolytic agents in thrombocytopenic cancer patients [1].

Name, *Identifier*	**Study Design** *(Status)*	**Interventions** [2]	**Study Population** [3]	**Primary Outcome**	**Time Frame**	**Planned Completion**
Antifibrinolytics in Thrombocytopenia						
TRial to EvaluAte Tranexamic Acid Therapy in Thrombocytope-nia (TREATT), NCT03136445	Interventional Randomized Phase 3 *(recruiting)*	*Arm A*: TXA 1 g q8hrs IV; *Arm B*: TXA 1.5 g q8hrs PO.	Thrombocytopenic patients (platelet count of $\leq 10 \times 10^9/L$ for ≥ 5 days) with hematological malignancies ($n = 616$)	Death or bleeding (WHO grade ≥ 2)	30 days	March 2021
PRevention of BLeeding in hEmatological Malignancies with Antifibrinolytic (PROBLEMA), NCT02074436	Interventional Randomized Phase 2 *(recruiting)*	*Arm A*: EACA 1000 mg q12hrs; *Arm B*: standard prophylactic platelet transfusion	Thrombocytopenic patients (platelet count $< 20 \times 10^9/L$) with hematological malignancies ($n = 100$)	Major bleeding episodes (WHO grades 3–4)	6 mo.	May 2021
Evolution of Thromboelastog-raphy During Tranexamic Acid Treatment (TTRAP-Bleeding), NCT03801122	Interventional Randomized Phase 2 *(recruiting)*	*Arm A*: TXA 3 g/day; *Arm B*: TXA 1.5 g/day; *Arm C*: No TXA	Thrombocytopenic patients (platelet count of $\leq 10 \times 10^9/L$ for ≥ 5 days) with hematological malignancies ($n = 18$)	Level of clot amplitude in thrombo-elastography	30 days	1 April 2022

[1] Interventional phase 2 and 3 studies shown, as identified in https://www.clinicaltrials.gov/ (accessed on 31 January 2021). [2] The ratio between intervention arms is 1:1 or 1:1:1 unless otherwise specified. [3] All participants are aged 18 years or older, unless otherwise specified. EACA, epsilon aminocaproic acid; IV, intravenous; PLT, platelet count ($\times 10^9/L$); TXA, tranexamic acid.

Up until recently, only three small RCTs evaluating TXA in hematological malignancies had been published (1989 thru 1995) including patients with acute leukemia, APL, aplastic anemia and myelodysplastic syndrome (MDS) [61–63]. TXA was associated with fewer bleeding episodes and fewer transfusion requirements in two of these studies [61,62]. In the third pilot study evaluating eight patients with MDS and aplastic anemia, TXA did not appear to be efficacious [63]. It should be noted that only three patients completed the randomized portion of this study and that patients were used as their own control. In addition, a prospective single arm study published in 1990 demonstrated a significant reduction in platelet transfusion with prophylactic TXA during induction and consolidation treatment in acute leukemia, compared to historical controls [64]. Of concern is a case series of three allogenic hematopoietic stem cell transplant patients who developed veno-occlusive disease (VOD) shortly after receiving TXA. The authors postulated a role for plasminogen activator inhibitor-1 in the development of hepatic VOD and that TXA could trigger or accelerate this process [65].

Accordingly, a systematic review and meta-analysis of antifibrinolytics for the prevention of bleeding in patients with hematological disorders concluded that there is uncertainty whether antifibrinolytics reduce the risk of bleeding in such patients, due to the small number of participants and low quality of evidence [66]. The question whether or not antifibrinolytics increase the risk of thromboembolic events or other adverse events could not be answered. A subsequent meta-analysis published in 2017 evaluated the safety and efficacy of lysine analogues in a total of 1177 cancer patients (both hematological and solid tumors) [67]. No increased risk of venous thromboembolism was observed among patients receiving lysine analogues compared to controls, and their use significantly decreased blood loss and transfusion risk.

The results of the randomized controlled A-TREAT trial, assessing prophylactic TXA administration in addition to routine platelet transfusion, were recently presented and published in abstract form [68]. The study included 165 patients in each arm and demonstrated that prophylactic TXA did not decrease the rate of WHO grade 2+ bleeding and did not change platelet and blood cell transfusions rates. Of note, the rate of central line occlusions was increased in the TXA arm. This preliminary publication suggests that TXA should not be currently used for preventing bleeding in addition to prophylactic platelet transfusions. The results of the sister TREAT-T trial conducted in the UK and Australia are eagerly anticipated (Table 1) [69]. Knowledge gaps not currently addressed by published or ongoing trials that we are aware of, include the use of antifibrinolytic therapy for breakthrough bleeding and as prophylaxis in patients with platelet transfusion refractoriness.

2.2. Thrombopoeitin Receptor Agonists in Cancer and Thrombocytopenia

Thrombopoetin receptor agonists (TPO-RAs), such as eltrombopag and romiplostim, increase platelet production through interactions with the thrombopoietin receptor on megakaryocytes. Eltrombopag is a small molecule agonist, while romiplostim is a peptibody (i.e., fusion of a novel peptide and antibody) that can stimulate the TPO receptor. The binding of romiplostim to the distal domain of the thrombopoietin receptor or binding of eltrombopag to the transmembrane region of the receptor triggers a number of signal transduction pathways, including activation of the JAK-STAT signaling pathway, which induce proliferation and differentiation of megakaryocytes [70]. Eltrombopag and romipostim were both licensed in the United States for the treatment of immune thrombocytopenia in 2008. Eltrombopag is also licensed for the treatment of aplastic anemia and the treatment of thrombocytopenia in patients with hepatitis C receiving interferon-based therapy [71].

Recombinant IL-11 (oprelvekin) is the only approved treatment in the United States for CIT. However, its use is very limited because of side effects [72]. Clinical development of recombinant human thrombopoietins (rhTPO) and pegylated recombinant megakaryocyte growth and development factor (PEG-rhMGDF) have stopped due to the development of neutralizing antibodies to PEG-rhMGDF [73]. The rhTPO, TPIAO™, is widely used to treat CIT in China and is unavailable elsewhere [74].

TPO-RAs have been studied for two major implications in cancer related thrombocytopenia. In the field of hematological disorders, they were mainly studied for MDS and acute myeloid leukemia (AML), in order to treat severe thrombocytopenia and avoid platelet transfusions, as summarized in Table 2. In the field of solid tumors, they were used to prevent CIT and enable scheduled anti-cancer treatment. Prevention was either primary, before anti-cancer treatment, or secondary, after the development of thrombocytopenia. Selected studies on TPO-RAs in CIT are detailed in Table 3.

2.2.1. Low-Intermediate Risk MDS

Giagouinidis et al. included 250 patients with low to intermediate (low-int) risk MDS to receive romiplostim or placebo (2:1) [75]. This study was terminated early because of an increase in peripheral blasts in the romiplostim group. Despite this initial signal, there was no increased risk of progression to AML in the romiplostim group [75], including in an analysis after five years follow-up [76]. Romiplostim increased platelet counts, and decreased platelet transfusions and overall bleeding, but did not affect clinically significant bleeding rates. Initial similar results were published for eltrombopag in low-int MDS [77]. That study reported improved quality of life in patients who received eltrombopag. The full study has not been published yet. Eltrombopag was also shown to increase white blood cell counts and hemoglobin levels in some patients in a small study of low-int risk MDS patients [78].

2.2.2. High Risk MDS/AML

In a phase 1/2 study of advanced MDS or AML, eltrombopag was well tolerated in 64 patients, and no difference in the percentage of blasts was observed [79]. In a phase 3 trial of intermediate-high risk MDS treated with azacitidine, eltrombopag did not reduce the need for platelet transfusions. In fact, this study was terminated early due to inferiority of the eltrombopag/azacitidine arm (16% vs. 31%) and a trend towards increased progression to AML [80]. Furthermore, in a phase 2 placebo controlled trial of eltrombopag in patients with AML undergoing induction chemotherapy, eltrombopag did not decrease the time to platelet recovery, while more serious adverse events and numerically higher death rates were observed in the eltrombopag group [81].

2.2.3. After Bone Marrow Transplantation

Persistent thrombocytopenia is a common complication after allogeneic hematopoietic cell transplantation. In a phase 1/2 single arm study, romiplostim given to patients after allogeneic stem cell transplantation who had persistent severe thrombocytopenia $<20 \times 10^9$/L (median of 84 days after transplantation), was effective in most patients. The median time to platelet counts $>50 \times 10^9$/L was 45 days [82]. Eltrombopag was also reported to achieve good platelet response in approximately 60% of patients in three small retrospective studies [83–85].

2.2.4. High Grade Lymphoma

In a phase 1/2 open label in patients with Hodgkin or non-Hodgkin lymphoma, who experienced grade 3–4 thrombocytopenia ($<50 \times 10^9$/L), romiplostim given one day after chemotherapy did not have a beneficial effect on platelet nadir [86]. In contrast, in patients receiving the RHyper-CVAD/RArac-MTX protocol, romiplostim, given 5 days before and after chemotherapy, significantly (for a total of 2 doses) increased the platelet nadir and decreased the duration of thrombocytopenia [87].

Table 2. Summary of studies on TPO-RAs in MDS and AML.

Design	Population	PLT, 10^9/L	Intervention	TPO-RA Dose	Participants, n	Primary Outcome	Follow up	Results	Comments	Ref.
Phase 2 randomized	Low-int 1 MDS	<20	Romiplostim or placebo	250–1000 µg (750 µg start)	n(romi) = 167; n(placebo) = 83	CSBE	58 wks.	No difference in CSBE. Decreased overall bleeding. PLT increased. Transfusion reduced.	Early termination due to transient increase in peripheral blasts with romi. No increase in AML (18% vs. 20.5%)	[75]
					n(romi) = 139; n(placebo) = 83	OS and leukemic progression	5 years	No difference in OS or leukemic progression		[76]
Phase I of single blind randomized phase 2 trial	Low-Int 1 MDS	<30	Eltrombopag or placebo	50–300 mg	n(el-pag) = 59; n(placebo) = 39	Platelet response	11 wks. (median)	47% platelet response. Less bleeding	No difference in AML progression	[77]
Phase 2	Low risk MDS	<30	Eltrombopag	50–150 mg	25	Hematologic response	16 wks.	44% response	24% bi-lineage response	[78]
Phase 1/2	Advanced MDS or AML	<30	Eltrombopag or placebo	50–300 mg	n(el-pag) = 64; n(placebo) = 34	Safety & tolerability	6 mo. (optional 6 mo. extension)	Acceptable safety profile	No increase in marrow or peripheral blasts	[79]
Phase 3	Int-High risk MDS receiving azacitidine	<75	Eltrombopag or placebo	200–300 mg	n(el-pag) = 179; n(placebo) = 177	Platelet transfusion free	Cycles 1–4	More transfusion free with placebo (31%) than eltrombopag (16%). Worse PLT recovery	Terminated early due to futility and safety. Trend to AML progression.	[80]
Phase 2 double blind randomized	AML induction		Eltrombopag or placebo	200 mg	n(el-pag) = 74; n(placebo) = 74	Safety & tolerability	Until PLT > 200 or 42 days post-induction	More SAEs with eltrombopag	Numerically more deaths with eltrombopag. Same VTE rates.	[81]

AML, acute myeloid leukemia; CSBE, clinically significant bleeding events; el-pag, eltrombopag; MDS, myelodysplastic syndrome; OS, overall survival; PLT, platelet count; romi, romiplostim; SAE. Serious adverse events; TPO-RA, thrombopoietin receptor agonists; VTE, venous thromboembolism; wk, week.

2.2.5. CIT in Solid Tumors

CIT in solid tumors is defined as platelet count below $100 \times 10^9/L$ with no other reason for thrombocytopenia. CIT may carry a risk of bleeding and may delay anti-cancer treatment and, therefore, it could potentially affect patients' prognosis. A recent Cochrane review assessed the effects of TPO-RAs to treat and prevent CIT [88]. No certain conclusions could be made due to the weak available data. Selected studies for treatment of CIT are presented in Table 3. These were mostly retrospective studies that reported off-label use of romiplostim for this indication as well as several phase 2 studies. The main type of tumor was of gastrointestinal origin. Romiplostim rapidly increased platelet counts and could enable the scheduled anti-cancer treatments in most patients (Table 3). In the largest retrospective study to date, predictors of non-response to romiplostim included bone marrow tumor invasion, prior pelvic irradiation and exposure to temozolomide [89]. Nonetheless, in an open label phase II study of romiplostim in patients with glioblastoma receiving temozolomide, 60% of patients had good response and only 20% had no response [90]. The rate of thrombotic complications in patients who received romiplostim was reported between 5–15% (Table 3). Most of the events were VTE and only a small number of arterial events were reported. It is unclear whether TPO-RAs increase thrombosis in patients with cancer since no comparison group was included in most of the studies. A phase 3 study of avatrombopag vs. placebo in cancer patients who experienced grade 3–4 thrombocytopenia, was recently terminated due to futility, but is yet to be published. The press release reported that although avatrombopag increased platelet counts relative to placebo as expected, the study did not meet the composite primary endpoint of avoiding platelet transfusions, chemotherapy dose reductions by $\geq 15\%$, and chemotherapy dose delays by ≥ 4 days [91,92].

2.2.6. Summary

TPO-RA studies in cancer are mainly retrospective or phase 2 trials. In these trials, both romiplostim and eltrombopag showed a potential benefit in patients experiencing severe thrombocytopenia related to low risk MDS and post allogeneic transplantation. In patients receiving chemotherapy for solid tumors TPO-RAs may improve platelet counts and the ability to prescribe scheduled anti-cancer treatments. The only two phase 3 trials of eltrombopag in patients with high risk MDS and avatrombopag in solid tumors did not meet the primary outcome. TPO-RAs may carry a risk in patients with advanced MDS in combination with azacitidine and in patients with AML undergoing induction chemotherapy. More phase 3 trials are indicated to investigate the role of TPO-RAs in cancer patients, some of which are planned or underway, as detailed in Table 4.

Table 3. Selected studies on TPO-RAs for preventing or treating CIT in solid tumors.

Design	Cancer Type	PLT, 10⁹/L	Intervention	TPO-RA Dose	Participants, n	Primary Outcome	Follow up	Key Results	Comments	Ref
Retrospective cohort	Wide range, mostly GI	75 (median)	Romiplostim	3 µg/kg/wk (median starting)	22	ChemoRx dose delay and/or reduction	NR	Reduced dose delay (36% vs. 94%) and reduction	No thrombosis	[93]
Retrospective cohort	Wide range	<100 for ≥6 weeks (mean 58; range 3–97)	Romiplostim	2.9 µg/kg/wk (mean)	20	PLT > 100; ChemoRx delay	NR	95% PLT >100; 75% resumed ChemoRx without TCP	3 DVT patients (15%) could continue ChemoRx	[94]
Retrospective cohort	Wide range, mostly GI	<100	Romiplostim	2 µg/kg/wk (median starting)	37	PLT > 100; ChemoRx continued	18 wk (median)	95% PLT < 100; 92% continued ChemoRx	14% (n = 6) thrombosis. Mostly in pancreatic cancer (5/6)	[95]
Phase 2 randomized open label	Wide range, mostly GI	<100	Romiplostim or placebo	1 µg/kg/wk (starting)	n(romi) = 15; n(placebo) = 8; n(open-label-romi) = 37	PLT > 100 within 3 wks	6 wk	Overall response (n = 54) 85%	10% VTE	[96]
Phase 2	NSCLC with Gemcitabine and carboplatin/cisplatin Rx	<50–100	Romiplostim or placebo	250–750 µg/wk	n(romi) = 50; n(placebo) = 12	Adverse events	≤5 cycles	Well tolerated. No effect on PLT or dose reduction	6% thrombosis	[97]
Retrospective cohort	Wide range	<100 for 3 weeks	Romiplostim	3 µg/kg/wk (median starting)	153	PLT response = Median PLT >75 or baseline +30	NR	71% response. 79% avoided dose delays or reduction	Less bleeding. 5.2% VTE (similar to historical controls)	[89]
Phase 2 open label single arm	Glioblastoma	<50	Romiplostim	750 µg/wk (starting; dose adjusted)	20	Proportion completing 6 cycles	6 cycles	60% completed 6 cycles	5% lower limb ischemia; 5% VTE	[90]
Phase 2	Advanced solid tumors, with Gemcitabine ± Carboplatin Rx	<150	Eltrombopag or placebo	100 mg/day	n(el-pag) = 53; n(placebo) = 23	PLT pre + post ChemoRx	6 cycles	Less time to PLT recovery; Fewer dose delays or reduction	Reduced rates of anemia and leukopenia	[98]

Table 3. Cont.

Design	Cancer Type	PLT, 10^9/L	Intervention	TPO-RA Dose	Participants, n	Primary Outcome	Follow up	Key Results	Comments	Ref
Phase 3	Ovarian, small cell lung cancer, NSCLC, bladder cancer	<50 in a previous treatment cycle	Avatrombopag or placebo	60 mg/day (5 days pre and post Rx)	122 (ava-pag:placebo, 2:1)	PLT transfusion or dose delays or reduction		No difference between ava-pag and placebo	Higher PLT in ava-pag group	[91, 92]

ava-pag, avatrombopag; *ChemoRx*, chemotherapy; *CIT*, chemotherapy-induced thrombocytopenia; *DVT*, deep vein thrombosis; *el-pag*; eltrombopag; *GI*, gastrointestinal; *NR*, not reported; *NSCLC*, non-small cell lung cancer; *PLT*, platelet count; *romi*; romiplostim; *Rx*, treatment; *TCP*, thrombocytopenia; *TPO-RA*, thrombopoietin receptor agonists; *VTE*, venous thromboembolism; *wk*, week.

Table 4. Ongoing and planned clinical trials of TPO-RAs in thrombocytopenia and cancer [1].

Name, *Identifier*	Study Design (*Status*)	Interventions [2]	Study Population [3]	Primary Outcome	Time Frame	Planned Completion
TPO-RAs in Hematological Malignancies						
Eltrombopag for the Treatment of Thrombocytopenia Due to Low- and Intermediate Risk Myelodysplastic Syndromes, *NCT02912208*	Interventional Randomized Phase 2 (*recruiting*)	>*Arm A*: eltrombopag 50–300 mg/day; *Arm B*: placebo	Stable low or int 1 MDS with PLT < 3C ineligible to receive other treatment options (n = 174)	Platelet response rate (complete or any)	6 mo.	August 2019
Phase II Study of Lenalidomide and Eltrombopag in Patients with Symptomatic Anemia in Low or Intermediate I Myelodysplastic Syndrome (MDS), *NCT01772420*	Interventional non-randomized Phase 2 with parallel assignment (*recruiting*)	*Arm A* if PLT > 50: lenalidomide and eltrombopag; *Arm B* if PLT < 50: eltrombopag until PLT > 50 for 2 wks. Then, Arm A.	Low-int 1 MDS or chronic myel-monocytic leukemia (n = 60)	Hematologic improvement as defined by the IWG 2006 criteria	8 weeks	January 2020
Eltrombopag in Myelodysplastic Syndrome (MDS) Patients with Thrombocytopenia, *NCT01286038*	Interventional single arm Phase 1–2 (*active, not recruiting*)	Eltrombopag	MDS after hypomethylating agent failure and PLT < 50 (n = 37)	Maximum tolerated dose	24 mo.	September 2021

Table 4. Cont.

Name, *Identifier*	Study Design (*Status*)	Interventions [2]	Study Population [3]	Primary Outcome	Time Frame	Planned Completion
Validation of a predictive model of response to romiplostim in patients with IPSS low or intermediate-1 risk MDS and thrombocytopenia (EUROPE-trial),	Interventional non-randomized Phase 2 with parallel assignment (*recruiting*)	Romiplostim stratified using TPO-based model to **Arm A** (score +3), **Arm B** (−1 or −2), **Arm C** (−6)	Low or int 1 MDS with PLT < 30 or PLT < 50 and bleeding (n = 84)	Hematologic improvement of platelets (HI-P) after 4 months on therapy	12 mo.	December 2021
Eltrombopag Olamine in Treating Thrombocytopenia in Patients with Chronic Myeloid Leukemia or Myelofibrosis Receiving Tyrosine Kinase Therapy, *NCT01428635*	Interventional single arm Phase 2 (*active, not recruiting*)	Eltrombopag	CML or MF patients with platelets <50 × 10^9/L (CML) or <100 × 10^9/L (MF) after 3 mo. of TKIs (n = 39)	Complete platelet response	30 days after last dose of eltrombopag	31 January 2022
Using Romiplostim to Treat Low Platelet Counts Following Chemotherapy and Autologous Hematopoietic Cell Transplantation in People with Blood Cancer, *NCT04478123*	Interventional single arm Phase 2 (*recruiting*)	Romiplostim 3 μg/kg on day 1+ after transplant (start dose)	Patients with multiple myeloma or lymphoma undergoing high dose chemotherapy with autologous stem cell transplant (n = 60)	No. of days post-transplant requiring platelet transfusions or grade 4 thrombocytopenia	42 days	July 2022
Using Romiplostim to Treat Low Platelet Counts during Chemotherapy in People with Lymphoma, *NCT04673266*	Interventional single arm Phase 2 (*recruiting*)	3 μg/kg/wk. on day 1 of chemotherapy cycle, titrated weekly	Lymphoma patients receiving chemotherapy, with grade 4 thrombocytopenia during previous cycle or PLT < 50 on day 1 of current cycle (n = 20)	PLT indication for dose delay (see definition)	1 year	December 2022
Study Impact on Outcome of Eltrombopag in Elderly Patients with Acute Myeloid Leukemia Receiving Induction Chemotherapy (EPAG2015), *NCT03603795*	Interventional Randomized Phase 2 (*recruiting*)	**Arm A**: eltrombopag 200 mg/day; **Arm B**: placebo	Patients aged ≥ 60yrs with de novo AML eligible for intensive induction chemotherapy (n = 110)	Overall survival rate	12 mo.	September 2024

Table 4. Cont.

Name, Identifier	Study Design (Status)	Interventions [2]	Study Population [3]	Primary Outcome	Time Frame	Planned Completion
TPO-RAs for CIT in solid tumors						
A Study of Romiplostim to Prevent Low Platelet Counts in Children and Young Adults Receiving Chemotherapy for Solid Tumors, NCT04671901	Interventional single arm Phase 2 (recruiting)	3 μg/kg/wk. from cycle 4, titrated weekly	Patients aged ≤21 years with a primary solid tumor undergoing N8/EFT chemotherapy treatment (n = 30)	No. of platelet transfusions	6 mo.	10 December 2022
Study of Romiplostim for Chemotherapy-induced Thrombocytopenia in Adult Subjects with Gastrointestinal, Pancreatic, or Colorectal Cancer (RECITE), NCT03362177	Randomized double-blind placebo controlled Phase 3 (recruiting)	**Arm A**: romiplostim 3 μg/kg/wk., titrated weekly; **Arm B**: placebo (2:1 ratio)	Patients receiving oxaliplatin-based chemotherapy for gastrointestinal/colorectal/pancreatic cancer, with PLT < 75 at or after scheduled start of next cycle (n = 162)	Thrombocytopenia-induced chemotherapy dose modification during the second or third on study chemotherapy cycles	48 days	1 June 2023
Study of Romiplostim for Chemotherapy-induced Thrombocytopenia in Adult Subjects with Non-small Cell Lung Cancer (NSCLC), Ovarian Cancer, or Breast Cancer, NCT03937154	Randomized double-blind placebo controlled Phase 3 (recruiting)	**Arm A**: romiplostim; **Arm B**: placebo (2:1 ratio)	Patients receiving carboplatin-based chemotherapy for locally advanced or metastatic non-small cell lung cancer, ovarian cancer, or breast cancer, with PLT < 75 at or after scheduled start of next cycle (n = 162)	Chemotherapy dose delay or reduction	48 days	28 June 2023
Avatrombopag on the Treatment of Thrombocytopenia Induced by Chemotherapy of Malignant Tumors, NCT04609891	Interventional single arm Phase 2 (recruiting)	Avatrombopag 40 mg or 60 mg, depending on PLT. Duration differs between prevention and treatment	Patients with solid tumors receiving chemotherapy, and 10 < PLT < 75 after the last cycle (n = 80)	Chemotherapy dose delay or reduction, or platelet transfusion	2 mo.	31 August 2021

[1] Interventional phase 2 and 3 studies shown, as identified on https://www.clinicaltrials.gov/ (accessed on 31 January 2021). [2] The ratio between intervention arms is 1:1 or 1:1:1 unless otherwise specified. [3] All participants are aged 18 years or older, unless otherwise specified. AML, acute myeloid leukemia; CIT, chemotherapy induced thrombocytopenia; CML, chronic myeloid leukemia; MDS, myelodysplastic syndrome; MF, myelofibrosis; mo., months; PLT, platelet count (x10⁹/L); TKI, tyrosine kinase inhibitor; TPO-RA, thrombopoietin receptor agonist.

3. Managing Antithrombotic Therapy in Thrombocytopenic Patients

Cancer is associated with an increased risk of both venous and arterial thrombosis [99–101]. Moreover, contemporary anticancer therapy and supportive care allow for the treatment of older patients with comorbid cardiovascular disease. This means that cancer patients, who are also at risk of thrombocytopenia, often have an indication for antithrombotic therapy (i.e., anticoagulation or antiplatelet therapy) before or after cancer diagnosis. Thrombocytopenic cancer patients remain at risk of venous and arterial thrombosis, since thrombocytopenia does not afford protection and is associated with adverse outcomes [102–108]. Multiple mechanisms, not dependent on the platelet compartment, contribute to cancer associated thrombosis, as recently reviewed [109]. These include tumor-driven increases in procoagulant activity and inhibition of fibrinolytic and natural anticoagulant pathways which lead to increased thrombin generation, as well as effects on leukocytes and endothelial cells. On the other hand, cancer patients are at increased risk of anticoagulation-associated bleeding [110,111], which is complicated by thrombocytopenia and other hemostatic defects [26–28]. Therefore, balancing the thrombotic and bleeding risk in thrombocytopenic risk remains a clinical challenge. Unfortunately, prospective data are scarce, meaning that management is currently informed mainly by expert opinion [112] and retrospective studies on VTE and ischemic heart disease [102,106,113–116], since clinical trials of anticoagulants in cancer-associated VTE exclude patients with thrombocytopenia (<50–100 × 10^9/L) [117–121].

3.1. Management Concepts

We generally manage antithrombotic medication within the framework of international guidelines for treatment of VTE in thrombocytopenic cancer patients [122]. Importantly, these recommendations do not apply to other indications such as atrial fibrillation or antiplatelet medication, which generally lack specific guidelines. Therefore, we adjust management after considering context-specific evidence (see Sections 3.2 and 3.3) and the risk-benefit ratio for the individual patient, bearing in mind the low level of evidence driving these recommendations.

3.1.1. Risk Assessment

We always reevaluate the indication for antithrombotic therapy, and assess the associated thrombotic risk. We then estimate the anticipated duration of platelet counts below 50×10^9/L, which may range from days to weeks in case of CIT or months to years for chronic disease-related thrombocytopenia, such as in MDS or graft versus host disease. Of note, the vast majority of evidence pertains to short-term thrombocytopenia. We also identify additional factors associated with higher bleeding risk in this setting, including a history of bleeding, hematological malignancy and increasing bilirubin, creatinine, and prothrombin time [113,114]. An important concept guiding management decisions is that these patients have a high short-term risk of clinically significant bleeding, especially with full anticoagulation [22,24,102,113,123–125]. Accordingly, the thrombotic risk should be sufficiently high to justify anticoagulation.

3.1.2. Management Plan

Using the above information, we formulate a clear management plan, to be reassessed frequently, often on a daily basis. We first decide whether to continue or hold the antithrombotic medication. If continued, we consider changes in the dose and/or class of antithrombotic medication, and modifications in platelet transfusion thresholds. When anticoagulation is discontinued, mechanical measures to possibly mitigate thrombotic risk are considered on a case-by-case basis. These include inferior vena cava filter placement for acute lower extremity deep vein thrombosis (DVT) [122] or removal of the central venous catheter in case of catheter-related DVT [126]. Finally, once the platelet count is consistently above the threshold for full antithrombotic medication, we consider restarting full antithrombotic therapy, even between treatment cycles, if the indication remains [123].

3.2. Anticoagulation

Changes in anticoagulation management are generally recommended when platelets are <50 × 10^9/L [112,122,127], since the bleeding risk appears to increase below this threshold [102,123]. The two main indications for therapeutic anticoagulation in this setting are VTE and atrial fibrillation. The evidence and guidelines relate almost exclusively to low-molecular weight heparin (LMWH). The lack of data on direct oral anticoagulants with platelets <50 × 10^9/L, and increased bleeding risk even with prophylactic doses indicate that they should currently be avoided in this setting [119,121,122,128]. Retrospective cohort studies of VTE patients show varying bleeding and thrombotic rates, as summarized in a prior review [109].

The first month of anticoagulation for VTE is a high risk period for both recurrent bleeding and thrombosis [110], with higher rates of recurrent VTEs in populations enriched with acute VTE (i.e., within 30 days) [109]. Higher VTE burden (e.g., pulmonary embolism or proximal lower extremity DVT) is also considered to carry a higher thrombotic risk [122]. The CHA_2DS_2VASC score may be used to assess the thrombotic risk in patients with atrial fibrillation. Lower thrombotic risk scenarios where full-dose anticoagulation may not be justified include non-acute VTE (especially in autologous hematopoietic stem cell transplantation), catheter-related thrombosis and low risk atrial fibrillation [114,125,126,129]. Strategies for mitigating the high bleeding risk associated with continued anticoagulation include increased platelet transfusion threshold (e.g., 40–50 × 10^9/L) and anticoagulation dose reductions, but evidence proving the safety and efficacy of both approaches is lacking [130].

Current guidelines use VTE acuity, risk of thrombus progression and platelet count to direct decisions regarding anticoagulation in thrombocytopenic cancer patients with VTE [122]. In case of acute VTE, high risk of thrombus progression and platelets <50 × 10^9/L, increased platelet transfusion thresholds are recommended to enable full-dose anticoagulation. In patients with acute VTE and a lower risk of thrombus progression or those with non-acute VTE, LMWH dose reduction by 50% or prophylactic LMWH doses are recommended when platelets are 25–50 × 10^9/L. Anticoagulation should generally be discontinued at platelet counts below 25 × 10^9/L.

A recent study of 774 hypothetical case vignettes managed by 168 physicians suggested that the management process was compatible with these guidelines but that management varied according to physician characteristics and practice setting [131]. Of note, prior major bleeding and the type of hematological disease and treatment influenced management, and may be considered in the decision-making process, although not incorporated in the guidelines. Two recent retrospective analyses suggest that current management may achieve a reasonable balance between bleeding and thrombotic risk in VTE patients [116,129], but this remains to be confirmed prospectively by ongoing observational studies [132].

3.3. Antiplatelet Therapy

We generally discontinue aspirin used for primary prevention of arterial disease in patients with thrombocytopenia. The platelet threshold requiring changes in aspirin management appears lower than 50 × 10^9/L, but the exact threshold is unknown [106,115]. There are sufficient data to suggest that aspirin use in acute myocardial infarction in thrombocytopenic patients (especially if platelets >30 × 10^9/L) should be considered [106], but evidence on other indications is lacking.

Formal ischemic heart disease and stroke guidelines do not provide recommendations for management of thrombocytopenic cancer patients. In a consensus statement from the Society for Cardiovascular Angiography and Interventions (SCAI), aspirin was recommended when platelet counts were >10 × 10^9/L, while dual antiplatelet therapy was reserved for platelets >30 × 10^9/L [133]. A recent review, not specific to cancer, provided higher platelet thresholds (aspirin >50 × 10^9/L; dual antiplatelet therapy >100 × 10^9/L) [134].

A case vignette study assessing the decision-making process among 145 physicians across three countries, outlined the patient and physician factors influencing management.

This study indicated that physicians considered ST elevation myocardial infarction to be a high-risk thrombotic scenario that warrants dual antiplatelet therapy despite thrombocytopenia [135]. Furthermore, platelet transfusion was used in 34% of cases continuing antiplatelet therapy to theoretically mitigate the risk of bleeding; however, there is no evidence to support this practice.

4. Summary

The main take home messages regarding antifibrinolytics, TPO-RAs and antithrombotic medication in thrombocytopenic patients are shown in Figure 2. Platelet transfusion remains the cornerstone of managing thrombocytopenia in cancer, while we eagerly await the results of ongoing studies on antifibrinolytics and TPO-RAs.

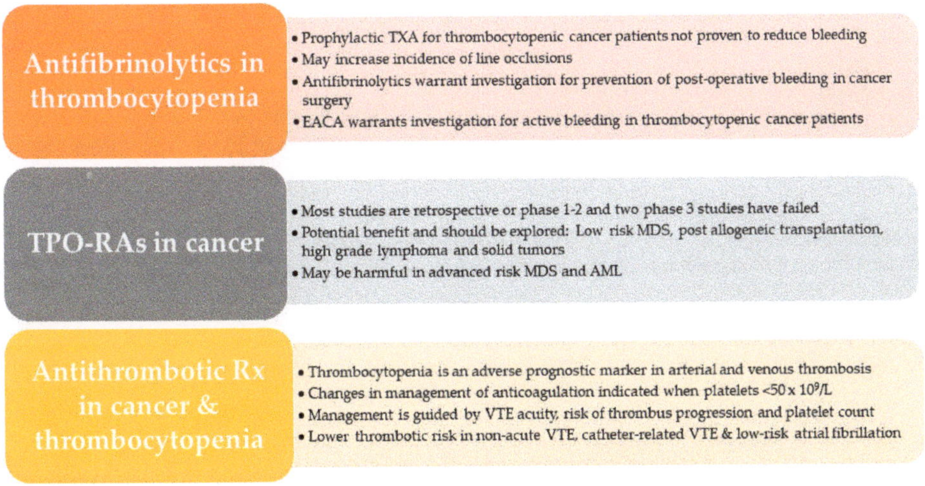

Antifibrinolytics in thrombocytopenia
- Prophylactic TXA for thrombocytopenic cancer patients not proven to reduce bleeding
- May increase incidence of line occlusions
- Antifibrinolytics warrant investigation for prevention of post-operative bleeding in cancer surgery
- EACA warrants investigation for active bleeding in thrombocytopenic cancer patients

TPO-RAs in cancer
- Most studies are retrospective or phase 1-2 and two phase 3 studies have failed
- Potential benefit and should be explored: Low risk MDS, post allogeneic transplantation, high grade lymphoma and solid tumors
- May be harmful in advanced risk MDS and AML

Antithrombotic Rx in cancer & thrombocytopenia
- Thrombocytopenia is an adverse prognostic marker in arterial and venous thrombosis
- Changes in management of anticoagulation indicated when platelets <50 x 10^9/L
- Management is guided by VTE acuity, risk of thrombus progression and platelet count
- Lower thrombotic risk in non-acute VTE, catheter-related VTE & low-risk atrial fibrillation

Figure 2. Take-home messages. *AML*, acute myeloid leukemia; *EACA*, epsilon aminocaproic acid; *MDS*, myelodysplastic syndrome; *TPO-RA*, thrombopoietin receptor agonists; *TXA*, tranexamic acid; *VTE*, venous thromboembolism.

Author Contributions: Literature review, writing—original draft preparation, writing—review and editing, A.L., L.H., G.S. All authors have read and agreed to the published version of the manuscript.

Funding: This research received no external funding.

Conflicts of Interest: A.L. declares personal fees for consultancy and scientific advisory boards from Bayer, Novartis, Pfizer, Sanofi, outside the scope of this manuscript; G.S. declares personal fees for consultancy and scientific advisory from Bayer, Boehringer Ingelheim, Medison, Novartis, Pfizer, Sanofi, outside the scope of this manuscript. L.H. declares no conflict of interest.

References

1. Liebman, H.A. Thrombocytopenia in cancer patients. *Thromb. Res.* **2014**, *133*, 63. [CrossRef]
2. McManus, P.M.; Weiss, L. Busulfan-induced chronic bone marrow failure: Changes in cortical bone, marrow stromal cells, and adherent cell colonies. *Blood* **1984**, *64*, 1036–1041. [CrossRef] [PubMed]
3. Dezern, A.E.; Petri, M.; Drachman, D.B.; Kerr, D.; Hammond, E.R.; Kowalski, J.; Tsai, H.L.; Loeb, D.M.; Anhalt, G.; Wigley, F.; et al. High-dose cyclophosphamide without stem cell rescue in 207 patients with aplastic anemia and other autoimmune diseases. *Medicine* **2011**, *90*, 89–98. [CrossRef] [PubMed]
4. Zhang, H.; Nimmer, P.M.; Tahir, S.K.; Chen, J.; Fryer, R.M.; Hahn, K.R.; Iciek, L.A.; Morgan, S.J.; Nasarre, M.C.; Nelson, R.; et al. Bcl-2 family proteins are essential for platelet survival. *Cell Death Differ.* **2007**, *14*, 943–951. [CrossRef] [PubMed]
5. Suvarna, V.; Singh, V.; Murahari, M. Current overview on the clinical update of Bcl-2 anti-apoptotic inhibitors for cancer therapy. *Eur. J. Pharmacol.* **2019**, *862*, 172655. [CrossRef]
6. Zhang, W.; Zhao, L.; Liu, J.; Du, J.; Wang, Z.; Ruan, C.; Dai, K. Cisplatin induces platelet apoptosis through the ERK signaling pathway. *Thromb. Res.* **2012**, *130*, 81–91. [CrossRef]

7. Tullemans, B.M.E.; Heemskerk, J.W.M.; Kuijpers, M.J.E. Acquired platelet antagonism: Off-target antiplatelet effects of malignancy treatment with tyrosine kinase inhibitors. *J. Thromb. Haemost.* **2018**, *16*, 1686–1699. [CrossRef]
8. Zeuner, A.; Signore, M.; Martinetti, D.; Bartucci, M.; Peschle, C.; De Maria, R. Chemotherapy-induced thrombocytopenia derives from the selective death of megakaryocyte progenitors and can be rescued by stem cell factor. *Cancer Res.* **2007**, *67*, 4767–4773. [CrossRef]
9. Lonial, S.; Waller, E.K.; Richardson, P.G.; Jagannath, S.; Orlowski, R.Z.; Giver, C.R.; Jaye, D.L.; Francis, D.; Giusti, S.; Torre, C.; et al. Risk factors and kinetics of thrombocytopenia associated with bortezomib for relapsed, refractory multiple myeloma. *Blood* **2005**, *106*, 3777–3784. [CrossRef]
10. Bishton, M.J.; Harrison, S.J.; Martin, B.P.; McLaughlin, N.; James, C.; Josefsson, E.C.; Henley, K.J.; Kile, B.T.; Prince, H.M.; Johnstone, R.W. Deciphering the molecular and biologic processes that mediate histone deacetylase inhibitor—Induced thrombocytopenia. *Blood* **2011**, *117*, 3658–3668. [CrossRef]
11. Michot, J.M.; Lazarovici, J.; Tieu, A.; Champiat, S.; Voisin, A.L.; Ebbo, M.; Godeau, B.; Michel, M.; Ribrag, V.; Lambotte, O. Haematological immune-related adverse events with immune checkpoint inhibitors, how to manage? *Eur. J. Cancer* **2019**, *122*, 72–90. [CrossRef] [PubMed]
12. Curtis, B.R.; Kaliszewski, J.; Marques, M.B.; Saif, M.W.; Nabelle, L.; Blank, J.; McFarland, J.G.; Aster, R.H. Immune-mediated thrombocytopenia resulting from sensitivity to oxaliplatin. *Am. J. Hematol.* **2006**, *81*, 199–201. [CrossRef] [PubMed]
13. Leach, M.; Parsons, R.M.; Reilly, J.T.; Winfield, D.A. Autoimmune thrombocytopenia: A complication of fludarabine therapy in lymphoproliferative disorders. *Clin. Lab. Haematol.* **2000**, *22*, 175–178. [CrossRef]
14. Thomas, M.; Scully, M. How I Treat Microangiopathic Hemolytic Anemia in Patients with Cancer. *Blood* **2021**. [CrossRef]
15. Zupancic, M.; Shah, P.C.; Shah-Khan, F.; Nagendra, S. Gemcitabine-associated thrombotic thrombocytopenic purpura. *Lancet Oncol.* **2007**, *8*, 634–641. [CrossRef]
16. Dimopoulos, M.A.; Goldschmidt, H.; Niesvizky, R.; Joshua, D.; Chng, W.J.; Oriol, A.; Orlowski, R.Z.; Ludwig, H.; Facon, T.; Hajek, R.; et al. Carfilzomib or bortezomib in relapsed or refractory multiple myeloma (ENDEAVOR): An interim overall survival analysis of an open-label, randomised, phase 3 trial. *Lancet Oncol.* **2017**, *18*, 1327–1337. [CrossRef]
17. Gandolfi, S.; Laubach, J.P.; Hideshima, T.; Chauhan, D.; Anderson, K.C.; Richardson, P.G. The proteasome and proteasome inhibitors in multiple myeloma. *Cancer Metastasis Rev.* **2017**, *36*, 561–584. [CrossRef] [PubMed]
18. Shi, D.S.; Smith, M.C.P.; Campbell, R.A.; Zimmerman, P.W.; Franks, Z.B.; Kraemer, B.F.; Machlus, K.R.; Ling, J.; Kamba, P.; Schwertz, H.; et al. Proteasome function is required for platelet production. *J. Clin. Invest.* **2014**, *124*, 3757–3766. [CrossRef] [PubMed]
19. Cengiz Seval, G.; Beksac, M. The safety of bortezomib for the treatment of multiple myeloma. *Expert Opin. Drug Saf.* **2018**, *17*, 953–962. [CrossRef]
20. Slichter, S.J.; Kaufman, R.M.; Assmann, S.F.; McCullough, J.; Triulzi, D.J.; Strauss, R.G.; Gernsheimer, T.B.; Ness, P.M.; Brecher, M.E.; Josephson, C.D.; et al. Dose of prophylactic platelet transfusions and prevention of hemorrhage. *N. Engl. J. Med.* **2010**, *362*, 600–613. [CrossRef]
21. Stanworth, S.J.; Hudson, C.L.; Estcourt, L.J.; Johnson, R.J.; Wood, E.M. Risk of bleeding and use of platelet transfusions in patients with hematologic malignancies: Recurrent event analysis. *Haematologica* **2015**, *100*, 740–747. [CrossRef]
22. Stanworth, S.J.; Estcourt, L.J.; Powter, G.; Kahan, B.C.; Dyer, C.; Choo, L.; Bakrania, L.; Llewelyn, C.; Littlewood, T.; Soutar, R.; et al. A No-Prophylaxis Platelet-Transfusion Strategy for Hematologic Cancers. *N. Engl. J. Med.* **2013**, *368*, 1771–1780. [CrossRef]
23. Wandt, H.; Schaefer-Eckart, K.; Wendelin, K.; Pilz, B.; Wilhelm, M.; Thalheimer, M.; Mahlknecht, U.; Ho, A.; Schaich, M.; Kramer, M.; et al. Therapeutic platelet transfusion versus routine prophylactic transfusion in patients with haematological malignancies: An open-label, multicentre, randomised study. *Lancet* **2012**, *380*, 1309–1316. [CrossRef]
24. Uhl, L.; Assmann, S.F.; Hamza, T.H.; Harrison, R.W.; Gernsheimer, T.; Slichter, S.J. Laboratory predictors of bleeding and the effect of platelet and RBC transfusions on bleeding outcomes in the PLADO trial. *Blood* **2017**, *130*, 1247–1258. [CrossRef]
25. Webert, K.; Cook, R.J.; Sigouin, C.S.; Rebulla, P.; Heddle, N.M. The risk of bleeding in thrombocytopenic patients with acute myeloid leukemia. *Haematologica* **2006**, *91*, 1530–1537.
26. Estcourt, L.J.; Stanworth, S.J.; Harrison, P.; Powter, G.; McClure, M.; Murphy, M.F.; Mumford, A.D. Prospective observational cohort study of the association between thromboelastometry, coagulation and platelet parameters and bleeding in patients with haematological malignancies-The ATHENA study. *Br. J. Haematol.* **2014**, *166*, 581–591. [CrossRef] [PubMed]
27. Heubel-Moenen, F.C.J.I.; Henskens, Y.M.C.; Verhezen, P.W.M.; Wetzels, R.J.H.; Schouten, H.C.; Beckers, E.A.M. Fibrinolysis in patients with chemotherapy-induced thrombocytopenia and the effect of platelet transfusion. *J. Thromb. Haemost.* **2019**, *17*, 1073–1084. [CrossRef] [PubMed]
28. Ypma, P.F.; van Geloven, N.; Kerkhoffs, J.L.H.; te Boekhorst, P.; Zwaginga, J.J.; Beckers, E.A.M.; Brand, A.; van der Meer, P.F.; Eikenboom, J.C.J. The association between haemorrhage and markers of endothelial insufficiency and inflammation in patients with hypoproliferative thrombocytopenia: A cohort study. *Br. J. Haematol.* **2020**, *189*, 171–181. [CrossRef] [PubMed]
29. Schiffer, C.A.; Bohlke, K.; Delaney, M.; Hume, H.; Magdalinski, A.J.; McCullough, J.J.; Omel, J.L.; Rainey, J.M.; Rebulla, P.; Rowley, S.D.; et al. Platelet Transfusion for Patients With Cancer: American Society of Clinical Oncology Clinical Practice Guideline Update. *J. Clin. Oncol. Off. J. Am. Soc. Clin. Oncol.* **2018**, *36*, 283–299. [CrossRef] [PubMed]
30. Juskewitch, J.E.; Norgan, A.P.; De Goey, S.R.; Duellman, P.M.; Wakefield, L.L.; Gandhi, M.J.; Stubbs, J.R.; Kreuter, J.D. How do I... manage the platelet transfusion–refractory patient? *Transfusion* **2017**, *57*, 2828–2835. [CrossRef]

31. Pereira, J.; Phan, T. Management of bleeding in patients with advanced cancer. *Oncologist* **2004**, *9*, 561–570. [CrossRef]
32. Cai, J.; Ribkoff, J.; Olson, S.; Raghunathan, V.; Al-Samkari, H.; DeLoughery, T.G.; Shatzel, J.J. The many roles of tranexamic acid: An overview of the clinical indications for TXA in medical and surgical patients. *Eur. J. Haematol.* **2020**, *104*, 79–87. [CrossRef]
33. Roberts, I.; Shakur-Still, H.; Afolabi, A.; Akere, A.; Arribas, M.; Brenner, A.; Chaudhri, R.; Gilmore, I.; Halligan, K.; Hussain, I.; et al. Effects of a high-dose 24-h infusion of tranexamic acid on death and thromboembolic events in patients with acute gastrointestinal bleeding (HALT-IT): An international randomised, double-blind, placebo-controlled trial. *Lancet* **2020**, *395*, 1927–1936. [CrossRef]
34. Squizzato, A.; Hunt, B.J.; Kinasewitz, G.T.; Wada, H.; ten Cate, H.; Thachil, J.; Levi, M.; Vicente, V.; D'Angelo, A.; Di Nisio, M. Supportive management strategies for disseminated intravascular coagulation: An international consensus. *Thromb. Haemost.* **2016**, *115*, 896–904. [CrossRef]
35. Levi, M.; Scully, M. How I treat disseminated intravascular coagulation. *Blood* **2018**, *131*, 845–854. [CrossRef]
36. Celebi, N.; Celebioglu, B.; Selcuk, M.; Canbay, O.; Karagoz, A.H.; Aypar, U. The role of antifibrinolytic agents in gynecologic cancer surgery. *Saudi Med. J.* **2006**, *27*, 637–641. [CrossRef]
37. Zhang, H.Z.; Dong, L.; Wang, H.M.; Hu, F.; Shao, Q.; Chen, X.; Chen, L. Safety and efficacy of tranexamic acid in spinal canal tumors: A retrospective cohort study. *Br. J. Neurosurg.* **2020**, *34*, 313–315. [CrossRef] [PubMed]
38. Das, A.; Chattopadhyay, S.; Mandal, D.; Chhaule, S.; Mitra, T.; Mukherjee, A.; Mandal, S.K.; Chattopadhyay, S. Does the preoperative administration of tranexamic acid reduce perioperative blood loss and transfusion requirements after head neck cancer surgery? A randomized, controlled trial. *Anesth. Essays Res.* **2015**, *9*, 384–390. [CrossRef] [PubMed]
39. Wu, C.-C.; Ho, W.-M.; Cheng, S.-B.; Yeh, D.-C.; Wen, M.-C.; Liu, T.-J.; P'eng, F.-K. Perioperative parenteral tranexamic acid in liver tumor resection: A prospective randomized trial toward a "blood transfusion"-free hepatectomy. *Ann. Surg.* **2006**, *243*, 173–180. [CrossRef]
40. Crescenti, A.; Borghi, G.; Bignami, E.; Bertarelli, G.; Landoni, G.; Casiraghi, G.M.; Briganti, A.; Montorsi, F.; Rigatti, P.; Zangrillo, A. Intraoperative use of tranexamic acid to reduce transfusion rate in patients undergoing radical retropubic prostatectomy: Double blind, randomised, placebo controlled trial. *BMJ* **2011**, *343*, d5701. [CrossRef] [PubMed]
41. Lundin, E.S.; Johansson, T.; Zachrisson, H.; Leandersson, U.; Bäckman, F.; Falknäs, L.; Kjølhede, P. Single-dose tranexamic acid in advanced ovarian cancer surgery reduces blood loss and transfusions: Double-blind placebo-controlled randomized multicenter study. *Acta Obstet. Gynecol. Scand.* **2014**, *93*, 335–344. [CrossRef]
42. Amar, D.; Grant, F.M.; Zhang, H.; Boland, P.J.; Leung, D.H.; Healey, J.A. Antifibrinolytic therapy and perioperative blood loss in cancer patients undergoing major orthopedic surgery. *Anesthesiology* **2003**, *98*, 337–342. [CrossRef]
43. Damade, C.; Tesson, G.; Gilard, V.; Vigny, S.; Foulongne, E.; Gauthé, R.; Ould-Slimane, M. Blood loss and perioperative transfusions related to surgery for spinal tumors. Relevance of tranexamic acid. *Neurochirurgie.* **2019**, *65*, 377–381. [CrossRef]
44. Vel, R.; Udupi, B.P.; Satya Prakash, M.V.S.; Adinarayanan, S.; Mishra, S.; Babu, L. Effect of low dose tranexamic acid on intra-operative blood loss in neurosurgical patients. *Saudi J. Anaesth.* **2015**, *9*, 42–48. [CrossRef] [PubMed]
45. Kulkarni, A.P.; Chaukar, D.A.; Patil, V.P.; Metgudmath, R.B.; Hawaldar, R.W.; Divatia, J.V. Does tranexamic acid reduce blood loss during head and neck cancer surgery? *Indian J. Anaesth.* **2016**, *60*, 19–24. [CrossRef] [PubMed]
46. De Boer, W.A.; Koolen, M.G.; Roos, C.M.; Ten Cate, J.W. Tranexamic acid treatment of hemothorax in two patients with malignant mesothelioma. *Chest* **1991**, *100*, 847–848. [CrossRef]
47. Kaufman, B.; Wise, A. Antifibrinolytic therapy for haemoptysis related to bronchial carcinoma. *Postgrad. Med. J.* **1993**, *69*, 80. [CrossRef]
48. Prokopchuk-Gauk, O.; Brose, K. Tranexamic Acid to Treat Life-threatening Hemorrhage in Prostate Cancer Associated Disseminated Intravascular Coagulation with Excessive Fibrinolysis. *Cureus* **2015**, *7*, e428. [CrossRef] [PubMed]
49. Dean, A.; Tuffin, P. Fibrinolytic inhibitors for cancer-associated bleeding problems. *J. Pain Symptom Manag.* **1997**, *13*, 20–24. [CrossRef]
50. Gardner, F.H.; Helmer III, R.E. Aminocaproic Acid: Use in Control of Hemorrhage in Patients With Amegakaryocytic Thrombocytopenia. *JAMA* **1980**, *243*, 35–37. [CrossRef] [PubMed]
51. Garewal, H.S.; Durie, B.G. Anti-fibrinolytic therapy with aminocaproic acid for the control of bleeding in thrombocytopenic patients. *Scand. J. Haematol.* **1985**, *35*, 497–500. [CrossRef]
52. Chakrabarti, S.; Varma, S.; Singh, S.; Kumari, S. Low dose bolus aminocaproic acid: An alternative to platelet transfusion in thrombocytopenia? *Eur. J. Haematol.* **1998**, *60*, 313–314. [CrossRef]
53. Kalmadi, S.; Tiu, R.; Lowe, C.; Jin, T.; Kalaycio, M. Epsilon aminocaproic acid reduces transfusion requirements in patients with thrombocytopenic hemorrhage. *Cancer* **2006**, *107*, 136–140. [CrossRef]
54. Wassenaar, T.; Black, J.; Kahl, B.; Schwartz, B.; Longo, W.; Mosher, D.; Williams, E. Acute promyelocytic leukaemia and acquired alpha-2-plasmin inhibitor deficiency: A retrospective look at the use of epsilon-aminocaproic acid (Amicar) in 30 patients. *Hematol. Oncol.* **2008**, *26*, 241–246. [CrossRef]
55. Cornelissen, L.L.; Caram-Deelder, C.; Meier, R.T.; Zwaginga, J.J.; Evers, D. Platelet transfusion and tranexamic acid to prevent bleeding in outpatients with a hematological disease: A Dutch nationwide survey. *Eur. J. Haematol.* **2020**. [CrossRef]
56. Gallardo, R.L.; Gardner, F.H. Antifibrinolytic therapy for bleeding control during remission induction for acute leukemia. *Blood* **1983**, *62*, 202a.

57. Antun, A.G.; Gleason, S.; Arellano, M.; Langston, A.A.; McLemore, M.L.; Gaddh, M.; el Rassi, F.; Bernal-Mizrachi, L.; Galipeau, J.; Heffner, L.T.J.; et al. Epsilon aminocaproic acid prevents bleeding in severely thrombocytopenic patients with hematological malignancies. *Cancer* **2013**, *119*, 3784–3787. [CrossRef]
58. Marshall, A.; Li, A.; Drucker, A.; Dzik, W. Aminocaproic acid use in hospitalized patients with hematological malignancy: A case series. *Hematol. Oncol.* **2016**, *34*, 147–153. [CrossRef]
59. Juhl, R.C.; Roddy, J.V.F.; Wang, T.-F.; Li, J.; Elefritz, J.L. Thromboembolic complications following aminocaproic acid use in patients with hematologic malignancies. *Leuk. Lymphoma* **2018**, *59*, 2377–2382. [CrossRef] [PubMed]
60. NCT02074436 Prevention of Bleeding in hEmatological Malignancies With Antifibrinolytic (Epsilon Aminocaproic Acid). Available online: https://clinicaltrials.gov/ct2/show/NCT02074436 (accessed on 24 January 2021).
61. Shpilberg, O.; Blumenthal, R.; Sofer, O.; Katz, Y.; Chetrit, A.; Ramot, B.; Eldor, A.; Ben-Bassat, I. A controlled trial of tranexamic acid therapy for the reduction of bleeding during treatment of acute myeloid leukemia. *Leuk. Lymphoma* **1995**, *19*, 141–144. [CrossRef] [PubMed]
62. Avvisati, G.; ten Cate, J.W.; Büller, H.R.; Mandelli, F. Tranexamic acid for control of haemorrhage in acute promyelocytic leukaemia. *Lancet* **1989**, *2*, 122–124. [CrossRef]
63. Fricke, W.; Alling, D.; Kimball, J.; Griffith, P.; Klein, H. Lack of efficacy of tranexamic acid in thrombocytopenic bleeding. *Transfusion* **1991**, *31*, 345–348. [CrossRef] [PubMed]
64. Ben-Bassat, I.; Douer, D.; Ramot, B. Tranexamic acid therapy in acute myeloid leukemia: Possible reduction of platelet transfusions. *Eur. J. Haematol.* **1990**, *45*, 86–89. [CrossRef] [PubMed]
65. Mori, T.; Aisa, Y.; Shimizu, T.; Yamazaki, R.; Mihara, A.; Yajima, T.; Hibi, T.; Ikeda, Y.; Okamoto, S. Hepatic veno-occlusive disease after tranexamic acid administration in patients undergoing allogeneic hematopoietic stem cell transplantation. *Am. J. Hematol.* **2007**, *82*, 838–839. [CrossRef] [PubMed]
66. Estcourt, L.J.; Desborough, M.; Brunskill, S.J.; Doree, C.; Hopewell, S.; Murphy, M.F.; Stanworth, S.J. Antifibrinolytics (lysine analogues) for the prevention of bleeding in people with haematological disorders. *Cochrane Database Syst. Rev.* **2016**, *3*, CD009733. [CrossRef]
67. Montroy, J.; Fergusson, N.A.; Hutton, B.; Lavallée, L.T.; Morash, C.; Cagiannos, I.; Cnossen, S.; Fergusson, D.A.; Breau, R.H. The Safety and Efficacy of Lysine Analogues in Cancer Patients: A Systematic Review and Meta-Analysis. *Transfus. Med. Rev.* **2017**, *31*, 141–148. [CrossRef]
68. Gernsheimer, T.B.; Brown, S.P.; Triulzi, D.J.; Key, N.S.; El Kassar, N.; Herren, H.; May, S. Effects of Tranexamic Acid Prophylaxis on Bleeding Outcomes in Hematologic Malignancy: The a-TREAT Trial. *Blood* **2020**, *136*, 1–2. [CrossRef]
69. Estcourt, L.J.; McQuilten, Z.; Powter, G.; Dyer, C.; Curnow, E.; Wood, E.M.; Stanworth, S.J. The TREATT Trial (TRial to EvaluAte Tranexamic acid therapy in Thrombocytopenia): Safety and efficacy of tranexamic acid in patients with haematological malignancies with severe thrombocytopenia: Study protocol for a double-blind randomised controlled tr. *Trials* **2019**, *20*, 592. [CrossRef]
70. Gonzalez-Porras, J.R.; Bastida, J.M. Eltrombopag in immune thrombocytopenia: Efficacy review and update on drug safety. *Ther. Adv. Drug Saf.* **2018**, *9*, 263–285. [CrossRef]
71. Ghanima, W.; Cooper, N.; Rodeghiero, F.; Godeau, B.; Bussel, J.B. Thrombopoietin receptor agonists: Ten years later. *Haematologica* **2019**, *104*, 1112–1123. [CrossRef] [PubMed]
72. Kirley Neumann, T.A.; Foote, M. Megakaryocyte growth and development factor (MGDF): An Mpl ligand and cytokine that regulates thrombopoiesis. *Cytokines Cell. Mol. Ther.* **2000**, *6*, 47–56. [CrossRef] [PubMed]
73. Vadhan-Raj, S. Management of Chemotherapy-Induced Thrombocytopenia: Current Status of Thrombopoietic Agents. *Semin. Hematol.* **2009**, *46*. [CrossRef] [PubMed]
74. Consensus on clinical diagnosis, treatment and prevention management of chemotherapy induced thrombocytopenia in China. *Zhonghua Zhong Liu Za Zhi* **2018**, *40*, 714–720. [CrossRef]
75. Giagounidis, A.; Mufti, G.J.; Fenaux, P.; Sekeres, M.A.; Szer, J.; Platzbecker, U.; Kuendgen, A.; Gaidano, G.; Wiktor-Jedrzejczak, W.; Hu, K.; et al. Results of a randomized, double-blind study of romiplostim versus placebo in patients with low/intermediate-1-risk myelodysplastic syndrome and thrombocytopenia. *Cancer* **2014**, *120*, 1838–1846. [CrossRef] [PubMed]
76. Kantarjian, H.M.; Fenaux, P.; Sekeres, M.A.; Szer, J.; Platzbecker, U.; Kuendgen, A.; Gaidano, G.; Wiktor-Jedrzejczak, W.; Carpenter, N.; Mehta, B.; et al. Long-term follow-up for up to 5 years on the risk of leukaemic progression in thrombocytopenic patients with lower-risk myelodysplastic syndromes treated with romiplostim or placebo in a randomised double-blind trial. *Lancet Haematol.* **2018**, *5*, e117–e126. [CrossRef]
77. Oliva, E.N.; Alati, C.; Santini, V.; Poloni, A.; Molteni, A.; Niscola, P.; Salvi, F.; Sanpaolo, G.; Balleari, E.; Germing, U.; et al. Eltrombopag versus placebo for low-risk myelodysplastic syndromes with thrombocytopenia (EQoL-MDS): Phase 1 results of a single-blind, randomised, controlled, phase 2 superiority trial. *Lancet Haematol.* **2017**, *4*, e127–e136. [CrossRef]
78. Vicente, A.; Patel, B.A.; Gutierrez-Rodrigues, F.; Groarke, E.M.; Giudice, V.; Lotter, J.; Feng, X.; Kajigaya, S.; Weinstein, B.; Barranta, E.; et al. Eltrombopag monotherapy can improve hematopoiesis in patients with low to intermediate risk-1 myelodysplastic syndrome. *Haematologica* **2020**, *105*, 2785–2794. [CrossRef]
79. Platzbecker, U.; Wong, R.S.M.; Verma, A.; Abboud, C.; Araujo, S.; Chiou, T.J.; Feigert, J.; Yeh, S.P.; Götze, K.; Gorin, N.C.; et al. Safety and tolerability of eltrombopag versus placebo for treatment of thrombocytopenia in patients with advanced

myelodysplastic syndromes or acute myeloid leukaemia: A multicentre, randomised, placebo-controlled, double-blind, phase 1/2 trial. *Lancet Haematol.* **2015**, *2*, e417–e426. [CrossRef]
80. Dickinson, M.; Cherif, H.; Fenaux, P.; Mittelman, M.; Verma, A.; Portella, M.S.O.; Burgess, P.; Ramos, P.M.; Choi, J.; Platzbecker, U. Azacitidine with or without eltrombopag for first-line treatment of intermediate- or high-risk MDS with thrombocytopenia. *Blood* **2018**, *132*, 2629–2638. [CrossRef]
81. Frey, N.; Jang, J.H.; Szer, J.; Illés, Á.; Kim, H.J.; Ram, R.; Chong, B.H.; Rowe, J.M.; Borisenkova, E.; Liesveld, J.; et al. Eltrombopag treatment during induction chemotherapy for acute myeloid leukaemia: A randomised, double-blind, phase 2 study. *Lancet Haematol.* **2019**, *6*, e122–e131. [CrossRef]
82. De Latour, R.P.; Chevret, S.; Ruggeri, A.L.; Suarez, F.; Souchet, L.; Michonneau, D.; De Fontbrune, F.S.; Coman, T.; Dhedin, N.; Rubio, M.T.; et al. Romiplostim in patients undergoing hematopoietic stem cell transplantation: Results of a phase 1/2 multicenter trial. *Blood* **2020**, *135*, 227–229. [CrossRef] [PubMed]
83. Tanaka, T.; Inamoto, Y.; Yamashita, T.; Fuji, S.; Okinaka, K.; Kurosawa, S.; Kim, S.W.; Tanosaki, R.; Fukuda, T. Eltrombopag for Treatment of Thrombocytopenia after Allogeneic Hematopoietic Cell Transplantation. *Biol. Blood Marrow Transplant.* **2016**, *22*, 919–924. [CrossRef] [PubMed]
84. Halahleh, K.; Gale, R.P.; Da'na, W.; Ma'koseh, M.; Saadeh, S.; Alan, W.; Yousef, D.; AL-Far, R.; Muradi, I.; Abujazar, H.; et al. Therapy of posttransplant poor graft function with eltrombopag. *Bone Marrow Transplant.* **2021**, *56*, 4–6. [CrossRef] [PubMed]
85. Marotta, S.; Marano, L.; Ricci, P.; Cacace, F.; Frieri, C.; Simeone, L.; Trastulli, F.; Vitiello, S.; Cardano, F.; Pane, F.; et al. Eltrombopag for post-transplant cytopenias due to poor graft function. *Bone Marrow Transplant.* **2019**, *54*, 1346–1353. [CrossRef] [PubMed]
86. Fanale, M.; Stiff, P.; Noonan, K.; McCoy, J.; Rutstein, M.; Moskowitz, C. 9209 Safety of romiplostim for treatment of severe chemotherapy induced thrombocytopenia (CIT) in patients with lymphoma receiving multi-cycle chemotherapy: Results from an open-label dose- and schedule-finding study. *Eur. J. Cancer Suppl.* **2009**, *7*, 563. [CrossRef]
87. Vadhan-Raj, S.; Hagemeister, F.; Fayad, L.E.; Zhou, X.; ORoark, S.S.; Ames, K.; Rodriguez, M.A.; Fanale, M.A.; Pro, B.; Johnson, M.M.; et al. Randomized, Double-Blind, Placebo-Controlled, Dose and Schedule-Finding Study of AMG 531 In Chemotherapy-Induced Thrombocytopenia (CIT): Results of a Phase I/II Study. *Blood* **2010**, *116*, 1544. [CrossRef]
88. Zhang, X.; Chuai, Y.; Nie, W.; Wang, A.; Dai, G. Thrombopoietin receptor agonists for prevention and treatment of chemotherapy-induced thrombocytopenia in patients with solid tumours. *Cochrane Database Syst. Rev.* **2017**, *2017*. [CrossRef]
89. Al-Samkari, H.; Parnes, A.D.; Goodarzi, K.; Weitzman, J.I.; Connors, J.M.; Kuter, D.J. A multicenter study of romiplostim for chemotherapy-induced thrombocytopenia in solid tumors and hematologic malignancies. *Haematologica* **2020**. [CrossRef] [PubMed]
90. Le Rhun, E.; Devos, P.; Houillier, C.; Cartalat, S.; Chinot, O.; Di Stefano, A.L.; Lepage, C.; Reyns, N.; Dubois, F.; Weller, M. Romiplostim for temozolomide-induced thrombocytopenia in glioblastoma: The PLATUM trial. *Neurology* **2019**, *93*, e1799–e1806. [CrossRef]
91. Sobi Announces Topline Phase 3 Data of Avatrombopag for the Treatment of Chemotherapy-Induced Thrombocytopenia | Sobi. Available online: https://www.sobi.com/en/press-releases/sobi-announces-topline-phase-3-data-avatrombopag-treatment-chemotherapy-induced (accessed on 29 January 2021).
92. Avatrombopag for the Treatment of Chemotherapy-Induced Thrombocytopenia in Adults With Active Non-Hematological Cancers—Full Text View—ClinicalTrials.gov. Available online: https://clinicaltrials.gov/ct2/show/NCT03471078 (accessed on 30 January 2021).
93. Al-Samkari, H.; Marshall, A.L.; Goodarzi, K.; Kuter, D.J. The use of romiplostim in treating chemotherapy-induced thrombocytopenia in patients with solid tumors. *Haematologica* **2018**, *103*, e169–e172. [CrossRef]
94. Parameswaran, R.; Lunning, M.; Mantha, S.; Devlin, S.; Hamilton, A.; Schwartz, G.; Soff, G. Romiplostim for management of chemotherapy-induced thrombocytopenia. *Support. Care Cancer* **2014**, *22*, 1217–1222. [CrossRef]
95. Miao, J.; Leblebjian, H.; Scullion, B.; Parnes, A. A single center experience with romiplostim for the management of chemotherapy-induced thrombocytopenia. *Am. J. Hematol.* **2018**, *93*, E86–E88. [CrossRef]
96. Soff, G.A.; Miao, Y.; Bendheim, G.; Batista, J.; Mones, J.V.; Parameswaran, R.; Wilkins, C.R.; Devlin, S.M.; Abou-Alfa, G.K.; Cercek, A.; et al. Romiplostim treatment of chemotherapy-induced thrombocytopenia. *J. Clin. Oncol.* **2019**, *37*, 2892–2898. [CrossRef] [PubMed]
97. Natale, R.; Charu, V.; Schütte, W.; Albert, I.; Tehenes, S.; McCoy, J.; Berger, D. 9248 Safety of romiplostim for treatment of chemotherapy-induced thrombocytopenia (CIT) in patients with advanced non-small cell lung cancer (NSCLC). *Eur. J. Cancer Suppl.* **2009**, *7*, 574. [CrossRef]
98. Winer, E.S.; Safran, H.; Karaszewska, B.; Bauer, S.; Khan, D.; Doerfel, S.; Burgess, P.; Kalambakas, S.; Mostafa Kamel, Y.; Forget, F. Eltrombopag for thrombocytopenia in patients with advanced solid tumors receiving gemcitabine-based chemotherapy: A randomized, placebo-controlled phase 2 study. *Int. J. Hematol.* **2017**, *106*, 765–776. [CrossRef] [PubMed]
99. Donnellan, E.; Khorana, A.A. Cancer and Venous Thromboembolic Disease: A Review. *Oncologist* **2017**, *22*, 199–207. [CrossRef]
100. Navi, B.B.; Reiner, A.S.; Kamel, H.; Iadecola, C.; Okin, P.M.; Elkind, M.S.V.; Panageas, K.S.; DeAngelis, L.M. Risk of Arterial Thromboembolism in Patients With Cancer. *J. Am. Coll. Cardiol.* **2017**, *70*, 926–938. [CrossRef]
101. Navi, B.B.; Reiner, A.S.; Kamel, H.; Iadecola, C.; Okin, P.M.; Tagawa, S.T.; Panageas, K.S.; DeAngelis, L.M. Arterial thromboembolic events preceding the diagnosis of cancer in older persons. *Blood* **2018**, *133*, 781–789. [CrossRef]

102. Khanal, N.; Bociek, R.G.; Chen, B.; Vose, J.M.; Armitage, J.O.; Bierman, P.J.; Maness, L.J.; Lunning, M.A.; Gundabolu, K.; Bhatt, V.R. Venous thromboembolism in patients with hematologic malignancy and thrombocytopenia. *Am. J. Hematol.* **2016**, *91*, E468–E472. [CrossRef]
103. Labrador, J.; Lopez-Anglada, L.; Perez-Lopez, E.; Lozano, F.S.; Lopez-Corral, L.; Sanchez-Guijo, F.M.; Vazquez, L.; Perez Rivera, J.A.; Martin-Herrero, F.; Sanchez-Barba, M.; et al. Analysis of incidence, risk factors and clinical outcome of thromboembolic and bleeding events in 431 allogeneic hematopoietic stem cell transplantation recipients. *Haematologica* **2013**, *98*, 437–443. [CrossRef]
104. Gerber, D.E.; Segal, J.B.; Levy, M.Y.; Kane, J.; Jones, R.J.; Streiff, M.B. The incidence of and risk factors for venous thromboembolism (VTE) and bleeding among 1514 patients undergoing hematopoietic stem cell transplantation: Implications for VTE prevention. *Blood* **2008**, *112*, 504–510. [CrossRef]
105. Hakim, D.A.; Dangas, G.D.; Caixeta, A.; Nikolsky, E.; Lansky, A.J.; Moses, J.W.; Claessen, B.; Sanidas, E.; White, H.D.; Ohman, E.M.; et al. Impact of baseline thrombocytopenia on the early and late outcomes after ST-elevation myocardial infarction treated with primary angioplasty: Analysis from the Harmonizing Outcomes with Revascularization and Stents in Acute Myocardial Infarction (HORIZONS-AMI). *Am. Heart J.* **2011**, *161*, 391–396. [CrossRef]
106. Feher, A.; Kampaktsis, P.N.; Parameswaran, R.; Stein, E.M.; Steingart, R.; Gupta, D. Aspirin Is Associated with Improved Survival in Severely Thrombocytopenic Cancer Patients with Acute Myocardial Infarction. *Oncologist* **2017**, *22*, 213–221. [CrossRef]
107. Del Prete, C.; Kim, T.; Lansigan, F.; Shatzel, J.; Friedman, H. The Epidemiology and Clinical Associations of Stroke in Patients With Acute Myeloid Leukemia: A Review of 10,972 Admissions From the 2012 National Inpatient Sample. *Clin. Lymphoma. Myeloma Leuk.* **2018**, *18*, 74–77.e1. [CrossRef]
108. Wang, T.Y.; Ou, F.-S.; Roe, M.T.; Harrington, R.A.; Ohman, E.M.; Gibler, W.B.; Peterson, E.D. Incidence and prognostic significance of thrombocytopenia developed during acute coronary syndrome in contemporary clinical practice. *Circulation* **2009**, *119*, 2454–2462. [CrossRef]
109. Leader, A.; ten Cate, H.; Spectre, G.; Beckers, E.A.M.; Falanga, A. Antithrombotic medication in cancer-associated thrombocytopenia: Current evidence and knowledge gaps. *Crit. Rev. Oncol. Hematol.* **2018**, *132*, 76–88. [CrossRef] [PubMed]
110. Prandoni, P.; Lensing, A.W.A.; Piccioli, A.; Bernardi, E.; Simioni, P.; Girolami, B.; Marchiori, A.; Sabbion, P.; Prins, M.H.; Noventa, F.; et al. Recurrent venous thromboembolism and bleeding complications during anticoagulant treatment in patients with cancer and venous thrombosis. *Blood* **2002**, *100*, 3484–3488. [CrossRef] [PubMed]
111. Melloni, C.; Shrader, P.; Carver, J.; Piccini, J.P.; Thomas, L.; Fonarow, G.C.; Ansell, J.; Gersh, B.; Go, A.S.; Hylek, E.; et al. Management and outcomes of patients with atrial fibrillation and a history of cancer: The ORBIT-AF registry. *Eur. Hear. J. Qual. Care Clin. Outcomes* **2017**, *3*, 192–197. [CrossRef] [PubMed]
112. Napolitano, M.; Saccullo, G.; Marietta, M.; Carpenedo, M.; Castaman, G.; Cerchiara, E.; Chistolini, A.; Contino, L.; De Stefano, V.; Falanga, A.; et al. Platelet cut-off for anticoagulant therapy in thrombocytopenic patients with blood cancer and venous thromboembolism: An expert consensus. *Blood Transfus.* **2019**, *17*, 171–180. [CrossRef]
113. Kopolovic, I.; Lee, A.Y.Y.; Wu, C. Management and outcomes of cancer-associated venous thromboembolism in patients with concomitant thrombocytopenia: A retrospective cohort study. *Ann. Hematol.* **2015**, *94*, 329–336. [CrossRef] [PubMed]
114. Li, A.; Davis, C.; Wu, Q.; Li, S.; Kesten, M.F.; Holmberg, L.A.; Gopal, A.K.; Garcia, D.A. Management of venous thromboembolism during thrombocytopenia after autologous hematopoietic cell transplantation. *Blood Adv.* **2017**, *1*, 707–714. [CrossRef] [PubMed]
115. Iliescu, C.; Balanescu, D.V.; Donisan, T.; Giza, D.E.; Muñoz Gonzalez, E.D.; Cilingiroglu, M.; Song, J.; Mukerji, S.S.; Lopez-Mattei, J.C.; Kim, P.Y.; et al. Safety of Diagnostic and Therapeutic Cardiac Catheterization in Cancer Patients With Acute Coronary Syndrome and Chronic Thrombocytopenia. *Am. J. Cardiol.* **2018**, *122*, 1465–1470. [CrossRef] [PubMed]
116. Lecumberri, R.; Ruiz-Artacho, P.; Trujillo-Santos, J.; Brenner, B.; Barillari, G.; Ruiz-Ruiz, J.; Lorente, M.A.; Verhamme, P.; Vázquez, F.J.; Weinberg, I.; et al. Management and outcomes of cancer patients with venous thromboembolism presenting with thrombocytopenia. *Thromb. Res.* **2020**, *195*, 139–145. [CrossRef] [PubMed]
117. Lee, A.Y.Y.; Kamphuisen, P.W.; Meyer, G.; Bauersachs, R.; Janas, M.S.; Jarner, M.F.; Khorana, A.A. Tinzaparin vs Warfarin for Treatment of Acute Venous Thromboembolism in Patients With Active Cancer: A Randomized Clinical Trial. *JAMA* **2015**, *314*, 677–686. [CrossRef] [PubMed]
118. Lee, A.Y.Y.; Levine, M.N.; Baker, R.I.; Bowden, C.; Kakkar, A.K.; Prins, M.; Rickles, F.R.; Julian, J.A.; Haley, S.; Kovacs, M.J.; et al. Low-molecular-weight heparin versus a coumarin for the prevention of recurrent venous thromboembolism in patients with cancer. *N. Engl. J. Med.* **2003**, *349*, 146–153. [CrossRef] [PubMed]
119. Raskob, G.E.; Van Es, N.; Verhamme, P.; Carrier, M.; Di Nisio, M.; Garcia, D.; Grosso, M.A.; Kakkar, A.K.; Kovacs, M.J.; Mercuri, M.F.; et al. Edoxaban for the treatment of cancer-associated venous thromboembolism. *N. Engl. J. Med.* **2018**, *378*, 615–624. [CrossRef] [PubMed]
120. Agnelli, G.; Becattini, C.; Meyer, G.; Muñoz, A.; Huisman, M.V.; Connors, J.M.; Cohen, A.; Bauersachs, R.; Brenner, B.; Torbicki, A.; et al. Apixaban for the treatment of venous thromboembolism associated with cancer. *N. Engl. J. Med.* **2020**, *382*, 1599–1607. [CrossRef]
121. Young, A.M.; Marshall, A.; Thirlwall, J.; Chapman, O.; Lokare, A.; Hill, C.; Hale, D.; Dunn, J.A.; Lyman, G.H.; Hutchinson, C.; et al. Comparison of an Oral Factor Xa Inhibitor With Low Molecular Weight Heparin in Patients With Cancer With Venous Thromboembolism: Results of a Randomized Trial (SELECT-D). *J. Clin. Oncol. Off. J. Am. Soc. Clin. Oncol.* **2018**, *36*, 2017–2023. [CrossRef]

122. Samuelson Bannow, B.T.; Lee, A.; Khorana, A.A.; Zwicker, J.I.; Noble, S.; Ay, C.; Carrier, M. Management of cancer-associated thrombosis in patients with thrombocytopenia: Guidance from the SSC of the ISTH. *J. Thromb. Haemost. JTH* **2018**. [CrossRef]
123. Samuelson Bannow, B.T.; Walter, R.B.; Gernsheimer, T.B.; Garcia, D.A. Patients treated for acute VTE during periods of treatment-related thrombocytopenia have high rates of recurrent thrombosis and transfusion-related adverse outcomes. *J. Thromb. Thrombolysis* **2017**, *44*, 442–447. [CrossRef]
124. Houghton, D.E.; Key, N.S.; Zakai, N.A.; Laux, J.P.; Shea, T.C.; Moll, S. Analysis of anticoagulation strategies for venous thromboembolism during severe thrombocytopenia in patients with hematologic malignancies: A retrospective cohort. *Leuk. Lymphoma* **2017**, 1–9. [CrossRef]
125. Livneh, N.; Braeken, D.; Drozdinsky, G.; Gafter-Gvili, A.; Seelig, J.; Rozovski, U.; Raanani, P.; Falanga, A.; ten Cate, H.; Spectre, G.; et al. Anticoagulation management and outcomes in thrombocytopenic cancer patients with atrial fibrillation. *Res Pr. Thromb Haemost* **2019**, *3*, PB0909.
126. Shatzel, J.J.; Mart, D.; Bien, J.Y.; Maniar, A.; Olson, S.; Liem, T.K.; DeLoughery, T.G. The efficacy and safety of a catheter removal only strategy for the treatment of PICC line thrombosis versus standard of care anticoagulation: A retrospective review. *J. Thromb. Thrombolysis* **2019**, *47*, 585–589. [CrossRef] [PubMed]
127. Easaw, J.C.; Shea-Budgell, M.A.; Wu, C.M.J.; Czaykowski, P.M.; Kassis, J.; Kuehl, B.; Lim, H.J.; MacNeil, M.; Martinusen, D.; McFarlane, P.A.; et al. Canadian consensus recommendations on the management of venous thromboembolism in patients with cancer. Part 2: Treatment. *Curr. Oncol.* **2015**, *22*, 144–155. [CrossRef] [PubMed]
128. Carrier, M.; Abou-Nassar, K.; Mallick, R.; Tagalakis, V.; Shivakumar, S.; Schattner, A.; Kuruvilla, P.; Hill, D.; Spadafora, S.; Marquis, K.; et al. Apixaban to Prevent Venous Thromboembolism in Patients with Cancer. *N. Engl. J. Med.* **2019**, *380*, 711–719. [CrossRef] [PubMed]
129. Htun, K.T.; Ma, M.J.Y.; Lee, A.Y.Y. Incidence and outcomes of catheter related thrombosis (CRT) in patients with acute leukemia using a platelet-adjusted low molecular weight heparin regimen. *J. Thromb. Thrombolysis* **2018**, *46*, 386–392. [CrossRef]
130. Samuelson Bannow, B.R.; Lee, A.Y.; Khorana, A.A.; Zwicker, J.I.; Simon, N.; Cihan, A.; Marc, C. Management of anticoagulation for cancer-associated thrombosis in patients with thrombocytopenia: A systematic review. *Res. Pract. Thromb. Haemost.* **2018**, *0*. [CrossRef]
131. Leader, A.; Hamulyák, E.N.; Carney, B.J.; Avrahami, M.; Knip, J.J.; Rozenblatt, S.; Beenen, L.F.; Yust-Katz, S.; Coppens, M.; Raanani, P.; et al. Intracranial Hemorrhage with Direct Oral Anticoagulants in Patients with Brain Metastases [abstract]. *Res. Pr. Thromb. Haemost.* **2020**, *4*, 6291–6297.
132. Leader, A.; Spectre, G.; ten Cate, H.; Falanga, A.; for the MATTER investigators. Prospective Cohort Study on Management and Outcomes in Thrombocytopenic Patients Receiving Antithrombotic Therapy. In Proceedings of the 27th International Society of Thrombosis and Haemostasis (ISTH) Congress and 65rd Annual Scientific and Standardization Committee (SSC) Meeting, Melbourne, Australia, 6–10 July 2019.
133. Iliescu, C.; Grines, C.L.; Herrmann, J.; Yang, E.H.; Cilingiroglu, M.; Charitakis, K.; Hakeem, A.; Toutouzas, K.; Leesar, M.A.; Marmagkiolis, K. SCAI expert consensus statement: Evaluation, management, and special considerations of cardio-oncology patients in the cardiac catheterization laboratory (Endorsed by the Cardiological Society of India, and Sociedad Latino Americana de Cardiologıa Interve. *Catheter. Cardiovasc. Interv. Off. J. Soc. Card. Angiogr. Interv.* **2016**, *87*, 895–899. [CrossRef]
134. McCarthy, C.P.; Steg, G.; Bhatt, D.L. The management of antiplatelet therapy in acute coronary syndrome patients with thrombocytopenia: A clinical conundrum. *Eur. Heart J.* **2017**, *38*, 3488–3492. [CrossRef]
135. Leader, A.; Ten Cate, V.; Ten Cate-Hoek, A.J.; Spectre, G.; Beckers, E.A.M.; Raanani, P.; Giaccherini, C.; Pereg, D.; Schouten, H.C.; Falanga, A.; et al. Managing Anti-Platelet Therapy in Thrombocytopaenic Patients with Haematological Malignancy: A Multinational Clinical Vignette-Based Experiment. *Thromb. Haemost.* **2019**, *119*, 163–174. [CrossRef] [PubMed]

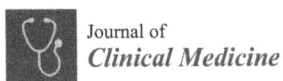

Journal of Clinical Medicine

Review

Thrombocytopenia and Hemostatic Changes in Acute and Chronic Liver Disease: Pathophysiology, Clinical and Laboratory Features, and Management

Rüdiger E. Scharf [1,2]

1. Program in Cellular and Molecular Medicine, Boston Children's Hospital, Harvard Medical School, Boston, MA 02115, USA
2. Division of Experimental and Clinical Hemostasis, Hemotherapy, and Transfusion Medicine, Blood and Hemophilia Comprehensive Care Center, Institute of Transplantation Diagnostics and Cell Therapy, Heinrich Heine University Medical Center, D-40225 Düsseldorf, Germany; rscharf@uni-duesseldorf.de

Citation: Scharf, R.E. Thrombocytopenia and Hemostatic Changes in Acute and Chronic Liver Disease: Pathophysiology, Clinical and Laboratory Features, and Management. *J. Clin. Med.* **2021**, *10*, 1530. https://doi.org/10.3390/jcm10071530

Academic Editor: Hugo ten Cate

Received: 1 February 2021
Accepted: 24 March 2021
Published: 6 April 2021

Publisher's Note: MDPI stays neutral with regard to jurisdictional claims in published maps and institutional affiliations.

Copyright: © 2021 by the author. Licensee MDPI, Basel, Switzerland. This article is an open access article distributed under the terms and conditions of the Creative Commons Attribution (CC BY) license (https://creativecommons.org/licenses/by/4.0/).

Abstract: Thrombocytopenia, defined as a platelet count <150,000/µL, is the most common complication of advanced liver disease or cirrhosis with an incidence of up to 75%. A decrease in platelet count can be the first presenting sign and tends to be proportionally related to the severity of hepatic failure. The pathophysiology of thrombocytopenia in liver disease is multifactorial, including (*i*) splenomegaly and subsequently increased splenic sequestration of circulating platelets, (*ii*) reduced hepatic synthesis of thrombopoietin with missing stimulation both of megakaryocytopoiesis and thrombocytopoiesis, resulting in diminished platelet production and release from the bone marrow, and (*iii*) increased platelet destruction or consumption. Among these pathologies, the decrease in thrombopoietin synthesis has been identified as a central mechanism. Two newly licensed oral thrombopoietin mimetics/receptor agonists, avatrombopag and lusutrombopag, are now available for targeted treatment of thrombocytopenia in patients with advanced liver disease, who are undergoing invasive procedures. This review summarizes recent advances in the understanding of defective but at low level rebalanced hemostasis in stable cirrhosis, discusses clinical consequences and persistent controversial issues related to the inherent bleeding risk, and is focused on a risk-adapted management of thrombocytopenia in patients with chronic liver disease, including a restrictive transfusion regimen.

Keywords: advanced liver disease; bleeding risk; cirrhosis; hemostasis; thrombocytopenia; thrombopoietin receptor agonists/mimetics

1. Introduction

Complex disorders of the hemostatic apparatus are present in acute and chronic liver disease, involving combined abnormalities of the megakaryocyte-platelet system, coagulation, and fibrinolysis. Apart from coagulation defects (international normalized ratio, INR > 1.5) due to reduced hepatocellular synthetic capacity, thrombocytopenia of variable extent is a frequent feature both in acute and chronic liver disease. Importantly, a decrease in platelet count tends to occur prior to clinical manifestations associated with progressive liver failure and decompensation. Thus, thrombocytopenia can be a sensitive noninvasive biomarker of liver disease and be used as a clinical diagnostic tool.

This review covers several aspects of platelet pathology in the context of a defective but at low level rebalanced hemostasis in stable cirrhosis, addresses clinical features and controversial issues, and discusses progress in the management of patients with chronic liver disease and associated risks.

2. Incidence of Thrombocytopenia

An analysis by the Acute Liver Failure Study Group, enrolling 1600 patients, documented that the median platelet count on admission was approximately 130,000/μL; 60% of patients had platelets counts <150,000/μL, 35% <100,000/μL, and 10% <50,000/μL [1]. Despite a perceived hemorrhagic diathesis, clinically significant bleeding is rather uncommon in acute liver disease. This observation is confirmed by a recent analysis on adult 1770 patients with acute liver failure by a Dutch Study Group [2]. Despite a median INR of 2.7 and platelet count of 96,000/μL on admission, hemorrhagic complications occurred in only 187 patients (11%), including 173 spontaneous and 22 postprocedural bleeding events. However, 20 subjects among this patient cohort experienced an intracranial hemorrhage [2]. Progressive thrombocytopenia in acute liver disease can be an indicator of impending multi-organ failure, as documented in a retrospective study [3]. Specifically, an early decrease in platelets (during days 1 to 7 after admission) was proportional to the grade of hepatic encephalopathy, requirement for treatment with vasopressor agents, and kidney replacement therapy [3].

In patients with advanced fibrosis or liver cirrhosis, the prevalence of thrombocytopenia ranges between 15 and 75% [4–6]. A progressive decrease in platelet count is considered as a noninvasive indicator for the development of portal hypertension due to severe liver fibrosis or cirrhosis [7]. Overall, the degree of thrombocytopenia appears to be proportionally related to the severity of liver disease but is not associated with spontaneous bleeding, unless platelets counts decrease to <50,000–60,000/μL [8–13].

3. Is Thrombocytopenia a Predictive Parameter of the Bleeding Risk in Chronic Liver Disease?

Several investigators have suggested that thrombocytopenia may be of predictive validity regarding hemorrhagic events in patients with cirrhosis. However, data on the overall significance of lowered platelet counts among this patient population are equivocal. Thus, a number of studies indicate severe thrombocytopenia (<50,000/μL) to be a predictor of major bleeding and re-bleeding in the peri-interventional setting [14], while others cannot confirm an explicit correlation between low platelet counts and the incidence of periprocedural hemorrhage [6,15]. The conflicting conclusions result, at least in part, from differences in study populations and procedures.

4. Pathophysiology

Thrombocytopenia in liver disease results from increased splenic sequestration due to portal hypertension and subsequent hypersplenism [7,8,13,16], decreased thrombopoietin (TPO) production [6,17–19], and/or from toxic or virus-induced suppression of megakaryocytopoiesis [6,19–21]. In the past, low platelet counts in liver disease were mainly attributed to splenic pooling and/or consumption. By contrast, autoantibody-mediated platelet destruction is of minor importance in most cases with chronic liver disease, but may be relevant in hepatitis C-induced cirrhosis [6]. In these patients, antiplatelet antibodies are detectable, often at high levels [22]. More recently, the impact of abnormal rheological conditions, resulting from enhanced portal pressure, is also discussed as an additional mechanism of increased platelet destruction in chronic liver disease [19]. It is hypothesized that platelets, upon exposure to high shear stress and subsequent activation, are rapidly eliminated from the circulation, thereby potentiating thrombocytopenia. However, this contention is distinct from established high-shear conditions resulting in bleeding complications due to loss of high-molecular-weight von Willebrand factor [23].

During the past decades, detailed exploration of the association between hepatic synthesis of TPO and residual hepatic function allowed a more specific insight into the pathophysiology of thrombocytopenia in liver disease. In fact, TPO levels are near-normal or even increased in acute hepatic disease [18]. This is in contrast to patients with chronic liver disease, in whom TPO serum levels are significantly decreased and therefore thought to be a central pathomechanism to thrombocytopenia in cirrhosis [6,24]. TPO is predominantly synthesized in hepatocytes and, consequently, reduced upon damage to or destruction of liver cell mass. Importantly, among other cytokines involved, TPO is the only one, driving both megakaryocytopoiesis and thrombocytopoiesis at all stages of differentiation and maturation (i.e., from stem cell to multipotent progenitor committed megakaryocyte progenitor cell, immature and mature megakaryocyte to the formation and release of platelets) [25]. The availability of TPO receptor agonists in patients with chronic liver disease and severe thrombocytopenia has therefore been highly anticipated [26,27]. Details on the use of the agents are discussed in the Management Section 9.

5. "Low-Level" Hemostasis—A Defective but Rebalanced System in Liver Disease

Despite the multifaceted hemostatic defects, bleeding episodes due to compromised hemostasis are relatively infrequent in patients with liver disease. Based on clinical and systematic laboratory findings, we hypothesized as early as the mid-1980s that a balanced *low-level* hemostatic equilibrium due to a *concordant* reduction in pro- and anti-hemostatic components is present in stable liver cirrhosis [8,16]. However, this balance is extremely labile and thus can be easily destabilized by various triggers (e.g., infection, variceal bleeding, decompensated liver cirrhosis, invasive procedures, or inadequate hemotherapy with prothrombotic components such fresh-frozen plasma, activated prothrombin complex concentrates, or recombinant factor VIIa). More recent studies have confirmed our contention of a *rebalanced* hemostasis (Figure 1), resulting from a commensurate decline in pro- and anti-hemostatic factors both in patients with acute and chronic liver disease [28–30].

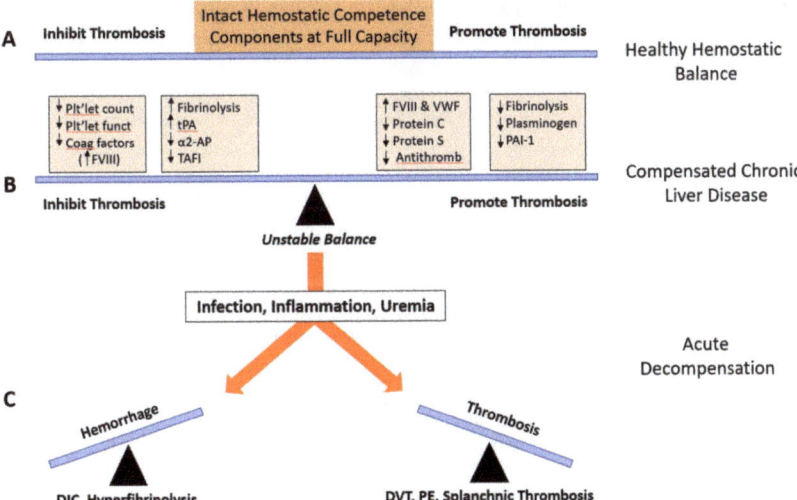

Figure 1. The concept of rebalanced hemostasis in patients with liver disease. In healthy subjects (**A**), hemostasis is in stable equilibrium. In patients with liver disease (**B**), concomitant changes in pro- and antihemostatic components and pathways result in rebalance of the hemostatic apparatus despite the quantitative and qualitative disease-related defects, affecting platelets (primary hemostasis), coagulation (secondary hemostasis), and fibrinolysis. Thus, hemostasis is rebalanced at low level, but the equilibrium now is extremely labile. In patients with decompensated liver disease (**C**) and comorbidities, various stimuli can lead to destabilization and tip the balance toward either bleeding or thrombosis [29]. Modification of a scheme, taken from Eby and Caldwell [31]. Abbreviations: α_2-AP, α_2-antiplasmin; Antithromb, antithrombin; DIC, disseminated intravascular coagulation; DVT, deep vein thrombosis; F, factor; PAI-1, plasminogen activator inhibitor-1; PE, pulmonary embolism; Plt'let, platelet; TAFI, thrombin activatable fibrinolysis inhibitor; t-PA, tissue-type plasminogen activator; VWF, von Willebrand factor.

Moreover, despite decreased procoagulant coagulation factors, thrombocytopenia and suspected platelet dysfunction, patients with acute or chronic liver disease can display hypercoagulable features, which may explain, at least in part, that thrombotic complications are more common than spontaneous bleeding complications [28–30]. For example, apart from normal or even enhanced thrombin generation in liver cirrhosis [12,32,33], Stravitz et al., have shown increased levels of highly procoagulant platelet-derived microparticles [34].

In addition, elevated plasma levels of von Willebrand factor (VWF), typically observed in chronic liver disease, can compensate for the low numbers of circulating platelets [35] and may restore primary hemostasis [28,30,32]. Concomitantly, concentrations of ADAMTS13, a plasma metalloprotease that cleaves high-molecular-weight VWF species into smaller and less prohemostatic VWF multimers, are decreased in patients with cirrhosis and thus support VWF-mediated platelet adhesion to the subendothelium at sites of vascular lesions [32,36]. However, these compensatory mechanisms fail to operate in patients with end-stage liver disease (Figure 1), in whom prominent bleeding complications remain a serious concern [32].

6. Platelet Dysfunction in Liver Cirrhosis

Concomitant platelet function defects, as suggested in chronic liver disease, are less well defined [23]. Generally, it has been assumed that platelet function deteriorates with the severity of liver disease. Older studies have described in vitro aggregation abnormalities in response to several agonists [37,38]. Some of the platelet aggregation defects were attributed to elevated levels of fibrinogen/fibrin degradation products or dysfibrinogenemia, both of which are rather common in chronic hepatitis and cirrhosis. Combined α- and δ-granule storage pool deficiency, as reported in a small series of patients [39], can impair platelet function and favor a hemorrhagic diathesis in chronic liver disease. However, platelets from patients with severe but stable cirrhosis display a normal content of α- and δ-granule constituents [8,16]. Thus, if at all, storage pool deficiency does not appear to play a significant role in the pathogenesis of platelet defects in cirrhotic patients. Importantly, toxic effects of ethanol may also contribute to platelet dysfunction [20]. Other possible mechanisms include defects in the glycoprotein (GP) Ib of the GPIb-IX-V complex [40], decreased availability of arachidonic acid and consequently reduced biosynthesis of thromboxane A_2 [41], increased cholesterol content of the platelet plasma membrane, impaired transmembrane signaling [41], elevated sialic acid concentration of circulating platelets, and hypersialylated fibrinogen [8].

Platelet defects resulting from various mechanisms, as outlined above, may remain compensated and clinically inapparent as long as platelet function (and/or coagulation) is not inhibited pharmacologically [42]. Therefore, drug-induced platelet dysfunction is a major concern, specifically in thrombocytopenic patients with liver cirrhosis.

By contrast, antiplatelet antibodies, rather infrequently found in patients with acute or chronic viral liver disease, appear to be of minor relevance in this setting with regard to qualitative or quantitative platelet disorders [4]. The diagnosis of impending disseminated intravascular coagulation (DIC) in patients with liver disease is often difficult to ascertain because of the multiple hemostatic alterations.

7. Clinical Features of Bleeding in Liver Disease

Bleeding is common among patients with liver disease but less frequent than generally assumed and also emphasized in traditional textbooks. Hemorrhagic diathesis includes spontaneous hematomas, oozing from oropharyngeal mucosa, and bleeding upon dental extraction, skin puncture, or from biopsy sites. Compared with age-matched individuals, the incidence of non-variceal upper gastrointestinal hemorrhage in patients with liver disease is estimated to be twice as high as in the general population (50–100 per 100,000 person per year) [43]. By contrast, intracranial bleeding is rare.

Given the fact that about 50% of cirrhotic patients develop gastroesophageal varices (and that one-third will experience variceal hemorrhage), patients with chronic liver disease are at risk for bleeding complications. This is illustrated by a high in-hospital mortality rate of approximately 15% for each episode of acute gastrointestinal hemorrhage, and variceal bleeding is the cause of death for approximately 6% of patients with liver cirrhosis [31]. Predictors of a first upper gastrointestinal bleeding in cirrhotic patients include presence of varices, elevated variceal pressure, and laboratory evidence of decreased hepatocellular synthesis (with or without manifest coagulopathy), and thrombocytopenia.

Moderate or severe bleeding complications reported after percutaneous liver biopsy are consistently low with rates of 0.5 to 0.7% in large contemporary series [31,44]. However, these findings should be considered with caution since most of the data from these studies are derived from patients in relatively stable or compensated condition of advanced liver disease. This is also true for attempts to correlate hemostasis test results with clinical outcome or prediction of bleeding in the setting of invasive procedures.

Drugs represent the most common cause of acquired platelet dysfunction in our overmedicated society. Apart from typical antiplatelet agents such as aspirin, adenosine diphosphate receptor antagonists, and integrin αIIbβ3 (GPIIb-IIIa) receptor blockers, other widely used agents, including non-steroidal anti-inflammatory drugs, antibiotics, cardiovascular and lipid-lowering drugs, selective serotonin reuptake inhibitors, and a plethora of miscellaneous agents, diets, and food additives or spices can affect platelet function and cause or aggravate a hemorrhagic diathesis [42].

8. Laboratory Assessment of Bleeding Risk in Liver Disease

8.1. Hemostasis Screening Tests—Often Inconclusive

Analysis of hemostasis in patients with advanced liver disease remains crucial for correct diagnosis, management decisions, assessment of bleeding risk, and monitoring of treatment, specifically of hemotherapy. However, most routine laboratory hemostasis tests are not really suitable to predict bleeding. For example, prolongation of bleeding time is found in about 40% of cirrhotic patients but a poor predictor of hemorrhage after percutaneous liver biopsy [31]. Moreover, screening coagulation tests are imprecise and display potentially misleading results in advanced liver disease. In particular, prothrombin time (INR) is of limited predictive value with regard neither to the bleeding nor to the thrombotic risk in a given patient. Thus, an elevated INR only reflects a reduction in procoagulant coagulation factors due to decreased hepatocellular synthesis but not the concomitant decline in anticoagulant activity of the protein C pathway. Alternative methods such as thrombin generation assays might not be routinely available and have not been sufficiently validated to be recommended as replacements for INR. This is in contrast to thromboelastography (TEG), a viscoelastic assay that more closely reflects global hemostasis in vivo. Importantly, TEG may overcome some of the limitations or shortcomings of standard coagulation tests in patients with acute and chronic liver disease [45].

8.1.1. Thromboelastography

TEG allows to dissect the kinetic conversion of fibrinogen into fibrin, the dynamics of fibrin- and platelet-driven clot formation, and the assessment of clot strength and clot stability. TEG can also be helpful for detecting abnormal fibrinolysis.

TEG is now widely used in patients with acute and chronic liver disease, specifically in subjects undergoing liver transplantation to guide replacement therapy with hemostatic factor concentrates (during the pre-anhepatic and anhepatic phases) and to monitor treatment of hyperfibrinolysis. However, neither the TEG method nor the hemotherapeutic consequences for correction of TEG parameters are consistently standardized across transplantation centers [45].

Interestingly, patients with cirrhosis secondary to cholestatic liver disease such as primary biliary cirrhosis (PBC) or primary sclerosing cholangitis (PSC) have been found to be hypercoagulable by TEG when compared to patients with noncholestatic entities [46,47]. This difference may be due to higher levels of fibrinogen and a still intact platelet function in the cholestatic stetting despite similar degrees of portal hypertension in the different patient populations [48]. Taken together, these observations may explain the lower rates of bleeding complications and fewer transfusion needs during liver transplantation in patients with PBC or PSC than in those with end-stage liver disease of other etiology. Moreover, several studies have demonstrated that TEG parameters indicative of hypocoagulation and/or thrombocytopenia are associated with liver disease severity and outcomes [49–51].

8.1.2. Standardization and Validation of Whole Blood Viscoelastic Assays

Most investigations suggest that analysis of patients with acute and chronic liver disease by TEG provides a more reliable assessment of the hemorrhagic risk than standard coagulation assays and determination of the bleeding time. However, only a few studies have directly compared the results of standard coagulation and viscoelastic assays. Overall, a poor correlation between test parameters of both approaches was reported [52].

During the past years, attempts have been made to implement standardization of viscoelastic testing in a variety of clinical conditions including acute and chronic liver disease [53]. Two commercially devices are currently used: the TEG^{TM} (TEG500 and TEG6s) and ROTEM (with a number of different modules including ROTEM platelet). The clinical utility and reliability of thromboelastography have recently been assessed in a prospective validation study [54]. Moreover, thromboelastographic reference ranges within a population of cirrhotic patients undergoing liver transplantation are now proposed [55].

8.2. MELD Score

The model for end-stage liver disease (MELD), initially created in 2000 by investigators from the Mayo Clinic to predict survival in patients with portal hypertension undergoing placement of transjugular intrahepatic portosystemic shunts (TIPS) [56], and subsequent refinement modifications of the MELD score are being broadly used to predict survival and bleeding complications in a variety of patient cohorts with liver disease of different etiology and distinct interventions [57,58]. MELD incorporates three widely available variables (INR, serum creatinine, and serum bilirubin). Thus, the score is affected by variability and interlaboratory variation of INR determinations [31], which in turn specifically limits its application to predict bleeding complications along with invasive procedures [59]. Consequently, most physicians are left in the difficult position of relying on clinical assessment of the individual bleeding risk when deciding whether or not to administer potentially harmful hemotherapy or hemostatic treatment.

8.3. Platelet Thresholds—Not Based on High-Quality Data

By contrast to screening coagulation tests, thrombocytopenia can be an indicator of increased hemorrhagic risk in patients with liver disease. As documented by a number of retrospective case series [31,60,61], bleeding complication rates after percutaneous liver biopsies are higher at platelet counts <50,000/μL. Based on these data, most recognized centers in Europe require preprocedural platelet counts >80,000/μL, whereas a survey of US centers showed a preference for a platelet threshold of >50,000/μL [60]. Thus, the evidence for a valid "cutoff" value remains scanty.

A very recent re-evaluation of published studies has revealed the paucity of data to recommend a "safe" minimum platelet number for invasive procedures in patients with chronic liver disease [61]. Importantly, in a large retrospective study of patients having percutaneous liver biopsy, implementation of less stringent preprocedural hemostasis parameters (INR < 2.0, platelet counts >25,000/μL) was associated with fewer hemorrhagic complication rates and a decrease in preprocedural administration of fresh-frozen plasma and platelet concentrates in comparison with using "historical" cut-off levels (INR < 1.5, platelet counts > 50,000/μL) [62]. A possible explanation for this apparent contradiction is that INR and platelet counts are surrogate markers of liver fibrosis and/or portal hypertension, which per se may be risk factors for bleeding. Such a contention would provide a plausible reason that attempts to correct hemostatic changes can increase the hemorrhagic risk since defective hemostasis is not necessarily the underlying cause of bleeding, and increasing the intravascular volume is likely to be counterproductive [61]. As discussed below, transfusion-associated circulatory overload is a major concern in the management of patients with chronic liver disease.

9. Management of Thrombocytopenia in Patients with Liver Disease

Generally, the approach to bleeding in patients with acute or chronic hepatic disease can be divided into supportive measures, prophylactic treatment prior to invasive procedures, and in rescue therapy for active bleeding. In particular, management of thrombocytopenia in cirrhotic patients is a challenging task for physicians both in the in- and out-patient setting.

9.1. Hemotherapy with Platelet Concentrates

Until recently, transfusion of platelets has been a gold standard for the management of thrombocytopenia in liver disease patients. Generally, two types of platelet concentrates are available for hemotherapy: single-donor apheresis platelet concentrates (SDAPC) and pooled whole blood-derived platelet concentrates (PPC) that are obtained from 4 to 6 donors and prepared either using the platelet rich plasma (PRP-PC) or the buffy coat (BC-PC) method [63–65]. There is ongoing debate on whether or not SDAPC are superior to PPC, specifically with regard to individuals, who frequently require multiple platelet transfusions such as cirrhotic patients [66–70]. Of note, SDAPC are preferentially used in France, Germany, and the UK, whereas in the USA more than 90% of platelet transfusions are performed using pooled PRP-PC.

9.2. Limitations of Platelet Transfusions

Despite advances in pathogen safety, platelet collection, preparation technologies, and storage modalities, potential risks associated with hemotherapy persist, including infection, alloimmunization, febrile non-hemolytic effects, hemolysis, and transfusion-related acute lung injury (TRALI). Refractoriness to platelet transfusions resulting from HLA alloimmunization is a serious complication in up to 50% of patients, who permanently require hemotherapy with platelets. Another concern in cirrhotic patients results from the fact that transfused platelets are rapidly sequestered in the spleen leading to low increments. Consequently, transfusion therapy is only effective in the short term.

9.3. Prophylactic or "On-Demand" Platelet Transfusions

Facing with low platelet counts and the hemorrhagic risk, most physicians are inclined to reach "near-normal" platelet levels in patients with acute or chronic liver disease. Thus, prophylactic platelet transfusions are common practice "to warrant safety and optimal care". However, as outlined above (Section 8 Laboratory Assessment), no evidence-based "trigger" for platelet transfusions exists. Consequently, guidelines from various societies provided only weak recommendations with regard to platelet count threshold levels at which "platelet transfusions should be considered" prior to scheduled invasive procedures. Very recent guidelines from the British Society of Gastroenterology, the Royal College of Radiologists, and the Royal College of Pathology and from the American Gastroenterology Association now define a uniform but still empirical "cut-off" with a platelet count of $>50,000/\mu L$ as threshold needed prior to high-risk procedures/interventions [61,71]. Outside the interventional setting, no prophylactic platelet transfusions should be initiated to prevent patients from being subjected to unnecessary transfusions that provide no additional benefit [72].

By contrast, treatment with SDAPC or PPC remains a cornerstone of rescue therapy for active bleeding in patients with hepatic failure. As discussed below, additional plasma-derived or recombinant products such as fibrinogen concentrate or activated factor VIIa (rFVIIa) may be required to control severe hemorrhagic complications in the majority of patients.

9.4. Thrombopoietin (TPO) Receptor Agonists

The use of TPO receptor agonists/mimetics has provided substantial progress in the treatment of acquired thrombocytopenia in various conditions, including liver disease [25,73–79]. Among the four available agents, two of them, avatrombopag and lusutrombopag, received approval in 2018 by the Food and Drug Administration for treating thrombocytopenia in patients with chronic liver disease needing a scheduled invasive procedure [80,81]. Both second-generation TPO receptor agonists are orally administered drugs.

9.4.1. Avatrombopag

In two seminal, identically designed, double-blind, randomized, placebo-controlled phase-3 trials, ADAPT-1 and ADAPT-2, avatrombopag was demonstrated to be superior to placebo in reducing the need for platelet transfusions or any rescue therapy for bleeding in 435 patients with thrombocytopenia and chronic liver disease undergoing a scheduled invasive procedure [82]. In both studies, patients were stratified into two groups based on lower (<40,000/μL) or higher (>40,000/μL to <50,000/μL) baseline platelet count levels. The efficacy of avatrombopag was documented in both cohorts with a significantly greater proportion in drug-treated than in corresponding placebo groups (Table 1). Upon administration of the TPO receptor agonist (40 or 60 mg daily for 5 days), platelet counts increased with a peak effect between days 10 and 13 and returned to baseline levels by day 35 [82]. The overall safety profile was similar for avatrombopag and placebo, except for hyponatremia reported as the most serious adverse effect.

Table 1. Efficacy of second-generation TPO receptor agonists for the treatment of thrombocytopenia in patients with chronic liver disease scheduled for invasive procedures. Synopsis of results from four multicentric, randomized, double-blind, placebo-controlled phase-3 trials [82–84].

Agent	Trial	N of Patients (Drug/Placebo)	Dosing	Baseline Platelet Count	Outcome Percentage of Responders *	
Avatrombopag					Drug	Placebo
	ADAPT-1	n = 231 (149/82)	60 mg/d for 5 d	<40,000/L	65.6%	22.9%
			40 mg/d for 5 d	≧40,000/μL to <50,000/μL	88.1%	38.2%
	ADAPT-2	n = 204 (128/76)	60 mg/d for 5 d	<40,000/L	68.6%	34.9%
			40 mg/d for 5 d	≧40,000/μL to <50,000/μL	87.9%	33.3%
Lusutrombopag					Drug	Placebo
	L-PLUS-1	n = 96 (48/48)	3 mg/d for 7 d	<50,000/μL	79%	12.5%
	L-PLUS-2	n = 215 (108/107)	3 mg/d for 7 d	<50,000/μL	64.8%	29.0%

* Responders were defined as patients not requiring platelet transfusion or rescue therapy for bleeding through 7 days after the invasive procedure.

9.4.2. Lusutrombopag

Efficacy and safety of lusutrombopag were assessed in two randomized, double-blind, placebo-controlled trails, L-PLUS-1 and L-PLUS-2, enrolling 96 and 215 cirrhotic patients undergoing invasive interventions, respectively [83,84]. Key endpoints of the studies were avoidance of preprocedure platelet transfusions (L-PLUS-1 and -2), avoidance of rescue therapy for bleeding (L-PLUS-2), and number of days with platelet counts >50,000/μL (L-PLUS-2). Both trials showed that lusutrombopag (3 mg once daily for up to 7 days) was effective in achieving and maintaining the target platelet count in patients with thrombocytopenia (<50,000/μL) and chronic liver disease (Table 1). The median time to reach peak levels in platelet counts was 12 days, and the median duration of platelet levels over the threshold lasted 19 days [84]. No significant safety concerns were raised in both trials. The most common adverse effect of lusutrombopag was headache, while the most common serious adverse event was portal-vein thrombosis [84]. However, the number of thrombotic complications did not differ between drug- and placebo-treated patients (two in each group).

9.4.3. Treatment Algorithm for the Management of Thrombocytopenia in Liver Disease

In the light of new options given by the availability of safe and efficacious agents, Saab and Brown recently proposed a treatment algorithm [25] based on the original version by Gangireddy et al. [85]. Core elements of the updated modification (Figure 2) include (*i*) stratification of patients according to their degree of thrombocytopenia (with a "wait and re-examine" strategy for those with mild decrease in platelet count), (*ii*) administration of a TPO receptor agonist as first-line, and (*iii*) transfusion of platelet concentrates as second-line treatment or "back-up" option for high-risk patients, major surgery, or rescue therapy for patients with active hemorrhage.

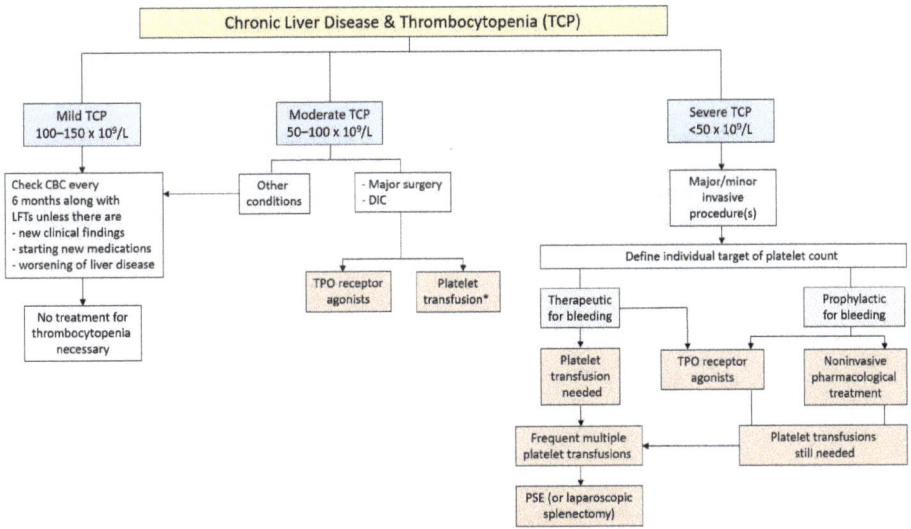

Figure 2. Proposed management of mild, moderate, and severe thrombocytopenia in patients with chronic liver disease. Displayed is the compilation of a treatment algorithm, originally designed by Gangireddy et al. [85] and subsequently adapted by Saab and Brown [25]. In this modification, administration of plasma products (e.g., fibrinogen concentrate, activated factor VII, prothrombin complex concentrate) as rescue therapy for active bleeding is omitted for clarity. To confirm no need for treatment, patients with mild thrombocytopenia should have periodic re-examination including complete blood screening. Of note, for moderate and severe thrombocytopenia, the use of TPO receptor agonists is now considered as first-choice treatment option, whereas platelet transfusions are restricted to major surgery and control of active hemorrhage. The star indicates that, upon platelet transfusion, a target platelet count >100,000/µL is aimed at. Abbreviations: CBC, complete blood cell count; DIC, disseminated intravascular coagulation; LFT, liver function testing; PSE, partial splenic embolization; TCP, thrombocytopenia; TPO, thrombopoietin.

It must be stressed, however, that the proposed treatment algorithm displayed in Figure 2 should be considered as a provisional recommendation, which requires careful evaluation and validation before becoming clinical practice. Specifically, caution is advised at this time regarding the use of TPO receptor agonists in patients with moderate thrombocytopenia when in critical conditions such as intracranial bleeding.

9.4.4. Thrombotic Risk in Chronic Liver Disease Patients upon Treatment with TPO Receptor Agonists

Thrombotic events are a key safety concern with the use of either platelet transfusions or the administration of TPO receptor agonist to raise platelet counts in cirrhotic patients with severe thrombocytopenia. For example, a phase-3 trial using eltrombopag in this condition prior to invasive procedures was prematurely terminated because of an increased rate of thrombotic complications [27]. However, by contrast to subsequent trials evaluating second-generation TPO receptor agonists in chronic liver disease, eltrombopag was assessed by the ELEVATE (Eltrombopag Evaluated for its Ability to Overcome Thrombocytopenia and Enable Procedures) study group without abdominal imaging for splanchnic thrombosis at baseline. Thus, it is possible that some of the patients had a subclinical portal-vein thrombosis at study entry [27].

Several recent reviews and meta-analyses of studies (including more than 2200 patients in total) that compared the effect of three TPO receptor agonists (eltrombopag, avatrombopag, and lusutrombopag) and placebo in patients with chronic liver disease and thrombocytopenia reported on a trend toward increased risk of portal-vein thrombosis upon preprocedural treatment with the TPO receptor agonist (1.6% overall for the drugs vs. 0.6% for placebo) [25,86–88]. However, this difference was not statistically significant. Interestingly, a significant association between portal-vein thrombosis and TPO receptor agonist was shown for eltrombopag alone but not with avatrombopag or lusutrombopag treatments. In accord with these results, Michelson et al., reported that avatrombopag leads to an approximately two-fold increase in platelet counts but not in platelet activation among thrombocytopenic patients with liver disease [89].

Another analysis reviewed the number of arterial and venous thromboembolic events in more than 1700 patients treated with either eltrombopag or placebo in the preprocedural setting and identified a significantly higher rate of thromboembolic events in patients treated with eltrombopag (3.6%) than in those with placebo (1.1%) [25]. Overall, there are differences among oral TPO receptor agonists regarding their thrombotic potential, with eltrombopag carrying a significant thrombotic risk. However, this conclusion is questioned by others due to the fact that eltrombopag, as discussed above, was studied in the ELEVATE trial without appropriate pre-screening for portal-vein thrombosis [90].

9.4.5. Medico-Economic Evaluation of Treatment with TPO Receptor Agonists vs. Platelet Transfusion

Several studies have assessed the clinical effectiveness in relation to the estimated cost-effectiveness of avatrombopag, lusutrombopag, and platelet transfusions. Some results of these analyses are equivocal or conflicting [91–94]. For example, Mladsi et al., reported that avatrombopag reduced the need for platelet transfusions and thus produced cost-savings compared with platelet transfusion (80% fewer prophylactic platelet transfusions, USD 4250 lower costs) or lusutrombopag (42% fewer platelet transfusions, USD 5820 lower costs) [91,92]. Others concluded from their cost-effectiveness analysis that avatrombopag and lusutrombopag are more expensive than no TPO receptor agonist over lifetime, as savings from avoiding platelet transfusions are exceeded by the drug cost and appear to be without long-term health benefits [93]. However, such a contention disregards that platelet transfusions are inappropriate as a sustained management option in patients with chronic liver disease.

10. Management of Hemostasis in Patients with Liver Disease

10.1. General Supportive Measures

Several general measures should be considered to stabilize or improve hemostasis in patients with liver disease, specifically in those with decompensated cirrhosis. Among others, these measures include: (*i*) control of the viral load (hepatitis B, C, or E virus), (*ii*) prevention and appropriate treatment of bacterial infection(s), (*iii*) therapy of renal dysfunction, and, importantly, (*iv*) avoidance of volume extension to reduce any side-effects on portal pressure and collateral vessels, in particular, varices. Indeed, understanding that volume extension increases portal pressure and promotes or exacerbates manifest bleeding in cirrhotic patients has had a significant impact on their management. Overall, this contention has promoted the concept of a "low-volume" approach to patients with chronic liver disease [31].

10.2. Additional Options for Supportive Hemotherapy to Bleeding Patients with Liver Disease

In accord with the "low-volume" concept but by contrast to common practice, a restrictive transfusion regimen is required in patients with liver disease to avoid prohemostatic hemotherapy and treatment-induced thrombotic complications or alloimmunization with resulting platelet refractoriness. Consequently, recent UK and US guidelines strongly recommend that blood products should be used sparingly in patients with acute or chronic liver disease [61,71].

Apart from the hemotherapy-induced increase of portal pressure, the risk of transfusion-associated circulatory overload, transfusion-related acute lung injury (TRALI), transmission of pathogens, alloimmunization, and/or transfusion reactions are major concerns. For management of active bleeding or high-risk invasive procedures the following transfusion thresholds are currently recommended to improve hemostasis in advanced liver disease: hematocrit >25%, platelet count >50,000/μL, and fibrinogen >120 mg/dL [61]. Of note, previously used thresholds for correction of the INR are no longer recommended since target reductions of INR are not supported by evidence.

10.2.1. Fresh-Frozen Plasma (FFP)

Upon administration at common dosing (10 mL/kg), FFP has minimal effect on defective coagulation; only 10% of cirrhosis patients reach a reduction in INR [31]. The large volume of FFP required to reach an arbitrary INR target and to improve thrombin generation causes circulatory overload, thus limiting the indication and usefulness of FFP considerably.

10.2.2. Prothrombin Complex Concentrates (PCCs) and/or Fibrinogen Concentrates

Replacement therapy with 4-factor (F) PCCs containing FII, FIX, FVII, and FX along with variable amounts of proteins C, S, and Z offers an attractive option to restore vitamin K-dependent coagulation factors with minimal volume.

In addition, whenever indicated (e.g., FI levels < 80 mg/dL), targeted substitution of fibrinogen using fibrinogen concentrates (e.g., Haemocomplettan^{TM}, initial dosing 2 g or 30 mg/kg) should be considered and monitored by appropriate monitoring of coagulation and platelet function testing (e.g., by aggregometry). Two recent retrospective single-center studies confirm that hemotherapy with PCCs (and co-administration of fibrinogen concentrate) is safe and effective in patients with acute or chronic liver disease and liver transplantation [95,96]. Importantly, the rate of thromboembolic events in association with coagulation factor replacement therapy was less than 3% [95]. However, these treatment options must not be generalized.

By contrast, special caution and careful decision making are required. As discussed above (see Section 8 "Low Level" Hemostasis and Figure 1), patients with stable liver cirrhosis display a labile low-level equilibrium of pro- and anti-hemostatic components that is highly susceptible to pathogenic triggers such as inappropriate hemotherapy [8,16]. Specifically, decompensated liver disease can lead to increased consumption of coagulation factors, including progressive hypofibrinogenemia and progressive thrombocytopenia, often associated with hyperfibrinolysis [16,28]. Elevated levels of platelet, coagulation and fibrinolysis activation markers may be indicative of their defective clearance [29], mainly due to the reduced hepatocyte mass and a compromised monocyte-macrophage system, and/or reflect, in part, ongoing low-grade disseminated intravascular coagulation (DIC) [16,97]. Such a condition is prone to be boosted by inappropriate replacement therapy and eventually resulting in manifest DIC [11,97].

10.2.3. Recombinant Activated Factor VII (rFVIIa)

rFVIIa is successfully used in a variety of conditions, including chronic liver disease, to control active hemorrhage [98–100]. Main settings related to end-stage liver disease are upper gastrointestinal bleeding (mainly from esophageal varices) and major surgery such as hepatectomy and liver transplantation. According to Consensus European Guidelines on the use of rFVIIa, this agent should not be administered to patients with Child-Pugh A cirrhosis; moreover, treatment with rFVIIa of acute hemorrhage in advanced liver disease (Child-Pugh B or C cirrhosis) is uncertain [101]. In addition, a number of thrombotic complications (stroke, myocardial ischemia, and portal-vein thrombosis) have been reported in patients with advanced liver disease following administration of rFVIIa, thus raising concerns on its safety in this setting (for which no license of rFVIIa exists) [99].

10.2.4. Red Blood Cells (RBC)

Transfusion of packed RBC should also be managed restrictively due to adverse side effects on portal pressure, analogously to volume expansion upon administration of FFP, as outlined above. Current recommendations indicate a target hemoglobin of 7 to 8 g/dL [31]. Prior to scheduled invasive interventions, slightly higher hemoglobin levels (8.5 to 9.5 g/dL) should be achieved to improve hemostasis and thus reduce the risk of periprocedural complications [61].

10.3. Other Specific Agents

10.3.1. Vitamin K

Replacement therapy can be considered in liver disease patients with an increased INR, which may in part reflect vitamin K deficiency (causing abrogated γ-carboxylation of coagulation factors II, VII, IX, and X and of proteins C and S). However, vitamin K deficiency is rather uncommon in this setting, unless there is coexisting cholestasis, antibiotic therapy, recent malnutrition, or long-term intensive care. If used, vitamin K should be administered parenterally due to impaired oral or intestinal adsorption in patients with liver failure. Caution is required, as intravenous application of vitamin K carries the risk of anaphylaxis.

10.3.2. Desmopressin (1-Deamino-8-Arginine Vasopressin, DDAVP)

DDAVP is frequently used to improve hemostasis empirically. The agent can decrease prolonged bleeding time due to drug-induced acute release of von Willebrand factor from its endothelial storage organelles. The benefit of DDAVP administration in patients with liver disease is debated controversially. In fact, several randomized trials comparing DDAVP and placebo prior to invasive procedures (e.g., percutaneous liver biopsy; partial hepatectomy in patients with hepatocellular cancer) showed no difference in blood loss or transfusion requirements [31]. Overall, while side effects (e.g., headache, nausea, flush, diarrhea, or hyponatremia) from DDAVP are infrequent, and the agent is commonly used preprocedurally, its clinical efficacy has not been established in this setting.

10.3.3. Antifibrinolytics

Antifibrinolytics may be useful when cirrhosis-associated hyperfibrinolysis is suspected or proven. Two agents are available, ε-aminocaproic acid (EACA) and tranexamic acid (TA), both of which abrogate binding of plasminogen or plasmin to fibrin, thus inhibiting fibrinolysis. There are only small series of patients and a number of case reports, demonstrating the efficacy and safety of EACA or TA in liver failure and advanced cirrhosis [102,103]. A systematic review and meta-analysis of more than 20 randomized controlled trials (with a total of 1400 patients) documented a reduction in RBC transfusions during liver transplantation when comparing TA to placebo, while the efficacy of EACA remained unproven in this setting (due an unpowered study) [104]. Importantly, this meta-analysis did not provide evidence for an increased risk of thromboembolic events associated with antifibrinolytic treatment in liver transplantation [104]. Overall, antifibrinolytic agents appear to be safe and well tolerated in cirrhotic patients [31].

11. Conclusions

Hemostatic dysfunction in acute and chronic liver disease and novel therapeutic options to control thrombocytopenia are a prime example for the significant progress that has been made in recent years. According to traditional paradigms, liver cirrhosis was considered as the epitome of an acquired coagulopathy that in combination with thrombocytopenia and/or thrombopathy causes hemorrhagic complications. Based on recent findings, this contention has been revised fundamentally in several aspects.

Firstly, patients with liver failure are also prone to thrombotic events, which may be even more common than bleeding complications, except for end-stage liver disease. Secondly, the commensurate decrease in pro- and antihemostatic components can lead to a *rebalanced low-level* hemostatic equilibrium. The rebalanced hemostatic system is, however, labile and can be destabilized by various triggers, which in turn may explain the occurrence of both bleeding and thrombotic complications. Thirdly, thrombocytopenia in liver cirrhosis results from multifaceted causes; apart from splenic pooling, decreased production of TPO plays a major role, as documented by the correlation between TPO levels and residual hepatic function. Fourthly, defective platelet function as a concomitant cause of bleeding events in hepatic failure has been overestimated in the past. However, drug-induced platelet inhibition remains an ongoing concern in this setting. Fifthly, high levels of plasma von Willebrand factor can restore platelet-vessel wall interaction and thus rebalance primary hemostasis that may be compromised otherwise in chronic hepatic disease. Sixthly, rebalanced hemostasis and, all the more, hypercoagulable features in liver disease have a major impact on the prevention and management of both bleeding and thrombosis.

This, however, is a challenging demand, which remains difficult to accompl in clinical practice. Most of routinely available hemostasis screening tests are inconclusive and without predictive validity in patients with liver disease, and comprehensive hemostasis profiles have to be restricted in this population to those undergoing high-risk invasive procedures such as major surgery.

Currently, the platelet threshold required for thrombocytopenic patients, who are scheduled for higher-risk interventions, is rather "defined" empirically but not based on study data of appropriate quality. However, recent advances are likely to solve this issue: the two newly licensed TPO receptor agonists, avatrombopag and lusutrombopag, were shown to be safe and efficacious at increasing platelet levels and avoiding platelet transfusions for invasive procedures in patients with thrombocytopenia and chronic liver disease. It can be expected that both agents will evolve to be the new standard of care for managing thrombocytopenia in patients with chronic liver disease.

Funding: Work from the author's laboratory that is cited here was supported by grants from the Deutsche Forschungsgemeinschaft (Scha 358/3-1; Collaborative Research Center, SFB612). Funding of the author's research at Boston Children's Hospital by a grant from the Society of Thrombosis and Hemostasis Research (GTH) is also acknowledged.

Acknowledgments: The author is grateful to Dieter Häussinger, Düsseldorf, for stimulating discussion and careful review of the manuscript.

Conflicts of Interest: The author declares no conflict of interest.

References

1. U.S. Acute Liver Failure Study Group. Unpublished data. 2015.
2. Stravitz, R.T.; Ellerbe, C.; Durkalski, V.; Schilsky, M.; Fontana, R.J.; Peterseim, C.; Lee, W.M.; The Acute Liver Failure Study Group. Bleeding complications in acute liver failure. *Hepatology* **2018**, *67*, 1931–1942. [CrossRef]
3. Stravitz, R.T.; Ellerbe, C.; Durkalski, V.; Reuben, A.; Lisman, T.; Lee, W.M. Thrombocytopenia is associated with multi-organ system failure in patients with acute liver failure. *Clin. Gastroenterol. Hepatol.* **2016**, *14*, 613–620.e4. [CrossRef]
4. Giannini, E.G.; Savarino, V. Thrombocytopenia in liver disease. *Curr. Opin. Hematol.* **2008**, *15*, 473–480. [CrossRef]
5. Afdhal, N.; McHutchison, J.; Brown, R.; Jacobson, I.; Manns, M.; Poordad, F.; Weksler, B.; Esteban, R. Thrombocytopenia associated with chronic liver disease. *J. Hepatol.* **2008**, *48*, 1000–1007. [CrossRef]

6. Peck-Radosavljevic, M. Thrombocytopenia in chronic liver disease. *Liver Int.* **2016**, *37*, 778–793. [CrossRef]
7. Bashour, F.N.; Teran, J.C.; Mullen, K.D. Prevalence of peripheral blood cytopenias (hypersplenism) in patients with nonalcoholic chronic liver disease. *Am. J. Gastroenterol.* **2000**, *95*, 2936–2939. [CrossRef]
8. Scharf, R.E. Platelets and Microcirculatory Disturbances. Clinical and Experimental Investigations of Platelet Secretion and Arachidonic Acid Metabolism. Ph.D. Thesis, University of Düsseldorf, Dusseldorf, Germany, 1984.
9. Tripodi, A.; Primignani, M.; Chantarangkul, V.; Clerici, M.; Dell'Era, A.; Fabris, F.; Salerno, F.; Mannucci, P.M. Thrombin generation in patients with cirrhosis: The role of platelets. *Hepatology* **2006**, *44*, 440–445. [CrossRef]
10. Scharf, R.E. (Ed.) Acquired Platelet Function Defects: An Underestimated but Frequent Cause of Bleeding Complications in Clinical Practice. In *Progress and Challenges in Transfusion Medicine, Hemostasis, and Hemotherapy*; Karger: Freiburg, Germany, 2008; pp. 296–316.
11. Scharf, R.E. Acquired platelet function disorders: Pathogenesis, classification, frequency, diagnosis, clinical management. *Hämostaseologie* **2008**, *28*, 299–311.
12. Tripodi, A.; Primignani, M.; Chantarangkul, V.; Mannucci, P.M. More on: Enhanced thrombin generation in patients with cirrhosis-induced coagulopathy. *J. Thromb. Haemost.* **2010**, *9*, 612–613. [CrossRef]
13. Scharf, R.E. Molecular complexity of the megakaryocyte-platelet system in health and disease. *Hämostaseologie* **2016**, *36*, 159–160. [CrossRef]
14. Seeff, L.B.; Everson, G.T.; Morgan, T.R.; Curto, T.M.; Lee, W.M.; Ghany, M.G.; Shiffman, M.L.; Fontana, R.J.; Di Bisceglie, A.M.; Bonkovsky, H.L.; et al. Complication rate of percutaneous liver biopsies among persons with advanced chronic liver disease in the halt-c trial. *Clin. Gastroenterol. Hepatol.* **2010**, *8*, 877–883. [CrossRef]
15. Brown, R.S. Current Management of thrombocytopenia in chronic liver disease. *Gastroenterol. Hepatol.* **2019**, *15*, 155–157.
16. Scharf, R.E.; Schneider, W.; Heisig, S.; Schramm, W. Thrombocytopenia in liver cirrhosis. *Klini Wschr* **1983**, *61*, 703–708. [CrossRef]
17. Peck-Radosavljevic, M.; Wichlas, M.; Zacherl, J.; Stiegler, G.; Stohlawetz, P.; Fuchsjäger, M.; Kreil, A.; Metz-Schimmerl, S.; Panzer, S.; Steininger, R.; et al. Thrombopoietin induces rapid resolution of thrombocytopenia after orthotopic liver transplantation through increased platelet production. *Blood* **2000**, *95*, 795–801. [CrossRef]
18. Schiødt, F.V.; Balko, J.; Schilsky, M.; Harrison, M.E.; Thornton, A.; Lee, W.M. Thrombopoietin in acute liver failure. *Hepatology* **2003**, *37*, 558–561. [CrossRef]
19. Sigal, S.H.; Mitchell, O.; Feldman, D.M.; Diakow, M. The pathophysiology of thrombocytopenia in chronic liver disease. *Hepatic Med. Évid. Res.* **2016**, *8*, 39–50. [CrossRef]
20. Scharf, R.E.; Aul, C. Alcohol-induced disorders of the hematopoietic system. *Z. Gastroenterol.* **1988**, *26* (Suppl. 3), 75–83.
21. Bordin, G.; Ballaré, M.; Zigrossi, P.; Bertoncelli, M.C.; Paccagnino, L.; Baroli, A.; Brambilla, M.; Monteverde, A.; Inglese, E. A laboratory and thrombokinetic study of HCV-associated thrombocytopenia: A direct role of HCV in bone marrow exhaustion? *Clin. Exp. Rheumatol.* **1995**, *13* (Suppl. 13), S39–S43.
22. Pradella, P.; Bonetto, S.; Turchetto, S.; Uxa, L.; Comar, C.; Zorat, F.; De Angelis, V.; Pozzato, G. Platelet production and destruction in liver cirrhosis. *J. Hepatol.* **2011**, *54*, 894–900. [CrossRef]
23. Scharf, R.E. Acquired Disorders of Platelet Function. In *Platelets*, 4th ed.; Michelson, A.D., Cattaneo, M., Frelinger, A.L., Newman, P.J., Eds.; Academic Press: Cambridge, MA, USA, 2019; pp. 905–920.
24. Peck-Radosavljevic, M.; Giannini, E. Platelet dysfunction: Status of thrombopoietin in thrombocytopenia associated with chronic liver failure. *Semin. Thromb. Hemost.* **2015**, *41*, 455–461. [CrossRef] [PubMed]
25. Saab, S.; Brown, R.S. Management of thrombocytopenia in patients with chronic liver disease. *Dig. Dis. Sci.* **2019**, *64*, 2757–2768. [CrossRef]
26. McHutchison, J.G.; Dusheiko, G.; Shiffman, M.L.; Rodriguez-Torres, M.; Sigal, S.; Bourliere, M.; Berg, T.; Gordon, S.C.; Campbell, F.M.; Theodore, D.; et al. Eltrombopag for thrombocytopenia in patients with cirrhosis associated with Hepatitis C. *N. Engl. J. Med.* **2007**, *357*, 2227–2236. [CrossRef] [PubMed]
27. Afdhal, N.H.; Giannini, E.G.; Tayyab, G.; Mohsin, A.; Lee, J.-W.; Andriulli, A.; Jeffers, L.; McHutchison, J.G.; Chen, P.-J.; Han, K.-H.; et al. Eltrombopag before procedures in patients with cirrhosis and thrombocytopenia. *N. Engl. J. Med.* **2012**, *367*, 716–724. [CrossRef] [PubMed]
28. Tripodi, A. Liver disease and hemostatic (dys)function. *Semin. Thromb. Hemost.* **2015**, *41*, 462–467. [CrossRef]
29. Lisman, T.; Porte, R.J. Rebalanced hemostasis in patients with liver disease: Evidence and clinical consequences. *Blood* **2010**, *116*, 878–885. [CrossRef]
30. Stravitz, R.T.; Lisman, T. Rebalanced Hemostasis in Patients with Acute Liver Failure. *Semin. Thromb. Hemost.* **2015**, *41*, 468–473. [CrossRef]
31. Eby, C.S.; Caldwell, S.H. Hemostatic Challenges in Liver Disease. In *Hemostasis and Thrombosis. Basic Principles and Clinical Practice*, 6th ed.; Marder, V.J., Aird, W.C., Bennett, J.S., Schulman, S., White, G.C., Eds.; Wolters Kluwer Lippincott: Philadelphia, PA, USA, 2013; pp. 1481–1490.
32. Tripodi, A.; Mannucci, P.M. The coagulopathy of chronic liver disease. *N. Engl. J. Med.* **2011**, *365*, 147–156. [CrossRef]
33. Tripodi, A.; Salerno, F.; Chantarangkul, V.; Clerici, M.; Cazzaniga, M.; Primignani, M.; Mannucci, P.M. Evidence of normal thrombin generation in cirrhosis despite abnormal conventional coagulation tests. *Hepatology* **2005**, *41*, 553–558. [CrossRef]
34. Stravitz, R.T.; Bowling, R.; Bradford, R.L.; Key, N.S.; Glover, S.; Thacker, L.R.; Gabriel, D.A. Role of procoagulant microparticles in mediating complications and outcome of acute liver injury/acute liver failure. *Hepatology* **2013**, *58*, 304–313. [CrossRef]

35. Lisman, T.; Bongers, T.N.; Adelmeijer, J.; Janssen, H.L.; De Maat, M.P.; De Groot, P.G.; Leebeek, F.W. Elevated levels of von Willebrand Factor in cirrhosis support platelet adhesion despite reduced functional capacity. *Hepatology* **2006**, *44*, 53–61. [CrossRef]
36. Feys, H.B.; Canciani, M.T.; Peyvandi, F.; Deckmyn, H.; Vanhoorelbeke, K.; Mannucci, P.M. ADAMTS13 activity to antigen ratio in physiological and pathological conditions associated with an increased risk of thrombosis. *Br. J. Haematol.* **2007**, *138*, 534–540. [CrossRef] [PubMed]
37. Rubin, M.H.; Weston, M.J.; Bullock, G.; Roberts, J.; Langley, P.G.; White, Y.S.; Williams, R. Abnormal platelet function and ultrastructure in fulminant hepatic failure. *Q. J. Med.* **1977**, *46*, 339–352.
38. Weston, M.J.; Langley, P.G.; Rubin, M.H.; Hanid, M.A.; Mellon, P.; Williams, R. Platelet function in fulminant hepatic failure and effect of charcoal haemoperfusion. *Gut* **1977**, *18*, 897–902. [CrossRef]
39. Laffi, G.; Marra, F.; Gresele, P.; Romagnoli, P.; Palermo, A.; Bartolini, O.; Simoni, A.; Orlandi, L.; Selli, M.L.; Nenci, G.G.; et al. Evidence for a storage pool defect in platelets from cirrhotic patients with defective aggregation. *Gastroenterology* **1992**, *103*, 641–646. [CrossRef]
40. Sánchez-Roig, M.J.; Rivera, J.; Moraleda, J.M.; Garcia, V.V. Quantitative defect of glycoprotein ib in severe cirrhotic patients. *Am. J. Hematol.* **1994**, *45*, 10–15. [CrossRef]
41. Laffi, G.; Cominelli, F.; Ruggiero, M.; Fedi, S.; Chiarugi, V.P.; La Villa, G.; Pinzani, M.; Gentilini, P. Altered platelet function in cirrhosis of the liver: Impairment of inositol lipid and arachidonic acid metabolism in response to agonists. *Hepatology* **1988**, *8*, 1620–1626. [CrossRef]
42. Scharf, R.E. Drugs that affect platelet function. *Semin. Thromb. Hemost.* **2012**, *38*, 865–883. [CrossRef]
43. Kalafateli, M.; Triantos, C.K.; Nikolopoulou, V.; Burroughs, A. Non-variceal Gastrointestinal Bleeding in Patients with Liver Cirrhosis: A Review. *Dig. Dis. Sci.* **2012**, *57*, 2743–2754. [CrossRef]
44. Potretzke, T.A.; Saling, L.J.; Middleton, W.D.; Robinson, K.A. Bleeding complications after percutaneous liver biopsy: Do subcapsular lesions pose a higher risk? *Am. J. Roentgenol.* **2018**, *211*, 204–210. [CrossRef]
45. Stravitz, R.T. potential applications of thromboelastography in patients with acute and chronic liver disease. *Gastroenterol. Hepatol.* **2012**, *8*, 513–520.
46. Ben-Ari, Z.; Panagou, M.; Patch, D.; Bates, S.; Osman, E.; Pasi, J.; Burroughs, A. Hypercoagulability in patients with primary biliary cirrhosis and primary sclerosing cholangitis evaluated by thromboelastography. *J. Hepatol.* **1997**, *26*, 554–559. [CrossRef]
47. Krzanicki, D.; Sugavanam, A.; Mallett, S. Intraoperative hypercoagulability during liver transplantation as demonstrated by thromboelastography. *Liver Transplant.* **2013**, *19*, 852–861. [CrossRef] [PubMed]
48. Pihusch, R.; Rank, A.; Göhring, P.; Pihusch, M.; Hiller, E.; Beuers, U. Platelet function rather than plasmatic coagulation explains hypercoagulable state in cholestatic liver disease. *J. Hepatol.* **2002**, *37*, 548–555. [CrossRef]
49. Shin, K.-H.; Kim, I.-S.; Lee, H.J.; Kim, H.-H.; Chang, C.L.; Hong, Y.M.; Yoon, K.T.; Cho, M. Thromboelastographic evaluation of coagulation in patients with liver disease. *Ann. Lab. Med.* **2017**, *37*, 204–212. [CrossRef] [PubMed]
50. Kohli, R.; Shingina, A.; New, S.; Chaturvedi, S.; Benson, A.; Biggins, S.W.; Bambha, K. Thromboelastography parameters are associated with cirrhosis severity. *Dig. Dis. Sci.* **2019**, *64*, 2661–2670. [CrossRef]
51. Shamseddeen, H.; Patidar, K.R.; Ghabril, M.; Desai, A.P.; Nephew, L.; Kuehl, S.; Chalasani, N.; Orman, E.S. Features of blood clotting on thromboelastography in hospitalized patients with cirrhosis. *Am. J. Med.* **2020**, *133*, 1479–1487.e2. [CrossRef] [PubMed]
52. Mallett, S.V. Clinical utility of viscoelastic tests of coagulation (TEG/ROTEM) in patients with liver disease and during liver transplantation. *Semin. Thromb. Hemost.* **2015**, *41*, 527–537. [CrossRef]
53. Thomas, W.; Samama, C.-M.; Greinacher, A.; Hunt, B.J. The utility of viscoelastic methods in the prevention and treatment of bleeding and hospital-associated venous thromboembolism in perioperative care: Guidance from the SSC of the ISTH. *J. Thromb. Haemost.* **2018**, *16*, 2336–2340. [CrossRef]
54. Lloyd-Donald, P.; Churilov, L.; Cheong, B.; Bellomo, R.; McCall, P.R.; Mårtensson, J.; Glassford, N.; Weinberg, L. Assessing TEG6S reliability between devices and across multiple time points: A prospective thromboelastography validation study. *Sci. Rep.* **2020**, *10*, 7045. [CrossRef]
55. De Pietri, L.; Bianchini, M.; Rompianesi, G.; Bertellini, E.; Begliomini, B. Thromboelastographic reference ranges for a cirrhotic patient population undergoing liver transplantation. *World J. Transplant.* **2016**, *6*, 583–593. [CrossRef] [PubMed]
56. Malinchoc, M.; Kamath, P.S.; Gordon, F.D.; Peine, C.J.; Rank, J.; Ter Borg, P.C.J. A model to predict poor survival in patients undergoing transjugular intrahepatic portosystemic shunts. *Hepatology* **2000**, *31*, 864–871. [CrossRef] [PubMed]
57. Murad, S.D.; Kim, W.R.; De Groen, P.C.; Kamath, P.S.; Malinchoc, M.; Valla, D.-C.; Janssen, H.L. Can the model for end-stage liver disease be used to predict the prognosis in patients with Budd-Chiari syndrome? *Liver Transplant.* **2007**, *13*, 867–874. [CrossRef] [PubMed]
58. Kamath, P.S.; Kim, W.R.; Advanced Liver Disease Study Group. The model for end-stage liver disease (MELD). *Hepatology* **2007**, *45*, 797–805. [CrossRef]
59. Segal, J.B.; Dzik, W.H.; Transfusion Medicine/Hemostasis Clinical Trials Network. Paucity of studies to support that abnormal coagulation test results predict bleeding in the setting of invasive procedures: An evidence-based review. *Transfusion* **2005**, *45*, 1413–1425. [CrossRef]
60. Grant, A.; Neuberger, J. Guidelines on the use of liver biopsy in clinical practice. *Br. Soc. Gastroenterol. Gut* **1999**, *45* (Suppl. 4), iv1–iv11. [CrossRef]

61. Neuberger, J.; Patel, J.; Caldwell, H.; Davies, S.; Hebditch, V.; Hollywood, C.; Hubscher, S.; Karkhanis, S.; Lester, W.; Roslund, N.; et al. Guidelines on the use of liver biopsy in clinical practice from the British society of gastroenterology, the royal college of radiologists and the royal college of pathology. *Gut* **2020**, *69*, 1382–1403. [CrossRef]
62. Kitchin, D.R.; Del Rio, A.M.; Woods, M.; Ludeman, L.; Hinshaw, J.L. Percutaneous liver biopsy and revised coagulation guidelines: A 9-year experience. *Abdom. Radiol.* **2017**, *43*, 1494–1501. [CrossRef]
63. Gulliksson, H. Platelets from platelet-rich-plasma versus buffy-coat-derived platelets: What is the difference? *Rev. Bras. Hematol. Hemoter.* **2012**, *34*, 76–77. [CrossRef]
64. Berger, K.; Schopohl, D.; Wittmann, G.; Schramm, W.; Ostermann, H.; Rieger, C. Blood product supply in Germany: The impact of apheresis and pooled platelet concentrates. *Transfus. Med. Hemother.* **2016**, *43*, 389–394. [CrossRef]
65. Vassallo, R.R.; Murphy, S. A critical comparison of platelet preparation methods. *Curr. Opin. Hematol.* **2006**, *13*, 323–330. [CrossRef]
66. Schrezenmeier, H.; Seifried, E. Buffy-coat-derived pooled platelet concentrates and apheresis platelet concentrates: Which product type should be preferred? *Vox Sang.* **2010**, *99*, 1–15. [CrossRef]
67. Hitzler, W.E. Single-donor (apheresis) platelets and pooled whole-blood-derived platelets: Significance and assessment of both blood products. *Clin. Lab.* **2014**, *60*, S1–S39. [CrossRef]
68. Hitzler, W.; Hutschenreuter, G.; Wartensleben, H.; German Association of Blood Transfusion Services. Risk assessment of single-donor (apheresis) platelet concentrates and pooled whole-blood-derived platelet concentrates. *Clin. Lab.* **2015**, *61*, 869–875. [CrossRef]
69. Gürkan, E.; A Patah, P.; Saliba, R.M.; A Ramos, C.; Anderson, B.S.; Champlin, R.; De Lima, M.; Lichtiger, B. Efficacy of prophylactic transfusions using single donor apheresis platelets versus pooled platelet concentrates in AML/MDS patients receiving allogeneic hematopoietic stem cell transplantation. *Bone Marrow Transplant.* **2007**, *40*, 461–464. [CrossRef] [PubMed]
70. Van der Meer, P.F. Platelet concentrates, from whole blood or collected by apheresis? *Transfus. Apher. Sci.* **2013**, *48*, 129–131. [CrossRef] [PubMed]
71. O'Leary, J.G.; Greenberg, C.S.; Patton, H.M.; Caldwell, S.H. AGA Clinical practice update: Coagulation in cirrhosis. *Gastroenterology* **2019**, *157*, 34–43.e1. [CrossRef] [PubMed]
72. Blumberg, N.; Heal, J.M.; Phillips, G.L. Platelet transfusions: Trigger, dose, benefits, and risks. *F1000 Med. Rep.* **2010**, *2*, 5. [CrossRef]
73. Imbach, P.; Crowther, M. Thrombopoietin-receptor agonists for primary immune thrombocytopenia. *N. Engl. J. Med.* **2011**, *365*, 734–741. [CrossRef]
74. Young, N.S. Aplastic anemia. *N. Engl. J. Med.* **2018**, *379*, 1643–1656. [CrossRef] [PubMed]
75. Cooper, N.; Ghanima, W. Immune thrombocytopenia. *N. Engl. J. Med.* **2019**, *381*, 945–955. [CrossRef]
76. Ghanima, W.; Cooper, N.; Rodeghiero, F.; Godeau, B.; Bussel, J.B. Thrombopoietin receptor agonists: Ten years later. *Haematologica* **2019**, *104*, 1112–1123. [CrossRef]
77. Mahat, U.; Rotz, S.J.; Hanna, R. Use of thrombopoietin receptor agonists in prolonged thrombocytopenia after hematopoietic stem cell transplantation. *Biol. Blood Marrow Transplant.* **2020**, *26*, e65–e73. [CrossRef]
78. Miller, J.B.; Figueroa, E.J.; Haug, R.M.; Shah, N.L. Thrombocytopenia in Chronic Liver Disease and the Role of Thrombopoietin Agonists. *Gastroenterol. Hepatol.* **2019**, *15*, 326–332.
79. Khemichian, S.; Terrault, N.A. Thrombopoietin receptor agonists in patients with chronic liver disease. *Semin. Thromb. Hemost.* **2020**, *46*, 682–692. [CrossRef] [PubMed]
80. U.S. Food & Drug Administration. Avatrombopag. Available online: www.fda.gov/approveddrugs/ (accessed on 21 May 2018).
81. U.S. Food & Drug Administration. Lusutrombopag. Available online: www.fda.gov/approveddrugs/ (accessed on 31 July 2018).
82. Terrault, N.; Chen, Y.-C.; Izumi, N.; Kayali, Z.; Mitrut, P.; Tak, W.Y.; Allen, L.F.; Hassanein, T. Avatrombopag before procedures reduces need for platelet transfusion in patients with chronic liver disease and thrombocytopenia. *Gastroenterology* **2018**, *155*, 705–718. [CrossRef]
83. Hidaka, H.; Kurosaki, M.; Tanaka, H.; Kudo, M.; Abiru, S.; Igura, T.; Ishikawa, T.; Seike, M.; Katsube, T.; Ochiai, T.; et al. Lusutrombopag reduces need for platelet transfusion in patients with thrombocytopenia undergoing invasive procedures. *Clin. Gastroenterol. Hepatol.* **2019**, *17*, 1192–1200. [CrossRef] [PubMed]
84. Peck-Radosavljevic, M.; Simon, K.; Iacobellis, A.; Hassanein, T.; Kayali, Z.; Tran, A.; Makara, M.; Ben Ari, Z.; Braun, M.; Mitrut, P.; et al. Lusutrombopag for the treatment of thrombocytopenia in patients with chronic liver disease undergoing invasive procedures (L-PLUS 2). *Hepatology* **2019**, *70*, 1336–1348. [CrossRef]
85. Gangireddy, V.; Kanneganti, P.; Sridhar, S.; Talla, S.; Coleman, T. Management of thrombocytopenia in advanced liver disease. *Can. J. Gastroenterol. Hepatol.* **2014**, *28*, 558–564. [CrossRef]
86. Kim, K.; Ong, F.; Varadi, G.; Gupta, S.; Jorge, V.M. A Systematic Review and meta-analysis of safety and efficacy for pre-procedural use of thrombopoietin receptor agonists in hepatic cirrhosis patients. *Blood* **2019**, *134* (Suppl. 1), 1094. [CrossRef]
87. Jaglal, M.; Laber, D.A.; Patel, A.K.; Haider, M.; Eatrides, J.; Visweshwar, N.; Abowali, H. A meta-analysis on the efficacy of thrombopoietin (TPO) agonists in reducing the need of platelet transfusion before procedures in chronic liver disease patients. *Blood* **2019**, *134* (Suppl. 1), 2108. [CrossRef]
88. Loffredo, L.; Violi, F. Thrombopoietin receptor agonists and risk of portal vein thrombosis in patients with liver disease and thrombocytopenia: A meta-analysis. *Dig. Liver Dis.* **2019**, *51*, 24–27. [CrossRef] [PubMed]

89. Michelson, A.D.; Koganov, E.S.; Forde, E.E.; Carmichael, S.L.; Frelinger, A.L., 3rd. Avatrombopag increases platelet count but not platelet activation in patients with thrombocytopenia resulting from liver disease. *J. Thromb. Haemost.* **2018**, *16*, 2515–2519. [CrossRef] [PubMed]
90. Lindquist, I.; Olson, S.R.; Li, A.; Al-Samkari, H.; Jou, J.H.; Mccarty, O.J.T.; Shatzel, J.J. The efficacy and safety of thrombopoietin receptor agonists in patients with chronic liver disease undergoing elective procedures: A systematic review and meta-analysis. *Platelets* **2021**, 1–7. [CrossRef] [PubMed]
91. Allen, L.F.; Aggarwal, K.; Vredenburg, M.; Barnett, C.; Mladsi, D.; Kim, R. Cost-effectiveness of avatrombopag for the treatment of thrombocytopenia in patients with chronic liver disease. *Blood* **2019**, *134* (Suppl. 1), 3454. [CrossRef]
92. Mladsi, D.; Barnett, C.; Aggarwal, K.; Vredenburg, M.; Dieterich, D.; Kim, R. Cost- effectiveness of avatrombopag for the treatment of thrombocytopenia in patients with chronic liver disease. *Clin. Outcomes Res.* **2020**, *12*, 515–526. [CrossRef] [PubMed]
93. Armstrong, N.; Büyükkaramikli, N.; Penton, H.; Riemsma, R.; Wetzelaer, P.; Carrera, V.H.; Swift, S.; Drachen, T.; Raatz, H.; Ryder, S. Avatrombopag and lusutrombopag for thrombocytopenia in people with chronic liver disease needing an elective procedure: A systematic review and cost-effectiveness analysis. *Health Technol. Assess.* **2020**, *24*, 1–220. [CrossRef]
94. The National Institute for Health and Care Excellence (NICE). Lusutrombopag for Treating Thrombocytopenia in People with Chronic Liver Disease Needing a Planned Invasive Procedure. Available online: www.nice.org.uk/guidance/ta617/ (accessed on 8 January 2020).
95. Drebes, A.; De Vos, M.; Gill, S.; Fosbury, E.; Mallett, S.; Burroughs, A.; Agarwal, B.; Patch, D.; Chowdary, P. Prothrombin complex concentrates for coagulopathy in liver disease: Single-center, clinical experience in 105 patients. *Hepatol. Commun.* **2019**, *3*, 513–524. [CrossRef] [PubMed]
96. Hartmann, M.; Walde, C.; Dirkmann, D.; Saner, F.H. Safety of coagulation factor concentrates guided by ROTEM™-analyses in liver transplantation: Results from 372 procedures. *BMC Anesthesiol.* **2019**, *19*, 97. [CrossRef]
97. Carr, J.M. Disseminated intravascular coagulation in cirrhosis. *Hepatology* **1989**, *10*, 103–110. [CrossRef]
98. Zotz, R.B.; Scharf, R.E. Recombinant factor VIIa in patients with platelet function disorders or thrombocytopenia. *Hämostaseologie* **2007**, *27*, 251–262. [PubMed]
99. Mannucci, P.M.; Franchini, M. Recombinant factor VIIa as haemostatic therapy in advanced liver disease. *High Speed Blood Transfus. Equip.* **2012**, *11*, 487–490.
100. Hedner, U. Recombinant activated factor VII: 30 years of research and innovation. *Blood Rev.* **2015**, *29* (Suppl. 1), S4–S8. [CrossRef]
101. Vincent, J.-L.; Rossaint, R.; Riou, B.; Ozier, Y.; Zideman, D.; Spahn, N.R. Recommendations on the use of recombinant activated factor VII as an adjunctive treatment for massive bleeding—A European perspective. *Crit. Care* **2006**, *10*, R120. [CrossRef] [PubMed]
102. Gunawan, B.; Runyon, B. The efficacy and safety of epsilon-aminocaproic acid treatment in patients with cirrhosis and hyperfibrinolysis. *Aliment Pharmacol. Ther.* **2006**, *23*, 115–120. [CrossRef] [PubMed]
103. Kodali, S.; Holmes, C.E.; Tipirneni, E.; Cahill, C.R.; Goodwin, A.J.; Cushman, M. Successful management of refractory bleeding in liver failure with tranexamic acid: Case report and literature review. *Res. Pract. Thromb. Haemost.* **2019**, *3*, 424–428. [CrossRef]
104. Molenaar, I.Q.; Warnaar, N.; Groen, H.; Tenvergert, E.M.; Slooff, M.J.H.; Porte, R.J. Efficacy and safety of antifibrinolytic drugs in liver transplantation: A systematic review and meta-analysis. *Am. J. Transplant.* **2007**, *7*, 185–194. [CrossRef] [PubMed]

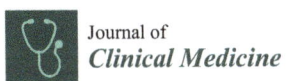

Review

Platelet Transfusion—Insights from Current Practice to Future Development

Annina Capraru [1,†], Katarzyna Aleksandra Jalowiec [1,†], Cesare Medri [1], Michael Daskalakis [1,2,‡], Sacha Sergio Zeerleder [1,2,3,‡] and Behrouz Mansouri Taleghani [1,*,‡]

1. Department of Hematology and Central Hematology Laboratory, Inselspital, Bern University Hospital, University of Bern, 3010 Bern, Switzerland; annina.capraru@insel.ch (A.C.); katarzynaaleksandra.jalowiec@insel.ch (K.A.J.); cesare.medri@insel.ch (C.M.); michael.daskalakis@insel.ch (M.D.); sacha.zeerleder@insel.ch (S.S.Z.)
2. Department of Biomedical Research, University of Bern, 3010 Bern, Switzerland
3. Department of Immunopathology, Sanquin Research and Landsteiner Laboratory, 1006 AD Amsterdam, The Netherlands
* Correspondence: behrouz.mansouri@insel.ch or Behrouz.MansouriTaleghani@insel.ch; Tel.: +41-31-632-8278; Fax: +41-31-632-3406
† Shared first-authorship.
‡ Shared last-authorship.

Citation: Capraru, A.; Jalowiec, K.A.; Medri, C.; Daskalakis, M.; Zeerleder, S.S.; Mansouri Taleghani, B. Platelet Transfusion—Insights from Current Practice to Future Development. *J. Clin. Med.* 2021, *10*, 1990. https://doi.org/10.3390/jcm10091990

Academic Editors: Hugo ten Cate and Bernhard Lämmle

Received: 3 March 2021
Accepted: 27 April 2021
Published: 6 May 2021

Publisher's Note: MDPI stays neutral with regard to jurisdictional claims in published maps and institutional affiliations.

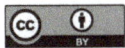

Copyright: © 2021 by the authors. Licensee MDPI, Basel, Switzerland. This article is an open access article distributed under the terms and conditions of the Creative Commons Attribution (CC BY) license (https://creativecommons.org/licenses/by/4.0/).

Abstract: Since the late sixties, therapeutic or prophylactic platelet transfusion has been used to relieve hemorrhagic complications of patients with, e.g., thrombocytopenia, platelet dysfunction, and injuries, and is an essential part of the supportive care in high dose chemotherapy. Current and upcoming advances will significantly affect present standards. We focus on specific issues, including the comparison of buffy-coat (BPC) and apheresis platelet concentrates (APC); plasma additive solutions (PAS); further measures for improvement of platelet storage quality; pathogen inactivation; and cold storage of platelets. The objective of this article is to give insights from current practice to future development on platelet transfusion, focusing on these selected issues, which have a potentially major impact on forthcoming guidelines.

Keywords: platelet transfusion guidelines; platelet transfusion alternatives; platelet additive solutions; platelet pathogen inactivation/reduction; cold stored platelet concentrates

1. Introduction

In 1910, William Duke discovered the link between platelet count and bleeding time of patients as well as cessation of bleeding in association with low platelet numbers after transfusion of fresh whole blood [1]. However, it took four more decades until selective platelet transfusion (PT) became available. PT relieved hemorrhagic complications of thrombocytopenic leukemia patients and hence confirmed the key role of thrombocytopenia in this context [2,3].

In the following years, PT was increasingly implemented in routine blood transfusion strategies in different clinical settings, either to stop (therapeutic strategy) or prevent (prophylactic strategy) actual bleeding. PT is consensually accepted for severely thrombocytopenic patients receiving chemotherapy or undergoing surgery or invasive exploration. However, all situations require different transfusion protocols, and individual decisions depend on the type of pathology and the patient's characteristics. Various national specific societies and/or competent authorities have published guidelines for platelet transfusion [4,5], but international and consensual guidelines are lacking. Therefore, transfusion protocols often vary from country to country, and—in spite of given national guidelines—still often also vary from hospital to hospital or even from team to team.

International variation of practice guidelines may in part be due to differences of platelet concentrates in use. For instance, according to given standards in different countries and regions of the world, single units of platelet concentrate (PC) may contain from 2 to 8×10^{11} platelets. Moreover, there are further differences, e.g., in preparation techniques, additive solutions in use, maximum storage duration, and implementation of pathogen reduction/inactivation processes. Therefore, it is often difficult to compare published results and recommendations, as the quantity and quality of platelets in a bag and the definition of a PC "unit" is not always mentioned and may vary extensively. Finally, as in all fields of therapy, current and upcoming advances will significantly affect present standards.

The objective of this article is to give insight into and discuss selected issues being currently debated and/or that have or may have a major impact on future guidelines for PT. At the end of each of the five sections (apheresis versus pool platelets/platelet storage media/platelet pathogen inactivation/cool storage and frozen platelets/alternatives to platelet transfusion), the reader will find a specific summary.

2. Methods

We searched for specific publications in PubMed and MEDLINE. We applied no restrictions to language and publication date. We performed the last search on 30 September 2020. Per topic, at least two authors screened the obtained references and selected those to be considered in this manuscript. Results per topic and their discussion are included in the following specific sections.

3. Results

3.1. Apheresis Versus Pool Platelets

There are three methods of platelet collection for transfusions. Two of them are based on the donation of whole blood (WB), which is subsequently centrifuged, resulting in separated blood components according to density. An initial soft-spin centrifugation step results in a product containing RBCs in the lower part and the platelet rich plasma (PRP) in the upper part of the collection bag. Using a hard-spin centrifugation step initially, three layers are obtained: the RBCs, the buffy coat (BC) (mainly leukocytes and platelets), and the plasma. After pooling the PRP or BC from 4–6 donors of the same AB0 blood group, a second hard-spin centrifugation of the PRP separates platelets from plasma (PRP-PC), whereas in the pooled BC a second soft-spin centrifugation separates the majority of leukocytes and RBCs from platelets. Finally, the gained BC-platelets are re-suspended in donors' plasma or in a mixture of additive solution and plasma (BC-PC). The BC-PC are the preferred pool PC in Europe and Canada, whereas PRP-PC is favoured in the U.S. and a few other countries [6,7]. The third method for platelet collection is the production of single-donor platelet concentrates by apheresis (A-PC). During this centrifugation-based cell separation process, the platelet-layer (including some amount of plasma) is collected, while the remaining blood constituents are returned to the donor. Storage of PLT in plasma is common in countries without or with low usage of pathogen reduction technology, while usage of additive solution is practiced in countries using pathogen-reduced APC or PPC. In Europe, all PC are leukocyte-depleted prior to storage in order to reduce side effects [8]. PRP-PC are leukocyte-depleted before or after storage. The usual shelf life of PC is 5 days and may be extended to 7 days in case of pathogen-inactivated products. There are countries like the U.S. or Germany, where pathogen inactivation is not yet routinely applied. The distribution of the different PCs varies in different countries. Kuwait and the Japanese Red Cross are using exclusively apheresis PCs; in the United States the distribution of apheresis platelets comprised 91.3% of all platelets in 2017 [9]. In Europe the distribution of whole blood PCs and apheresis PCs varies between different countries; e.g., the U.K. produces about 90% apheresis platelets, whereas countries like Finland, Denmark, The Netherlands, Croatia, Cyprus, and Israel have focused mainly on the production of whole-blood derived PCs [10].

According to, e.g., current American guidelines, available comparative studies consider these types of PCs to be clinically equivalent [4]. Thus, in routine circumstances, they can be used interchangeably. One acknowledged exception is single-donor platelets from selected donors, which are necessary for patients requiring HLA (human leukocyte antigen) compatible and/or HPA (human platelet antigen) compatible platelets, i.e., mainly those with platelet refractoriness due to HLA and/or HPA antibodies as well as in neonatal allo-immune thrombocytopenia (NAIT)). Nevertheless, some centres still prefer apheresis PCs for patients with haematological diseases, e.g., in order to reduce donor exposure. In many countries, pooled PCs are less costly, which may also have influence in opposite decision-making. In the following sections, we summarize current evidence for using pool or single-donor PCs.

There are various differences between apheresis and pool platelets and their potential significance, including the following:

- Several studies have shown that transfusion of apheresis platelets results in higher corrected count increments (CCIs) in vivo compared to BC- or PRP-PCs [11,12]. However, a higher CCI may not result in an improved haemostatic effect or bleeding prevention, as shown also in a different context by Triulzi et al. [13].
- The risk of bacterial contamination of PC may be lowest in A-PC, since the procedure implies only one donor and one venipuncture, in contrast to pooled PC, where four to six donors and venipunctures are necessary. However, the estimated contamination rates of the different platelet products partly overlapped and partly varied widely in the different studies, depending on the time of sampling and the bacterial detection method in use [12,14–17].
- Regarding the risk of transmission of viral infections, older studies reported at least a twofold increased risk for HIV (human immune deficiency virus), HCV (hepatitis C virus), and HBV (hepatitis B virus) associated with pooled PCs [17], whereas more recent data from the German National Blood Donor Surveillance System showed an overall comparable estimated residual risk of transmission for pooled and single-donor PCs for the years 2006–2012 [18]. The implementation of pathogen inactivation processes will equalize potential differences and sustainably reduce the rates in microbial transmission for the different PC products globally in the next decades (see separate section).
- Rhesus-D alloimmunization resulting from PC transfusion is of particular importance in female children and female adults of childbearing potential being treated with curative intent. The volume of contaminating RBCs is lower for A-PC compared to pool PCs. However, several studies have shown that neither cumulative PLT dose nor repeated exposure to Rhesus-D-positive platelet concentrates is associated with a higher rate of anti-D alloimmunization in none of the platelet products [19–23]. Prevention of RhD alloimmunization resulting from platelet transfusions to RhD-negative recipients can be achieved either through the exclusive use of platelet products collected from RhD-negative donors or via anti-D immunoprophylaxis [4].
- Platelets express HLA class I and HPA antigens. In the majority of cases, platelet refractoriness is caused by alloimmunization against HLA antigens; it is less frequently due to HPA-alloantibodies [24]. However, results of the "Trial to Reduce Alloimmunization to Platelets Study Group" did not show differences between leukoreduced pool PC and A-PC groups according the development of HLA antibodies or allo-immune platelet refractoriness [25]. The Study group could demonstrate that leukoreduction is the major factor associated with reduction of HLA alloimmunization after platelet transfusion and not the product type of platelets or the number of donors that the patient was exposed to.
- With regard to adverse events after platelet transfusion, several studies investigated the incidence of transfusion-related acute lung injury (TRALI) after platelet transfusion [26]. There was no evidence of an increased risk of TRALI caused by pool PCs compared to A-PCs in either of the reports [27,28]. Febrile non-hemolytic transfusion reactions (FNHTRs) are mainly due to the accumulation of leukocyte- and platelet-derived cytokines during platelet storage and also due to in vivo cytokine production caused by recipient antibodies to transfused donor's leukocytes. Several

studies demonstrate that the rate of FNHTRs is equal for both platelet products (pool PCs and A-PCs) when the products were leukoreduced [11].
- To investigate how PC characteristics (such as dose, source, and storage duration) influence the rate of transfusion-related adverse events (including allergic/hypersensitivity reaction, sinus bradycardia or tachycardia, hypertension, hypotension, dyspnoea, hypoxia, wheezing, cough, haemolysis, rigor/chills, fever, and infection), Kaufman et al. performed a sub-analysis of the before-mentioned study by Triulzi et al. The type of platelet product (pool PC versus A-PC) did not significantly influence the risk of adverse events; only the platelet dose was associated with the rate of adverse reactions [29].

In summary, BC-PC, PRP-PC, and A-PC reveal similar quality, haemostatic benefits, and adverse event profiles. Hence, they are considered clinically equivalent for most the patients. However, A-PC from selected donors remains essential when HLA/HPA compatible platelet transfusions are needed.

3.2. Platelet Storage Media

Historically, platelets were stored in plasma, in order to preserve their hemostatic and structural integrity during storage [30]. However, transfusion of plasma is always associated with a significant risk of allergic reactions, circulatory overload, and passive transfer of anti-A and anti-B-antibodies. In the 1980s, plasma was suspected to contain harmful enzymes that caused the so-called platelet storage lesion, which triggered the development of different types of platelet additive solutions (PASs) to replace plasma as the sole storage medium and reduce costs [31]. Currently used storage media typically contain 50–80% PAS, with a corresponding plasma-remainder of 20–50% [32]. Recent approaches successfully reduced the latter to 5% [33]. Transfusion of PC in PAS reduced the frequency of allergic transfusion reactions by nearly 50%. Because it also preserves adequate platelet increments, PAS has increasingly become the preferred storage medium [34]. Research is ongoing to define the optimal composition of platelet storage media in order to modulate the storage quality, facilitating the longest possible shelf life together with a minimal loss of functionality and effectiveness not inferior to plasma-only stored platelets.

3.2.1. Components of PAS

Platelet additive solutions aim to preserve platelet function over time and to prevent storage lesions [32]. All types of PAS contain NaCl to preserve osmolality, citrate to prevent calcium-induced clumping, and in almost all types, acetate to replace glucose as an additional source of energy for platelets. Acetate reduces synthesis of lactic acid and serves as a catcher of H+ ions from the environment, thus preventing the detrimental lowering of pH. Moreover, oxidation of acetate produces bicarbonate, which serves as an efficient buffer, further preventing a decrease in pH. Although glucose remains crucial for the metabolism of platelets, it is not added in all types of PAS, since the amount of glucose in the remainder plasma-fraction of currently used PASs (usually 20–50%) seems to be sufficient. Moreover, the addition of glucose increasingly provokes its caramelisation during steam sterilization that occurs as part of the manufacturing process of PASs. However, in the case of less than 15–20% plasma-fraction, the quantity of glucose becomes progressively insufficient for sustained preservation of the platelets' metabolism. The adding of phosphate also seems to prevent the decrease of pH (buffer) and to stimulate platelet glycolysis to increase production of lactic acid. Additionally to its effect on coagulation through the chelation of divalent cations such as calcium and magnesium, citrate may modify potassium efflux through the platelet membrane. The addition of electrolytes like potassium and magnesium to some types of PAS results in improved pH preservation and lowering of platelet activation markers [30].

3.2.2. Types of PAS

Present generations of PASs are categorized from A to G (PAS-A to PAS-G) based on their composition [32]. As an alternative, other names can be used, for instance InterSol for PAS-C, SSP+ for PAS-E, and Plasma Lyte A for PAS-F. This nomenclature was developed to define concentrations of citrate, phosphate, acetate, magnesium, potassium, gluconate, and glucose. Describing all types of PAS is beyond the scope of this study and is summarized in the referenced reviews. Here, we will focus on selected types of PAS and their most important properties. For PAS-B (containing only citrate and acetate) and PAS-C (containing citrate, acetate, and phosphate), corrected platelet count increments are lower as compared to PAS-E (containing citrate, phosphate, acetate, magnesium, and potassium) but comparable to plasma-only stored platelets. So far, platelet increment data is best for PAS-E. Studies using the recently developed PAS-F (containing acetate, magnesium, and potassium as key constituents) showed that platelets might be stored for 13 days with recovery and survival outcomes being equal or even superior to 7-day-stored platelets in plasma [35].

To summarise, an ideal storage medium does not exist to-date. There are myriad advantages and disadvantages of plasma vs. PAS stored platelets. Nevertheless, current PAS generations may extend shelf life up to 13 days, retaining adequate platelet increment in the case of PAS-E and recovery and survival data in the case of PAS-F. In addition, there is a decrease in adverse reactions related to plasma. Further development of PAS types should aim to assure even better platelet quality and to facilitate pathogen inactivation as well as cold storage of platelets. Because of preserved quality and efficiency, along with reduced transfusion-related adverse events as well as costs of PC manufacturing, PASs are steadily replacing plasma as the storage medium of platelets.

3.3. Pathogen Inactivation of Platelet Concentrates

Safety measures regarding the risk of pathogen transmission are implemented throughout the complete manufacturing process of blood components for transfusion [36]. This led to an overall impressive improvement in infectious risks of blood transfusion in the last two decades. However, in many countries bacterial contamination of platelet concentrates (PCs) remained as the most prevalent transfusion-associated infectious risk, being responsible for considerable morbidity and mortality in blood transfusion. The UN National Safety Network rated the frequency of septic transfusion reactions to one per 41,000 to 116,000 distributed PC between the years 2010 and 2016, with Staphylococcus and Streptococcus infections being the most often-detected pathogens [37].

The main reason for this is that, thus far, platelets are mainly stored at room temperature ($22 \pm 2\ °C$) (RT) to maintain their optimal viability and function. However, this provides a favorable environment for bacterial growth, with an increasing risk during their storage. Therefore, the shelf life of RT-PC is currently limited to 3–7 days, depending on the national specifications, usually stipulated by responsible authorities. The "cold storage" of platelet products is described in a separate section of this article; it may prolong storage time up to 21 days ($4\ °C$) or even two years ($-80\ °C$).

Bacterial detection methods are useful but not sufficiently sensitive because of the initial low bacterial concentration [38,39]. Furthermore, undetected bacteria may grow during storage time into health-threatening levels [40]. Therefore, the development of pathogen reduction technology systems are a major step in transfusion medicine by reducing the risk of transfusion-transmitted diseases. Currently, three commercial systems (Intercept®, Cerus, Concord, CA, USA; Mirasol®, Terumo BCT, Lakewood, CO, USA; and Theraflex®, Macopharma, Tourcoing, France) are approved by several national competent authorities and available for routine use. Recent in vitro experiments showed pathogen inactivation to be applicable in cold-stored PC (see separate section) and will probably be soon included in larger clinical trials [41].

Intercept Blood System (Cerus) (IBS) was the first approved pathogen inactivating system in clinical use. As described elsewhere, the procedure is based on the addition of the psoralen compound amotosalen HCl to the PC suspended in 65% PAS and 35% plasma, resulting in an amotosalen concentration of 150 µmol/L [42]. The amotosalen intercalates between the pyrimidine base pairs of nucleic acids. Upon UVA illumination with an energy of 3 J/cm^2 at 320–400 nm wavelength, it forms covalent bonds, preventing further replication and thus inactivating pathogens as well as residual leukocytes. A compound absorption device reduces the amotosalen residual content to <2 µmol/L in the final PC product for transfusion, which can be stored for up to 7 days [42,43]. National hemovigilance programs from Switzerland, France, and Belgium reported a significantly lower rate of septic reactions when using IBS pathogen-inactivated platelets between 2005 and 2016 [36].

One of the main and early concerns and topic of many studies was the assumed higher occurrence of bleeding events in patients transfused with IBS, or more generally, pathogen-inactivated platelets [44–46]. However, the most recent analyses found no significant difference between patients receiving pathogen-reduced (IBS and Mirasol) platelets and the control group, including the occurrence of clinically significant/severe bleedings, all-cause mortality, and even severe transfusion reactions [47,48]. Comparing IBS platelets with platelets in PAS and platelets in plasma showed that IBS platelets were non-inferior to platelets in PAS regarding bleeding events WHO Grade 2 or higher but were inferior to platelets in plasma [49]. Another meta-analysis investigated the efficacy of IBS platelets in patients with chronic cytopenia due to bone marrow failure, since this patient collective is transfusion-dependent and often immunosuppressed. The data described a lower increment in the thrombocyte count compared to untreated platelets but without a higher bleeding rate [50]. All data indicated that IBS treated platelets result in a lower platelet increment. Butler et al. additionally reported a 7% increase of IBS-PC transfusions and a shorter time interval between transfusions in their systematic review [51]. The already introduced meta-analysis of Estcourt et al. could reproduce all the results [47].

Trying to explain the reduced platelet increment and slightly higher bleeding rate of WHO Grade 2 or less, some groups studied IBS treated platelets extensively in vitro, including adhesion to collagen and vWF under flow and different proteomics analysis, showing impairment of platelets physiologic activity through IBS exposition. Treated platelets seem to have a reduced response to certain agonists (vWF, collagen, thrombin) due to loss of surface proteins, needed for interaction. IBS treated platelet transfusion in combined immune-deficient mice revealed a faster platelet degradation. IBS treated platelets have upregulated apoptosis pathways, which can explain their accelerated degradation [52].

Altogether, IBS reliably reduces infectious risks from platelet transfusion while maintaining adequate efficacy. Switzerland recently confirmed the above-mentioned study results by analyzing the data of their mandatory national hemovigilance system [42]. In 2011, it was the worldwide first country switching mandatorily from untreated platelets towards 100% IBS-PC in PAS. Between 2005 and 2011, there were 16 documented transfusion-transmitted bacterial infections, including three fatalities. Since 2011, there have been no reported bacterial-transmitted transfusion reactions; additionally, there has been a specific and overall statistically significant reduction of transfusion reactions. Even though there was an expected loss of 10–15% of average platelet content per unit, there was no increase in IBS-PC requirements, no increased bleeding complication, and no ineffectiveness of transfused IBS-PC reported [42].

In vitro comparison of cryopreserved IBS-PC and control PC showed that IBS-PC appeared slightly more susceptible to lesion effects by freezing than conventional PC, in particular in assays on day one after thawing. However, these differences were small in relation to the dramatic effects of the freezing process itself. Moreover, functional tests, including coagulometry and rotational thromboelastometry, showed similar results [53].

Mirasol Pathogen reduction technology system (TerumoBCT) (MPR) was FDA approved in 2007. It uses riboflavin (vitamin B2), which has a very high safety profile and a narrow spectrum UV light (280–360 nm), to inhibit proliferation of bacteria, viruses, and white blood cells [54,55]. The principle of action is similar to Psoralen, as Riboflavin intercalates with the DNA/RNA bases and becomes chemically active through UV light. Electron transfer and the production of singlet oxygen and hydrogen peroxide are the results of the provoked photochemical reactions, subsequently causing base damage and strand breaks [56]. There are several UV light spectra described as being successful pathogen inactivators. When analyzing the effectiveness and side-effect profile of narrow and broad UV light, it seems that narrow light is more suitable for bacterial and viral inactivation, while preserving platelet qualities and metabolism even though a significant reduction of platelet counts was observed. Light energy should also be chosen wisely, since increased light energy effectively inactivates pathogens, while causing a higher degradation of platelets. Thus, the latter is not recommended [57,58].

One of the main questions regarding MPR technology is its degree of negative impact on the physiologic hemostatic function of platelets, which may result in increased frequency of bleedings of WHO Grade 2 or higher. A recent non-inferiority multicenter controlled trial compared the transfusion of MPR-PC and standard PC in plasma. The primary outcome parameter was the proportion of transfusion treatment periods in which the patient had Grade 2 or higher bleeding, as defined by WHO criteria. There was a 3% absolute difference in Grade 2 or higher bleeding in the intention-to-treat analysis: 51% of the transfusion treatment periods in the control arm and 54% in the intervention arm, with significance for non-inferiority (p = 0.012). However, in the per-protocol analysis, the difference in Grade 2 or higher bleeding was 8%: 44% in the control arm and 52% in the intervention arm, with a failed significance of p = 0.19 for non-inferiority [59]. Therefore, the study indicated a slightly higher incidence of bleedings of WHO Grade 2 or higher in the MPR-PC group. MPR-PC had a lower platelet increment than the untreated control group. The transfusion increment was about 50% lower in the MPR thrombocyte treated group compared to the control group [58]. Similar biochemical findings are reported for MPR- and IBS-PC. MPR seems to activate apoptosis pathways, responsible for earlier destruction of platelets [60].

Alloimmunization is one of the main problems for multiple transfused patients, causing a decreased increment after transfusion and thus higher bleeding risk. The question thus arises whether pathogen reduced platelets are prone to trigger alloimmunization as part of the pathomechanisms of lowered platelet increment. A multivariate study analyzed this question by measuring anti HLA Class I and II antibodies before and after transfusion of MPR platelets and untreated control platelets. All patients lacked alloantibodies at randomization. HLA Class I antibodies were detected more often after transfusion of MPR platelets, while HLA Class II antibodies were detected in both groups with similar frequencies. HLA Class I antibodies are probably caused by a platelet-mediated indirect immunization pathway. The differences between groups regarding high-titer Class I antibodies are less pronounced, so that the clinical implications of these findings are reduced and need further analysis. MPR-PC surely do not protect alloimmunization [61]. Another study of HLA Class I alloimmunization after transfusion of MRP-PC and control PC in plasma showed no significant difference between groups [58].

MPR has also been used successfully in cryopreserved platelets. In vitro testing showed that the platelets had a better hemostatic activity and fewer morphological changes than the untreated control group and maintained their function. On the other hand, they seemed to have a higher metabolic activity; further studies are under way [62].

Theraflex UV-Platelet System (MacoPharma) is the most recently introduced pathogen inactivation technology. It differs from the former two by using ultraviolet C light (UVC) only, i.e., without the need for a photoactive substance to interfere with the nucleic acids. UVC interacts directly with nucleic acids, resulting in the dimerization of pyrimidine bases, thus preventing further replication of the DNA/RNA. Theraflex inactivates bacteria, viruses, and protozoa replication as well as contaminating white blood cells. Available studies showed a broad effectiveness, with a bacterial load reduction of 3–7 log [63]. It also effectively inactivates the majority of coated and non-coated viruses (including HIV) with $\geq$2 log [64].

Theraflex was very recently evaluated in a phase III clinical trial (CAPTURE), and the results were published online in February 2021 [65]. In a randomized, controlled, double blind, multicenter, non-inferiority trial, the group compared the efficacy and safety of UVC-treated platelets (UVC-PC) to that of untreated platelets in thrombocytopenic patients with hematologic-oncologic diseases. The primary objective was to determine the non-inferiority of UVC-PC, assessed by the 1 h corrected count increment (CCI) in up to eight per-protocol platelet transfusion episodes. The defined non-inferiority margin of 30% of UVC-PC was narrowly missed, as the mean differences in 1 h CCI between standard platelets versus UVC-PC for intention-to-treat and per-protocol analyses were 18.2% (95% confidence interval [CI]: 6.4%; 30.1%) and 18.7% (95% CI: 6.3%; 31.1%), respectively. Moreover, the UVC group had a 19.2% lower mean 24 h CCI and received about 25% more PC units, but the average number of days to next platelet transfusion did not differ significantly between treatment groups. The frequency of low-grade adverse events was slightly higher in the UVC-PC group, and the frequencies of refractoriness to platelet transfusion, platelet alloimmunization, severe bleeding events, and red blood cell transfusions were comparable between groups. The study suggests that transfusion of pathogen-reduced platelets produced with the UVC technology is safe; however, non-inferiority was not demonstrated.

Hepatitis E virus is one of the non-enveloped viruses with increasing incidence in industrialized countries and may have serious clinical courses with chronic hepatitis and neurological complications, particularly in immunocompromised patients [66]. Mini pool nucleic acid amplification testing is currently used in blood manufacturing establishments for screening, but it can only detect high viremia [67]. IBS was reported to be ineffective to neutralize hepatitis E virus [68,69]. MPR has been proven effective, showing a reduction of viral load of 2–3 log [70]. The UVC method was highly effective, since the standard dose decreased the viral load below the standard of detection [63].

Initial in vitro studies have already showed the effectiveness of this method in cryopreserved platelets. Blood group AB0 matched pool PC were treated with Theraflex before freezing. In vitro analysis after thawing showed that pathogen-inactivated platelets and untreated controls expressed similar amounts of adhesion molecules, but treated platelets expressed a higher level of activated GPIIb/IIIa, which may indicate a higher susceptibility to damage during cryopreservation. Nevertheless, the treated platelets showed no difference to the controls regarding aggregometry, thromboelastography, and thrombin generation assays [71].

To summarise, there are three pathogen reduction technologies for PC, with two of them (IBS and MPR) being available in some countries for more than a decade for routine use. This approach is increasingly becoming the new paradigm in transfusion safety, as the described technologies are capable of diminishing or neutralizing infectious threats, including those that are not addressed or may not be detected by standard screening techniques. In addition, gamma or X-ray irradiation of platelet units for GvHD-prophylaxis becomes superfluous, because all described technologies already inactivate white blood cells efficiently.

3.4. Cold and Frozen Storage of Platelet Products

Platelet concentrates are currently mainly stored in gas-permeable bags with increased surface at 22 ± 2 °C (room temperature, RT) and constant agitation. Depending on the country, the accepted shelf life is limited to 3–7 days, mainly due to bacterial proliferation risk and progressive metabolic processes. However, even in the case of accepting a shelf life of 7 days, supply and logistic challenges and problems remain significant. To address and overcome the obvious limitations, alternative storage methods, including lyophilized (freeze-drying), cryopreserved (freezing with DMSO at -80 °C), and cold-stored platelets (CSPs), are currently being studied in clinical trials.

Until 1980, platelets (PLTs) were stored at 4 °C ("cold stored platelets"). However, this method was abandoned in light of a study conducted by Murphy et al., demonstrating that the half-life of cold-stored platelets after transfusion was markedly reduced in blood circulation (1.3 days compared to 3.9 days of RT stored PLTs) and that they undergo morphological distortions [72]. The latter are described as cold storage lesions and comprise irreversible disc-to-sphere transformation, apoptosis, signs of activation with increased expression of both P-selectin and GPIba, and increased production of thromboxane A2 [73]. This led to a paradigm shift towards storage of PC at RT. However, because the cold storage lesions include PLT pre-activation, cold stored PLTs may have a better hemostatic effectiveness for treating active hemorrhage than RT stored PLTs. Becker et al. demonstrated that CSPs were not inferior to RT PLTs, showing even greater reduction of bleeding time in healthy volunteers treated with aspirin [74]. In 2017, the US Food and Drug Administration (FDA) stated that apheresis PLTs stored at 4 °C for up to 72 h could be used for the treatment of active hemorrhage.

Two recent studies addressed the characteristics of CSPs in more detail. Nair et al. demonstrated that CSPs form a significantly stiffer and stronger blood clot with more crosslinks as well as thinner, denser, and straighter fibers compared to RT stored PLTs [75]. Additionally, cold-induced binding of plasma factor XIII to the platelet surface resulted in enhanced mechanical clot strength by increased crosslinking [74]. The study of Johnson et al. focused on the biochemical and morphological changes platelets undergo during cold storage [76]. CSPs had a lower metabolic activity, using ATP mainly for shape changes from disc to sphere. According to the maintained metabolic reserves and shape-change capacity, CSPs were at least non-inferior in comparison with RT-PC [75]. Both studies agree that CSPs are a useful alternative to RT platelets and could be even more effective in a post-traumatic context, where speed and strength of clot formation has priority. A recent pilot trial supports the feasibility of platelets stored cold for up to 14 days and provides critical guidance for future pivotal trials in high-risk cardiothoracic bleeding patients [77].

Cryopreserved Platelets (CPPs) carry minimal bacterial contamination risk and can be stored at −80 °C for several years. Stored as platelet pellets at −15 °C, the first application of CPPs was in pediatric patients with thrombocytopenia and resulted in a moderate success [78]. After invention of the dimethyl sulfoxide (DMSO) method by Valeri and colleagues in 1974 [79] and its modifications [80–82], CPPs can be stored at −80 °C, resulting in a more standardized and frequent manufacturing of CPPs, particularly used by military services. Further investigations showed that freezing and thawing affects the morphology and surface marker expression of CPPs, resulting in a pre-activation state [75]. In several trials in bleeding patients, CPPs revealed equivalent or even slightly improved hemostatic effectiveness when compared to RT-stored PLTs [41,83–85]. Serious adverse events, including an increased risk of thrombo-embolism, could not be found. However, there is an increased release of biological response modifiers in CPPs, which may be a potential further clinical risk of these products [86]. Combining IBS pathogen inactivation and cryopreservation did not affect the release of immunomodulatory factors more than cryopreservation alone [87]. CPPs showed lower posttransfusion increments and reduced 24 h recovery, making them more applicable for resuscitation of active hemorrhage and less suitable for prophylactic transfusion in thrombocytopenic patients.

In highly alloimmunized thrombocytopenic patients after chemotherapy, autologous CPPs can serve as an additional source of HLA-compatible units. A Swiss group used autologous CPPs for thrombocytopenic alloimmunized and PLT-refractory patients undergoing chemotherapy. They reported a significantly higher median 1 h PLT count increment compared to RT-stored, AB0-matched, but HLA-unselected PCs [88].

The largest and most recent randomized, double blind, multicenter pilot study of CPPs to date, the CLIP-I trial, investigated the effects of CPPs versus RT stored PLTs in 121 cardiac surgery patients [89]. The trial's primary endpoint of feasibility was met, and investigators found neither significant differences between the two patient cohorts in blood loss or RBC use nor in adverse event rates [86].

In summary, CPPs could be a useful addition for certain patient settings and populations. Frequent usage in frontline military surgical units and in rural hospitals as well as "back-up units" in busy urban trauma centers are reasonable scenarios. For HLA-alloimmunized patients, autologous and allogeneic CPPs could expand the number and variety of appropriate PCs.

The production of lyophilized (synonymous: freeze-dried) platelets (LPs) was already attempted in the 1950s. However, the rehydrated PLT units showed no hemostatic effectiveness [90]. In 1995, Read and colleagues reported an improvement of the lyophilization procedure by stabilizing the PLTs with paraformaldehyde (pLPs) before freeze-drying [91]. In vitro testing of rehydrated pLPs revealed normal morphology, with adhesive properties remaining largely intact. Even though activation and aggregation functions are impaired, they retain the ability to facilitate coagulation [92–94]. In animal studies, the infusion of pLPs improved bleeding time and showed no difference with respect to transfusion requirements, PLT increment, adverse effects, or survival in comparison to fresh PLTs [88,95]. There is no evidence supporting an increased risk of pro-thrombotic complications after transfusion of pLPs. In vivo studies showed that pLPs have minimal adhesion to intact endothelium and are rapidly cleared from blood circulation if they are not bound immediately to the site of injury after transfusion [96,97].

In 2001, Wolkers and colleagues described another procedure, where PLTs were loaded with trehalose before lyophilization [98]. After rehydration, these PLTs showed a recovery rate of ca. 80%, and about 40% of the cells showed characteristics of pre-activation [99]. Compared to fresh PLTs, their clot formation time was similar, with an aggregation rate ca. 80% and aggregation speed ca. 40%.

The current LPs have inferior hemostatic properties compared to fresh PLTs, but they may be an alternative if fresh PLTs are not available, especially in the setting of acute hemorrhage. Due to their rapid clearance from blood circulation, they are not an alternative for prophylactic transfusions in thrombocytopenic patients.

In summary, cold and frozen stored platelet products could be an efficient substitute or at least supplementation of RT-stored PCs. In vitro results demonstrate that their clotting and hemostatic properties could exceed those of conventional PCs, though sufficient evidence based on clinical studies in routine use is still pending. It has reasonably been postulated that the "one size fits all" strategy, where only RT-stored PCs are used for both prophylaxis and therapeutic needs, may be neither cost effective nor the best choice for the single patient. The task of switching from "RT PC only" supply to a dual inventory with CSP and RT PC is obviously huge. However, recent pilot studies have shown the feasibility of building and maintaining a dual inventory and the efficacy of CSPs in patients undergoing complex cardiothoracic surgery [76]. The challenge of a dual inventory may be mitigated by storing platelets at room temperature until they are close to the expiration date and only then refrigerating them [100].

The data for cryopreserved and lyophilized platelets are currently not sufficient to suggest a paradigm shift but are extremely promising and interesting, suggesting that further studies should be done to assess the efficacy and feasibility of these fascinating blood products.

3.5. Alternatives to Platelet Transfusions

The increasing demand for platelet products, in combination with their limited storage time, outpaces the availability of donors, resulting in a high economic burden and product shortage. In addition to the potential transmission of viruses and bacteria, platelet transfusion is associated with potentially life-threatening complications, such as allergic and febrile reactions. In addition, alloimmunization after repetitive platelet transfusion may result in platelet refractoriness and hence with increased risk for hemorrhagic complications for affected patients due to a significantly constricted number of compatible products. Recent attempts to produce platelets devoid of HLA Class I molecules are promising. Such an approach would offer a solution to prevent alloimmunization and reduce the risk of refractoriness [101]. However, this will not provide a solution to meet the increasing needs of platelet products and hence platelet donors. Therefore, it may be prudent to find substitutes for platelets products.

Alternatives to platelet transfusion in clinical use include auxiliary therapeutic strategies to support plasma coagulation. Such strategies are of special value in the treatment of bleeding complications of thrombocytopenic patients, since clots with low platelet contents are more prone to lysis. Platelets contain plasminogen activator inhibitor-1 (PAI-1) and Factor XIII, which inhibit fibrin degradation and stabilize the clot firmness through fibrin cross-linking, respectively [102].

Thrombopoietin (TPO) mimetics are used off label in a wide range of malignant diseases with impaired thrombocyte production due to the disease itself and/or the therapy applied. Their extended indication may be an appropriate approach to avoid or at least reduce platelet transfusions. For example, there is some evidence for the usage of TPO agonists in myelodysplastic syndromes. A meta-analysis including 384 patients described a lower bleeding and transfusion rate in TPO treated patients compared to placebo [103]. However, this treatment is expensive, and some authors assume an increased risk of thrombosis upon TPO agonist treatment [104]. TPO agonists are most suitable to increase platelet count in the long term (i.e., days to weeks). Hence, they are not appropriate for the treatment of acute bleedings in thrombocytopenic patients.

Research activities focusing on alternatives to platelet transfusion have shifted into the foreground in the last decades. They attempt to find an effective "off the shelf" product, with optimal storage properties, that can mimic the biochemical platelet mechanisms (adhesion, aggregation, and coagulation) even after prolonged storage, but with no need for blood group typing and a reduced risk of side effects. In 1992, an autologous, semiartificial alternative to platelet transfusion, called "Thromboerythrocytes", was reported. Peptide sequences containing the specific recognition sequence, containing arginine-glycine-aspartic acid (RGD) as found in the extracellular matrix and in fibrinogen, were cross-linked to amino groups on erythrocytes. The coupled RGD sequences revealed interaction with the GPIIb/IIIa receptor in fluid phase as well as binding to activated platelets adherent to collagen. The authors reported of their in vitro studies, indicating that 50 mL of processed thromboerythrocytes may be equivalent to at least two PC units [105]. Although a very attractive concept, thromboerythrocytes have not found their way into the clinic thus far. A comparable approach by means of membrane modification, called "Plateletsomes", was successfully used in rat experiments. In this case, platelet membrane fractions, including relevant platelet-receptors such as GPIb, GPIIb-IIIa, and GPIV/III, were extracted from platelets and incorporated into liposome membranes. These plateletsomes reduced tail bleeding in thrombocytopenic rats by 67% [106].

Given the fact that even small membrane fragments seem to have comparable hemostatic qualities to intact platelets, Cypress Bioscience Incorporated (San Diego, CA, USA) developed concentrates of platelet fragments of non-viable platelets, called Infusible Platelet Membranes (IPMs). First, fresh, or even expired platelet concentrates are centrifuged and washed to remove plasma and contaminating white and red blood cells. Subsequently, they are pasteurized to reduce bacterial contamination. Finally, their sonication yields spherical vesicles. When stored at 4 °C, the IPM product is stable over two years. In healthy volunteers, IPM did not alter coagulation parameters, was tolerated well, and importantly did not show any immunogenicity. Indeed, administration of IPM resulted in an improvement or cessation of bleeding in thrombocytopenic patients with moderate bleeding. Interestingly, a patient refractory to platelet transfusion, who did not respond to IPM, showed a platelet increment after consecutive platelet transfusions. There has been no phase III clinical trial for this product and no FDA approval due to difficulties in demonstrating its efficacy [107,108]. The lack of provable efficacy in patients has been attributed to its lack of GPIIb/IIIa epitopes in IPM preparations.

An attempt to improve the IPM idea resulted in "Thrombosomes", entire membranes extracted from outdated platelets. However, in contrast to IPM, thrombosomes express platelet surface receptors, including GPIb, GPIIb/IIIa, and Annexin V. They efficiently adhere to collagen exposed in the subendothelial matrix, activate the tenase complex, and form a stable clot. In animal models for bleeding, thrombosomes reduced blood loss by 80% [109]. Thrombosomes are currently evaluated in clinical trials. One of the main technical challenges so far is the significant loss of relevant platelet glycoprotein receptors and hence functionality during thrombocyte membrane processing.

Another possible alternative to thrombocytes are liposomes, containing ADP and synthetic fibrinogen derived γ-chain inclosing a dodecapeptide motif. The liposomes accumulate at the intravascular lesion site and interact with platelets by binding of the fibrinogen γ-chain dodecapeptide sequence to GPIIb/IIIa and inducing the release of stored ADP, thereby further promoting platelet aggregation [110]. The efficacy of this synthetic platelet replacement has been demonstrated in thrombocytopenic rabbits: 60% of the animals were rescued after a potentially fatal liver hemorrhage. Treating thrombocytopenic rabbits before the induction of the liver hemorrhage showed a 100% survival rate. Importantly, no thromboembolic complications occurred [111,112]. Furthermore, in a bleeding model in rats, the liposomes accumulated at the venous lesion of the tails of thrombocytopenic rats, leading to reduced bleeding [107]. Pharmacokinetic studies in rats showed a predominant localization of the synthetic liposomes in the liver and spleen after 24 h, and after 7 days there was a complete clearance from all organs [113].

SynthoPlate are synthetic platelet nanoconstructs that integrate, in a heteromultivalent approach, the adhesion and aggregation process of platelets. SynthoPlate consists of a biocompatible liposomal membrane with, on one hand, von Willebrand Factor-binding peptide and collagen-binding peptide to mimic platelet adhesion, and on the other hand, GPIIb/IIIa to mimic platelet aggregation. The efficacy of SynthoPlate was demonstrated in a mouse model for liver injury and in a trauma model in pigs. SynthoPlate reduced blood loss, stabilized blood pressure, and improved survival [114,115].

A comparable approach finally resulted in the idea of completely synthetic "platelets" made from polymers incorporating both platelet properties—adhesion and aggregation. The nanospheres are composed of PLGA-PLL nanoparticles (poly(lactic-co-glycolicacid)-poly-L-lysine), conjugated to polyethylene glycol (PEG) and surface-bound fibrinogen-derived RGD peptides, with additional flanking amino acids to enhance adhesion. By binding through specific integrins like GPIIb/IIIa, activated platelets bind to RGD sequences [116]. In vitro assays show a high specificity of binding of the synthetic platelets to inactivated physiologic platelets, which might be an indicator for a low risk of thrombotic complications in vivo. In a traumatic bleeding model in rats, the administration of synthetic platelets before injury was proven approximately 25% more effective than recombinant Factor VIIa, which is currently used in uncontrolled hemorrhage [117,118]. The same kind of synthetic platelets improved survival in a mouse model with blast trauma [119].

HAPPI, an injectable hemostatic agent via polymer peptide interfusion, is one of the most recent developments. It is a polymer-based hemostatic agent that binds selectively to activated platelets and promotes their accumulation at the injury site. HAPPI consists of a hyaluronic acid backbone conjugated with a collagen-binding peptide and a von Willebrand factor-binding peptide. It is designed to bind to vWF and collagen on activated platelets, thus recruiting and activating additional platelets. Through lyophilization, HAPPI is stable at room temperature for several months. Administration of HAPPI in a thrombocytopenic mouse model with tail-vein laceration significantly reduced bleeding time and blood loss as compared to untreated mice. In rats with traumatic hemorrhage due to inferior vena cava rupture, HAPPI showed an almost threefold improvement in survival compared to those treated with saline [120].

A future-oriented strategy to reduce the shortness of platelet products is to propagate the in vitro production of thrombocytes through forward programming of human pluripotent stem cells to megakaryocytes using exogenously expressed transcription factors GATA1, LFI1, and TAL1. This approach is highly efficient, with a yield of up to 2×10^5 megakaryocytes per activated human pluripotent stem cell. This technique could yield sufficient HLA-matched platelets to cover the needs for platelets [121]. The limitations of the technique are the high production costs and scarce availability of human embryonic stem cells [122,123].

In summary, current and upcoming advances will significantly affect present standards. In particular, B-PC and A-PC are considered clinically equivalent, revealing similar quality, effectiveness, and adverse event profiles. However, A-PC from selected donors remains essential when HLA/HPA compatibility of PC is needed. Current PAS generations may extend the shelf life of PC up 13 to days while retaining adequate platelet increment as well as platelet recovery and survival and decreasing adverse reactions. Because manufacturing costs are reduced simultaneously, PASs are steadily replacing plasma as the storage medium of platelets. There are three pathogen reduction technologies for PC, with two of them being available in some countries for routine use for many years. This approach is increasingly becoming the new paradigm in transfusion safety, because it safeguards against the majority of the remaining associated infectious threats and makes X-ray/gamma irradiation of PC (for prevention of GvHD) superfluous. Cold stored platelet products could be an efficient substitute or at least supplementation of PCs stored at $22 \pm 2\,°C$. The in vitro hemostatic properties of these products may exceed those of the conventional PCs, at least in the therapeutic setting, i.e., the bleeding patients. Recent pilot studies have shown the feasibility of building and maintaining a dual inventory and the efficacy of the cold stored platelets in patients undergoing complex cardiothoracic surgery, but sufficient evidence based on clinical studies in routine use is still pending. The data about cryopreserved and lyophilized platelets are extremely promising, but further studies have to assess the efficacy and feasibility of these fascinating blood products. Several promising approaches are underway to find safe and effective alternatives to platelet transfusions, including auxiliary therapeutic strategies to support plasma coagulation, thrombopoietin mimetics, "Thromboerythrocytes", "Plateletsomes", "Infusible Platelet Membranes", "Thrombosomes", liposomal constructs, SynthoPlate® (Haima Therapeutics, Cleveland, OH, USA) completely synthetic "platelets", HAPPI (hemostatic agent via polymer peptide interfusion), and in vitro production of thrombocytes.

Altogether, several promising approaches are underway to find safe and effective improvements and/or alternatives to platelet transfusions. The reviewed issues are expected to have a major impact on current practices of platelet transfusion as soon as their efficacy and safety are revealed in current and upcoming clinical studies.

Author Contributions: S.S.Z., M.D. and B.M.T. developed the frame and focus, supervised, and contributed to the manuscript. A.C., K.A.J. and C.M. contributed equally to the manuscript, while A.C. focused on sections on pathogen reduction/inactivation and platelet alternatives, K.A.J. focused on platelet storage solutions and buffy-coat versus apheresis platelets, and C.M. focused on cold and frozen stored platelet products. B.M.T. merged and meshed the manuscript. All authors have read and agreed to the published version of the manuscript.

Funding: This work received no external funding.

Institutional Review Board Statement: Not applicable.

Informed Consent Statement: Not applicable.

Data Availability Statement: Not applicable.

Conflicts of Interest: The authors declare no conflict of interest.

References

1. Duke, W.W. The relation of blood platelets to hemorrhagic disease: Description of a method for determining the bleeding time and coagulation time and report of three cases of hemorrhagic disease relieved by transfusion. *JAMA* **1910**, *55*, 1185–1192. [CrossRef]
2. Hersh, E.M.; Bodey, G.P.; Nies, B.A.; Freireich, E. Causes of death in acute leukemia: A ten-year study of 414 patients from 1954–1963. *JAMA* **1965**, *193*, 105–109. [CrossRef]
3. Han, T.; Stutzman, L.; Cohen, E.; Kim, U. Effect of platelet transfusion on hemorrhage in patients with acute leukemia: An autopsy study. *Cancer* **1966**, *19*, 1937–1942. [CrossRef]
4. Schiffer, C.A.; Bohlke, K.; Delaney, M.; Hume, H.; Magdalinski, A.J.; McCullough, J.J.; Omel, J.L.; Rainey, J.M.; Rebulla, P.; Rowley, S.D.; et al. Platelet Transfusion for Patients With Cancer: American Society of Clinical Oncology Clinical Practice Guideline Update. *J. Clin. Oncol.* **2018**, *36*, 283–299. [CrossRef]

5. Estcourt, L.J.; Birchall, J.; Allard, S.; Bassey, S.J.; Hersey, P.; Kerr, J.P.; Mumford, A.D.; Stanworth, S.J.; Tinegate, H. British Committee for Standards in Haematology: Guidelines for the use of platelet transfusions. *Br. J. Haematol.* **2017**, *176*, 365–394. [CrossRef]
6. Murphy, S.; Heaton, W.A.; Rebulla, P. Platelet production in the Old World—And the New. *Transfusion* **1996**, *36*, 751–754. [CrossRef]
7. Garraud, O.; Cognasse, F.; Tissot, J.-D.; Chavarin, P.; Laperche, S.; Morel, P.; Lefrère, J.-J.; Pozzetto, B.; Lozano, M.; Blumberg, N.; et al. Improving platelet transfusion safety: Biomedical and technical considerations. *Blood Transfus.* **2016**, *14*, 109–122.
8. Heddle, N.M.; Klama, L.; Meyer, R.; Walker, I.; Boshkov, L.; Roberts, R.; Chambers, S.; Podlosky, L.; O'Hoski, P.; Levine, M. A randomized controlled trial comparing plasma removal with white cell reduction to prevent reactions to platelets. *Transfusion* **1999**, *39*, 231–238. [CrossRef]
9. Jones, J.M.; Sapiano, M.R.P.; Savinkina, A.A.; Haass, K.A.; Baker, M.L.; Henry, R.A.; Berger, J.J.; Basavaraju, S.V. Slowing decline in blood collection and transfusion in the United States—2017. *Transfusion* **2020**, *60* (Suppl. 2), S1–S9. [CrossRef]
10. World Health Organization. *Global Status Report on Blood Safety and Availability 2016*; World Health Organization: Geneva, Switzerland, 2017.
11. Heddle, N.M.; Arnold, D.M.; Boye, D.; Webert, K.E.; Resz, I.; Dumont, L.J. Comparing the efficacy and safety of apheresis and whole blood-derived platelet transfusions: A systematic review. *Transfusion* **2008**, *48*, 1447–1458. [CrossRef]
12. Ness, P.M.; Campbell-Lee, S.A. Single donor versus pooled random donor platelet concentrates. *Curr. Opin. Hematol.* **2001**, *8*, 392–396. [CrossRef] [PubMed]
13. Triulzi, D.J.; Assmann, S.F.; Strauss, R.G.; Ness, P.M.; Hess, J.R.; Kaufman, R.M.; Granger, S.; Slichter, S.J. The impact of platelet transfusion characteristics on posttransfusion platelet increments and clinical bleeding in patients with hypoproliferative thrombocytopenia. *Blood* **2012**, *119*, 5553–5562. [CrossRef]
14. Lafeuillade, B.; Eb, F.; Ounnoughene, N.; Petermann, R.; Daurat, G.; Huyghe, G.; Vo Mai, M.-P.; Caldani, C.; Rebibo, D.; Weinbreck, P. Residual risk and retrospective analysis of transfusion-transmitted bacterial infection reported by the French National Hemovigilance Network from 2000 to 2008. *Transfusion* **2015**, *55*, 636–646. [CrossRef]
15. Kuehnert, M.J.; Roth, V.R.; Haley, N.R.; Gregory, K.R.; Elder, K.V.; Schreiber, G.B.; Arduino, M.J.; Holt, S.C.; Carson, L.A.; Banerjee, S.N.; et al. Transfusion-transmitted bacterial infection in the United States, 1998 through 2000. *Transfusion* **2001**, *41*, 1493–1499. [CrossRef] [PubMed]
16. Jacobs, M.R.; Good, C.E.; Lazarus, H.M.; Yomtovian, R.A. Relationship between bacterial load, species virulence, and transfusion reaction with transfusion of bacterially contaminated platelets. *Clin. Infect. Dis.* **2008**, *46*, 1214–1220. [CrossRef] [PubMed]
17. Vamvakas, E.C. Relative safety of pooled whole blood-derived versus single-donor (apheresis) platelets in the United States: A systematic review of disparate risks. *Transfusion* **2009**, *49*, 2743–2758. [CrossRef]
18. Van der Heiden, M.; Ritter, S.; Hamouda, O.; Offergeld, R. Estimating the residual risk for HIV, HCV and HBV in different types of platelet concentrates in Germany. *Vox Sang.* **2015**, *108*, 123–130. [CrossRef] [PubMed]
19. Cid, J.; Carbassé, G.; Pereira, A.; Sanz, C.; Mazzara, R.; Escolar, G.; Lozano, M. Platelet transfusions from D+ donors to D- patients: A 10-year follow-up study of 1014 patients. *Transfusion* **2011**, *51*, 1163–1169. [CrossRef]
20. Shaz, B.H.; Hillyer, C.D. Residual risk of D alloimmunization: Is it time to feel safe about platelets from D+ donors? *Transfusion* **2011**, *51*, 1132–1135. [CrossRef]
21. O'Brien, K.L.; Haspel, R.L.; Uhl, L. Anti-D alloimmunization after D-incompatible platelet transfusions: A 14-year single-institution retrospective review. *Transfusion* **2014**, *54*, 650–654. [CrossRef]
22. Cid, J.; Lozano, M.; Ziman, A.; West, K.A.; O'Brien, K.L.; Murphy, M.F.; Wendel, S.; Vázquez, A.; Ortín, X.; Hervig, T.A.; et al. Biomedical Excellence for Safer Transfusion collaborative: Low frequency of anti-D alloimmunization following D+ platelet transfusion: The Anti-D Alloimmunization after D-incompatible Platelet Transfusions (ADAPT) study. *Br. J. Haematol.* **2015**, *168*, 598–603. [CrossRef] [PubMed]
23. Curtis, G.; Scott, M.; Orengo, L.; Hendrickson, J.E.; Tormey, C.A. Very low rate of anti-D development in male, primarily immunocompetent patients transfused with D-mismatched platelets. *Transfusion* **2018**, *58*, 1568–1569. [CrossRef]
24. Stanworth, S.J.; Navarrete, C.; Estcourt, L.; Marsh, J. Platelet refractoriness—Practical approaches and ongoing dilemmas in patient management. *Br. J. Haematol.* **2015**, *171*, 297–305. [CrossRef]
25. The Trial to Reduce Alloimmunization to Platelets Study Group. Leukocyte reduction and ultraviolet B irradiation of platelets to prevent alloimmunization and refractoriness to platelet transfusions. *N. Engl. J. Med.* **1997**, *337*, 1861–1869. [CrossRef] [PubMed]
26. Tariket, S.; Sut, C.; Hamzeh-Cognasse, H.; Laradi, S.; Pozzetto, B.; Garraud, O. Cognasse: Transfusion-related acute lung injury: Transfusion, platelets and biological response modifiers. *Expert Rev. Hematol.* **2016**, *9*, 497–508. [CrossRef]
27. Eder, A.F.; Herron, R.; Strupp, A.; Dy, B.; Notari, P.E.; Chambers, L.A.; Dodd, R.Y.; Benjamin, R.J. Transfusion-related acute lung injury surveillance (2003–2005) and the potential impact of the selective use of plasma from male donors in the American Red Cross. *Transfusion* **2007**, *47*, 599–607. [CrossRef]
28. Gajic, O.; Rana, R.; Winters, J.L.; Yilmaz, M.; Mendez, J.L.; Rickman, O.B.; O'Byrne, M.M.; Evenson, L.K.; Malinchoc, M.; DeGoey, S.R.; et al. Transfusion-related acute lung injury in the critically ill: Prospective nested case-control study. *Am. J. Respir. Crit. Care Med.* **2007**, *176*, 886–891. [CrossRef]
29. Kaufman, R.M.; Assmann, S.F.; Triulzi, D.J.; Strauss, R.G.; Ness, P.; Granger, S.; Slichter, S.J. Transfusion-related adverse events in the Platelet Dose study. *Transfusion* **2015**, *55*, 144–153. [CrossRef]

30. van der Meer, P.F. PAS or plasma for storage of platelets? A concise review. *Transfus. Med.* **2016**, *26*, 339–342. [CrossRef] [PubMed]
31. Holme, S.; Heaton, W.A.; Courtright, M. Improved in vivo and in vitro viability of platelet concentrates stored for seven days in a platelet additive solution. *Br. J. Haematol.* **1987**, *66*, 233–238. [CrossRef] [PubMed]
32. Gulliksson, H. Platelet storage media. *Vox Sang.* **2014**, *107*, 205–212. [CrossRef]
33. Radwanski, K.; Wagner, S.J.; Skripchenko, A.; Min, K. In vitro variables of apheresis platelets are stably maintained for 7 days with 5% residual plasma in a glucose and bicarbonate salt solution, PAS-5. *Transfusion* **2012**, *52*, 188–194. [CrossRef]
34. Tobian, A.A.; Fuller, A.K.; Uglik, K.; Tisch, D.J.; Borge, P.D.; Benjamin, R.J.; Ness, P.M.; King, K.E. The impact of platelet additive solution apheresis platelets on allergic transfusion reactions and corrected count increment (CME). *Transfusion* **2014**, *54*, 1523–1529. [CrossRef]
35. van der Meer, P.F.; de Korte, D. Platelet Additive Solutions: A Review of the Latest Developments and Their Clinical Implications. *Transfus. Med. Hemother.* **2018**, *45*, 98–102. [CrossRef]
36. Benjamin, R.J.; Braschler, T.; Weingand, T.; Corash, L.M. Hemovigilance monitoring of platelet septic reactions with effective bacterial protection systems. *Transfusion* **2017**, *7*, 2946–2957. [CrossRef]
37. Haass, K.A.; Sapiano, M.R.P.; Savinkina, A.; Kuehnert, M.J.; Basavaraju, S.V. Transfusion-Transmitted Infections Reported to the National Healthcare Safety Network Hemovigilance Module. *Transfus. Med. Rev.* **2019**, *33*, 84–91. [CrossRef]
38. Blajchman, M.A. Bacterial contamination of cellular blood components: Risks, sources and control. *Vox Sang.* **2004**, *87*, 98–103. [CrossRef] [PubMed]
39. Abela, M.A.; Fenning, S.; Maguire, K.A.; Morris, K.G. Bacterial contamination of platelet components not detected by BacT/ALERT(®). *Transfus. Med.* **2018**, *28*, 65–70. [CrossRef] [PubMed]
40. Schmidt, M.; Hourfar, M.K.; Sireis, W.; Pfeiffer, U.; Göttig, S.; Kempf, V.A.; McDonald, C.P.; Seifried, E. Evaluation of the effectiveness of a pathogen inactivation technology against clinically relevant transfusion-transmitted bacterial strains. *Transfusion* **2015**, *55*, 2104–2112. [CrossRef]
41. Bohonek, M.; Kutac, D.; Landova, L.; Koranova, M.; Sladkova, E.; Staskova, E.; Voldrich, M.; Tyll, T. The use of cryopreserved platelets in the treatment of polytraumatic patients and patients with massive bleeding. *Transfusion* **2019**, *59*, 1474–1478. [CrossRef] [PubMed]
42. Jutzi, M.; Mansouri Taleghani, B.; Rueesch, M.; Amsler, L.; Buser, A. Nationwide Implementation of Pathogen Inactivation for All Platelet Concentrates in Switzerland. *Transfus. Med. Hemother.* **2018**, *45*, 151–156. [CrossRef] [PubMed]
43. Lin, L.; Cook, D.N.; Wiesehahn, G.P.; Alfonso, R.; Behrman, B.; Cimino, G.D.; Corten, L.; Damonte, P.B.; Dikeman, R.; Dupuis, K.; et al. Photochemical inactivation of viruses and bacteria in platelet concentrates by use of a novel psoralen and long-wavelength ultraviolet light. *Transfusion* **1997**, *37*, 423–435. [CrossRef]
44. Snyder, E.; Raife, T.; Lin, L.; Cimino, G.; Metzel, P.; Rheinschmidt, M.; Baril, L.; Davis, K.; Buchholz, D.H.; Corash, L.; et al. Recovery and life span of 111indium-radiolabeled platelets treated with pathogen inactivation with amotosalen HCl (S-59) and ultraviolet A light. *Transfusion* **2004**, *44*, 1732–1740. [CrossRef]
45. Slichter, S.J.; Raife, T.J.; Davis, K.; Rheinschmidt, M.; Buchholz, D.H.; Corash, L.; Conlan, M.G. Platelets photochemically treated with amotosalen HCl and ultraviolet A light correct prolonged bleeding times in patients with thrombocytopenia. *Transfusion* **2006**, *46*, 731–740. [CrossRef]
46. Vamvakas, E.C. Meta-analysis of the studies of bleeding complications of platelets pathogen-reduced with the Intercept system. *Vox Sang.* **2012**, *102*, 302–316. [CrossRef] [PubMed]
47. Estcourt, L.J.; Malouf, R.; Hopewell, S.; Trivella, M.; Doree, C.; Stanworth, S.J.; Murphy, M.F. Pathogen-reduced platelets for the prevention of bleeding. *Cochrane Database Syst. Rev.* **2017**, *7*, CD009072. [CrossRef] [PubMed]
48. Lanteri, M.C.; Santa-Maria, F.; Laughhunn, A.; Girard, Y.A.; Picard-Maureau, M.; Payrat, J.M.; Irsch, J.; Stassinopoulos, A.; Bringmann, P. Inactivation of a broad spectrum of viruses and parasites by photochemical treatment of plasma and platelets using amotosalen and ultraviolet A light. *Transfusion* **2020**, *60*, 1319–1331. [CrossRef] [PubMed]
49. Garban, F.; Guyard, A.; Labussière, H.; Bulabois, C.E.; Marchand, T.; Mounier, C.; Caillot, D.; Bay, J.O.; Coiteux, V.; Schmidt-Tanguy, A.; et al. Comparison of the Hemostatic Efficacy of Pathogen-Reduced Platelets vs. Untreated Platelets in Patients With Thrombocytopenia and Malignant Hematologic Diseases: A Randomized Clinical Trial. *JAMA Oncol.* **2018**, *4*, 468–475. [CrossRef]
50. Cid, J.; Escolar, G.; Lozano, M. Therapeutic efficacy of platelet components treated with amotosalen and ultraviolet A pathogen inactivation method: Results of a meta-analysis of randomized controlled trials. *Vox Sang.* **2012**, *103*, 322–330. [CrossRef]
51. Butler, C.; Doree, C.; Estcourt, L.J.; Trivella, M.; Hopewell, S.; Brunskill, S.J.; Stanworth, S.; Murphy, M.F. Pathogen-reduced platelets for the prevention of bleeding. *Cochrane Database Syst. Rev.* **2013**, Cd009072. [CrossRef]
52. Stivala, S.; Gobbato, S.; Infanti, L.; Reiner, M.F.; Bonetti, N.; Meyer, S.C.; Camici, G.G.; Lüscher, T.F.; Buser, A.; Beer, J.H. Amotosalen/ultraviolet A pathogen inactivation technology reduces platelet activatability, induces apoptosis and accelerates clearance. *Haematologica* **2017**, *102*, 1650–1660. [CrossRef]
53. Meinke, S.; Wikman, A.; Gryfelt, G.; Hultenby, K.; Uhlin, M.; Höglund, P.; Sandgren, P. Cryopreservation of buffy coat-derived platelet concentrates photochemically treated with amotosalen and UVA light. *Transfusion* **2018**, *58*, 2657–2668. [CrossRef] [PubMed]
54. Keil, S.D.; Bengrine, A.; Bowen, R.; Marschner, S.; Hovenga, N.; Rouse, L.; Gilmour, D.; Duverlie, G.; Goodrich, R.P. Inactivation of viruses in platelet and plasma products using a riboflavin-and-UV-based photochemical treatment. *Transfusion* **2015**, *55*, 1736–1744. [CrossRef] [PubMed]

55. Goodrich, R.P.; Doane, S.; Reddy, H.L. Design and development of a method for the reduction of infectious pathogen load and inactivation of white blood cells in whole blood products. *Biologicals* **2010**, *38*, 20–30. [CrossRef] [PubMed]
56. Kumar, V.; Lockerbie, O.; Keil, S.D.; Ruane, P.H.; Platz, M.S.; Martin, C.B.; Ravanat, J.L.; Cadet, J.; Goodrich, R.P. Riboflavin and UV-light based pathogen reduction: Extent and consequence of DNA damage at the molecular level. *Photochem. Photobiol.* **2004**, *80*, 15–21. [CrossRef]
57. Reikvam, H.; Marschner, S.; Apelseth, T.O.; Goodrich, R.; Hervig, T. The Mirasol Pathogen Reduction Technology system and quality of platelets stored in platelet additive solution. *Blood Transfus.* **2010**, *8*, 186–192. [PubMed]
58. Yin, Y.; Li, L.; Gong, L.; Xu, H.; Liu, Z. Effects of riboflavin and ultraviolet light treatment on pathogen reduction and platelets. *Transfusion* **2020**, *60*, 2647–2654. [CrossRef] [PubMed]
59. van der Meer, P.F.; Ypma, P.F.; van Geloven, N.; van Hilten, J.A.; van Wordragen-Vlaswinkel, R.J.; Eissen, O.; Zwaginga, J.J.; Trus, M.; Beckers, E.A.M.; Te Boekhorst, P.; et al. Hemostatic efficacy of pathogen-inactivated vs. untreated platelets: A randomized controlled trial. *Blood* **2018**, *132*, 223–231. [CrossRef]
60. Chen, Z.; Schubert, P.; Culibrk, B.; Devine, D.V. p38MAPK is involved in apoptosis development in apheresis platelet concentrates after riboflavin and ultraviolet light treatment. *Transfusion* **2015**, *55*, 848–857. [CrossRef] [PubMed]
61. Saris, A.; Kerkhoffs, J.L.; Norris, P.J.; van Ham, S.M.; Ten Brinke, A.; Brand, A.; van der Meer, P.F.; Zwaginga, J.J. The role of pathogen-reduced platelet transfusions on HLA alloimmunization in hemato-oncological patients. *Transfusion* **2019**, *59*, 470–481. [CrossRef] [PubMed]
62. Bohonek, M.; Kutac, D.; Acker, J.P.; Seghatchian, J. Optimizing the supply of whole blood-derived bioproducts through the combined implementation of cryopreservation and pathogen reduction technologies and practices: An overview. *Transfus. Apher. Sci.* **2020**, *59*, 102754. [CrossRef]
63. Gravemann, U.; Handke, W.; Müller, T.H.; Seltsam, A. Bacterial inactivation of platelet concentrates with the THERAFLEX UV-Platelets pathogen inactivation system. *Transfusion* **2019**, *59*, 1324–1332. [CrossRef]
64. Praditya, D.; Friesland, M.; Gravemann, U.; Handke, W.; Todt, D.; Behrendt, P.; Müller, T.H.; Steinmann, E.; Seltsam, A. Hepatitis E virus is effectively inactivated in platelet concentrates by ultraviolet C light. *Vox Sang.* **2020**, *115*, 555–561. [CrossRef] [PubMed]
65. Brixner, V.; Bug, G.; Pohler, P.; Krämer, D.; Metzner, B.; Voß, A.; Casper, J.; Ritter, U.; Klein, S.; Alakel, N.; et al. Efficacy of UVC-treated, pathogen-reduced platelets versus untreated platelets: A randomized controlled non inferiority trial. *Haematologica* **2021**, *106*, 1086. [CrossRef] [PubMed]
66. Goel, A.; Vijay, H.J.; Katiyar, H.; Aggarwal, R. Prevalence of hepatitis E viraemia among blood donors: A systematic review. *Vox Sang.* **2020**, *115*, 120–132. [CrossRef]
67. Kamp, C.; Blümel, J.; Baylis, S.A.; Bekeredjian-Ding, I.; Chudy, M.; Heiden, M.; Henseler, O.; Keller-Stanislawski, B.; de Vos, A.S.; Funk, M.B. Impact of hepatitis E virus testing on the safety of blood components in Germany—Results of a simulation study. *Vox Sang.* **2018**, *113*, 811–813. [CrossRef]
68. Hauser, L.; Roque-Afonso, A.M.; Beylouné, A.; Simonet, M.; Deau Fischer, B.; Burin des Roziers, N.; Mallet, V.; Tiberghien, P.; Bierling, P. Hepatitis E transmission by transfusion of Intercept blood system-treated plasma. *Blood* **2014**, *123*, 796–797. [CrossRef] [PubMed]
69. Mallet, V.; Sberro-Soussan, R.; Roque-Afonso, A.M.; Vallet-Pichard, A.; Deau, B.; Portal, A.; Chaix, M.L.; Hauser, L.; Beylouné, A.; Mercadier, A.; et al. Transmission of Hepatitis E Virus With Plasma Exchange in Kidney Transplant Recipients: A Retrospective Cohort Study. *Transplantation* **2018**, *102*, 1351–1357. [CrossRef]
70. Owada, T.; Kaneko, M.; Matsumoto, C.; Sobata, R.; Igarashi, M.; Suzuki, K.; Matsubayashi, K.; Mio, K.; Uchida, S.; Satake, M.; et al. Establishment of culture systems for Genotypes 3 and 4 hepatitis E virus (HEV) obtained from human blood and application of HEV inactivation using a pathogen reduction technology system. *Transfusion* **2014**, *54*, 2820–2827. [CrossRef] [PubMed]
71. Waters, L.; Padula, M.P.; Marks, D.C.; Johnson, L. Cryopreservation of UVC pathogen-inactivated platelets. *Transfusion* **2019**, *59*, 2093–2102. [CrossRef]
72. Murphy, S.; Gardner, F.H. Effect of storage temperature on maintenance of platelet viability—Deleterious effect of refrigerated storage. *N. Engl. J. Med.* **1969**, *280*, 1094–1098. [CrossRef]
73. Wood, B.; Padula, M.P.; Marks, D.C.; Johnson, L. Refrigerated storage of platelets initiates changes in platelet surface marker expression and localization of intracellular proteins. *Transfusion* **2016**, *56*, 2548–2559. [CrossRef] [PubMed]
74. Becker, G.A.; Tuccelli, M.; Kunicki, T.; Chalos, M.K.; Aster, R.H. Studies of platelet concentrates stored at 22 C and 4 C. *Transfusion* **1973**, *13*, 61–68. [CrossRef]
75. Nair, P.M.; Pandya, S.G.; Dallo, S.F.; Reddoch, K.M.; Montgomery, R.K.; Pidcoke, H.F.; Cap, A.P.; Ramasubramanian, A.K. Platelets stored at 4 degrees C contribute to superior clot properties compared to current standard-of-care through fibrin-crosslinking. *Br. J. Haematol.* **2017**, *178*, 119–129. [CrossRef]
76. Johnson, L.; Tan, S.; Wood, B.; Davis, A.; Marks, D.C. Refrigeration and cryopreservation of platelets differentially affect platelet metabolism and function: A comparison with conventional platelet storage conditions. *Transfusion* **2016**, *56*, 1807–1818. [CrossRef]
77. Strandenes, G.; Sivertsen, J.; Bjerkvig, C.K.; Fosse, T.K.; Cap, A.P.; Del Junco, D.J.; Kristoffersen, E.K.; Haaverstad, R.; Kvalheim, V.; Braathen, H.; et al. A Pilot Trial of Platelets Stored Cold versus at Room Temperature for Complex Cardiothoracic Surgery. *Anesthesiology* **2020**, *133*, 1173–1183. [CrossRef]
78. Klein, E.; Toch, R.; Farber, S.; Freemen, G.; Fiorentino, R. Hemostasis in thrombocytopenic bleeding following infusion of stored, frozen platelets. *Blood* **1956**, *11*, 693–699. [CrossRef]

79. Valeri, C.R.; Feingold, H.; Marchionni, L.D. A simple method for freezing human platelets using 6 per cent dimethylsulfoxide and storage at −80 °C. *Blood* **1974**, *43*, 131–136. [CrossRef]
80. Valeri, C.R.; Ragno, G.; Khuri, S. Freezing human platelets with 6 percent dimethyl sulfoxide with removal of the supernatant solution before freezing and storage at −80 °C without postthaw processing. *Transfusion* **2005**, *45*, 1890–1898. [CrossRef] [PubMed]
81. Slichter, S.J.; Jones, M.; Ransom, J.; Gettinger, I.; Jones, M.K.; Christoffel, T.; Pellham, E.; Bailey, S.L.; Corson, J.; Bolgiano, D. Review of in vivo studies of dimethyl sulfoxide cryopreserved platelets. *Transfus. Med. Rev.* **2014**, *28*, 212–225. [CrossRef] [PubMed]
82. Cohn, C.S.; Dumont, L.J.; Lozano, M.; Marks, D.C.; Johnson, L.; Ismay, S.; Bondar, N.; T'Sas, F.; Yokoyama, A.P.H.; Kutner, J.M.; et al. Vox Sanguinis International Forum on platelet cryopreservation: Summary. *Vox Sang.* **2017**, *112*, 684–688. [CrossRef] [PubMed]
83. Schiffer, C.A.; Aisner, J.; Dutcher, J.P.; Daly, P.A.; Wiernik, P.H. A clinical program of platelet cryopreservation. *Prog. Clin. Biol. Res.* **1982**, *88*, 165–180. [PubMed]
84. Khuri, S.F.; Healey, N.; MacGregor, H.; Barnard, M.R.; Szymanski, I.O.; Birjiniuk, V.; Michelson, A.D.; Gagnon, D.R.; Valeri, C.R. Comparison of the effects of transfusions of cryopreserved and liquid-preserved platelets on hemostasis and blood loss after cardiopulmonary bypass. *J. Thorac. Cardiovasc. Surg.* **1999**, *117*, 172–183; discussion 183–184. [CrossRef]
85. Slichter, S.J.; Dumont, L.J.; Cancelas, J.A.; Jones, M.L.; Gernsheimer, T.B.; Szczepiorkowski, Z.M.; Dunbar, N.M.; Prakash, G.; Medlin, S.; Rugg, N.; et al. Safety and efficacy of cryopreserved platelets in bleeding patients with thrombocytopenia. *Transfusion* **2018**, *58*, 2129–2138. [CrossRef] [PubMed]
86. Johnson, L.; Tan, S.; Jenkins, E.; Wood, B.; Marks, D.C. Characterization of biologic response modifiers in the supernatant of conventional, refrigerated, and cryopreserved platelets. *Transfusion* **2018**, *58*, 927–937. [CrossRef]
87. Tynngård, N.; Wikman, A.; Uhlin, M.; Sandgren, P. Haemostatic responsiveness and release of biological response modifiers following cryopreservation of platelets treated with amotosalen and ultraviolet A light. *Blood Transfus.* **2020**, *18*, 191–199.
88. Gerber, B.; Alberio, L.; Rochat, S.; Stenner, F.; Manz, M.G.; Buser, A.; Schanz, U.; Stussi, G. Safety and efficacy of cryopreserved autologous platelet concentrates in HLA-alloimmunized patients with hematologic malignancies. *Transfusion* **2016**, *56*, 2426–2437. [CrossRef] [PubMed]
89. Reade, M.C.; Marks, D.C.; Bellomo, R.; Deans, R.; Faulke, D.J.; Fraser, J.F.; Gattas, D.J.; Holley, A.D.; Irving, D.O.; Johnson, L.; et al. A randomized, controlled pilot clinical trial of cryopreserved platelets for perioperative surgical bleeding: The CLIP-I trial. *Transfusion* **2019**, *9*, 2794–2804. [CrossRef] [PubMed]
90. Jackson, D.P.; Sorensen, D.K.; Cronkite, E.P.; Bond, V.P.; Fliedner, T.M. Effectiveness of transfusions of fresh and lyophylized platelets in controlling bleeding due to thrombocytopenia. *J. Clin. Investig.* **1959**, *38*, 1689–1697. [CrossRef]
91. Read, M.S.; Reddick, R.L.; Bode, A.P.; Bellinger, D.A.; Nichols, T.C.; Taylor, K.; Smith, S.V.; McMahon, D.K.; Griggs, T.R.; Brinkhous, K.M. Preservation of hemostatic and structural properties of rehydrated lyophilized platelets—potential for long-term storage of dried platelets for transfusion. *Proc. Natl. Acad. Sci. USA* **1995**, *92*, 397–401. [CrossRef]
92. Fischer, T.H.; Merricks, E.P.; Bode, A.P.; Bellinger, D.A.; Russell, K.; Reddick, R.; Sanders, W.E.; Nichols, T.C.; Read, M.S. Thrombus formation with rehydrated, lyophilized platelets. *Hematology* **2002**, *7*, 359–369. [CrossRef] [PubMed]
93. Valeri, C.R.; Macgregor, H.; Barnard, M.R.; Summaria, L.; Michelson, A.D.; Ragno, G. In vitro testing of fresh and lyophilized reconstituted human and baboon platelets. *Transfusion* **2004**, *44*, 1505–1512. [CrossRef]
94. Fischer, T.H.; Bode, A.P.; Parker, B.R.; Russell, K.E.; Bender, D.E.; Ramer, J.K.; Read, M.S. Primary and secondary hemostatic functionalities of rehydrated, lyophilized platelets. *Transfusion* **2006**, *46*, 1943–1950. [CrossRef] [PubMed]
95. Bode, A.P.; Lust, R.M.; Read, M.S.; Fischer, T.H. Correction of the bleeding time with lyophilized platelet infusions in dogs on cardiopulmonary bypass. *Clin. Appl. Thromb. Hemost.* **2008**, *14*, 38–54. [CrossRef]
96. Inaba, K.; Barmparas, G.; Rhee, P.; Branco, B.C.; Fitzpatrick, M.; Okoye, O.T.; Demetriades, D. Dried platelets in a swine model of liver injury. *Shock* **2014**, *41*, 429–434. [CrossRef]
97. Fischer, T.H.; Merricks, E.; Bellinger, D.A.; Hayes, P.M.; Smith, R.S.; Raymer, R.; Read, M.S.; Nichols, T.C.; Bode, A.P. Splenic clearance mechanisms of rehydrated, lyophilized platelets. *Artif. Cells Blood Substit. Immobil. Biotechnol.* **2001**, *29*, 439–451. [CrossRef]
98. Wolkers, W.F.; Walker, N.J.; Tablin, F.; Crowe, J.H. Human platelets loaded with trehalose survive freeze-drying. *Cryobiology* **2001**, *42*, 79–87. [CrossRef]
99. Wang, J.X.; Yang, C.; Wan, Y.; Liu, M.X.; Ren, S.P.; Quan, G.B.; Hanet, Y. Stability of lyophilized human platelets loaded with small molecule carbohydrates. *Cryoletters* **2011**, *32*, 123–130. [PubMed]
100. Wood, B.; Johnson, L.; Hyland, R.A.; Marks, D.C. Maximising platelet availability by delaying cold storage. *Vox Sang.* **2018**, *113*, 403–441. [CrossRef]
101. Gras, C.; Schulze, K.; Goudeva, L.; Guzman, C.A.; Blasczyk, R.; Figueiredo, C. HLA-universal platelet transfusions prevent platelet refractoriness in a mouse model. *Hum. Gene Ther.* **2013**, *24*, 1018–1028. [CrossRef]
102. Desborough, M.; Estcourt, L.J.; Doree, C.; Trivella, M.; Hopewell, S.; Stanworth, S.J.; Murphy, M.F. Alternatives, and adjuncts, to prophylactic platelet transfusion for people with haematological malignancies undergoing intensive chemotherapy or stem cell transplantation. *Cochrane Database Syst. Rev.* **2016**, Cd010982. [CrossRef]

103. Prica, A.; Sholzberg, M.; Buckstein, R. Safety and efficacy of thrombopoietin-receptor agonists in myelodysplastic syndromes: A systematic review and meta-analysis of randomized controlled trials. *Br. J. Haematol.* **2014**, *167*, 626–638. [CrossRef]
104. Weber, E.; Moulis, G.; Mahévas, M.; Guy, C.; Lioger, B.; Durieu, I.; Hunault, M.; Ramanantsoa, M.; Royer, B.; Default, A.; et al. Thrombosis during thrombopoietin receptor agonist treatment for immune thrombocytopenia. A French multicentric observational study. *Rev. Med. Interne* **2017**, *38*, 167–175. [CrossRef] [PubMed]
105. Coller, B.S.; Springer, K.T.; Beer, J.H.; Mohandas, N.; Scudder, L.E.; Norton, K.J.; West, S.M. Thromboerythrocytes. In vitro studies of a potential autologous, semi-artificial alternative to platelet transfusions. *J. Clin. Investig.* **1992**, *89*, 546–555. [CrossRef]
106. Rybak, M.E.; Renzulli, L.A. A liposome based platelet substitute, the plateletsome, with hemostatic efficacy. *Biomater. Artif. Cells Immobil. Biotechnol.* **1993**, *21*, 101–118. [CrossRef]
107. Alving, B.M.; Reid, T.J.; Fratantoni, J.C.; Finlayson, J.S. Frozen platelets and platelet substitutes in transfusion medicine. *Transfusion* **1997**, *37*, 866–876. [CrossRef]
108. Nasiri, S. Infusible platelet membrane as a platelet substitute for transfusion: An overview. *Blood Transfus.* **2013**, *11*, 337–342.
109. Fitzpatrick, G.M.; Cliff, R.; Tandon, N. Thrombosomes: A platelet-derived hemostatic agent for control of noncompressible hemorrhage. *Transfusion* **2013**, *53* (Suppl. 1), 100s–106s. [CrossRef] [PubMed]
110. Okamura, Y.; Takeoka, S.; Eto, K.; Maekawa, I.; Fujie, T.; Maruyama, H.; Ikeda, Y.; Handa, M. Development of fibrinogen gamma-chain peptide-coated, adenosine diphosphate-encapsulated liposomes as a synthetic platelet substitute. *J. Thromb. Haemost.* **2009**, *7*, 470–477. [CrossRef] [PubMed]
111. Hagisawa, K.; Nishikawa, K.; Yanagawa, R.; Kinoshita, M.; Doi, M.; Suzuki, H.; Iwaya, K.; Saitoh, D.; Seki, S.; Takeoka, S.; et al. Treatment with fibrinogen γ-chain peptide-coated, adenosine 5'-diphosphate-encapsulated liposomes as an infusible hemostatic agent against active liver bleeding in rabbits with acute thrombocytopenia. *Transfusion* **2015**, *55*, 314–325. [CrossRef]
112. Nishikawa, K.; Hagisawa, K.; Kinoshita, M.; Shono, S.; Katsuno, S.; Doi, M.; Yanagawa, R.; Suzuki, H.; Iwaya, K.; Saitoh, D.; et al. Fibrinogen γ-chain peptide-coated, ADP-encapsulated liposomes rescue thrombocytopenic rabbits from non-compressible liver hemorrhage. *J. Thromb. Haemost.* **2012**, *10*, 2137–2148. [CrossRef]
113. Taguchi, K.; Ujihira, H.; Ogaki, S.; Watanabe, H.; Fujiyama, A.; Doi, M.; Okamura, Y.; Takeoka, S.; Ikeda, Y.; Handa, M.; et al. Pharmacokinetic study of the structural components of adenosine diphosphate-encapsulated liposomes coated with fibrinogen γ-chain dodecapeptide as a synthetic platelet substitute. *Drug Metab. Dispos.* **2013**, *41*, 1584–1591. [CrossRef]
114. Hickman, D.A.; Pawlowski, C.L.; Shevitz, A.; Luc, N.F.; Kim, A.; Girish, A.; Marks, J.; Ganjoo, S.; Huang, S.; Niedoba, E.; et al. Intravenous synthetic platelet (SynthoPlate) nanoconstructs reduce bleeding and improve 'golden hour' survival in a porcine model of traumatic arterial hemorrhage. *Sci. Rep.* **2018**, *8*, 3118. [CrossRef] [PubMed]
115. Dyer, M.R.; Hickman, D.; Luc, N.; Haldeman, S.; Loughran, P.; Pawlowski, C.L.; Sen Gupta, A.; Neal, M.D. Intravenous administration of synthetic platelets (SynthoPlate) in a mouse liver A. injury model of uncontrolled hemorrhage improves hemostasis. *J. Trauma Acute Care Surg.* **2018**, *84*, 917–923. [CrossRef]
116. Pytela, R.; Pierschbacher, M.D.; Ginsberg, M.H.; Plow, E.F.; Ruoslahti, E. Platelet membrane glycoprotein IIb/IIIa: Member of a family of Arg-Gly-Asp–specific adhesion receptors. *Science* **1986**, *231*, 1559–1562. [CrossRef] [PubMed]
117. Benharash, P.; Bongard, F.; Putnam, B. Use of recombinant factor VIIa for adjunctive hemorrhage control in trauma and surgical patients. *Am. Surg.* **2005**, *71*, 776–780. [CrossRef]
118. Bertram, J.P.; Williams, C.A.; Robinson, R.; Segal, S.S.; Flynn, N.T.; Lavik, E.B. Intravenous hemostat: Nanotechnology to halt bleeding. *Sci. Transl. Med.* **2009**, *1*, 11ra22. [CrossRef] [PubMed]
119. Lashof-Sullivan, M.M.; Shoffstall, E.; Atkins, K.T.; Keane, N.; Bir, C.; VandeVord, P.; Lavik, E.B. Intravenously administered nanoparticles increase survival following blast trauma. *Proc. Natl. Acad. Sci. USA* **2014**, *111*, 10293–10298. [CrossRef]
120. Gao, Y.; Sarode, A.; Kokoroskos, N.; Ukidve, A.; Zhao, Z.; Guo, S.; Flaumenhaft, R.; Gupta, A.S.; Saillant, N.; Mitragotri, S. A polymer-based systemic hemostatic agent. *Sci. Adv.* **2020**, *6*, eaba0588. [CrossRef]
121. Moreau, T.; Evans, A.L.; Vasquez, L.; Tijssen, M.R.; Yan, Y.; Trotter, M.W.; Howard, D.; Colzani, M.; Arumugam, M.; Wu, W.H.; et al. Large-scale production of megakaryocytes from human pluripotent stem cells by chemically defined forward programming. *Nat. Commun.* **2016**, *7*, 11208. [CrossRef]
122. Matsunaga, T.; Tanaka, I.; Kobune, M.; Kawano, Y.; Tanaka, M.; Kuribayashi, K.; Iyama, S.; Sato, T.; Sato, Y.; Takimoto, R.; et al. Ex vivo large-scale generation of human platelets from cord blood CD34+ cells. *Stem Cells* **2006**, *24*, 2877–2887. [CrossRef] [PubMed]
123. Takayama, N.; Nishikii, H.; Usui, J.; Tsukui, H.; Sawaguchi, A.; Hiroyama, T.; Eto, K.; Nakauchi, H. Generation of functional platelets from human embryonic stem cells in vitro via ES-sacs, VEGF-promoted structures that concentrate hematopoietic progenitors. *Blood* **2008**, *111*, 5298–5306. [CrossRef] [PubMed]

MDPI
St. Alban-Anlage 66
4052 Basel
Switzerland
Tel. +41 61 683 77 34
Fax +41 61 302 89 18
www.mdpi.com

Journal of Clinical Medicine Editorial Office
E-mail: jcm@mdpi.com
www.mdpi.com/journal/jcm

www.ingramcontent.com/pod-product-compliance
Lightning Source LLC
LaVergne TN
LVHW070202100526
838202LV00015B/1983